This book is due for return not later than the
last date stamped below, unless recalled sooner.

OCCUPATIONAL HYGIENE

Occupational Hygiene

EDITED BY

J. M. HARRINGTON
CBE, BSc, MSc, MD, FRCP, FFOM

AND

K. GARDINER
BSc, PhD, Dip. Occup. Hyg., MIOH, MIOSH

Both at
Institute of Occupational Health
The University of Birmingham
Edgbaston, Birmingham

SECOND EDITION

b

Blackwell
Science

© 1980, 1995 by
Blackwell Science Ltd
Editorial Offices:
Osney Mead, Oxford OX2 0EL
25 John Street, London WC1N 2BL
23 Ainslie Place, Edinburgh EH3 6AJ
238 Main Street, Cambridge
  Massachusetts 02142, USA
54 University Street, Carlton
  Victoria 3053, Australia

Other Editorial Offices:
Arnette Blackwell SA
  1, rue de Lille, 75007 Paris
France

Blackwell Wissenschafts-Verlag GmbH
  Kurfürstendamm 57
  10707 Berlin, Germany

  Feldgasse 13, A-1238 Wien
  Austria

First published 1980
Second edition 1995

Set by Setrite Typesetters, Hong Kong
Printed and bound in Great Britain
at the Bath Press, Bath, Avon

DISTRIBUTORS

Marston Book Services Ltd
PO Box 87
Oxford OX2 0DT
(*Orders*: Tel: 01865 791155
         Fax: 01865 791927
         Telex: 837515)

North America
  Blackwell Science, Inc.
  238 Main Street
  Cambridge, MA 02142
  (*Orders*: Tel: 800 215-1000
           617 876-7000
           Fax: 617 492-5263)

Australia
  Blackwell Science Pty Ltd
  54 University Street
  Carlton, Victoria 3053
  (*Orders*: Tel: 03 9347-0300
           Fax: 03 9349-3016)

A catalogue record for this title
is available from the British Library

ISBN 0-632-03734-2

Library of Congress
Cataloging-in-Publication Data

Occupational hygiene. — 2nd ed./edited by
J.M. Harrington and K. Gardiner.
      p.   cm.
    Includes bibliographical references and index.
    ISBN 0-632-03734-2
    1. Industrial hygiene. 2. Industrial
  toxicology.   I. Harrington, J.M. (John Malcolm)
  II. Gardiner, K.
  [DNLM: 1. Occupational Health.
  2. Occupational Diseases — prevention & control.
  3. Accidents, Occupational — prevention & control.
  WA 440 015 1995]
  RC963.0224 1995
  613.6′2 — dc20
  DNLM/DLC
  for Library of Congress   94-45425

Contents

List of Contributors

T-C. Aw MB PhD FRCP FFOM, *Institute of Occupational Health, The University of Birmingham, Edgbaston, Birmingham, B15 2TT*

L. M. Brosseau ScD CIH, *Division of Environmental and Occupational Health, School of Public Health, University of Minnesota, Box 807 Mayo, 420 Delaware Street SE, Minneapolis, MN 55455, USA*

R. H. Brown MA MSc PhD FRSC CChem, *Health and Safety Laboratory, Broad Lane, Sheffield, S3 7HQ*

R. F. Clayton LRSC, *18 Hendred Way, Abingdon, Oxfordshire, OX14 2AN*

I. S. Foulds MB ChB MRCP MFOM, *The Skin Hospital, George Road, Edgbaston, Birmingham, B15 1RP*

K. Gardiner BSc PhD Dip. Occup. Hyg. MIOH MIOSH, *Institute of Occupational Health, The University of Birmingham, Edgbaston, Birmingham, B15 2TT*

F. S. Gill BSc MSc CEng MIMinE FIOH FFOM(Hon), *Stone House, Bowyers, Liss, Hampshire, GU33 6LJ*

M. J. Griffin BSc PhD, *Institute of Sound and Vibration, University of Southampton, Highfield, Southampton, SO17 1BJ*

J. M. Harrington CBE BSc MSc MD FRCP FFOM, *Institute of Occupational Health, The University of Birmingham, Edgbaston, Birmingham, B15 2TT*

R. F. Herrick ScD CIH, *Division of Surveillance, Health Effects and Field Studies, NIOSH MS R12, 4676 Columbia Parkway, Cincinnati, OH 45226, USA*

R. M. Howie Grad. Inst. P. Dip. Occup. Hyg., *12 Morningside Road, Edinburgh, EH10 4DB*

M. J. Lever BA DPhil, *Centre for Biological and Medical Systems, Imperial College of Science, Technology and Medicine, London, SW7 2BX*

B. J. Maddock MA PhD CPhys FInstP CEng FIEE, *1A Clifford Manor Road, Guildford, GU4 8AG*

D. Mark BSc MPhil, *AEA Technology, Aerosol Science Centre, B401.8, Harwell, Didcot, Oxfordshire, OX11 0RA*

D. McBride TD MB ChB MFOM, *Institute of Occupational Health, The University of Birmingham, Edgbaston, Birmingham, B15 2TT*

A. J. Newman-Taylor OBE MSc FRCP FFOM, *Department of Occupational and Environmental Medicine, National Heart and Lung Institute, Brompton Hospital, Fulham Road, London, SW3 6HP*

D. Oakes PhD, *Department of Statistics, University of Rochester, Rochester, NY 14627, USA*

K. C. Parsons BSc PhD F. Erg. S., *Department of Human Sciences, Loughborough University, Loughborough, Leicestershire, LE11 3TU*

R. C. Schroter PhD FCGI FIChemE CEng, *Centre for Biological and Medical Systems, Imperial College of Science, Technology and Medicine, London, SW7 2BX*

N. A. Smith BA, *20 Valiant Gardens, Sprotbrough, Doncaster, DN5 7RU*

T. J. Smith PhD CIH, *Department of Environmental Health, Harvard School of Public Health, 665 Huntingdon Avenue, Boston, MA 02115, USA*

P. A. Stewart PhD CIH, *Occupational Studies Section, National Cancer Institute, 6130 Executive Boulevard, EPN 418 Rockville, MD 20892, USA*

J. H. Vincent BSc PhD DSc, *Division of Environmental and Occupational Health, School of Public Health, University of Minnesota, Box 807 Mayo, 420 Delaware Street SE, Minneapolis, MN 55455, USA*

S. C. Whitaker RGN RMN OHNC MIOSH MMedSc, *Institute of Occupational Health, The University of Birmingham, Edgbaston, Birmingham, B15 2TT*

A. Youle MA PhD CEng MCIBSE MInstE, *CUBE, Ravelin House, Museum Road, Portsmouth, PO1 2QQ and Adams Green Ltd, Consulting Engineers, 4 Carlton Crescent, Southampton, SO15 2EY*

Preface

The first edition of this book was published 15 years ago and, at that time, was one of the few general introductory texts in occupational hygiene. Many more books have appeared in the intervening years on various aspects of occupational health but there is still little choice for the reader wishing to acquire general information on the recognition, evaluation and control of work environments. Meanwhile, the subject has advanced greatly and the first edition seemed to warrant an update.

It is regretted that Tony Waldron was unable to help with this edition but the inclusion of a professional hygienist as editor helps to ensure the correct treatment of the subject that two physicians might perhaps not achieve.

Compared with the earlier version, this edition is much expanded and the American contribution is greater. In some cases, the authors have been changed; in others, new chapters have been added where significant advances in the subject demand. Where the authors have remained the same, they have thoroughly revised and updated their chapters. In the case of Chapter 4, one of us revised Tony Waldron's earlier and excellent text. Chapter 9 has also been revised by one of us from the previous version by the late Ivan King. There is inevitable overlap between certain chapters which we hope has been kept to a minimum but, where it does occur, it should serve to emphasize the importance of approaching certain subjects from both the engineering and medical perspective.

Despite the book's expanded size and scope we hope it remains a primer for students following degree courses in this subject as well as being a useful guide for other health professionals who need an understanding of occupational hygiene. We also hope that the new text has a greater international appeal as reference to national legislation is more for the purposes of exposition than a reflection of the origin of the editors.

We would welcome comments and criticisms from readers in case, at a later date, the publishers have the temerity to suggest a further edition. Such a prospect is unlikely to be greeted with enthusiasm by two people, Jayne Grainger and Julie Tucker, who have worked tirelessly and in good humour with the mountains of paper, the many revisions and the unenviable task of 'chasing up' some of the slower contributors. We are indebted to them for their work and for remaining our secretaries despite everything.

J. M. HARRINGTON
K. GARDINER
Birmingham, 1994

CHAPTER 1

The Structure and Function
of the Lungs

J.M. Harrington and A.J. Newman-Taylor

INTRODUCTION

The primary function of the lungs is to secure the exchange of gases — oxygen and carbon dioxide — between air and blood. The structure of the lungs effects this function and allows air to be conducted through a series of branching tubes (bronchi) to the sites of gas exchange: the alveoli.

STRUCTURE

The lungs are composed of a number of topographical units called bronchopulmonary segments which are roughly pyramidal in shape, with their apices directed inwards and their bases lying on the surface of the lung. Each lung is composed of 10 such segments grouped together into lobes. The right lung has three distinct lobes: upper, middle and lower, but on the left there are only two, since the rudimentary third lobe (the lingula) has become incorporated into the upper lobe. Each lower lobe contains five segments: the right middle lobe (and the lingula), two; and the upper lobes, three.

The airways

Air is conducted into the lungs through a system of branching tubes. The first of these is the trachea which is attached above to the larynx. It is a tube about 15 cm long lying directly in front of the oesophagus, and held open by C-shaped rings of cartilage in its walls. At the back it is joined together by a sheet of muscle fibres (the trachealis muscle) which, by contraction, diminishes the diameter of the tube. The muscle probably has the function of preventing overdistension of the trachea when the pressure inside it is raised, for example during the act of coughing.

The trachea divides into the left and right main bronchi which themselves give rise to the segmental bronchi (Fig. 1.1) and branching continues within each segment. A bronchus is defined as an airway which contains cartilage within its walls; divisions of the airways which contain no cartilage are termed bronchioles. The smaller bronchi contain less cartilage in their walls than do the trachea and the large bronchi. Instead their walls, and those of the bronchioles, are supported by elastic fibres and also by dense connective tissue. Moreover, they have two spiral layers of smooth muscle fibres surrounding their lumen which contract under the influence of nervous (or other) stimuli, thus lessening the calibre of the airway and altering the rate of flow of air into and out of the lungs.

When discussing the structure of the lungs it is usual to describe the airways in terms of the number of divisions, or generations, which separate them from the main bronchus. Thus, the segmental bronchus is counted as the first generation, and its first branch as the second generation, and so on. In this classification, the bronchi comprise about 15 generations, the first five of which are 'large' bronchi, having a plentiful supply of cartilage in their walls. The sixth to fifteenth generations are 'small' bronchi whose walls contain only a sparse amount of cartilage. There are about 10 generations of bronchioles which ultimately open into the alveolar ducts from which the alveoli originate. By definition the bronchiolus which opens into the alveolar duct is a respiratory bronchiole whilst the

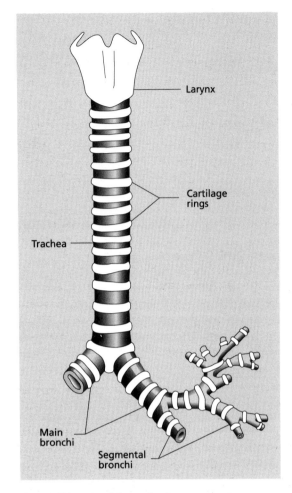

Fig. 1.1 Diagram of the main airways.

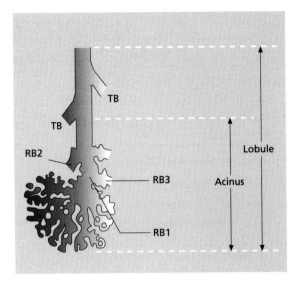

Fig. 1.2 Diagram of an acinus. TB, terminal bronchiolus; RB, respiratory bronchiolus. Note that RB has several generations (RB1, RB2, RB3 . . .).

one immediately proximal to it is a terminal bronchiole.

The acinus

The acinus is all that part of the lung distal to a terminal bronchiole. It includes up to eight generations of respiratory bronchioles and their associated alveoli, and it is approximately 0.5 – 1 cm in diameter.

The lobule is the term used to describe the three to five terminal bronchioles, together with their acini, which cluster together at the end of any airway (Fig. 1.2).

The consequences of branching

The consequence of branching within the airways is greatly to increase their total cross-sectional area whilst decreasing the rate of airflow through them. Thus by the time air has reached the terminal bronchioles, bulk flow of air has ceased leaving diffusion down concentration gradients as the method of transport. This has relevance and importance for dust deposition. This is well illustrated by the data in Table 1.1.

The alveolus

The alveolus is the part of the lung in which gas exchange occurs. There are 200–600 million alveoli in the fully developed adult lung which offer a surface area of some $100-200 \, m^2$ over which gas can diffuse. The alveolus is about 250 mm in diameter and its walls are lined by two types of epithelial cells: the type 1 and type 2 pneumocytes. The alveolar wall is typically less than 0.5 mm thick, but the epithelial lining is continuous throughout, and is composed of the cytoplasm of the pneumocytes. The alveolar wall is surrounded by, and in intimate contact with, the endothelial

Table 1.1 Cross-sectional area of the airways, and rate of airflow

	Area (cm²)	Flow rate (cm s⁻¹)*
Trachea	2.0	50
Terminal bronchioles	80	1.25
Respiratory bronchioles	280	0.36
Alveoli	$10-20 \times 10^5$	Negligible

*For a volume flow of $100 \, \text{ml s}^{-1}$.

cells of the capillaries of the pulmonary vascular bed (Fig. 1.3).

The type 1 pneumocyte is a large flat cell (like a fried egg!) covering a much greater area of the alveolar wall than the type 2 cell, although it is less numerous than the latter. The type 2 cell, which is usually found in corners of the alveolus, is a small cell containing characteristic lamellated inclusion bodies within its cytoplasm. These inclusion bodies are the origin of surfactant, a lipoprotein which lines the surface of the alveoli and acts to stabilize their size. The alveoli may be thought of as small bubbles, the surface tension of which is inversely related to the radius. The forces acting to keep the alveolar radius constant are less than one would predict and this is due to the presence of surfactant, which reduces the surface tension within the alveolus. A number of other cells are also encountered in association with the alveoli, including phagocytes called alveolar macrophages, which often contain carbon pigment taken up from the smoke-laden air. They are present in the alveolar space, connective tissue cells and some blood cells. The walls also contain elastic and collagen fibres which help support them. Having taken up the foreign material, the macrophages travel up the airways aided by the cilia in the epithelial lining (see below). Upon reaching the larynx, they and their contents are either coughed out with the sputum or swallowed. Foreign material cleared from the lungs and swallowed may be subsequently absorbed from the gut.

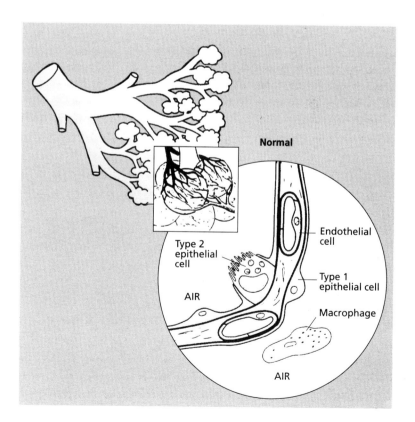

Fig. 1.3 Diagram of a section of alveoli showing the relationship between the various cell types.

The blood−gas barrier

The epithelial lining cells of the alveolar wall, together with the endothelial cells of the capillaries (each with their own basement membrane) and the tissue fluid in the spaces between, make up what is known as the blood−gas barrier. This is the 'thin' side of the alveolus where the basement membranes of type 1 epithelial cells and capillary endothelial cells are fused. It is the distance which gas molecules, or indeed any other material, must cross when passing into or out of the alveolus. The total distance involved is probably less than 0.001 mm.

The lining of the airways

The airways are lined with a ciliated epithelium which contains a number of different types of cell (Fig. 1.4). In the large airways, the epithelium is pseudostratified, that is, it has the appearance of being composed of more than one layer. This is due to the fact that the basal cells do not reach the surface of the epithelium, although all the other cells do reach the basement membrane which is a permeable layer of material synthesized by the cells, acting to stick the cells together. In the smaller airways there is only one layer of cells, each of which reaches the surface. The goblet cells secrete mucus which spreads out to form a layer on the surface of the airway where it traps particulate matter. Mucus is also secreted by the submucosal glands and is constantly being moved up towards the larynx by the synchronous beating of the cilia, carrying with it material trapped in the airways, together with the alveolar macrophages containing material scavenged from the alveoli. This so-called mucociliary escalator is one of the most important mechanisms through which the airways are cleared of particulate matter. Ciliated cells are found down as far as the respiratory bronchioles so that this mechanism operates continuously from the bronchiolo-alveolar junction to the larynx.

The function of the brush cells is unclear at present, but the structure and dimensions of the microvilli on the surface of the cells, from which they take their name, suggest that they could be concerned with the absorption of fluids from the airways and hence with the control of fluid balance.

The blood supply to the lungs

The lungs have two arterial blood supplies and two sets of venous drainage. Their arterial supply is from the pulmonary and bronchial arteries, whilst venous blood is conducted away by the pulmonary and bronchial veins.

The left and right pulmonary arteries arise from the right ventricle of the heart and convey to the lungs blood which has been returned from the

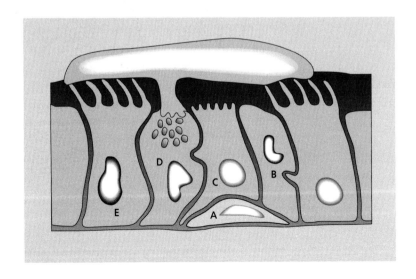

Fig. 1.4 Diagram of the epithelial lining of the trachea with its various cell types. A = basal cell; B = non-ciliated cell; C = brush cell; D = goblet cell (secreting muscle); E = ciliated cell.

tissues into the right atrium. Thus the blood in the pulmonary arteries, unlike that in all other arteries, has a low partial pressure of oxygen. It is also under much less pressure than blood in the other arteries, the pressure in the pulmonary artery being about one-tenth of the pressure in the systemic arterial circulation.

Both airways and blood vessels are low resistance systems allowing equivalent flow of air and blood to either side of an alveolar capillary. The pulmonary artery supplies the capillary bed surrounding the alveoli and at any one time approximately 80 ml of blood is in contact with the alveolar air (out of the total of 400 ml in the pulmonary circulation). The pulmonary artery divides each time the airway divides, but in addition, other arteries arise to supply the alveoli around the airway. These additional arteries are called the supernumerary branches and they outnumber the so-called conventional branches by about three to one.

The pulmonary veins run at the periphery of the bronchopulmonary segments and return blood with a high partial pressure of oxygen to the left side of the heart from whence it is pumped around the body.

The bronchial arteries are branches of the aorta and supply oxygenated blood to the capillary beds in the walls of the airways. Blood from the capillaries drains back through the pulmonary veins, and the bronchial veins receive blood only from the large airways, the lymph nodes and the pleura, which they convey to the azygos vein for return to the right atrium.

Lymphatics

Lymph vessels convey interstitial fluid from the tissue spaces back to the thoracic duct which opens into the confluence of the left internal jugular and subclavian veins. After the mucociliary escalator, this drainage system from the centre of acini is the second major route by which alveolar macrophages, laden with dust particles, leave the lung. The lymph vessels drain at intervals through lymph nodes which may be regarded, simply, as filters which trap particulate matter travelling in the lymph. Cells present in the lymph may also be arrested in the lymph nodes, and if these cells happen to have

broken away from a tumour developing within the lung, they may divide and multiply within the nodes, causing them to enlarge.

Lymph vessels are abundant in the pleura, the connective tissue septa between the bronchopulmonary segments, and in the walls of the airways and blood vessels; they do not appear in the walls of the alveoli. The lymph drains from the periphery towards the hilum of the lung, and through the nodes situated there (Fig. 1.5).

The pleura

The lungs are completely covered by a fibro-elastic membrane called the visceral pleura. Lining the inside of the thoracic cavity is a complementary membrane, the parietal pleura. The opposing pleural faces are covered with a layer of cells which secrete a serous fluid into the space between them. This fluid acts as a lubricant between the two pleural layers and allows the lungs to move easily over the parietal pleura during respiration.

The two pleural layers are continuous around

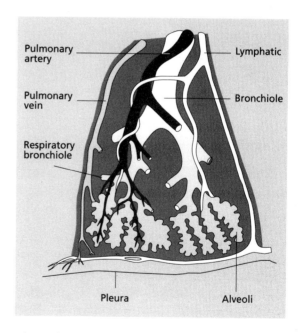

Fig. 1.5 Diagram of a bronchopulmonary segment. The sizes of the vessels and the airways are not to scale. Note that for clarity, the lymphatics are shown only on the right and the blood vessels only on the left.

the root of the lungs (Fig. 1.6). The space between the two layers of pleura is known as the pleural cavity and under normal conditions it contains only a thin film of fluid. For this reason, it is only a potential space, although under some abnormal conditions it may become filled with fluid, and thus become a real space.

FUNCTION

Introduction

Only a brief outline of lung function is provided here. Emphasis is placed on the main aspects of pulmonary function and on the more commonly used measures. Patterns of disordered function that are characteristic of the commoner occupational lung diseases are appended. More extensive reviews of the subject are listed at the end of the chapter.

The main function of the lungs is to allow exchange of gas between air and blood. At a cellular level this is achieved by means of the blood. Oxygen is carried to the cells primarily by the red cell pigment haemoglobin whilst carbon dioxide is removed from the cells using the same transport mechanism. The lungs, therefore, act rather like a bellows, transporting oxygen in the air to the alveoli where it is exchanged for carbon dioxide. The blood leaving the lungs via the pulmonary veins has a higher oxygen concentration and a lower carbon dioxide concentration than the blood entering through the pulmonary arteries. The rate of ventilation controls these concentrations within narrow limits in the presence of wide variations in the demand for oxygen and for the removal of carbon dioxide by responding to carbon dioxide concentration.

The pathway from air to body cell involves several steps. Firstly, the air has to reach the alveolar–capillary membrane, then the oxygen has to cross this membrane and reach the red blood cell. The final step is the uptake of oxygen by the tissue cells

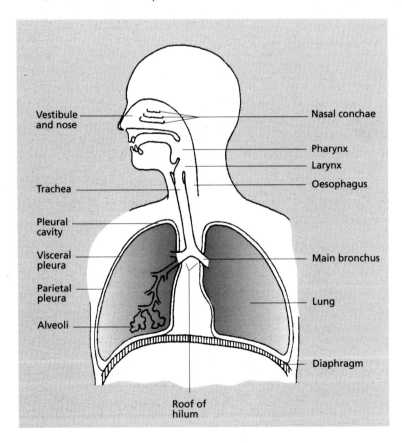

Fig. 1.6 Diagram of the respiratory tract showing the relation of the pleura to the other parts.

from the circulating blood. Carbon dioxide is transported in the opposite direction. This chapter is mainly concerned with the first two steps in the pathway.

The propelling force for the first step is the alternating pressure changes produced in the lungs by breathing — which is itself controlled by the respiratory muscles. Resistance to these pressure changes comes from the conducting airways themselves and from the inherent elasticity of the lung and chest wall tissues. Disordered function of this first step results from reduced ventilatory capacity, which can be due to respiratory muscle weakness, decreased lung compliance or damaged airways.

The second step, across the alveolar-capillary membrane, is short compared with the first step (300 μm compared to 50 cm). However, gas transport can be disrupted at this stage by thickening of the alveolar-capillary membrane such as occurs in diffuse pulmonary fibrosis. Such thickening impedes the flow of oxygen and carbon dioxide which is governed by the partial pressure differences of these two gases across the membrane. As carbon dioxide is much more water soluble than oxygen, the main effect of such fibrosis is failure to transport oxygen. Carbon dioxide retention in the body is much more likely to be due to poor ventilation than to pulmonary fibrosis.

Efficient ventilation and undamaged alveolar–capillary membranes are of no value unless the perfusion of the lung with blood is efficient as well. Ventilation perfusion imbalance is a major cause of impaired gas exchange. This can be illustrated, *reductio ad absurdam*, by stating that death rapidly supervenes if the right main bronchus is blocked and the left pulmonary artery is occluded! Under normal circumstances about 4 l of air are exposed to about 5 l of blood in the lungs giving an overall ventilation : perfusion (V : Q) ratio of around 0.9. Deviation in either direction from this figure of 0.9 can cause serious deficiences in tissue cell oxygenation.

Therefore, the processes involved in gaseous exchange can be sub-divided into:

1 ventilation;
2 gas transfer;
3 blood gas transport.

These sub-divisions can also be used to outline lung function tests in common usage. None of these measures of lung function is diagnostic in itself, and the degree of accuracy and sophistication used in measuring lung function depends on many factors, including the facilities available (for example a cardiothoracic unit) and the needs of the patient and the investigator. In this chapter, emphasis is placed on the simpler tests used in occupational health practice, either to monitor an individual worker or as a measure of lung function in a clinical epidemiological survey of a factory population. It is worth noting, however, that although tests of lung volume, ventilation, gas distribution and gas transfer may be useful in differing circumstances, the basic spirometric measures of ventilatory capacity described below are indispensable in all investigations.

Ventilation

The rhythmic contraction of the inspiratory muscle produces expansion of the thorax and lungs. This ventilation is controlled by the brain stem to maintain the partial pressure of carbon dioxide. In order to produce lung expansion, the inspiratory muscles must be capable of overcoming the inherent elastic recoil of the lung tissues and the resistance of the airways to the flow of air consequent upon these pressure changes.

The *ventilatory capacity* of the lungs is frequently assessed by using either a peak flow meter or a spirometer. Peak flow readings are not equivalent to spirometer readings, nor are they as valuable. If a single test of lung function is to be used, most authorities would advocate the use of a spirometer to measure *forced* vital capacity (FVC) and *forced* expiratory volume in 1 s (FEV_1).

Typical tracings obtained by such a machine are illustrated in Fig. 1.7. As these measures are frequently done by non-physiologists, it is essential that the techniques used are standardized to minimize inter- and intra-observer error. All such tests should be accompanied by information on the subject's age, height, sex, ethnic group and smoking habit. Prediction formulae incorporating the first four of these variables are available. Results are frequently expressed as a percentage of the predicted value.

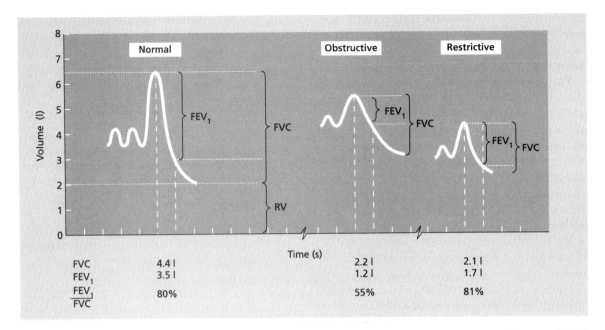

Fig. 1.7 Spirograms to illustrate the differences in forced expiratory volume in 1 s (FEV$_1$) and forced vital capacity (FVC) in health, airways obstruction and restrictive defects (such as diffuse lung fibrosis or severe spinal deformity). Inspiration is upwards and expiration downwards. Although the vital capacity is reduced in both obstructive and restrictive lung disease, the proportion expired in one second shows considerable differences. RV, residual volume.

Total lung capacity at full inspiration is governed to a large extent by body size. In normal subjects this correlates well with height. Chest deformities, inspiratory muscle weakness and increased lung stiffness (loss of compliance) will reduce this volume. During maximal expiration, some air is left in the lungs — the residual volume. The physiological event which limits expiration is closure of the intrathoracic airways. Their patency depends not only on the elastic tissues of the lungs holding them open but also on the strength and integrity of their walls and on the presence or absence of fluid (oedema) or muscle spasm which may narrow the airways. For example, in asthma and bronchitis, the airways tend to close prematurely because of disease in the walls of the airways.

In normal subjects, 75% or more of the vital capacity can be expired in 1 s and the remaining 25% takes a further 2–3 s. Diffuse airways obstruction, as in asthma, bronchitis or emphysema, causes irregular and premature airways closure during expiration. Therefore, not only do these patients frequently have a reduced vital capacity

(VC) but they may be unable to expire a large portion of this air in the first second (Fig. 1.7). FEV$_1$ is reduced in all lung diseases which reduce the VC, but the ratio FEV$_1$: VC is reduced only in airways obstruction. When the subject has restrictive lung disease, for example in diffuse pulmonary fibrosis, although the VC and FEV$_1$ are reduced, the ratio is normal. Variable airways obstruction is a characteristic feature of asthma and can be assessed by measuring the FEV$_1$: FVC ratio before and after the administration of bronchodilator drugs.

Increased attention has been paid to so-called 'small airways' disease which seems to be an early sign of impaired ventilatory capacity. Frequently, it is not distinguishable on the standard spirometer measurement recounted above. It can, however, be estimated by measuring the rate of expiratory flow during the middle of expiration. Consequently, some respiratory physiologists have turned to the forced mid-expiratory flow rate (FMF) to reveal early airways disease. This measure is sometimes referred to as the FEF$_{25-75}$. The fashion has diminished somewhat recently because of the low 'signal to noise' ratio. The standard spirometric reading can be used to calculate this value and is illustrated in Fig. 1.8. A more accurate assessment can be achieved using a flow–volume pneumotachograph.

The *mechanical properties* of the lung may also need to be studied. This includes not only the ability of the respiratory muscles and rib cage to perform their tasks but also the physical (visco-elastic) properties of the lungs themselves. 'Elasticity' in this sense strictly means the ability of a structure or substance to return to its original shape and dimensions after a deforming force has been removed. It is not synonymous with 'stretchability'. 'Compliance' is the term often used to describe this property of lung tissue, but it is not the only elastic force in operation. Surface tension of the liquid lining the alveolus, for example, is estimated to provide about half of the lung's elastic recoil. In addition, there is impedance to airflow through the airways associated with viscous (non-elastic resistance) properties of the lung.

The estimation of compliance and non-elastic resistance of the lungs requires the measurement of the pressure differences between the alveoli and the lung surface, and between the alveoli and the mouth, respectively. The first of these parameters requires the measurement of intra-oesophageal pressure and is beyond the scope of this book. However, an apparently satisfactory measure of non-elastic resistance is the pressure difference between mouth and alveoli per unit rate of airflow. This can be achieved using the body plethysmograph. The subject sits in an airtight box and measurements are made of the subject's rate of airflow and the mouth pressures with and without blockage of the airway at the mouth by means of a shutter. Although the body plethysmograph is unsuitable for most field surveys, it does have the advantage of measuring residual volume and total lung capacity as well as non-elastic resistance. Similar measurements can also be achieved using chest X-rays.

Gas transfer

The effective exchange of oxygen and carbon dioxide in the lung depends upon three processes:
1 the correct distribution of ventilated lung to blood-perfused lung;
2 the efficient diffusion of gases across the alveolar-capillary membrane;
3 the appropriate uptake and release of the gases by the red cell.

Ventilation–perfusion measures are primarily research tools and frequently involve the inhalation of inert gases and the subsequent measurement of the exhaled concentrations. Alternatively, radio-active gases can be used and lung scanning techniques employed to show the distribution of the inhaled gas in the lung.

Diffusion of gases across the alveolar capillary membrane is, likewise, a laboratory technique. However, the measurement of the gas transfer factor (TL) using carbon monoxide is so widely employed in assessing diffusion defects (as may occur in asbestosis and other fibrotic diseases of the lung) that it is worthy of note here.

TL_{CO} is defined as the quantity of pure carbon monoxide which crosses the alveolar capillary membrane in 1 min when the difference between the concentration of carbon monoxide in the lung and the blood is 1 mmHg tension. Three measurements are required: the volume of carbon monoxide taken up by the pulmonary capillary blood, the partial pressure of carbon monoxide in the alveolar

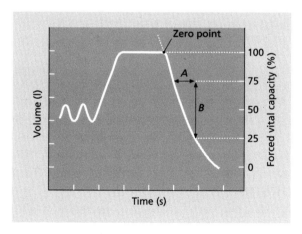

Fig. 1.8 Spirogram showing the measurement of the forced vital capacity (FVC) and the derivation of the forced mid-expiratory flow rate (FMF). This is calculated from the rate of flow between the 75% and 25% points on the FVC scale and can be calculated from A/B and corrected to 1 BTPS per second.

air and the partial pressure of carbon monoxide in the pulmonary capillary blood. The procedure involves breathing a known concentration of carbon monoxide and air or oxygen (usually with helium in order to assess the dilution effect of the residual volume).

It must be noted, however, that the TL_{CO} is not solely governed by the thickness of the alveolar capillary membrane. Many other factors are involved — ventilation–perfusion inequalities and haemoglobin concentration in the blood being amongst the more important. Nevertheless, the TL_{CO} remains the most useful, convenient and widely quoted measure of diffusing capacity.

Blood gas transport

The final step in getting oxygen to the tissues and transporting the carbon dioxide in the opposite direction involves the blood. An estimate of the efficiency of blood gas transport requires the measurement of the concentration of alveolar carbon dioxide as well as arterial oxygen, carbon dioxide and pH. Blood gas tensions and pH are rarely measured in occupational health practice, though they are frequently vital in the management of respiratory failure in hospital practice.

Factors influencing lung function

Before outlining some of the lung function abnormalities present in the common occupationally induced lung diseases, it is pertinent to consider non-occupational factors which can influence lung function. Of these, the most important are age and smoking habits.

Age

As a person gets older, and especially past middle age, the alveolar volume decreases and the airway volume increases. In addition, the respiratory muscles weaken and the elastic recoil of the lung becomes reduced. This results in a rise in the residual volume : total lung capacity (RV : TLC) ratio and a fall in the TL_{CO}. It is essential, therefore, that age is taken into account when comparing lung function results in survey populations. The effect on FEV_1, for example, is a loss of about $25-30\,ml\,yr^{-1}$ from the third decade onwards.

Smoking

Tobacco smoke, particularly cigarette smoke, has a serious adverse effect on lung function, leading to an accelerated decline in FEV_1, as great as $90-100\,ml\,year^{-1}$ (cf. age effect of $25-30\,ml\,year^{-1}$). The acute effect of smoking is increased airways resistance, whilst habitual smoking leads to a chronic airways obstruction in both sexes and all age groups. It causes a narrowing of small airways and alveolar destruction (emphysema) as well as small airway narrowing. In lung function terms this leads to a lowered FEV_1, FVC and FEV_1 : FVC ratio, and a raised TL and RV. The TL_{CO} is normal unless emphysema supervenes when it falls.

The effects of smoking are so marked that failure to consider this in estimating occupational factors that might be influencing lung function can vitiate the whole investigation. It should also be remembered that the carcinogenic effect of some inhaled occupational hazards may be greatly enhanced by smoking. In some cases this effect may be multiplicative.

Other functions

Lung size, sex, ethnic group, height (rather than weight), skeletal deformity, posture, exercise tolerance, observer and instrument error, diurnal variation and ambient temperatures can all influence the results obtained from lung function tests. Many of these can be either controlled or allowed for using standard techniques and consulting nomograms of normal (predicted) values.

Occupational lung disease and disordered function

Lung disease can be arbitrarily divided into subgroups on the basis of the nature of the inhaled noxious agent. These are:
1 mineral dusts;
2 organic dusts;
3 irritant gases and vapours;
4 radiations.

Table 1.2 Occupational lung diseases and their functional impairment

Agent	Type of respiratory impairment	Pathology
DUSTS		
Mineral		
Iron, barium, tin	None	Dust accumulation
Coal (early effects)	None (usually), occasionally obstructive	Focal emphysema
Coal (late effects)	Obstructive, restrictive, diffusion	Nodular fibrosis
Silica	Restrictive, obstructive, diffusion	Nodular fibrosis
Beryllium	Restrictive, diffusion	Interstitial fibrosis (granulomas)
Aluminium	?Restrictive, diffusion	Interstitial fibrosis
Cobalt	Restrictive, diffusion	Interstitial fibrosis
Asbestos	Restrictive, obstructive, ?diffusion	Interstitial fibrosis, pleural thickening
Talc	Obstructive	Chronic bronchitis, ?some fibrosis
Organic		
Cotton, hemp, sisal, mouldy hay, barley, bagasse and straw, pigeon droppings, certain insects, animal hairs, bacterial products and drugs	Restrictive, diffusion (chronic) (immunological tests may be helpful)	Interstitial fibrosis (granulomas) in some cases Asthma (in some cases)
GASES AND VAPOURS*		
Nitrogen dioxide	Obstructive…diffusion	Acute bronchitis, pulmonary oedema
Sulphur dioxide, ammonia, chlorine, phosgene	Obstructive, restrictive, diffusion	Bronchopneumonia, pulmonary oedema, mild to severe tissue damage
Cadmium oxide	Restrictive, diffusion	Interstitial fibrosis and emphysema
Isocyanates, platinum salts	Obstructive, ??diffusion (late effect)	Asthma (in some cases)
Hairspray	?None	
RADIATION		
Ionizing radiation	Restrictive, diffusion	?Intestinal fibrosis, pulmonary oedema (early)—intestinal fibrosis (late)

*Obstruction or restriction depends on solubility of gas and on site of injury.

Table 1.2 summarizes the common occupational pulmonary diseases and their pattern of functional disorder. A detailed description of the deposition of materials in the lung and the effects of inhaled materials appears in Chapters 3 and 4 respectively.

FURTHER READING

Newman-Taylor, A.J. (1991). Occupational aspects of pulmonary disease. In *Recent Advances in Respiratory Medicine*, (5th edn), (ed. D.M. Mitchell). Churchill Livingstone, Edinburgh.

Parkes, W.R. (ed.) (1994). *Occupational Lung Disorders*, (3rd edn). Butterworth, London.

West, J.B. (1990). *Respiratory Physiology — the Essentials*, (4th edn). Williams and Wilkins, Baltimore.

CHAPTER 2

Organ Structure and Function: the Skin

I.S. Foulds

INTRODUCTION

The skin is one of the largest organs in the body, having a surface area of $1.8\,m^2$ in an adult and making up approximately 16% of the body weight. It has many functions, the most important of which is as a barrier to protect the body from noxious external factors and to keep the internal body systems intact.

The skin is composed of three layers: the epidermis; the dermis; and the subcutis (Fig. 2.1). There are two main kinds of human skin: glabrous skin (found on the palms and soles) and hairy skin.

The skin is a metabolically active organ with vital functions including the protection and homeostasis of the body (Table 2.1).

EPIDERMIS

The epidermis is defined as a stratified squamous epithelium which is about 0.1 mm thick, although the thickness is greater (0.4−1.4 mm) on the glabrous skin of the palms and soles. Its main function

Table 2.1 Functions of the skin

Presents barrier to physical agents
Protects against mechanical injury
Prevents loss of body fluids
Reduces penetration of ultraviolet radiation
Helps regulate body temperature
Acts as a sensory organ
Affords a surface for grip
Plays a role in vitamin production
Acts as an outpost for immune surveillance
Cosmetic association

is to act as a protective barrier. The main cell of the epidermis is the keratinocyte, which produces the protein keratin. The four layers of the epidermis — the basal; prickle; granular cell layers; and the horny layer (stratum corneum) (Fig. 2.1) — represent the stages of maturation of the keratin by keratinocytes.

The differentiation of basal cells into dead, but functionally important, corneocytes is a unique feature of the skin. The horny layer is important in preventing all manner of agents from entering the skin, including micro-organisms, water and particulate matter. The epidermis also prevents the body's fluids from getting out.

Epidermal cells undergo the following sequence during keratinocyte maturation.

1 Undifferentiated cells in the basal layer (stratum basale) and the layer immediately above divide continuously. Half of these cells remain in place and half progress upwards and differentiate.

2 In the prickle cell layer (stratum spinosum) cells change from being columnar to polygonal. Differentiating keratinocytes synthesize keratins which aggregate to form tonofilaments. The desmosomes are the connections between keratinocytes which are condensations of tonofilaments. Desmosomes distribute structural stresses throughout the epidermis and maintain a distance of 20 nm between adjacent cells.

3 Enzymes in the granular cell layer (stratum granulosum) induce degradation of nuclei and organelles. Keratohyalin granules mature the keratin and provide an amorphous protein matrix for the tonofilaments. Membrane-coating granules attached to the cell membrane release an impervious

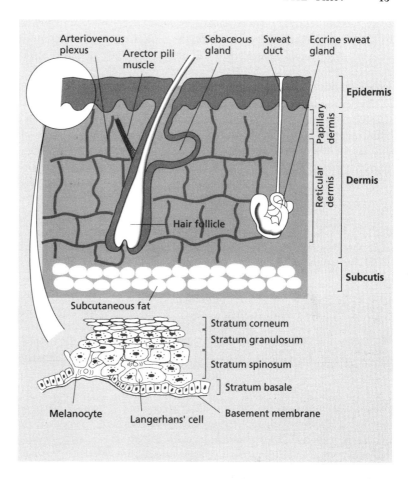

Arteriovenous plexus
Arector pili muscle
Sebaceous gland
Sweat duct
Eccrine sweat gland
Epidermis
Papillary dermis
Reticular dermis
Dermis
Hair follicle
Subcutis
Subcutaneous fat
Stratum corneum
Stratum granulosum
Stratum spinosum
Stratum basale
Melanocyte
Langerhans' cell
Basement membrane

Fig. 2.1 A cross-section of normal skin.

lipid-containing cement which contributes to cell adhesion and to the horny layer barrier.

4 In the horny layer (stratum corneum) the dead, flattened corneocytes have developed thickened cell envelopes encasing a matrix of keratin tonofibrils. The strong disulphide bonds of the keratin provide strength to the stratum corneum but the layer is also flexible and can absorb up to three times its own weight in water. However, if it dries out with the water content falling below 10%, pliability fails.

5 The corneocytes are eventually shed from the skin surface.

Rate of maturation

Kinetic studies show that, on average, the dividing basal cells replicate every 200–400 h and the result-

ant differentiating cells take about 14 days to reach the stratum corneum and a further 14 days to be shed. The cell turnover time is considerably shortened in keratinization disorders such as psoriasis.

DERMIS

The dermis is defined as a tough, supportive connective tissue matrix, containing specialized structures, which is found immediately below, and intermittently connected with, the epidermis. It varies in thickness, being thin (0.6 mm) on the eyelids and thicker (3 mm or more) on the back, palms and soles. Collagen fibres make up 70% of the dermis and impart a toughness in strength to the structure. Elastin fibres are loosely arranged in all directions in the dermis and provide elasticity to the skin. They are more numerous near hair follicles and sweat glands and less so in the papillary dermis. The ground substance of the dermis is a semi-solid matrix of glycosaminoglycans (GAG) which allows dermal structures some movement.

The dermis contains fibroblasts which synthesize collagen, elastin and other connective tissue, and GAG. In addition the dermis contains dermal dendrocytes (dendritic cells) with a probable immune function, mast cells, macrophages and lymphocytes.

SUBCUTANEOUS LAYER

The subcutis consists of loose connective tissue and fat (up to 3 cm thick on the abdomen).

DERIVATIVES OF THE SKIN

Hair

Hairs are found over the entire surface of the skin, with the exception of the glabrous skin of the palms, soles, glans penis and vulva. The density of the follicles is greatest on the face. Embryologically the hair follicle has an input from the epidermis, which is responsible for the matrix cells and the hair shaft, and the dermis, which contributes the papilla with its blood vessels and nerves.

There are three types of hair and these are listed below.
1 *Lanugo hairs* are fine and long and are formed in the fetus at 20 weeks' gestation. They are normally shed before birth but may be seen in premature babies.
2 *Vellus hairs* are the short, fine, light coloured hairs that cover most of the body surfaces.
3 *Terminal hairs* are longer, thicker and darker and are found on the scalp, eyebrows, eyelashes and also on the pubic, axillary and beard areas. They originate as vellus hair; differentiation is stimulated at puberty by androgens.

In most mammals hair or fur plays an essential role in survival, especially in the conservation of heat; this is not the case in nude man. Scalp hair in humans does function as a protection against the cancer-inducing effects of ultraviolet radiation; it also protects against minor injury. However, the main role of hair in human society is as an organ of sexual attraction and therein lies its importance to the cosmetics industry.

Nails

The nail is a phylogenetic remnant of the mammalian claw and consists of a plate of hardened and densely packed keratin. It protects the fingertips and facilitates grasping and tactile sensitivity in the finger pulp.

SEBACEOUS GLANDS

Sebaceous glands are found associated with hair follicles, especially those of the scalp, face, chest and back, and are not found on non-hairy skin. They are formed from epidermis-derived cells and produce an oily sebum, the function of which is uncertain.

The glands are small in the child but become large and active at puberty, being sensitive to androgens. Sebum is produced by holocrine secretion in which the cells disintegrate to release their lipid cytoplasm.

SWEAT GLANDS

Sweat glands are like coiled tubes, located within the epidermis, which produce a watery secretion. There are two separate types: eccrine and apocrine.

Eccrine sweat glands

Eccrine sweat glands develop from down-budding of the epidermis. The secretory portion is a coiled structure in the deep reticular dermis; the excretory duct spirals upwards to open onto the skin surface. An estimated 2.5 million sweat ducts are present on the skin surface. They are universally distributed but are most profuse on the palms, soles, axillae and forehead where the glands are under both psychological and thermal control (those elsewhere being under thermal control only). Eccrine sweat glands are innervated by sympathetic (cholanergic) nerve fibres.

Apocrine glands

These are also derived from the epidermis. Apocrine sweat glands open into hair follicles and are larger than eccrine glands. They are most numerous around the axillae, perineum and areolae. The secretion is odourless when produced although an odour develops after the action of skin bacteria. Sweating is controlled by sympathetic (adrenergic) innervation. The apocrine glands represent a phylogenetic remnant of the mammalian sexual scent gland.

OTHER STRUCTURES IN THE SKIN

Nerve supply

The skin is richly innervated, with the highest density of nerves being found in areas such as the hands, face and genitalia. All nerve supplies in the skin have their cell bodies in the dorsal root ganglia. Both myelinated and non-myelinated fibres are found. Free sensory nerve endings occur in the dermis and also encroaching on the epidermis where they may abut onto Merkel cells. These nerve endings detect pain, irritation and temperature. Specialized corpuscular receptors are distributed in the dermis, such as Pacini's corpuscles detecting pressure and vibration, and touch-sensitive Meissner's corpuscles which are mainly seen in the dermal papillae of the feet and hands.

Autonomic nerves supply the blood vessels, sweat glands and arrector pili muscles. The nerve supply is dermatomal with some overlap.

BLOOD AND LYMPHATIC VESSELS

The skin also has a rich and adaptive blood supply. Arteries in the subcutis branch upwards forming a superficial plexus at the papillary–reticular dermal boundary. Branches extend to the dermal papillae, each of which has a single loop of capillary vessels, one arterial and one venous. Veins drain from the venous side of this loop to form the mid-dermal and subcutaneous venous networks. In the reticular and papillary dermis there are arteriovenous anastomoses which are well innervated and are concerned with thermoregulation.

The lymphatic drainage of the skin is important. Abundant meshes of lymphatics originate in the papillary dermis and assemble into larger vessels which ultimately drain into the regional lymph nodes.

Melanocyte function

Melanocytes (located in the basal layer) produce the pigment melanin in elongated, membrane-bound organelles known as melanosomes. These are packaged into granules which are moved down dendritic processes and transferred by phagocytosis to adjacent keratinocytes. Melanin granules form a protective cap over the outer part of keratinocyte nuclei in the inner layers of the epidermis. In the stratum corneum, they are uniformly distributed to form an ultraviolet absorbing blanket which reduces the amount of radiation penetrating the skin.

Ultraviolet radiation, mainly the wavelengths of 290–320 nm (ultraviolet B), darkens the skin firstly by immediate photo-oxidation of preformed melanin, and secondly over a period of days by stimulating melanocytes to produce more melanin. Ultraviolet radiation also induces keratinocyte proliferation, resulting in thickening of the epidermis.

Variations in racial pigmentation are not due to differences in melanocyte numbers, but to the number and size of melanosomes produced. Red-haired people have phaeomelanin, not the more usual eumelanin, and their melanosomes are spherical rather than oblong.

Thermoregulation

The maintenance of a near constant body core temperature of 37°C is a great advantage to humans, allowing a constancy to many biochemical reactions which would otherwise fluctuate widely with temperature changes. Thermoregulation depends on several factors, including metabolism and exercise, but the skin plays an important part in control through the evaporation of sweat and by direct heat loss from the surface.

Blood flow

Skin temperature is highly responsive to skin blood flow. Dilatation or contraction of the dermal blood vessels results in vast changes in blood flow which can vary from 1 to 100 ml min^{-1} per 100 g of skin for the fingers and forearms. Arteriovenous anastamoses under the control of the sympathetic nervous system shunt blood to or from the superficial venous plexus, affecting skin temperature. Local factors, both chemical and physical, can also have an effect.

SWEAT

The production of sweat cools the skin through evaporation. The minimum secretion per day is 0.5 l and the maximum is 10 l, with a maximum output of about 2 l h^{-1}. Men sweat more than women.

Watery isotonic sweat, produced in the sweat gland, is modified in the excretory portion of the duct so that the fluid delivered to the skin surface has:
1 a pH of between 4 and 6.8;
2 a low concentration of sodium (32–70 mEq l^{-1}) and chlorine (30–70 mEq l^{-1});
3 a high concentration of potassium (up to 5 mEq l^{-1}), lactate (4–14 mEq l^{-1}), urea, ammonia and some amino acids.
Only small quantities of toxic substances are lost.

Sweating may also occur in response to emotion and after eating spicy foods. In addition to thermoregulation sweat also helps to maintain the hydration of the horny layer and improves grip on the palms and soles.

DEFENCE MECHANISMS OF THE SKIN

The skin achieves protection through a variety of mechanisms. The outermost layer of the skin, known as the horny layer or stratum corneum, acts as a barrier against chemicals. Therefore with the stratum corneum being relatively thin on the backs of the hands compared to the palms, it is often the backs of the hands which are initially affected by dermatitis. The presence of pigment cells (melano-

cytes) provides protection against the damaging effects of ultraviolet light, and the sweat glands and sebaceous glands help maintain hydration and suppleness of the skin. The skin is able to resist shearing stresses due to elastic tissue and collagen. A continual upward movement of cells in the epidermis provides continual replacement from wear and tear, and at the same time discourages growth of bacteria on the surface of the skin. The skin is able to resist (buffer) the effects of mild acids but does not buffer alkalis effectively and does not tolerate strong acids, alkalis or solvents.

THE SKIN AS A BARRIER

Penetration of the skin is a passive process that occurs unaided by the cells within the skin. With different chemical substances the penetration rate may vary fourfold. In addition, damage or disease may affect the barrier and result in increased percutaneous absorption. Percutaneous absorption involves a series of processes. Molecules of the chemical must be absorbed at the surface of the stratum corneum and then diffuse through the flattened cell layers. After that the compound must enter the viable epidermis and then the dermis until it reaches a capillary where it can enter the systemic circulation. Water can penetrate the skin at an average of 0.2–0.4 mg cm^{-2} h^{-1} at 30°C. Hydrophilic chemicals generally penetrate the skin more slowly than does water.

Cell membranes and intercellular spaces contain lipids, and therefore lipophilic compounds can also penetrate the skin. When chemical compounds penetrate the skin, local toxicity may occur, for example with caustic, allergenic or phototoxic agents or compounds that can cause skin cancer.

Chemicals absorbed through the skin rather than through the oral route may be more toxic to the body as detoxification by the liver may be bypassed. However the skin also contains many different enzyme systems, some of which are similar to the liver and therefore some detoxification may be possible. An example of this is when organophosphorus pesticides are applied to the skin and a large proportion are metabolized during their passage through the skin. Conversely, aryl hydrocarbon hydroxylase in the skin may convert non-carcinogenic benzo-alpha-pyrene into a potent carcinogen that could cause effects within the skin or elsewhere. Therefore, first-pass metabolism may increase or decrease the systemic bioavailability of a compound.

In theory compounds may also penetrate through the appendages of the skin (sweat, sebaceous and apocrine glands and beside hair follicles). In practice this route accounts for less than 6% chemical penetration.

IRRITANT CONTACT DERMATITIS

Over 90% of industrial dermatitis is due to irritant contact factors. Irritants are substances which damage the skin by direct toxic action. Their effect is proportional to the nature of the chemical, the length of exposure and the individual's skin protection and tolerance.

Irritants can be divided into absolute and relative irritants. Absolute irritants are chemicals which produce irritation in everyone by direct tissue destruction if the concentration and exposure time are adequate. Concentrated acids or alkalis are examples of absolute irritants.

Relative irritants are milder substances which will produce inflammatory changes in most individuals provided there is repeated exposure; for example, paraffin and solvents. A fuller list of potential irritants in certain occupations can be found in standard dermatology texts (see Further Reading). Moreover, certain factors can increase the susceptibility of the skin to irritants. Dermatitis that has healed, or a burn, may remain more susceptible to irritants for several months. This is due to a lower threshold of resistance, which is also one of the reasons why those with previous atopic eczema are more susceptible to the effects of irritants. Extremes of humidity and temperature, friction, pressure, sweating and occlusion may also contribute to irritant damage by allowing relatively bland substances to cause irritation.

This can be more easily understood in simple graphical terms (Fig. 2.2). Exposure to an irritant may cause some damage to the skin (point A), but no clinical abnormality is present. Repeated exposure to this irritant or to other irritants over a period of time (B, C, D) will produce further damage to the skin, but still no clinical abnormality. However, with further exposure to an irritant (E), dermatitis (inflammation of the skin) develops once the threshold is crossed, as a result of the cumulative effect of damage by irritants. This process may take a considerable time to develop. Many workers will state that they have worked with a particular substance for years with no trouble until the present time. This is a typical story of an individual suffering from irritant contact dermatitis due to repeated insults occurring to the skin.

In practice the threshold for the development of

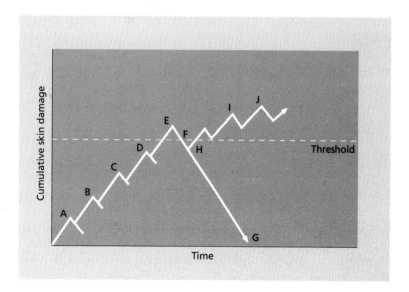

Fig. 2.2 A model of irritant contact dermatitis. After Malten (1981).

dermatitis varies in individuals, and those with a pre-existing skin disease or previous history of atopic eczema will have a lower threshold of susceptibility. Once the dermatitis has started it can appear to improve clinically (F), but to achieve full recovery (G) may take months or possibly even years. In practice, once dermatitis appears to have improved, individuals tend to revert to exposing themselves to irritants, and at this stage (H) a minimum amount of irritation will result in a recurrence of the dermatitis. With continuing exposure to irritants (I, J, etc.) the dermatitis may never heal.

The clinical course of irritant contact dermatitis

Once irritant contact dermatitis develops then all exposure to irritant factors must be reduced, not only at work but also at home, if clinical clearance is to be achieved and maintained. All too often an employee is signed off work with no particular advice for irritant avoidance at home, the dermatitis clears, a return to work follows with re-exposure to irritants and the dermatitis recurs. When recurrence occurs repeatedly on returning to work the employees may be forced to stop working, but if all potential irritants were carefully identified, clearance of dermatitis could be achieved and maintained. Every effort must therefore be made to reduce overall exposure to irritants, which should enable an individual to remain in gainful employment.

However, repeated daily exposure to irritants may induce toughening and resistance, allowing repeated contact without further evidence of irritation. This process is called 'hardening' and is an individually acquired resistance, providing only local protection, with short periods away from work resulting in decreased resistance. This cannot therefore, be relied on as a means of protection against irritants.

Water is a potential irritant. It penetrates relatively easily through the stratum corneum and prolonged exposure is a well recognized cause of dermatitis amongst housewives, bartenders, nurses and mechanics. The protective layer of the skin is diminished, and warmth, occlusion, bacteria, fungi and chemical exposure can further contribute to skin damage. Few claims are made for occupational dermatitis caused by water, as many affected are self-treated with no loss of time from work.

The stratum corneum accounts for the major diffusional resistance of the skin. Initially, on contact with water, a diffusion pathway exists through the hair follicles and sweat glands for a short period. With continued exposure a steady state is reached across the whole stratum corneum, with diffusion across this layer being the predominant pattern. In environments of relative humidities less than 60% water binds directly to keratin fibrils. At relative humidities from 60% to 94% water interacts with the fibrillar bound water. At humidities greater than 94% water content increases rapidly as 'free water' not bound to keratin fibrils, and the stratum corneum begins to break down mechanically.

Solvents, which are mixtures of fluids capable of dissolving substances to produce other compounds, are estimated to be responsible for up to 20% of industrial dermatitis. The physical properties of solvents influence the injurious effects they have on the skin. In general, the more poorly absorbed solvents cause the most skin damage and the least systemic symptoms. For example, saturated hydrocarbon solvents and the paraffin series of solvents are stronger skin irritants than those derived from the aromatic series. Solvents with a higher boiling point tend to have a less irritant effect.

The most frequent cause of solvent-induced industrial dermatitis is the practice of washing with solvents. As solvents are frequently used in industry as degreasing agents to remove oil, grease and stains from manufactured products, they are commonly use as hand cleansers because they are quick and effective. With repeated use cumulative irritation occurs, with the risk of irritant contact dermatitis developing. Painters use thinners and turpentine, printers use type-wash, plastic workers use acetone, mechanics use petrol or paraffin and dry-cleaners use trichloroethylene or perchloroethylene as soap substitutes.

Solvents dissolve and remove surface lipids, the lipid material within the stratum corneum, and the fatty fraction of cell membranes. With defatting of the skin there is increased percutaneous absorption of water and other substances.

Soaps and detergents are the major predisposing

or perpetuating factors in the majority of cases of hand dermatitis. The irritancy of soaps is due to the combination of alkalinity, degreasing action and direct irritancy of fatty acids, which with repeated water exposure damage the epidermal layers. In addition to this abrasive contact, the presence of additives may also contribute to irritation. Most bar soaps have alkaline builders such as sodium bicarbonate, sodium phosphate, ash, borax or silicate added to increase cleansing. These may additionally irritate the skin. Perfumes and colours increase the appeal, and germicidal agents help to prevent deterioration, but these may cause irritancy or sensitization. Abrasive agents are often incorporated into industrial cleansers to increase the mechanical cleansing action. These include inorganic agents such as pumice, chalk, sand or borax, and organic agents such as groundnut shells, cornmeal or wood flours.

In summary, the early recognition and appropriate institution of measures to reduce the overall exposure to irritants by an individual with irritant contact dermatitis will often enable continuation of employment.

IMMUNOLOGY OF THE SKIN

The skin is an important immunological organ and normally contains nearly all the elements of cellular immunity with the exception of B cells. Much of the original research into immunology was undertaken using the skin as a model.

Hypersensitivity reactions and the skin

'Hypersensitivity' is the term applied when an adaptive immune response is inappropriate or exaggerated to the degree that tissue damage results. The skin can exhibit all the main types of hypersensitivity response.

Type I (immediate)

Immunoglobulin E (IgE) is bound to the surface of mast cells by Fc receptors. On encountering an antigen (e.g. a housedust mite, food or pollen) the IgE molecules become cross-linked causing degranulation and the release of the inflammatory mediators. These include preformed mediators

(such as histamine) and newly formed ones (e.g. prostaglandins or leukotrienes). The result in the skin is urticaria, although massive histamine release can cause anaphylaxis — a life-threatening condition. The response occurs within minutes and individuals may react to many different chemical coming in contact with the skin. This results in a widespread itchy rash similar to a giant nettle rash (urticaria or hives). This may be caused by diverse substances, from rubber latex to amniotic fluid (Table 2.2). If the swellings affect the mouth, then the throat may also become affected and this can lead to suffocation.

Type II (antibody-dependent cytotoxicity)

Antibodies directed against an antigen on target skin cells or structures induce cytotoxicity by killer T cells or by complement activation. This type of hypersensitivity is not thought to be of significance in occupational health.

Type III (immune complex disease)

Immune complexes are formed by the combination of an antigen and antibodies in the blood and are deposited in the walls of small vessels, often those of the skin. Complement activation, platelet aggregation and the release of lysosomal enzymes from polymorphs cause vascular damage. Again this type of hypersensitivity is not thought to be of significance in occupational health.

Table 2.2 Agents causing contact urticaria

Foodstuffs and body fluids
Latex
Ammonium persulphate
Platinum salts
Cobalt chloride
Ammonia
Aliphatic polyamines
Sulphur dioxide
Aminothiazole
Lindane
Acrylic monomers
Exotic woods

Type IV (cell mediated or delayed)

Specifically sensitized T lymphocytes have secondary contact with the antigen when it is presented on the surface of the antigen-presenting cells. Cytokine release causes T cell activation and amplifies the reaction by recruiting other T cells and macrophages to the site. Tissue damage results which is maximal at 48–72 h after contact with T lymphocyte antigen. Allergic contact dermatitis and the tuberculin reaction to intradermally administered antigen are both forms of type IV reaction. This is the most important immunological reaction in the development of allergic dermatitis.

ALLERGIC CONTACT DERMATITIS

Clinically this form of dermatitis looks identical to irritant contact dermatitis, but it is caused by an individual developing a specific allergy to a substance. Whereas irritant contact dermatitis has the potential to affect all people, allergic contact dermatitis will only affect a small proportion of people exposed to the substance. Unfortunately it is not possible to predict which individuals may develop this problem.

For allergy to develop, repeated exposure to the substance over a period of time is required, usually months or years, until the skin becomes sensitized. For sensitization to occur, a potential allergen needs to penetrate the epidermis and therefore its molecular weight must be less than 500. More typically this falls in the range of 200–300. The chemical is then picked up by Langerhans' cells and transported to the regional lymph nodes where it is processed. In some individuals a pool of sensitized cells (lymphocytes) is then formed. In practice it usually takes months or even years of exposure for sensitization to occur.

Once sensitized, further exposure to the substance, even at low concentrations, and at any skin site will result in an outpouring of these cells from the lymph nodes to the site of exposure, causing inflammation (dermatitis) (Fig. 2.3). However the

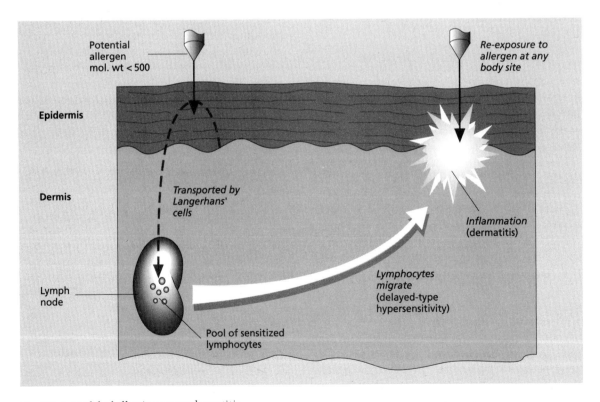

Fig. 2.3 A model of allergic contact dermatitis.

time of onset of dermatitis from re-exposure may take from one to five days as it takes time for the allergen to penetrate and for the sensitized cells to respond. Hence the name 'delayed-type hypersensitivity'. For this reason a cause and effect may not be realized by the sufferer. Once individuals becomes sensitized they remain sensitized for the rest of their lives, however a small proportion may lose their sensitivity with the passage of time.

If allergic sensitization is suspected then patch testing may be undertaken by dermatologists to identify the allergen. This involves trying to reproduce what is happening in the skin by applying the allergen to the skin at an appropriate concentration to try to induce an inflammatory reaction. The allergens are usually applied to the back and are left in place. After 48 h an initial reading is taken and a final reading is taken after 96 h.

Once an allergen has been identified for an individual then avoidance has to be instituted to prevent recurrences of the dermatitis. Allergic contact dermatitis accounts for about 5% of all industrial dermatitis whereas irritant contact dermatitis accounts for the rest.

BARRIER CREAMS

It should be recognized that there is no cream which actually provides a barrier preventing the penetration of substances into the skin. In fact, in some situations they may actually enhance penetration. There are numerous formulations available and these are intended for either dry or wet work. Those for dry work are water soluble and often contain polyethylene glycols. Those for wet work are water insoluble and are often based on lanolins, paraffins or silicones.

In practice the main benefit they offer is due to their bases, which may help to improve the hydration (suppleness) of the skin, with the result that, when cleansers are used, less degreasing of the skin occurs. In theory this may help to reduce irritant contact dermatitis from repeated hand washing. There is subjective evidence amongst those using barrier creams that the skin is easier to cleanse.

There is no evidence that barrier creams protect against sensitizers and occasionally sensitization to some of the constituents of the cream may occur. However the use of a barrier cream may give an employee a false sense of security and lead to increased abuse of the skin.

Provided their limitations are recognized barrier creams are of benefit overall by increasing the hydration of the skin, which may result in less harsh cleansers being required.

SKIN CLEANSING

If substances remain on the skin after the working day, the risk of irritation or sensitization is increased. The most efficient skin cleansers, however, are often the most irritant of substances because of their solvent or detergent content. If cleansers are too mild for the task, workers will often use degreasing agents used at work for industrial purposes, for example solvents or paraffins, to obtain adequate cleansing. Although these latter substances will clean, they are potentially very irritant if used repeatedly. It is often not appropriate to provide one type of cleanser for different jobs. These agents should be chosen to provide adequate cleaning in a short period of time without being too strong a degreasing agent.

Drying of the skin after cleansing is equally important, and disposable paper towels or a pull-down roller towel are preferable to a roller towel or rag which will become — and remain — wet or dirty.

AFTER-WORK CREAMS

Many companies now produce after-work creams, which in essence are moisturizers, but which have the benefit of increasing the hydration of the skin at the end of the day. They are of particular benefit in occupations where excessive drying of the skin may occur. In addition their use should be encouraged where hot-air driers are used as these tend to dry the skin excessively.

CONCLUSIONS

In the workplace, some skin contact with chemicals is almost inevitable. This cutaneous exposure may not necessarily constitute a health hazard, but

seemingly minimal contact with certain substances may lead to toxicity. Many factors play an
important role with regard to the rate and extent of
absorption through the skin. As a result of the
complexities, individual percutaneous absorption
cannot be predicted, even from working habits and
methods. This situation is therefore very different
from the more familiar respiratory reactions to
airborne chemical exposure. Therefore, for safe
working practices and for preventive purposes,
appropriate safeguards must be defined for each
specific exposure.

REFERENCE

Malten, K.E. (1981). Thoughts on irritant contact dermatitis. *Contact Dermatitis*, **7**, 238–42.

FURTHER READING

Fisher, A.A. (1986). *Contact Dermatitis*, (3rd edn). Lea
and Febiger, Philadelphia.

Foulds, I.S. (1987). Occupational skin disease. In *Textbook
of Occupational Medicine*, (ed. J.K. Howard and F.H.
Tyner). Churchill Livingstone, Edinburgh.

Fregert, S. (1981). *Manual of Contact Dermatitis*, (2nd
edn). Munksgaard, Copenhagen.

Rycroft, R.J.G. (1986). Occupational dermatoses. In *Text-
book of Dermatology*, (4th edn), (ed. A. Rook, D.S.
Wilkinson, F.J.G. Ebling, R.H. Champion and J.L.
Burton), pp. 569–86. Blackwell Scientific Publications,
Oxford.

Wilkinson, J.D. and Rycroft, R.J.G. (1986). Contact dermatitis. In *Textbook of Dermatology*, (4th edn), (ed. A.
Rook, D.S. Wilkinson, F.J.G. Ebling, R.H. Champion
and J.L. Burton), pp. 435–532. Blackwell Scientific
Publications, Oxford.

Wilkinson, J.D. and Rycroft, R.J.G. (1986). The principal
irritants and sensitizers. In *Textbook of Dermatology*,
(4th edn), (ed. A. Rook, D.S. Wilkinson, F.J.G. Ebling,
R.H. Champion and J.L. Burton), pp. 533–67. Blackwell
Scientific Publications, Oxford.

CHAPTER 3

Deposition of Inhaled Materials in the Respiratory Tract

M.J. Lever and R.C. Schroter

INTRODUCTION

The average adult inhales approximately 10 000 litres of air every day in order to exchange oxygen and carbon dioxide across the alveolar membrane. This delicate membrane has a vast area of approximately $100\,m^2$, and needs protection from the environmental air which is breathed. During inspiration the air is heated and humidified, so that on reaching the membrane it is at body temperature and saturated with water vapour. It is also important to protect the alveolar membrane from noxious substances in the atmosphere, both particulate and gaseous. This is achieved by deposition of particulate matter and scrubbing out of the gases on the walls of the upper airway and bronchial passages of the respiratory system. The mechanisms controlling these processes, which are the subject of this chapter, are extremely efficient and provide a powerful defence mechanism for the body.

The area of the lung presented to the inspired gas is very much greater than that of the skin covering the outer surface of the body which is only about $1.5-2\,m^2$. This indicates the enormous importance of the lung as the major route of entry of airborne foreign materials into the body. The fact that very large volumes of air are breathed each day means that, even if a pollutant is present in very low concentration, the potential toxicological burden in the lungs can be very high. In healthy subjects, particles that deposit on all but the smallest airway structures in the periphery of the lung are removed from the pulmonary system on a blanket of mucus by the mucociliary clearance system (see also Chapter 1). Although this process eliminates substances from the lung, it does not necessarily remove them from the body since once the mucus layer reaches the top of the larynx, it is swallowed and absorption can then occur within the gastrointestinal system. Similar ciliary clearance mechanisms also remove deposited material from the nasal passages, while saliva constantly washes the buccal surfaces.

Materials which are not removed in the larger airways may penetrate to the most peripheral parts of the lung where there are no cilia lining the airway surfaces. At these sites, soluble materials will dissolve and be absorbed into the lung tissue and the blood. Insoluble particles will be engulfed by macrophages which are present on the alveolar surface. They may then be carried across the membranes into the blood for elimination elsewhere in the body. Some deposited particles may be cytotoxic, killing the macrophages and causing inflammatory reactions which may lead to progressive scarring. If this occurs extensively, it will lead to pulmonary fibrosis.

Because all surfaces of the airways have a liquid lining, airborne particles that alight on them cannot be easily resuspended. Deposited particles and gases, particularly if they are irritants, can precipitate reflex actions causing sneezing or coughing, which are very effective methods of facilitating their rapid removal from the body. Elimination mechanisms are discussed more fully in Chapter 4.

The presence of pollutants in the air we breathe is not simply a consequence of modern industrial civilization. The atmosphere has long contained dusts and smoke from various sources, as well as toxic gases such as hydrogen sulphide, sulphur dioxide and ammonia resulting from the decay of biological material. The transport of pollen and fungal spores by the wind, and the existence of aerial bacteria and viruses, have always been causes of inconvenience to humans. However, the greatly elevated pollution levels resulting from industrial activities have provided an added burden to the defence mechanisms of the lung, both as an increase in the uptake, and the unusually high toxicity, of a number of substances. These products will obviously cause serious problems in the location where they are being produced, but an increasing number of studies are showing that whole human and animal populations are displaying adverse effects attributable to airborne agents, indicating their widespread release into the environment.

Gas and particle concentrations in the atmosphere may vary from parts per million to many per cent. Aerosols may consist of liquid droplets as in fogs, or solid particles as in smokes, and the particle size range of the aerosols we breathe is considerable. For instance, pollen and spores are typically in the size range $5-100\,\mu m$, while viruses can be as small as $0.005\,\mu m$. Industrial ashes, and grinding and crushing products are in the same approximate size range as pollen and spores. Metallurgical fumes can cover the vast range of less than $0.001\,\mu m$ to more than $100\,\mu m$. Tobacco smoke contains a wide mixture of particles, but the majority of particles are in the range $0.01-0.1\,\mu m$. Densities also vary widely from very low values for some spores to high values for metals and minerals.

Because they tend to persist for relatively long periods of time in the atmosphere, particles less than about $100\,\mu m$ are the ones of greatest importance when considering respiratory tract deposition. Particles with diameters more than about $10\,\mu m$ are effectively filtered out in the airways of the head and neck and so do not normally reach the lungs. For this reason they are sometimes classified as 'non-respirable dusts' in contrast to smaller particles constituting 'respirable dusts'. As will become apparent, such a distinction is not a clear one and some very large particles, in the form of fibres, can penetrate deeply into the lungs. Some aerosols, such as bacteria, pollen and fungal spores, are very uniform in size, but the majority tend to be polydisperse with a range of particle sizes depen-

dent on the manner in which they are formed. Assessment of the amount of an inhaled material which is retained within the lungs requires both a quantitative description of the size distribution and knowledge of the deposition probabilities for particles of each size.

Whilst early interest in the scientific principles underlying aerosol deposition in the lung was driven by concern about the potential toxic effects of inhaled substances, there has recently been a huge growth of interest in using inhalation as a means of delivering therapeutic drugs to the body. With increasing understanding of the deposition mechanisms, it is now proving possible to deliver materials in a controlled manner to quite specific locations within the respiratory tract. This mode of treatment can ensure that the inhaled drug acts locally within the lung at a desired airway site, or can be released in a controlled manner to all body tissues by its slow uptake into the blood.

Gases such as sulphur dioxide and the oxides of nitrogen are often present in the atmosphere at exceedingly low concentrations, of the order of a few parts per million. However, physiological effects can be demonstrated for exposure even to these low levels. Other gases and vapours, such as industrial solvents, are sometimes present at high concentrations in confined spaces. The chemical nature of a number of gases changes in the presence of water; thus the nitrogen oxides form nitric acid, and ozone breaks down. Such changes may occur in the air during humidification in the airways or on the surface lining of the bronchi.

A wide range of physical processes controls the deposition of materials in the respiratory tract and these depend not only upon the properties of the inhaled materials, but also on a number of factors related to the pattern of breathing and the geometry of the airway path. Anatomical factors, such as the geometry of the nasal turbinates and the way in which the airways branch and become progressively narrower, are extremely important, as are the pattern of breathing and the total ventilation, which are dictated by the metabolic needs of the body. Particle deposition and gas uptake in small people who are resting will be different from those in larger people engaged in heavy physical exercise. It is therefore appropriate to consider first those factors which will dictate the ventilation and flow patterns within the different major regions of the respiratory system.

DIVISIONS OF THE RESPIRATORY TRACT

As indicated above, the fate of inhaled material depends very strongly on where in the respiratory system it is taken up. Insoluble particles that deposit in the nasopharyngeal region are handled differently from those that deposit on the mucociliary escalator and from those that reach the alveoli. The fate of gases, and particles that are soluble, will also differ between these three principal sections. These anatomical regions are also quite distinct in their geometry and the patterns of airflow within them, and so the local mechanisms of gas absorption and particle deposition exhibit important differences. Additionally, the quantity of material which reaches each of these sections will not be the same, but will be determined by the amount of absorption occurring while the inhaled air traverses the upstream regions. The amount of deposition during exhalation will depend upon what happens during inhalation and during the residence of the gas in the alveolar regions.

For these reasons, it is appropriate to consider the three sections of the respiratory tract independently. Their morphology and main physiological features have been described in Chapter 1, and so attention will be focused only on those features pertinent to deposition processes. We will look first at conditions in the upper airway, which comprises all structures, including the larynx, above the trachea. Secondly we will discuss conditions within the tracheobronchial tree, which is the branching airway system as far as the terminal bronchioles, and includes all the airways with a ciliated lining. We will then consider the alveolar region, which comprises the non-ciliated respiratory bronchioles, alveolar ducts and associated alveoli.

The upper airway

Inhalation can occur either through the nose or the mouth, depending on habit, the presence or absence of upper respiratory infections, the ventilation rate and speech patterns. The pathway used will have a dramatic effect on how much material is extracted from the inspired air before it enters the lungs.

The oral pathway is a wide conduit covered in a relatively vascular layer. The surface contains no mucus secreting cells or cilia but is constantly washed by saliva. It joins the nasal pathway at the rear of the soft palate. In contrast with the buccal cavity of the mouth, the nasal pathway is very much more complex with two distinct regions, external and internal to the skull. The external nose has two parallel passages, the external nares which have relatively soft tissue, the ali, on either side and are separated by a more rigid nasal septum. They contain coarse nasal hairs which are very efficient at filtering out the largest inhaled particles. These external passages continue into the left and right internal nasal cavities, each of which has three vertically stacked, shelf-like structures — the nasal turbinates or conchae. These turbinates divide each main passageway into slit-like spaces through which the respired gas passes. The main physiological function of the turbinates is to warm and humidify the inspired gas to avoid cooling or dehydration of the lung. In addition, their large surface area and rich underlying vascular supply facilitates the local uptake and removal of soluble materials into the bloodstream. The upper part of the internal nasal cavities contains the olfactory organs and the nasal sinuses in which inhaled gas can remain trapped for considerable periods. The surface of the nasal cavities is covered by a ciliated epithelium which contains mucus secreting cells, and there is a continuous movement of the mucus layer backwards towards the throat.

The internal nares converge above the soft palate to form a single conduit which then joins the buccal cavity to form the pharynx. At the base of the tongue the pharynx enters the larynx, which contains two folds of tissue running from the front to the back, the ventricular folds, and beyond these, the vocal cords which form an elongated fissure, the glottis. The glottis can be the narrowest segment of the upper airways. The width of its aperture can be altered by contraction of groups of muscles acting on cartilages around the larynx. Although the gap is fairly narrow during quiet breathing, it widens during deep inspiration, and its shape is dramatically modified during speech. The velocity of the air through the gap may be very high and influence the deposition of materials, both in the larynx itself and on downstream surfaces.

The tracheobronchial tree

This is a tree-like system of conducting airways from the trachea to the terminal bronchioles. In the human, the diameters of airways fall from approximately 2 cm at the trachea to about 200 μm at the level of the terminal bronchioles; model descriptions of the tree have commonly divided the branching system into approximately 25 generations of airways of decreasing size. However, it must be emphasized that, in the real lung, the branching properties of the tree produce a highly asymmetrical structure in which relatively small branches often originate from quite large airways. This results in tremendous variability in the distance which gas must travel from the top of the trachea to the alveoli. Whilst the average pathlength from trachea to respiratory bronchiole is about 13 cm in the adult, it can be as little as 8 cm (corresponding to about 8 generations), and up to about 22 cm (corresponding to 25 generations), for some other parts of the lung. Failure to recognize this asymmetry has led to considerable problems when attempting to use theoretical models to describe the deposition of inhaled materials.

The combined volume of the upper airway and tracheobronchial trees is often referred to as the anatomical dead space, which is typically 150–200 cm³ in adults. Because of the complexity of respiratory flow patterns, material inhaled in volumes which are much smaller than the dead space can penetrate very deeply into the lungs. Indeed inhaled volumes of aerosol-laden gas, even as small as 50 cm³, can result in the deposition of considerable quantities of material in the periphery of the lungs, far beyond the nominal depth of penetration.

The alveolar region

This is the region beyond the terminal bronchioles and it provides an enormous surface area for the deposition of particles and the uptake of gases which penetrate that far. It contains the largest volume of gas in the lung, and air which reaches an alveolus early in the breath will remain within it for most of the duration of the respiratory cycle. Since the radius of the expanded alveolus is about 100 μm, it may be traversed easily by inhaled substances within the period of a breath. As it does not have a ciliated epithelium for the rapid, efficient removal of particles, deposited materials may remain in this region of the tract for long periods.

AIRFLOW IN THE RESPIRATORY TRACT

To understand the processes which determine the behaviour of noxious gases and aerosols in the respiratory system, it is necessary to consider the manner in which the inspired gas moves in and out of the lungs. Breathing patterns show considerable variation between different people as well as for an individual, according to what tasks are being undertaken. Breathing is slower and deeper when sleeping than when awake, it increases during any form of exercise and has to be modulated in a complex way during speech. We may, however, make a number of generalizations about the time course and ventilation volumes for normal subjects.

During quiet breathing at rest, tidal volumes of between 400 and 700 cm³ are inhaled at a rate of 8–12 breaths min⁻¹, the minute ventilation being between 4 and 8 l min⁻¹. The inspired gas becomes mixed with approximately 2–3 l of residual gas (the functional residual capacity) which is present in the lung at the end of each expiration. Even on maximal exhalation, a residual volume of 0.5–1 l remains in the lung; this volume of gas is essential to prevent collapse of the airways.

At low ventilation levels, gas is inhaled more rapidly than it is exhaled and there is a short respiratory pause at the end of exhalation. When the ventilation requirement increases on exercise, there are changes in both the tidal volume and frequency of breathing. With gentle exercise there is first an abolition of the respiratory pause followed by an increase in the tidal volume causing rises in both inspiratory and expiratory flow rates. As ventilation increases further, and the tidal volume reaches 1–2 l, breathing frequency rises and the functional residual capacity is slightly elevated. These changes occur progressively in such a way as to minimize the work expended on breathing.

The highest levels at which ventilation can be sustained for long periods depend on lung size and on training but are usually between 50 and $80 \, \text{l} \, \text{min}^{-1}$ in fit adults, at a breathing frequency of about 50 breaths min^{-1}. Greater ventilation rates with both higher tidal volumes and frequencies may be achieved for brief periods but cannot be sustained indefinitely. Under these circumstances, tidal volumes can go up to $4 \, \text{l}$ and frequencies up to 150 breaths min^{-1}, but not usually at the same time. The fact that breathing is cyclical and ventilation levels vary so widely with exercise implies that there is a very wide range of flow conditions, not only in different parts of the lung but at any site within the airways, as a function of time.

Flow in the upper airway

At rest, when ventilation rates are low, the mouth is normally closed and breathing takes place through the nose. However, as inspiratory flow rates increase, the resistance to flow through the nose rises rapidly and, as can be observed when sniffing, the ali of the nose tend to collapse. Consequently, on exercise, when inspiratory flow rates exceed approximately $1 \, \text{l} \, \text{s}^{-1}$, the mouth route for respiration is preferred as it offers a far lower flow resistance. However, in consequence, the defences of the nasal hairs and the turbinates are then bypassed.

The complex geometry of the nasal passages makes it especially difficult to give a quantitative description of gas velocities and flow patterns within them. High velocities are always seen in the external nares, partly because of the small cross-section of this region, and partly because breathing tends to cycle between the two passages as the nasal turbinates of each side swell and shrink with a periodicity of $1-3 \, \text{h}$. At normal quiet ventilation rates, velocities in the nostrils, past the coarse hair filter, are in the region of $2-3 \, \text{m} \, \text{s}^{-1}$ and turbulent flow is generated on entry to the internal nose and turbinates. This turbulence helps to maintain high mass transfer rates between the respired air and mucosal surface, a factor important both for

humidification and warming of air, and the extraction of particles and soluble gases from it. Not all the inspired air passes over the turbinates however; a very small amount flows into the nasal sinuses and over the olfactory receptors. The residence time in the sinuses is very long, allowing adequate exchange between air and tissue. During expiration, some of the air is diverted over the same surfaces, flushing out the air entrained there during inspiration.

As air leaves the turbinates and proceeds to the curve of the nasopharynx, the velocity increases to about $4 \, \text{m} \, \text{s}^{-1}$ because the total cross-section for flow again decreases. On exit from the larynx further turbulence is generated because the air emerges as a jet into the trachea.

Flow in the tracheobronchial tree

Flow conditions in the bronchial airways have been much more extensively studied than those in the upper airway, by means of experiments on hollow casts of the lung and on simplified models of the airways. Because of asymmetry, both in branching and in airway diameter, air velocities and patterns of flow will vary considerably between generations; the use of 'typical' values of velocity, shown in Fig. 3.1, must be done with caution.

The majority of flow and transport models that have been developed for the human lung use the airway geometry presented in the classical simplified model developed by Weibel. However, this was produced on the basis of limited morphometric data and was presented in the form of a 'symmetrical' model. When the Weibel model predictions of the distribution of velocity along the tree are compared with more recent, and extensive, morphometric airway data, it can be seen that there are significant differences in the predicted flow rate within airways of different diameters. These differences result partly from actual differences in diameter of individual airways, but principally from the inherent asymmetry in the branching system.

Because the total cross-sectional area of the airways increases on moving towards the peripheral regions of the lungs, the gas velocity progressively falls, and changes occur in the patterns of flow as inertia becomes less dominant. A useful predictor

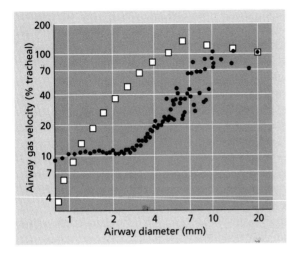

Fig. 3.1 Average airway velocity (as a percentage of tracheal value) in airways of different diameter down to 0.8 mm. □ represent data of Weibel's symmetrical model, ● represent directly measured anatomical data of Raabe *et al.* (1976). After Phillips, Kaye and Schroter (1994).

of likely flow patterns is the Reynolds number (*Re*) defined as:

$$Re = \frac{\bar{U}\rho d}{\eta} \qquad (3.1)$$

where ρ is the density and η the viscosity of gas, d is the diameter of the tube or airway and $\bar{U}$ is the mean gas velocity. (NB. η has been used throughout this book as the symbol for viscosity, however, μ is gaining in general usage.) For *Re* values above 1, inertial factors are increasingly important and flow in the airways is not axisymmetric and parabolic as once assumed, but of a complicated three-dimensional nature. Flow near the outer walls of

bifurcations can experience separation with low local velocities and long residence times. On inspiration, the curvature of each bifurcation produces strong secondary motions consisting of a pair of helices in each daughter airway. On expiration, strong secondary flows consisting of two pairs of helices are formed in the parent tube (Fig. 3.2). Although the flow appears to be disturbed, it follows predictable courses during inhalation and exhalation and can give rise to distinctive patterns of deposition of materials on the airway walls (Fig. 3.3). If *Re* is greater than about 2000, flow can become turbulent as happens at higher levels of ventilation in the trachea and the first few generations of bronchi. If very dense gases are breathed, as in diving, then *Re* is elevated even more.

In the most peripheral airways, the reduction of both the velocity of the air and the dimensions of the airways contributes to a rapid fall in *Re*. For values below 1, disturbances caused by bifurcations are very rapidly overcome and flow conditions become re-established within about one diameter, providing axisymmetrical flows by the end of an airway.

It is possible to gain some feeling for the range of flow properties along the tree by comparing *Re* in large and small airways on the basis of Fig. 3.1. For a flow rate of $21s^{-1}$ (about the highest velocity expected during heavy exercise) in a trachea of 2 cm diameter, *Re* is approximately 8500; in a 1 mm diameter airway, the local velocity is approximately 10% of the tracheal value and *Re* is around 40. In the very smallest airways of the order of 200 μm diameter, in which velocities are unlikely to exceed $1 \, cm \, s^{-1}$, the local *Re* will be less than approximately 0.1.

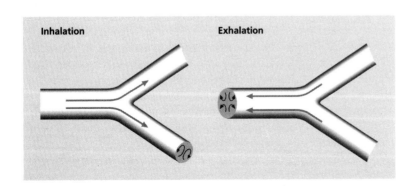

Fig. 3.2 Schematic view of a bifurcation showing the structure of the secondary motions caused by the junction on inhalation and exhalation. After Schroter and Sudlow (1969).

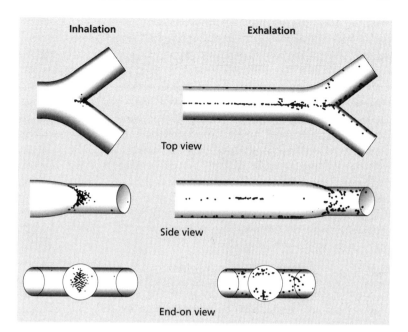

Fig. 3.3 The spatial distribution of the deposition of 10 µm particles in a bifurcation from flows with Reynolds numbers similar to those found in larger airways. During inhalation deposition occurs predominantly on the carina, but during exhalation deposition occurs at sites which are predictable from secondary flows. After Balashazy and Hoffman (1993).

The detailed geometry of a bifurcation strongly influences flow conditions and particle deposition. In normal subjects, flow dividers are almost always 'sharp', so far as the flow is concerned; the split between flows on inspiration is clean, with no backward motion of gas. However, the flow divider may be bluff in subjects with some forms of lung disease, in this case the divider acts as a stagnation zone causing reverse flows into the junction.

Flow in the alveolar region

On reaching the respiratory alveolar ducts and the alveoli, air velocities are very low, never exceeding about $1 \, \text{cm} \, \text{s}^{-1}$ even during heavy exercise. The alveoli accommodate most of the inspired gas, giving rise to the longest residence times within the respiratory tract. Despite low Re, flow conditions are somewhat complicated because of differences in the pattern of expansion and contraction of the alveoli during the respiratory cycle. Consequently, the flow within them is not reversible and air inspired during one breath becomes mixed with the residual air; as a result the mean residence time is greater than the time of a single respiratory cycle.

Mixing in the lung

Mixing between the inspired and residual gases in the lung is not restricted to the alveolar region but occurs continuously all along the respiratory tract throughout the respiratory cycle. As the fresh, inspired air flows through the airways behind the residual gas, the turbulence and secondary motions in the flow cause a distortion of the velocity profile. Considerable blurring of the interface occurs to produce a zone in which conditions change progressively from 'pure' inspired to 'residual' air. The distorted velocity profiles in the airways elongate the interface between the new and old gases. The gas flowing along the middle of the airway traverses it rapidly, whereas that near the wall moves slowly and is held back.

Consequently there is a radial concentration gradient between new and old gases — radial diffusion processes work to overcome and abolish this gradient. Gas molecules will diffuse away from the fast moving centre towards the slower moving region near the wall and thus will not be transported along the airways as rapidly as would be expected in the absence of radial diffusion. Clearly, the rate of such radial diffusion depends upon the diffusible properties of the gas molecules or particles which may then be transported along the airways at different rates and penetrate to different depths in the lung.

An additional mixing process is afforded by the beating of the heart. As it fills and empties of blood during the cardiac cycle, the heart deforms the lungs which surround it. This local movement causes some alveolar expansion and compression and thus enhances mixing in the airways as they are being further alternately compressed and expanded. Consequently, there is shunting of gases from one part of the lung to another — this is commonly known as 'pendelluft'.

Physiological effects on flow conditions

A number of physiological factors influence the flow conditions and distribution of ventilation in the lung. It is important to mention here those which would be likely to strongly influence particle deposition and noxious gas uptake by the lungs.

So far we have described the bronchial airways as though they were rigid tubes, however they are elastic structures and change size with lung volume. As a result, at low respiratory flow rates the majority of a tidal volume breath goes towards the base of the lung (or the apex if the subject is inverted). However, as the flow rate increases, this distribution imbalance is progressively overcome so that at high flow rates all regions of the lung achieve almost uniform ventilation.

It is also important to remember that the bronchial airways are not passive structures. They can react to the deposition of materials by constricting, which markedly increases their local flow resistance. This response can be demonstrated, even in normal subjects breathing chalk dust, and the effect on a subject liable to even mild asthma can be quite dramatic. Bronchoconstriction probably occurs in all generations of airways but can most easily be identified when occurring in the large airways as any diminution in their diameter can lead to a measurable increase in the resistance to breathing. If bronchoconstriction occurs at any time whilst breathing an aerosol or noxious gas then the uptake by the airways may change dramatically.

MECHANISMS OF PARTICLE DEPOSITION

When aerosol particles are suspended in still air, they are able to move independently by means of the processes of diffusion and gravitational sedimentation. By these mechanisms they can leave the gas phase and deposit onto surfaces.

Sedimentation

The gravitational force on a settling, airborne particle is counterbalanced by drag forces exerted by surrounding gas molecules. Stokes' law describes the final sedimentation velocity (V) which a particle will attain while falling through still air:

$$V = \frac{\rho \, g \, d^2}{18 \, \eta} \tag{3.2}$$

where ρ is the particle density, g is the acceleration due to gravity (approximately $9.8 \, \mathrm{m \, s^{-2}}$), d is the diameter of the particle and η is the viscosity of air (approximately $1.9 \times 10^{-5} \, \mathrm{N \, s \, m^{-2}}$. Particles smaller than about 1 μm diameter fall somewhat more rapidly than predicted by Stokes' law because they tend to slip between the air molecules as the particle diameter approaches the mean free pathlength of the gas molecules. Particles larger than about 30 μm sediment more slowly than expected because their higher inertia sets up complex eddies in the surrounding gas during their fall. Within the period of a typical breath, approximately 4 s, a 20 μm particle of unit density can fall 5 cm, a 10 μm particle can fall 1.2 cm and a 1 μm particle can fall 140 μm. These distances are comparable with the dimensions of different airways within the respiratory tract.

Most dust particles, such as those which are crystalline or produced by abrasion, are not spherical and so have a larger surface area than a sphere of the same mass. This increases the drag of the air on the moving particle and reduces the falling velocity. It is, therefore, necessary to consider the aerodynamic diameter of a particle when discussing its sedimentation characteristics. The aerodynamic diameter is defined as the diameter of a sphere of unit density which would sediment at the same velocity as the particle. It takes account of both density and drag in the application of Stokes' law and is invaluable in describing sedimentation properties. When a particle's shape deviates markedly from spherical, as in the case of a fibre, even a very large particle may have a relatively small aerodynamic diameter. A fibre of unit density, whose length is at least 10 times its diameter, will have an aerodynamic diameter only approximately three times greater than its physical diameter. Consequently, fibres can persist in the air very much longer than spherical particles of the same mass and therefore have a much greater likelihood of being inhaled.

Diffusion

Small particles are inherently mobile because of their own translational energy, and because of collision with surrounding gas molecules causing Brownian motion. This may bring particles into contact with any surface to which they can adhere; the liquid lining of the respiratory tract provides an excellent surface for such adhesion. Whilst particles which settle by gravitational sedimentation always fall onto upward facing surfaces, those moving by Brownian motion do so in random directions and can deposit on surfaces of any orientation. As particles deposit, a region of diminished concentration is created in the adjacent gas phase; for example, sedimenting particles may leave an upper particle-free space. This will create a concentration gradient for the diffusional flux of particles in the reverse (upward) direction. In the steady state, this diffusional flux J may be estimated using Fick's first law:

$$J = D \, A \, \frac{dC}{dx} \qquad (3.3)$$

where A is the area across which the flux is occurring and dC/dx is the concentration gradient of the particles. The diffusion coefficient (D) of the particle can be estimated using the Einstein equation:

$$D = \frac{k \, T}{3 \, \pi \, d \, \eta} \qquad (3.4)$$

where k is the Boltzmann constant, T is the absolute temperature, d is the particle diameter and η is the viscosity of air. The diffusion coefficient is independent of the density of the particle, but does depend on its shape, deviating progressively from the Einstein equation prediction as it becomes less spherical.

The equations given above will indicate the times of persistence of particles in the environment in conditions of still air and will also describe the behaviour of particles within the lung airways when the flow of air has stopped at the end of both inspiration or expiration. Although the net movement of small particles will be determined by the combination of both gravitational and diffusional processes, the sedimentation rate increases with the square of the particle diameter, whereas the diffusional flux decreases linearly with increasing diameter. The distance over which a particle can diffuse in a given time is proportional to the square root of that time, and thus a $0.1 \, \mu m$ diameter particle can diffuse up to $150 \, \mu m$ during a normal $4 \, s$ breath (i.e. the radius of a small airway), but a $1 \mu m$ diameter particle can only diffuse up to $30 \, \mu m$ in the same period.

Sedimentation and diffusion processes will also be occurring while the gas is moving; therefore for particles within the lung airways, we must additionally take account of the rate at which they are being convected by the gas. The residence time of the gas in an airway will determine the time available for local deposition by the mechanisms of sedimentation and diffusion. The complex flow patterns observed within airways may, however, increase the rate of transport of particles toward the airway wall and thus enhance both sedimentation and diffusional deposition.

Impaction

When air movement is initiated, as for example at the start of inhalation or exhalation, drag forces will be exerted on suspended particles causing them to move with the airstream. Because of the inertia of the particles, they will at first move more slowly than the air, but will progressively accelerate and may reach the velocity of the surrounding air. Because of their greater density and mass, the particles will then have greater momentum than the air, and their inertia will cause them to tend to continue in their original direction, even when that of the airflow changes. This is also the situation towards the end of an inhalation or exhalation when airborne particles will tend to keep moving relative to the surrounding air.

If the momentum of the particles is sufficiently great, they will impact onto the leading edges of obstructions and on the outer surfaces of curving airways. The most important sites for impaction are in the upper airways because there the air velocities, and hence the momentum, of the particles is greatest. Sites include the upstream surfaces of the nasal hairs and turbinates, the outer walls of curvature of the nose and mouth and the flow dividers of carinae of the larger bronchial bifurcations. Indeed, impaction at these sites is a major mechanism for scrubbing the inspired air of larger particles before it enters the lobes of the lung. Fibres, particularly those which are straight rather than coiled, tend to become aligned with streamlines and are therefore impacted less readily than compact particles of a similar mass.

The probability of deposition of particles by this impaction mechanism is given by:

$$P_I = \frac{\rho \, d^2 \, \bar{U} \sin\theta}{18 \, R \, \eta} \qquad (3.5)$$

where P_I is the probability of impaction on the outer surface of a tube of radius R which bends with an angle of curvature θ. $\bar{U}$ is the mean particle velocity (which may be that of the flowing air), d is the particle aerodynamic diameter, ρ is the particle density and η is the viscosity of air.

When airflow profiles are disturbed, as happens in the airways because of turbulence and secondary flows, streamlines are not aligned parallel to the airway wall and suspended particles are likely to be propelled towards the wall. It is likely that impaction will be increased under these circumstances. Studies of the deposition of $10 \, \mu m$ diameter particles in model bifurcations have demonstrated that uptake by the wall occurs preferentially at sites where the changing geometry and secondary flows would favour impaction (see Fig. 3.3).

Because the predominant mechanisms for deposition vary according to particle diameter, some authors have classified aerosols into three different size ranges. The *thermodynamic range* is defined by those particles depositing by diffusion. It includes particles of unit density with diameters less than $0.16 \, \mu m$ (for spheres of density $3 \, g \, cm^{-3}$ the upper limit is only $0.09 \, \mu m$). The *intermediate range* contains particles of $0.16-1 \, \mu m$ diameter $(0.09-0.058 \, \mu m$ for $3 \, g \, cm^{-3}$ particles). It includes particles for which diffusion and sedimentation occur in an interdependent manner. The *aerodynamic range* includes all larger particles for which sedimentation and impaction are the predominant deposition mechanisms.

DEPOSITION ALONG THE RESPIRATORY TRACT

The total mass of particulate matter taken into the respiratory system will depend on both the total number of particles within the inhaled air and on their size distribution, a disproportionate fraction of the total mass being present as larger particles. Deposition rates are normally expressed in terms of fractional deposition, that is the ratio of the number of particles deposited relative to the number inhaled, and will be strongly dependent on the size distribution. When particle-laden air is inhaled, the number of particles which arrive at any location in the respiratory tract will depend not only on the inhaled concentration, but also on the efficiency of deposition in structures upstream of the site. These will be the upper airways during inhalation or the deeper airways during exhalation.

The largest particles, particularly those in the form of fibres, may be too large to penetrate some of the passages between nasal hairs or the nasal turbinates and will be arrested at these sites by interception. Because air velocities are high in the upper airways during inhalation, there is a very high probability that most particles with aerodynamic diameters in excess of $10 \, \mu m$ will impact on airway surfaces in this region, with very few penetrating to the airways of the lungs. As a consequence, deposition in this region may account for a large fraction of the total mass of inhaled material that is deposited in the respiratory tract. Penetration of large particles beyond the upper airways will be very strongly dependent on the inspiratory flow rate and whether inhalation occurs through the nose or mouth.

Within the tracheobronchial tree, the fall in air

velocity, and the transition from turbulent to laminar flow, reduces the importance of impaction as the principal mode of deposition, except close to the flow dividers of bifurcations where the airflow is split during inspiration. As airway size decreases, the distances which particles must travel to reach the walls are shorter, and the probability of deposition by sedimentation and diffusion increases. The airways within the lung are oriented in all directions since the main bronchi enter the lungs well below the apices. There can, therefore, be considerable variation in the distance a particle has to fall to sediment on the airway surfaces.

Particles pass fairly rapidly along the lung airways and those which enter an alveolus early during inhalation will remain there as the alveolus expands during the breath. Residence times in the alveolar region can, therefore, be several seconds and consequently the deposition probability of particles which sediment or diffuse rapidly is very high. Particles which remain airborne at the end of inhalation are still able to deposit during exhalation, either by sedimentation or diffusion in the smaller airways, or by impaction in the larger airways. The sites at which particles deposit during exhalation may be different from those affected during inhalation.

Throughout the period of inhalation the tidal volume of inspired air is continually mixing with the residual gas remaining in the lungs at the end of the previous exhalation. Particles which move into the residual gas may not be exhaled immediately but remain airborne and either deposit, or be exhaled during subsequent breaths. In a study using $0.5\,\mu m$ diameter monodispersed aerosols, particles were detected in exhaled air for up to six breaths after breathing clean air, demonstrating persistence in the residual gas for more than half a minute.

THE ROLE OF PARTICLE PROPERTIES IN DEPOSITION

It is apparent from experimental observations that the aerodynamic diameter of particles is of prime importance in determining the likely sites and levels of deposition in the lung. The use of aerodynamic diameters takes account of differences between particle density and shape together, but each of these factors is independently very significant in determining particle deposition. Density can vary from much less than $0.1\,g\,cm^{-3}$ for certain dry spores, to more than $10\,g\,cm^{-3}$ for mineral dusts. Both impaction and sedimentation rates are directly proportional to particle density which will therefore be a particularly important factor in the deposition of particles greater than $0.5\,\mu m$ diameter. Deviations from sphericity which may influence particle behaviour vary, from those of compact particles which are approximately spherical but have very rough surfaces, to highly elongated fibrous particles. Such particles will have smaller aerodynamic diameters than those expected from their masses for the reasons explained above.

Because of the many adverse effects of fibrous materials, such as asbestos or fibreglass, on the lungs, much attention has been given to such aerosols. Fibres tend to become aligned with flow streamlines and they are not readily filtered from the inhaled air in the upper airways. Consequently they can penetrate to the periphery of the lung in larger numbers than would be expected if they were spherical. Fibres longer than $100\,\mu m$ have been found in alveoli on post-mortem examination. To reach this region they will have traversed airways whose diameters were not many times the fibre length. Because of secondary flows, fibrous material can, however, undergo rotational motion in the conducting airways and as a result can be intercepted by the walls. In airways with marked secondary motions, deposition appears to occur mainly at sites just downstream from bifurcations. The exact sites are somewhat different for uniaxial fibres, such as fibreglass, from those of branching fibres, such as chrysotile asbestos.

Many solid particles carry some electrical charge, particularly if they are formed or released into the atmosphere by shearing mechanisms. Highly charged particles will tend to be deposited in the lungs more readily than uncharged particles, but in most practical situations these effects are likely to be small. The deposition mechanisms are similar to those in electrostatic precipitators used for aerosal sampling from the atmosphere. Although the lung surface probably carries no inherent charge, an approaching charged particle can induce an opposing charge on the surface and the resulting attraction will enhance deposition. In addition, if the concentration of particles carrying similar charges is very high the repulsive forces between them may cause their precipitation onto adjacent surfaces.

Many materials, including all salts and many aerosolized drugs, absorb water on entering the respiratory tract because the inhaled air is rapidly humidified and heated. The alteration in size may be small, but if the material is miscible with water, or is water soluble, then the particles can grow in size indefinitely as they pass down the airways. The net effects of this growth on overall deposition is highly complex and will depend strongly on the original size of the inhaled particles, as discussed below.

Certain materials have properties which can exert physiological or pathological effects on the airways and thereby elicit changes in subsequent deposition patterns. Mention has already been made of particles which cause coughing and sneezing, but certain irritant materials can cause contraction of the bronchial smooth muscle, which is a component of the walls of all but the smallest airways. This results in a constriction of the airways and the consequent changes in dimensions and flow patterns will normally lead to enhanced uptake within them. These effects are particularly severe in sensitized subjects with hay fever or asthma. In addition, many particles, though inherently inert, will adsorb gases from the atmosphere onto their surface. In this way noxious gases which might otherwise be scrubbed in the nose may penetrate to the lungs in high enough concentrations to cause adverse effects.

EXPERIMENTAL STUDIES OF PARTICLE DEPOSITION

There have been a considerable number of experimental studies of deposition mechanics both in humans and in other animals. With the latter it has been possible to study both total and regional deposition, by post-mortem examination after inhalation of known concentrations of particles. Although they have yielded much information about the nature of the deposition mechanisms, their results cannot be extrapolated directly to humans

because of differences in airway geometry (including dimensions and patterns of branching) and differences in the dynamics of breathing.

The implications of differing airway dimensions and ventilatory patterns when attempting to extrapolate data obtained in inhalation studies in animals to the human is well illustrated in Fig. 3.4. Markedly different patterns of uptake of similarly sized particles are observed in humans and rats. Rats have much smaller upper airways than the human and therefore experience higher uptake rates in this region. Although the tracheobronchial tree of the rat has dimensions similar to the smaller airways of the human, deposition rates in this region are much smaller in rats. This is probably because of much higher breathing frequencies resulting in very short residence times.

Aerosol uptake in humans has usually been determined by indirect methods. Some direct studies have employed soluble materials which are rapidly absorbed and whose concentration can be measured in blood samples; others have used radioactively labelled particles. The commonest method of as-

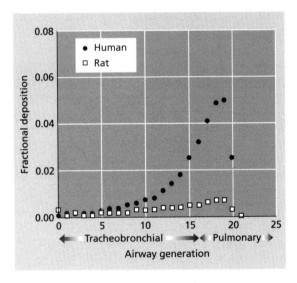

Fig. 3.4 Deposition of aerosol particles of 2.0 μm aerodynamic diameter along the respiratory tract of an adult human and rat. The fractional deposition in the trachea is slightly greater in the rat because of its smaller size, but is lower in the more peripheral airways because of shorter residence times. Data from Martonen, Zhang and Yang (1992).

sessing total deposition within the human respiratory tract involves measurements of the difference in the concentrations of particles in the inhaled and exhaled air. The concentration can be determined quantitatively using chemical analyses, by employing a variety of aerosol detectors including cascade impactors, or by using the light-scattering properties of aeorosols. To separate the inspired and exhaled gases it is often necessary to use breathing valves which may offer an additional site for aerosol deposition. The best methodology involves analyses at the mouth or the external nares where the gas enters and leaves the body.

Figure 3.5(a) shows the results of a set of studies with stable monodispersed aerosols breathed via the mouth, under carefully controlled conditions, in which deposition is expressed as a function of aerodynamic diameter. Small particles deposit most readily by diffusion whilst larger particles deposit both by sedimentation and impaction in the upper airways. Deposition rates of particles of all sizes are very sensitive to the pattern of breathing. The results obtained by mouth breathing may be compared with those for nose breathing (Fig. 3.6(a)) using the same experimental techniques. Deposition of the largest and smallest particle sizes

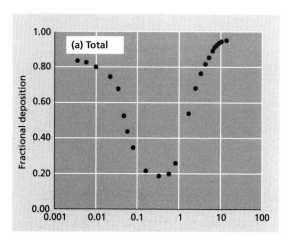

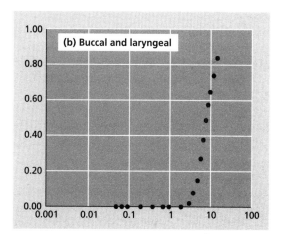

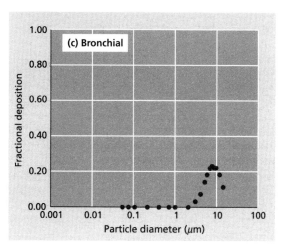

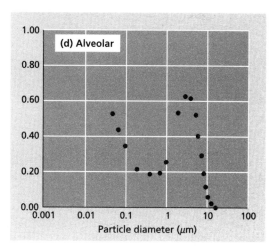

Fig. 3.5 Deposition of unit density spheres of different sizes (0.001–15 μm) in the adult human lung while mouth breathing at a controlled frequency of 8 breaths min^{-1} and a tidal volume of 1000 cm^3. Figure 3.5(a) gives the total deposition throughout the respiratory tract, and Figs 3.5(b)–(d) give data for the regional distribution of deposition for the larger particles. Data from Heyder *et al.* (1986).

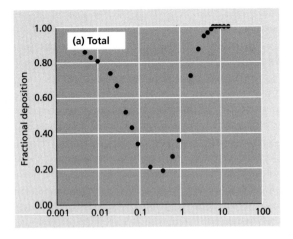

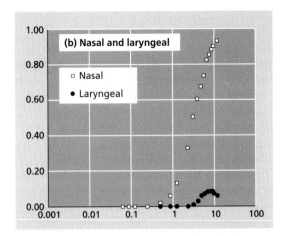

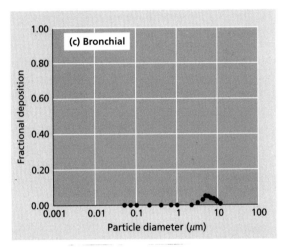

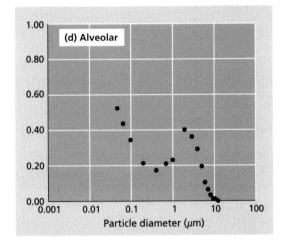

Fig. 3.6 Deposition of unit density spheres of different sizes (0.001–12 μm) in the adult human lung while breathing through the nose at a controlled frequency of 8 breaths min^{-1} and a tidal volume of 1000 cm^3 (as in Fig. 3.5). Figure 3.6(a) gives the total deposition throughout the respiratory tract, and Figs 3.6(b)–(d) give data for the regional distribution of deposition for the larger particles. Note that the total deposition for the larger particles is greater than during mouth breathing but the alveolar deposition of these particles is much lower because of their extraction in the nose. Data from Heyder *et al.* (1986).

is greater during nose breathing but is similar in the size range between 0.01 and 0.5 μm. Nasal hairs and the nasal passages are highly efficient at removing larger particles which therefore do not enter the lungs, but not only large particles are removed in the nose. Experiments in which gas is sampled in the trachea during inhalation through the nose demonstrates that at slow flow rates, up to 45% of particles of 0.01 μm diameter can be deposited within the nasal passages. This is presumably because sufficient time is available for diffusional

mechanisms to enhance capture by nasal hairs and the nasal mucosal surface.

Even in the most carefully controlled experiments, there is considerable variability in the deposition rates reported for particles of similar aerodynamic diameters. However, there is general agreement that minimal deposition occurs for particles in the size range 0.5–1.0 μm, the fractional deposition in this range varying from approximately 8 to 20%.

Regional patterns of uptake

As well as the total quantity of aerosol depositing within the respiratory system, it is very important to know the distribution between sites, since this will determine the fate of the particles and potentially their long-term effects. Except for materials which have local toxic effects such as certain metal fumes, deposition in the nasal passages normally causes only mild irritation. Similarly, materials landing on the mucociliary escalator, which covers the surfaces of all but the smallest airways, are effectively cleared from the lungs by being transported to the larynx. However, they may subsequently cause adverse systemic effects after they have been swallowed. Thus, whilst the total bulk of material deposited in the lungs may consist predominantly of larger particles, their effects may be much less than those of smaller particles which are not trapped in the larger airways but penetrate through to the non-ciliated alveolar region and are removed only slowly.

Regional patterns of uptake in humans become better understood with the introduction of gamma cameras and the employment of short-lived, relatively safe isotopes, such as technetium 99m, with which aerosol particles can be tagged. With these methods, it is particularly easy to assess the total quantity of material depositing within the head, since the neck and chest can be screened from the camera. Nasal deposition values, such as those shown in Fig. 3.6, can be obtained in this way. Similar methods can be used to investigate variations in deposition rates in different parts of the lungs. Problems arise in such studies though, because of non-uniformity in the thickness of the chest, and also because material deposited on the mucociliary escalator can appear very quickly in the stomach, which is radiologically difficult to differentiate from the lower lobes of the left lung.

Mouth and nasal deposition are shown in Figs 3.5(b) and 3.6(b). The nose is able to trap most inspired particles with an aerodynamic diameter greater than $10\,\mu m$, but because of the relatively larger dimensions of the upper airway passages, small particles are less effectively removed. When particles are inspired through the mouth, a greater proportion of the larger particles are able to pen-

etrate through to the lungs because air velocities are lower and there are fewer obstructions for impaction. There is insignificant deposition of particles smaller than approximately $1.0\,\mu m$ within either the nasal or the oral paths. An important exception is that extremely small particles, less than about $0.01\,\mu m$ diameter, are effectively removed in the nose at low inspiratory flow rates.

A considerable amount of information on nasal deposition has been obtained in experiments using casts of the human nasopharynx. Interestingly, deposition in the models commonly underestimates that which has been reported *in vivo*, suggesting that the exact pattern of inhalation may be very important in determining the filtering efficiency of this organ.

It is possible to distinguish the deposition characteristics of particles of different diameters within the lung by utilizing the differing rates of the various particle clearance mechanisms. Inert particles landing on the mucociliary blanket are generally cleared by ciliary action within $24\,h$ of deposition (although this time may be longer in smokers, whose clearance systems operate less effectively). Using radioactively tagged particles, the total quantity of material that has been deposited in the lung is measured by scanning the chest immediately after inhalation. A later scan, after $24\,h$, should show material which has deposited in airways beyond those that are ciliated, because the clearance mechanisms for insoluble particles from these distal regions are very slow. The difference between the quantities recorded in each scan indicates the quantity of material which has deposited on the tracheobronchial tree and in the alveolar region. The fractional deposition in the airway tree has been found, experimentally, to be low, rarely exceeding 5% of the inhaled quantity and to be comprised mainly of particles with diameters between 5 and $10\,\mu m$, or less than $0.1\,\mu m$. Most particles larger than $10-20\,\mu m$ (depending on whether breathing is through the nose or mouth) will have been removed by the upper airways. Residence times within the conducting airways are also rather short, giving little chance for sedimentation or diffusional deposition. Figures 3.5(c), (d) and 3.6(c), (d) illustrate measurements made of bronchial airway and alveolar deposition patterns for a range of particle sizes breathed through both the oral and nasal routes. The detailed differences in bronchial and alveolar uptake of particles inhaled orally and nasally reflect the relative efficiency with which the two upper airway paths remove large particles.

Because larger particles are lost by impaction or sedimentation, only those with diameters of less than 5 µm normally penetrate through to the alveoli. Exceptions are fibrous particles which can travel unimpeded along the conducting airways because of their alignment with the gas stream-lines. Clearance from the alveolar region by macrophages occurs only slowly, and so these particles may remain in the lung for very long periods and can give rise to a variety of adverse effects. For spherical particles with aerodynamic diameters between 0.5 and 5 µm there appears to be a maximal fractional deposition in the alveoli for those of about 3 µm. Particles with diameters less than 0.5 µm exhibit a very large increase in alveolar fractional deposition as size decreases because of the increase in the diffusion coefficient and because of the relatively long residence times of gas in this region. For particles less than 0.1 µm diameter, alveolar deposition normally exceeds 50% of that inhaled. There is insufficient time during transit through the bronchial tree for such small particles to reach the airway walls in large numbers. However, the relatively long time spent in the alveolar region, both during each breath and as the result of inter-breath mixing, enables these small particles to deposit efficiently in this region.

With the exception of extremely small particles with diameters less than 0.01 µm, there are no discernible differences in the alveolar handling of very small particles breathed through the mouth or nose. This is because the upper airway and bronchial airways are both inefficient at capturing particles in this size range at normal respiratory rates.

As well as considering deposition on a regional basis, as we have done so far, it is possible to consider more localized variations in sites of deposition. Velocities in the trachea can be very high and the carina at its bifurcation into the two main bronchi, and the bifurcation of the main bronchi into the lobar bronchi, are important sites for the impaction of larger particles. They are also sites to which material is carried by the mucociliary escalator from the deeper airways of the lungs. Consequently these branch points are common foci for the development of pathological lesions such as tumours. These sites correlate with those demonstrated in the model studies described above (see Fig. 3.3), showing a highly asymmetrical deposition of particles within an airway in the vicinity of a bifurcation.

THEORETICAL STUDIES OF DEPOSITION

Because the movement of aerosol particles can in principle be predicted by well-defined physical laws, there have been numerous attempts to describe aerosol deposition in the respiratory tract mathematically. A great stimulus to this approach arises from the ethical problem of experimental studies in human volunteers using potentially toxic aerosols. Early models applied equations describing impaction, sedimentation and diffusion to a series of tubes of dimensions appropriate to those of each generation of airways. These models failed to recognize, however, the complexity of the patterns of airflow within the airways and the highly asymmetrical nature of the tracheobronchial tree. Perhaps surprisingly, the models tended to overestimate deposition rates in the upper airways and tracheobronchial tree and in doing so they tended to underestimate deposition in the alveoli, the region of greatest importance because of the long retention times.

The ability to model aerosol deposition has improved over the last few years with the introduction of sophisticated modelling techniques. Use of computational fluid mechanics and Monte Carlo methods has enabled the prediction of the behaviour of a wide range of materials of different physical properties. Models now appear to be reliable for describing both total and regional deposition and have advanced to the point where they can predict the deposition of fibrous and hygroscopic aerosols. These improvements in theoretical modelling techniques are of great importance in that they help us to rely less and less upon both human and animal studies of deposition.

The fact that some particles can absorb water from the inhaled air in which they are suspended makes the prediction of their deposition characteristics very difficult because of the continuous changes in their diameter and the resultant changes in deposition efficiency by the different mechanisms. Nonetheless such behaviour can now be modelled by introducing terms describing the kinetics of particle growth as they pass down the airways. The predicted behaviour of hygroscopic salt particles is shown in Fig. 3.7. Hygroscopic particles whose initial diameter is larger than approximately 0.3 µm deposit to a greater extent than inert particles of the same nominal size. This is because, as the particle grows in size, the processes of sedimentation and impaction become more effective. In contrast, small hygroscopic particles whose initial size is less than approximately 0.3 µm show a reduction in deposition; this is because as they grow in size their diffusional mobility, and hence tendency to deposit, decreases.

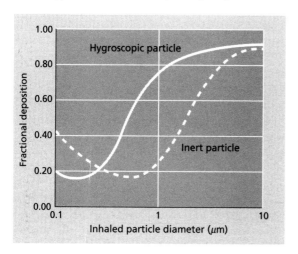

Fig. 3.7 Theoretically derived deposition curves for the whole respiratory tract during mouth breathing for hygroscopic salt particles and non-hygroscopic (inert) particles with unit density. The breathing frequency and tidal volume are the same as that for the experimental data in Fig. 3.5. Note that the deposition rates for hygroscopic particles smaller than 0.2 µm are less than those for the non-hygroscopic particles, since as they absorb water vapour, their diffusion velocities decrease. For hygroscopic particles larger than 0.3 µm the deposition rates are higher because of greater sedimentation and impaction rates. Data from Ferron *et al.* (1988).

PHYSIOLOGICAL FACTORS AFFECTING PARTICLE DEPOSITION

The lungs are not spherical and so although the assumption is often made that the orientation of airways is random, many of the larger airways have a preferred orientation to the vertical in an erect person. Inevitably this will result in changes in the sedimentation of particles with alterations of posture. In contrast, diffusional deposition will be unaffected by airway orientation.

During quiet breathing, gas is not delivered in equal proportions to all parts of the lungs, but goes preferentially to the lower lobes because these are inflated with least effort. They are supplied by relatively long conducting airways which offer a high probability for particle deposition on the mucociliary layer before the gas reaches the alveoli. Nonetheless, the total dose of material received by these lobes tends to be high. As the breathing rate increases, for example on exercise, the distribution of ventilation, and hence the distribution of aerosol deposition, becomes more uniform.

There are marked differences in the size of the lungs of different individuals. A subject's height and body surface area appear to be the best indices of lung volume, but the volumes of women are normally smaller than those of men of similar height. Airway dimensions are of course much smaller in children than in adults and their ventilation volumes and patterns are different. Data which have become available relatively recently suggest that children have somewhat higher fractional aerosol deposition rates than adults.

Even in individuals with similar-sized lungs, tremendous variation is observed between the deposition rates for similar particles, partly because of anatomical differences and partly because of inter-subject differences in the patterns of breathing. Even factors such as the shape of the nose have been shown to be important. The morphology of the nasal turbinates is also variable, as is the extent to which they respond to altered temperature and humidity. Deeper in the lung, the branching angles of bifurcations and the shape of the flow divider can also be quite different, giving rise to variability in the extent and pattern of deposition by impaction.

Changes in tidal volume, breathing frequency and the functional residual capacity can all be brought about by changes in the respiratory needs of the body. Elevated ventilation is invariably associated with an increase in tidal volume. In a given period of time, more particles are brought into the lungs from the atmosphere and a greater proportion of the inhaled gas passes to the alveoli. This will cause a rise in both total and fractional deposition (Fig. 3.8). Enhanced flow rates, associated with greater tidal volumes or increases in breathing frequency, cause more complex changes in deposition because of contrasting effects on different deposition mechanisms. The consequent rise in gas velocities increases the probability of impaction of larger particles in the upper airways and also in those regions of curvature in the smaller airways where impaction would be unlikely to occur at lower flow rates. There will also be an improvement in mixing between the tidal volume and the expiratory reserve gas which will transfer particles deeper into the lung. Set against these effects, which would all tend to favour deposition on increasing breathing frequency, there will be a decrease in the residence time of inhaled gas within the lung which will reduce the probability of deposition by diffusion and sedimentation. The net effect is normally an increase in the fractional deposition of particles with aerodynamic diameters greater than 5 μm but a decrease for particles less than 3 μm.

It should also be remembered that deposition patterns can be dramatically altered in individuals with any form of lung disease. These differences are additional to any relating to reduced efficiency of removal of particles by macrophages or ciliary action once they have been deposited. Upper airway infections, including rhinitis, invariably increase the likelihood of mouth breathing, even at low flow rates, thus leading to increased aerosol delivery to the lungs. Bronchoconstriction, resulting from asthma or other allergic conditions, increases particle impaction and gas mixing, and enhanced deposition rates are usually observed in such individuals, even during asymptomatic phases of the disease. Bronchitis causes an increase in the thickness of the mucous layer, thus diminishing airway calibre, and often leads to air trapping during expir-

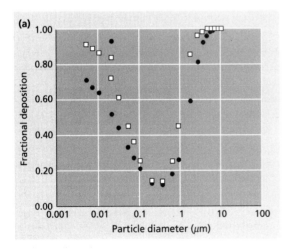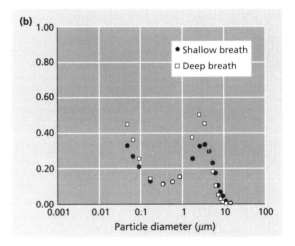

Fig. 3.8 Experimentally measured (a) total and (b) alveolar deposition during nose breathing under conditions simulating rest and exercise. In both cases the breathing frequency is 4 breaths min^{-1}, but the shallow breaths have a tidal volume of 500 cm^3 and the deep breaths a tidal volume of 1500 cm^3. With higher tidal volumes the deposition of small particles is enhanced by increased gas mixing and the presence of a larger fraction of the inhaled gas in the alveoli, while deposition of larger particles is enhanced by more impaction resulting from the threefold increase in flow rate. This causes a diminution of the alveolar deposition of the large particles. Note that the total deposition per unit time for all particles will be more than three times greater for the deeper breathing. Data from Heyder *et al.* (1986).

ation; both factors favour deposition. Highly disabling diseases, such as fibrosis and emphysema, involve dynamic changes in airway size, coupled with breathlessness and changes in ventilation patterns which invariably lead to increased mouth breathing, all of which generally enhance deposition.

UPTAKE OF GASES AND VAPOURS

Just as with particulate materials, the respiratory tract offers one of the most important routes for the absorption of soluble gases and vapours into the body. They may be absorbed throughout the tract, entering either the pulmonary circulation via the alveoli, or the systemic circulation through absorption on the surfaces of the upper airways and tracheobronchial tree. Whilst many noxious gases cause damage in other parts of the body following removal by the blood, others may cause diseases within the respiratory tract itself as the consequence of local direct action on the tissues of the airway walls. Despite the obvious importance of this uptake route into the body, relatively little information is available regarding the underlying physical processes. This is in marked contrast to our understanding of the mechanisms governing the deposition of particulate material.

The uptake of gases by the upper airway or tracheobronchial tree provides a very important defence mechanism for protection of the delicate alveolar membrane, but by doing so these airways can themselves be exposed to the risk of damage. This is particularly so in the case of transient exposure to highly soluble gases. Because of the rapidity of the absorption, the only surfaces encountering the gas on inhalation may be the upper airways and larger airways of the tracheobronchial tree.

Inhaled gases can have a wide range of physical properties and both their transport and uptake in the airways and alveoli are extremely complex. The processes in the gas phase involve diffusion and convection, which cause dispersion within the airway. Exchange between air and wall phases also involves gas–tissue solubility and diffusion within the wall phase. Simple gases, in low concentrations which do not react in solution, will obey Henry's law which states that the quantity of gas which dissolves is proportional to its partial pressure in the gas phase. Therefore, the amount of a gas extracted from the inhaled air by the conducting airways, or alveoli, is dependent on its partial pressure and its solubility coefficient in the tissue. However the vast majority of substances of interest, such as complex organic vapours that react with the tissues, do not obey this law and their detailed solubility characteristics in the tissue of interest are unknown.

The bulk of our direct knowledge of gas uptake within the human upper airway and tracheobronchial tree is based on clinical knowledge of chronic exposure to long-known industrial pollutants. For example, sulphur dioxide is well known to irritate the larger airways and oxidant gases such as ozone and nitrogen dioxide, whilst partially absorbed in the upper airway, appear to penetrate further into the bronchial tree, where they may cause pulmonary oedema, bronchopneumonia and emphysema. The particulate fumes of many metals, such as chromium, which may be inhaled industrially, are known to cause lung cancers, whereas chromium vapour causes ulceration of the nose, clearly being taken up at a different site. Acetaldehyde, a gaseous constituent of tobacco smoke, is highly soluble and may be involved in the development of cancers in the conducting airways. High local burdens of oxidants and nicotine within airway walls may also have disruptive effects on the mucociliary transport process and thereby modify the handling, and hence the toxic effects, of other materials — particularly particulates which may themselves carry absorbed gases.

Alveolar gas uptake

When a gas is not taken up by the conducting airways, because of low solubility in the wall or because the airway tissues have become saturated as after prolonged exposure, then it can penetrate to the alveoli. The gas can then diffuse across the alveolar membrane and absorption is mainly determined by the solubility of the gas in blood, pulmonary blood flow rate and the gas concentration in pulmonary arterial blood. Ultimately, an equilibrium will become established in which the rate of uptake of the gas is matched by the rate at which it is transported away by the blood flow and taken up by other target organs in the body.

Vapours like benzene and carbon tetrachloride are relatively insoluble in blood. Consequently, even though enough vapour dissolves to bring the pulmonary blood into equilibrium with the gas phase, only a small fraction of that which is inhaled is absorbed. Hence, after the few breaths required to mix the inhaled gas with the residual gas, an effectively steady state concentration will be obtained in the gas phase from which the vapour is continuously extracted into the flowing pulmonary blood.

In contrast, when a vapour like methanol, which is very soluble in blood, or a gas like carbon monoxide, which reacts with blood haemoglobin, enters the alveoli, a very large proportion of the material will be lost from the gas phase. Hence, alveolar concentration will fall markedly during the course of a breath and the rate of solution will also diminish. This will happen on successive breaths and so a steady concentration in the lung will not be attained rapidly and the time required to reach a steady concentration in the whole body will be retarded.

The quantity of material taken up from the lung within a breath is dependent on its concentration in the pulmonary arterial blood which is returning to the lungs from body tissues. Initially, this concentration will be very low because the gas carried in solution in arterial blood will be lost during its passage around the body, but it will rise as tissue levels increase. The uptake rate of soluble gases from the alveoli is also very dependent on the ventilation pattern and is greatly enhanced at high ventilation rates.

Fatty tissues have a high affinity for organic vapours such as benzene and carbon tetrachloride and so the venous blood which drains from such tissues will have a low concentration of such gases even after prolonged exposure. This helps to maintain a concentration gradient between lung gas and pulmonary blood for further uptake of gas, and it may therefore take several days for all the body tissues to reach equilibrium with respect to the inhaled concentration. If a gas reacts on entering solution, as does nitrogen dioxide or chlorine, or if

it reacts on entering the target tissues, then its concentration in the tissue and blood will be lower than that of a similar non-reacting gas and the diffusion gradient for uptake from the airspace will be enhanced.

Transient gas uptake

If the inhaled gas is soluble in the walls of the upper airway and tracheobronchial tree, then a significant fraction of the amount inhaled will be extracted by the conducting passages of the respiratory tract. Thus, on transient exposure they are able to protect the alveoli and reduce the effect of noxious gases on the alveolar-capillary membranes and entry into the blood.

Experimental studies on both humans and animals suggest that on transient exposure, the nasal passages are able to remove more than 95% of sulphur dioxide from the inspirate but only 45% of nitrous oxide which is a less soluble gas. Studies with ozone suggest that this gas is almost completely removed by the nasal passages. It has been demonstrated that the efficiency of uptake within the nose depends upon the detailed properties of the flow over the nasal surfaces. Experiments on acetone uptake by the nasal passages of dogs demonstrated that on increasing the flow rate from 2 to $5 \, l \, min^{-1}$, the efficiency of extraction of gas doubled, despite the marked reduction in the residence time of the inspirate in the nose.

The toxicological effects in humans of short-term exposure to most substances are estimated by extrapolation modelling from animal studies. This involves theoretical modelling of the transport processes involved. As is apparent from the description earlier in the chapter of the airflow in the respiratory tract, there will be significant differences between species in ventilation patterns and hence flow regimes within airways. Furthermore there are also marked differences in the geometry of the airways. In particular the branching of airways is clearly asymmetrical in the human, and even more so in animals, such as the dog and rat, which have been widely used for inhalation toxicological studies. The vast majority of theoretical models incorporating human airway geometry have, moreover, assumed that the tracheobronchial airways are a simple symmetrical system, rather than being asymmetrical, thereby departing even further from reality. There have been no useful models to extrapolate uptake within the upper airways, particularly the nose.

Current theoretical uptake models focus predominantly on describing the behaviour of poorly soluble gases. However the majority of gases of interest have a high solubility and it has been demonstrated that the transport characteristics of low and high solubility gases along the airways are likely to be very different, thus making it hard to draw conclusions about the behaviour of high solubility gases from available models.

For the application of extrapolation modelling to yield reliable information for use in humans, it will be necessary to incorporate the underlying physical processes and an adequate description of geometry into any description. This is not yet possible and much research in this area remains to be done.

REFERENCES

Balashazy, I. and Hoffman, W. (1993). Particle deposition in airway bifurcations I. Inspiratory flow, II. Expiratory flow. *Journal of Aerosol Science*, **24**, 745–86.

Ferron, G.A. *et al.* (1988). Inhalation of salt aerosol particles II. Growth and deposition in the human respiratory tract. *Journal of Aerosol Science*, **19**, 611–31.

Heyder, J., Gebhart, J., Rudolf, G., Schiller, C.F. and Stahlhofen, W. (1986). Deposition of particles in the human respiratory tract in the size range 0.005 to 15 μm. *Journal of Aerosol Science*, **17**, 811–25.

Martonen, T.B., Zhang, W. and Yang, Y. (1992). Interspecies modelling of inhaled particle deposition patterns. *Journal of Aerosol Science*, **23**, 389–406.

Phillips, C.G., Kaye, S.R. and Schroter, R.C. (1994). A diameter-based reconstruction of the branching pattern of the human bronchial tree. Part I. Description and application. *Respiration Physiology*, **98**, 193–217.

Raabe, O.G., Yeh, H.-C., Schum, G.H. and Phalen, R.F. (1976). *Tracheobronchial Geometry: Human, Dog, Rat, Hamster.* LF 53. Lovelace Foundation for Medical Education and Research, Albuquerque.

Schroter, R.C. and Sudlow, M.F. (1969). Flow patterns in models of the human bronchial airways. *Respiration Physiology*, **7**, 341–55.

FURTHER READING

Dodgson, J., McCallum, R.I., Bailey, M.R. and Fisher, D.R. (ed.) (1989). *Inhaled Particles VI.* Pergamon Press, Oxford.

Lee, D.H.K. (ed.) (1977). *Reactions to Environmental Agents. Handbook of Physiology — Respiration Section 9.* American Physiological Society, Bethesda, MD.

Marple, V.A. and Liu, B.Y.H. (ed.) (1983). *Aerosols in the Mining and Industrial Work Environment.* Ann Arbor Sciences, Ann Arbor.

Pedley, T.J., Schroter, R.C. and Sudlow, M.F. (1977). Gas flow and mixing in the airways. In *Bioengineering Aspects of the Lung.* Marcel Dekker Inc., New York.

Walton, W.H. (ed.) (1977). *Inhaled Particles and Vapours IV.* Pergamon Press, Oxford.

CHAPTER 4

The Effects of Inhaled Materials on Target Organs

J.M. Harrington

INTRODUCTION

Many hazardous substances encountered in the workplace gain entry to the body through inhalation. Some may be absorbed through the skin or ingested, although ingestion is rarely an important route of entry in occupational health. Inhaled materials may affect the lung directly, or they may be absorbed from the lung and affect other parts of the body. To have an effect outside the lungs, inhaled materials must be able to cross the blood–gas barrier (see Chapter 1) and efficiency with which this is achieved will depend, *inter alia*, on their particle size and their solubility in the tissue fluid of the alveolus (see Chapter 3).

Humans evolved in an environment in which the air was clean but in which food and water were likely to be contaminated. The result of this has been that a number of protective mechanisms have developed by which the uptake of materials from the gut is regulated, but none has developed in the lungs. Thus soluble materials which are capable of penetrating into the alveoli are likely to pass unimpeded into the pulmonary circulation. A large section of this chapter is devoted to the lung as it is the target organ of greatest importance.

THE LUNG

The lung, in common with the other organs of the body, has a limited capacity to respond to toxic materials. In general, the more specialized the organ, the fewer are the ways in which damage can be expressed. Harmful effects to the lung can be grouped into about six, more or less distinct,

categories which are discussed below (see also Table 1.2).

Irritation of the airways

A number of gases and fumes produce intense irritation of the airways and the most important of these are shown in Table 4.1. The resulting symptoms vary depending upon which parts of the airways are affected, and this is in turn a function of the solubility of the material under consideration. For example, highly soluble gases, such as ammonia, produce immediate effects on the upper respiratory tract (and the eyes), causing pain in the mouth, throat and eyes, due to the swelling and ulceration of the mucous membranes. These symptoms are so intensely unpleasant that affected individuals will make every effort to remove themselves from exposure as quickly as possible. Continual exposure, or a single exposure to a very high concentration, will result in the deeper airways becoming affected with an outpouring of tissue fluid and blood into the alveoli as a consequence of damage to the alveolar membranes and capillaries in the lung. The presence of fluid in the alveoli (known as pulmonary oedema) seriously interferes with gas exchange and causes severe symptoms if not adequately treated.

By contrast, a relatively insoluble gas such as phosgene produces no immediate effects on the upper respiratory tract, but does induce profound pulmonary oedema after a delay of several hours. Some of the pulmonary irritants will also cause permanent lung damage if exposure is particularly high or frequently repeated, whilst others appear to

Table 4.1 Irritant gases or fumes

Substance	Sources	Acute effects	Chronic effects
Ammonia	Production of fertilizers and explosives; refrigeration; manufacture of plastics	Pain in eyes, mouth and throat; oedema of mucous membranes; conjunctivitis; pulmonary oedema	Airways obstruction; usually clears in about a year
Chlorine	Manufacture of alkali, bleaches and disinfectants	Chest pain; cough; pulmonary oedema	Usually none; occasionally causes airways obstruction
Sulphur dioxide	Paper production; oil refining; atmospheric pollutant	As for ammonia	Chronic bronchitis
Nitrogen oxides	Silo filling; arc welding; combustion of nitrogen-containing materials	Pulmonary oedema after lag of 1 or 2 h; obliteration of bronchioles in severe cases after 2–3 weeks	Permanent lung damage with repeated exposure
Phosgene	Chemical industry; World War I gas	Pulmonary oedema after a lag of several hours	Chronic bronchitis
Ozone	Argon-shielded welding	Cough; tightness in the chest; pulmonary oedema in severe cases	None
Mercury	Chemical and metal industries	Cough and chest pain after lag of 3–4 h; acute pneumonia	Usually none; pulmonary fibrosis rarely
Osmium tetroxide	Chemical and metal industries; laboratories	Tracheitis; bronchitis; conjunctivitis	None
Vanadium pentoxide	Ash and soot from oil	Nasal irritation; chest pain; cough	Bronchitis; bronchopneumonia
Zinc chloride	Manufacture of dry cells; galvanizing	Tracheobronchitis	None

Table 4.2 Agents producing occupational asthma

Grain, flour, hops, tobacco dust
Beetles, locusts, cockroaches, grain mites
Laboratory animals, e.g. rats, mice
Avian feathers
Amoebas ('humidifier fever')
Fungi
Various woods, including cedars, boxwood
Various metals and their salts, including platinum, chromium, nickel
Vanadium
Formalin
Ethylene diamine
Chloramine T
Phthalic anhydride (epoxy resin hardener)
Colophony (soldering flux)
Certain dyes
Drugs, including penicillin, tetracycline and methyldopa
Enzymes, including *Bacillus subtilis* and pancreatic extracts
Isocyanates

predispose individuals to other conditions such as pneumonia or chronic bronchitis.

Obstructive airways disease

In this condition, the calibre of the airways is decreased, thus impeding the flow of gas. The obstruction may be reversible (in which case it is usually referred to as asthma) or irreversible, in which case it may progress to produce permanent impairment of lung function. Both kinds of obstructive disease are encountered as the result of exposure to the appropriate precipitating agent at work.

Asthma

The underlying mechanism of occupational asthma is an abnormal immunological response to foreign materials which act as antigens. The inhalation and absorption of the antigen provokes the production of specific antibodies which, in turn, set in motion a series of events culminating in the release from cells of histamine and other active materials which cause bronchial constriction.

Occupational agents which cause asthma have been somewhat arbitrarily divided into two types: high molecular weight protein antigens (rodent urine, shellfish protein, flour, grain, mite faeces) and low molecular weight chemicals (isocyanates, acid anhydrides, platinum salts). Agents in the former group are more likely to affect individuals who are atopic — that is, who have a past or present history of eczema or asthma. Atopy is not a risk factor for exposure to the latter group.

Asthmatic symptoms in industry may follow immediately upon exposure to the antigenic material, but more commonly there is a delay of several hours and symptoms may develop during the evening or at night. This often means that the relation of the symptoms to occupation is overlooked. Examples of agents responsible for occupational asthma are shown in Table 4.2. The list is long and still growing.

Byssinosis

This is the best example of an obstructive airways disease of occupational origin which may progress to produce irreversible impairment of pulmonary function. It is considered by many authorities to be a type of occupational asthma. The disease is due to the inhalation of cotton dust and probably has an immunological basis, although the precise mechanism is by no means clear. Characteristically, symptoms are first noted on Monday mornings when the cotton worker returns from a weekend away from exposure. There may be an interval of several years from first exposure to the onset of symptoms which, in the early stages, disappear on the second day back at work. If exposure continues, then the symptoms are noted for longer periods during the week, until finally they are present continuously throughout the week. On clinical grounds, the disease can be graded as shown in Table 4.3. This classification is of more than just academic interest since if the disease is caught in the early stages (Grade $\frac{1}{2}$–1), the symptoms will disappear if exposure to cotton dust is discontinued, whereas this may not happen if the worker progresses into later stages of the disease.

Pneumoconiosis

The term pneumoconiosis literally means 'dusty lungs' and, as such, conveys no connotation of harm. For medical purposes, however, the term should be confined to mean permanent alteration of lung structure following the inhalation of mineral dust, and the tissue reactions of the lung to its presence. Nevertheless, clinicians still refer to 'benign' pneumoconiosis which is an apparent contradiction in terms if the definition given above

Table 4.3 Grading of symptoms of byssinosis

Grade	Symptoms
$\frac{1}{2}$	Occasional tightness of the chest on Monday (or the day on which work is resumed)
1	Tightness of the chest and/or difficulty in breathing on Monday (or the day on which work is resumed)
2	Tightness of the chest and difficulty in breathing on the first and other days of the working week
3	Grade 2 symptoms accompanied by evidence of permanent respiratory impairment

is adhered to. The dusts which are most harmful to the lungs are silica (or quartz), coal dust and asbestos.

Silicosis. This follows exposure to fine crystalline silicon dioxide or quartz. It is probably the oldest of all the occupational diseases since there is little doubt that the Palaeolithic flint toolmakers would have suffered from it; however, there is no objective evidence that this is the case. During the last century the disease was common in many industries including mining, quarrying, the pottery industry, iron and steel foundries and sand blasting. In recent years the number of new cases has fallen sharply as the result of improved working practices and from the substitution of safer materials for silica wherever possible.

The presence of silica in the lung initiates a reaction which leads to the formation of small nodules of fibrotic tissue (*c.* 1 mm in diameter) which increase in size and coalesce as the disease progresses. These nodules are seen on a chest X-ray as small, round opacities scattered throughout the lung fields. The radiographic changes are often most prominent in the upper parts of the lung, and may be present before any symptoms of breathlessness appear. It should be realized that pneumoconiosis is essentially a radiological diagnosis since radiographic evidence of dust retention in the lungs is visible in all cases before symptoms appear. In the so-called 'benign' varieties of pneumoconiosis symptoms *never* appear.

Early diagnosis in cases of pneumoconiosis is essential, as the symptoms may progress even after exposure has ceased if a sufficiently large quantity of dust has been inhaled. The progression of the disease is marked by increasing difficulty in breathing, and death frequently results from combined heart and lung failure. An unexpectedly large number of patients with silicosis also develop tuberculosis, which does nothing to help their dismal prognosis.

Coalminers' pneumoconiosis. This produces a somewhat different picture and frequently has less severe sequelae as well as being less aggressively fibrotic. It may be sub-divided into simple pneumoconiosis and progressive massive fibrosis (PMF).

The diagnosis of simple pneumoconiosis is made on the finding of small, round opacities in the lung, presumably due to the presence of coal dust, and the radiographic changes bear a close relationship to the total amount of dust inhaled. Beyond a slight cough which produces blackish sputum there are virtually no symptoms attributable to coalminers' simple pneumoconiosis; its importance lies in the fact that it is the precursor of PMF. The reasons why simple pneumoconiosis progresses to PMF in a small proportion of miners are not clear, as is attested by the numerous explanations which have been put forward. The most recent explanation proposes that it is due to an antigen–antibody reaction in the lungs. However, the mechanism underlying this reaction remains obscure.

PMF is recognized on the chest X-ray by the presence of large opacities usually in the upper part of the lung and these are often irregular in shape. In the lung itself, these areas appear as hard, black masses often with a central cavity filled with jet-black fluid. Occasionally, the process may involve one of the larger airways and erode its wall, and the liquid contents of the lesion may be coughed up as inky black sputum. Moderate or severe forms of PMF produce destruction of a sufficient amount of lung tissue to disable the victim and can lead to premature death. Fortunately the number of cases of the severe form of the disease is declining rapidly as a result of better methods of dust suppression underground.

Asbestos exposure. This is associated with fibrotic changes in the lung (which may become extremely severe), with the development of cancer of the bronchus, and rarely, with the development of tumours of the pleura.

The development of pulmonary fibrosis mainly follows exposure to white asbestos (chrysotile), although blue (crocidolite) and brown (amosite) asbestos are also fibrogenic. This is the condition known as asbestosis. It manifests itself clinically by increasing shortness of breath, a dry cough and weight loss. The radiographic changes are usually confined to the lower parts of the lung and show up as linear shadows which become larger and more irregular as the disease progresses. Although patients may die from uncomplicated asbestosis, perhaps as many as 50% of those who die do so because of the development of cancer of the bronchus. Smoking and asbestos dust act in a synergistic way in the production of cancer of the lung and smokers who are exposed to asbestos are at a very much greater risk of developing lung cancer than are people who only smoke or only have asbestos exposure.

Pleural tumours (mesotheliomas) are rare and seem to occur almost entirely in those who have been exposed to blue asbestos (crocidolite). Some tumours have developed in women whose only exposure to asbestos occurred when they washed their husband's dirty overalls in the days when men were allowed to take them home. The tumour spreads from the pleura into the underlying tissues and is inevitably fatal. There may be a delay of up to 50 years between the first exposure and the symptoms of the tumour. Other tumours linked to asbestos exposure include mesothelioma of the abdominal cavity (peritoneum), cancer of the larynx and, perhaps, cancer of the ovary.

Asbestos bodies are commonly found in the sputum of individuals exposed to asbestos. They are rod-like structures, 20−150 mm in length, often with a beaded appearance. They are coated with an iron-containing protein which can be stained so that they are visible under the microscope. The presence of asbestos bodies in sputum can be taken as evidence of exposure to asbestos but it does not imply disease. Similarly, the calcified pleural plaques seen on a chest X-ray are a sign of exposure to asbestos, but are not by themselves indicative of ill-effects.

Benign pneumoconiosis

The presence of dust particles in the lung will be detected radiologically if the atomic number is greater than that of calcium. The higher the atomic number of the dust, the denser the shadow produced on the X-ray film. Unfortunately, it is too simplistic to assume that opacities on the X-ray are the inhaled particles as 'spotty' lungs can follow exposure to pure carbon particles. In truth, it is not entirely clear what constitutes the opacity in such pneumoconiosis.

The diagnosis of benign pneumoconiosis is entirely dependent upon radiological findings since, by definition, the patient is symptom-free. Some of the dusts which cause radiological changes in the absence of disease are shown in Table 4.4.

Extrinsic allergic alveolitis

Organic materials which are inhaled may have one or two distinct effects on the lungs: they may either induce asthma (as described above) or they may affect the alveoli and reduce gas transfer. The latter condition is referred to as 'extrinsic alveolitis' because the underlying mechanism is an allergic response to an external (extrinsic) antibody and the alveoli are affected. A wide range of organic materials may produce the disease (Table 4.5), the most common being fungal spores.

Many clinical varieties of the condition have been described, each due to one (or occasionally more than one) specific allergen, but the symptoms in each variety are similar. The individual types of the disease are usually named after the occupational group in which they were first discovered, or are most common. Farmer's lung is the predominant form in Britain. Symptoms typically appear 4−8h after exposure to mouldy hay after which time the patient develops a fever, tiredness, chills and generalized aches and pains. Shortness of breath and an unproductive cough are then noted but there is none of the wheeziness so typical of the patient with asthma. After removal from exposure, the symptoms can be expected to clear up within 12h. Repeated exposure, however, may result in the development of pulmonary fibrosis with permanent impairment of lung function and with X-ray changes most apparent in the upper part of the lung.

Table 4.4 Dusts producing benign pneumoconiosis

Dust	Condition
Antimony	
Barium	Baritosis
Iron	Siderosis
Tin	Stannosis

Table 4.5 Some types and causes of extrinsic allergic alveolitis

Clinical Condition	Due to exposure to:	Allergen
Farmer's lung	Mouldy hay	*Faeni rectivirgula*
		Thermoactinomyces vulgaris
Bird fancier's lung	Bird droppings	Protein in the droppings
Bagassosis	Mouldy sugar-cane	*T. vulgaris* and *I. sacchari*
Malt worker's lung	Mouldy malt or barley	*Aspergillus clavatus*
Suberosis	Mouldy cork dust	*Penicillium frequentans*
Maple bark stripper's lung	Infected maple dust	*Cryptostroma corticale*
Cheese washer's lung	Mouldy cheese	*Penicillium casei*
Wood pulp worker's lung	Wood pulp	*Alternaria* species
Wheat weevil disease	Wheat flour	*Sitophilus granarius*
Mushroom worker's lung	Mushroom compost	*F. rectivirgula*
Animal handler's lung	Dander, dried rodent urine	Serum and urine proteins
Pituitary snuff-taker's lung	Therapeutic pituitary snuff	Pig or ox protein
Air-conditioner disease	Dust or mist	*T. vulgaris*
		T. thapophilus and amoebas
		(various)

Malignant disease

The association between bronchial carcinoma and exposure to asbestos has already been mentioned but there are other occupations which predispose workers to an unduly high risk of this disease, the foremost being miners subjected to ionizing radiation. The radioactive source in mines is radon or its daughter products: polonium 218, 214 and 210. All these elements are gases which diffuse from the rock into the air in the mineshafts. They all emit alpha particles which have a penetration range in tissue cells of between 40 and 70 mm, which is just sufficient to enable them to damage the nuclear material in the basal cells of the bronchial epithelium and initiate the train of events which culminates in the proliferation of a clone of malignant cells (see also Chapter 14).

In the past, an excess of lung tumours occurred in men engaged in the manufacture of arsenical sheep dips and in nickel refining. Arsenical sheep dips have now been rendered obsolete by the development of other compounds, but arsenic is still encountered in other occupations and great care must be taken to avoid both its acute and chronic effects.

The risk of lung cancer in nickel refining disappeared when the process was altered in the 1920s and arsenic-free sulphuric acid was used to remove copper from the ore. Concurrent with this change, the levels of nickel dust in the atmosphere were reduced and it has never been determined unequivocally whether arsenic or nickel — or some other material — was the carcinogenic agent. Nickel dust itself is not suspected, but acidic and sulphidic oxides of nickel may have been the culprits. Recently it has been found that exposure to certain hexavalent, but not trivalent, chrome salts increases the likelihood of contracting lung cancer, although not so much as exposure to asbestos or radon. Excessive levels of lung cancer have been reported also in coke oven workers, particularly those on the oven tops, due to the presence of polynuclear aromatic hydrocarbons in the air in the vicinity of the ovens.

The only other tumour of the respiratory tract which is relevant here (apart from the pleural mesothelioma cancer by crocidolite) is the adenocarcinoma of the nasal sinuses. This was first described in woodworkers in the furniture industry in High Wycombe, and in leather workers in the Northampton shoe trade. This is an otherwise rare tumour, and came to light, as have a number of other occupationally induced tumours, when clinicians became aware that they were seeing an unusually large number of patients with uncommon diseases. Subsequent epidemiological studies were able to confirm the original clinical observations and identify the exposure sources but not the specific carcinogenic agents.

Recent epidemiological studies have shown a consistent excess of lung cancer in patients with silicosis. Whether silica alone or in combination with fibrosis and/or smoking is to blame remains unresolved at present.

EFFECTS ON OTHER TARGET ORGANS

Materials which are inhaled and absorbed from the lungs into the bloodstream are distributed to other organs of the body, the functions of which they may adversely affect either directly or after they have undergone some metabolic transformation, normally in the liver. Most of the metallic poisons are directly toxic: lead, cadmium and metallic mercury for example, whereas carbon tetrachloride becomes toxic only when it has been acted upon by a hydroxylation enzyme system to produce the highly reactive CCl_3 radical. Only cells containing the enzyme system with the capacity to perform this transformation are subject to the toxic effects of carbon tetrachloride. Similarly, it is generally considered that polynuclear aromatic hydrocarbons all require metabolic transformation before their carcinogenic potentials can be realized. The particular transformation in this case requires the molecule to be acted upon by the enzyme aryl hydrocarbon hydroxylase to form active epoxides.

Many toxic materials must be metabolized in the liver before they or their metabolites can be excreted in the urine, as the kidney can only excrete molecules which are water soluble. The principal role of the liver in this context is to transform insoluble molecules into those which are soluble, frequently by conjugation with glucuronic acid. The metabolism of trichloroethylene (TRI) will serve as an example of this process in action.

Following absorption, TRI is converted to chloral hydrate which is further metabolized via two routes. One of these involves a rapid reduction to trichloroethanol (TCE) and the other involves a slow oxidation to trichloroacetic acid (TCA). TCE is not water soluble and any which is not metabolized to TCA is conjugated with glucuronic acid and the conjugate is excreted by the kidney. TCA, being water soluble, is excreted direct. Exposure to TRI vapour can be monitored by the estimation of the rate of excretion of TCA and TCE in the urine.

Although there is a vast range of potentially harmful materials encountered in the environment, both at work and in the home, the response of the body to them tends to be limited, because the various organs and organ systems have a finite capacity to respond to damage. Therefore, it is simpler to consider toxic effects from the standpoint of the individual target organ, rather than catalogue the various effects of individual toxins, since this tends to make dreary and repetitious reading. In addition, as the individual affected worker will complain of target organ-based symptoms this approach has clinical validity. Further information on these clinical effects can be found in the texts listed at the end of the chapter.

THE NERVOUS SYSTEM

That part of the nervous system over which we have some control is conventionally, but somewhat artificially, divided into the central nervous system (CNS), comprising the brain and spinal cord, and the peripheral nervous system which is made up of the sensory and motor nerves which convey information to and from the brain. Reflex activity is controlled by the so-called autonomic nervous system which also has both central and peripheral components.

Depending upon which nerves are affected, materials damaging the peripheral nervous system produce defects in motor function, manifested by a partial or total decrease in muscular activity, or a loss of sensation, or both. The number of neurotoxic materials which are likely to be encountered in industry is far from small, as may be seen from Table 4.6, and, with the exception of lead, each produces a mixed motor and sensory loss. Lead is exceptional amongst the occupational neurotoxins in producing a pure motor neuropathy. In almost all cases, the alteration in nerve function is the consequence of structural damage which interferes with the normal conduction of the nerve impulses. The organophosphates produce their effects, however, not by damaging the integrity of the nerve cells but by prolonging the effect of acetylcholine, thus preventing the normal passage of the nerve impulses. There have been some reports that lead

Table 4.6 The most common neurotoxins

Organophosphate pesticides
Carbamate pesticides
Triorthocresyl phosphate
n-Hexane
Methylbutylketone
Acrylamide and/or dimethylaminoproprionitrile
(DMAPN)
Carbon disulphide
Mercury compounds (inorganic and organic)
Lead and its compounds (inorganic)
Arsenic
Thallium
Antimony

Table 4.7 Changes in central nervous system function due to industrial toxins

Symptom	Caused by:
Narcosis	Organic solvents
	Trichloroethylene
	Carbon tetrachloride
	Chloroform
	Benzene
	Carbon monoxide
	Carbon dioxide
	Hydrogen sulphide
Mental changes	Carbon disulphide
	Manganese
	Mercury
	Tetraethyl lead
Epilepsy	Chlorinated naphthalenes, e.g. aldrin, dieldrin, endrin
Defects in balance and vision	Methyl mercury
Parkinsonism	Manganese
	Carbon disulphide
	Carbon monoxide

and carbon disulphide may produce sub-clinical nerve damage, which means that impairment in function occurs of which the worker is unaware. Such change is detected by the use of sensitive tests, but its significance is not yet clear. Thus, it is not known whether sub-clinical changes progress to produce frank clinical effects with continued exposure, nor how far performance is affected. In the case of lead, there does not appear to be a strong correlation between sub-clinical neuropathy and impairment of performance in physiological or psychological tests and so its importance is open to doubt.

Some of the changes in the function of the CNS, together with the causative agents, are shown in Table 4.7. A general depression of the CNS results from exposure to a wide range of volatile organic solvents, the symptoms of which may vary from headache and dizziness to unconsciousness or death. The narcotic action of some organic compounds is harnessed to good effect by using them as anaesthetics, and trichloroethylene, one of the more widely used of all industrial solvents, is still used as an anaesthetic in obstetric practice. Other asphyxiant agents of importance in industry, such as the chemical asphyxiant carbon monoxide or the simple asphyxiant carbon dioxide, are in some ways more insidious than the organic compounds because they cannot be detected by smell and so give no warning of impending danger. The converse is true of hydrogen sulphide since the evil smell of this gas ensures that exposure is kept to the bare minimum — although 'smell fatigue' can set in.

The mental changes induced by carbon disulphide became apparent soon after the compound was introduced for the cold curing of rubber. Workers heavily exposed began to demonstrate bizarre behaviour and some took to throwing themselves through windows, with disastrous effects if the window happened to be above ground level. The manufacturers, alarmed by the occurrences, took steps to prevent these unnecessary deaths amongst their work force and put bars in the upper storey windows! In these more enlightened times, levels of exposure are minimized and frank psychotic syndromes are now unknown in carbon disulphide workers.

Mercury exposure as a cause of mental changes is also now only of historical and literary interest. During the last century, rabbit fur was dipped into hot mercuric nitrate and the pelters engaged in this process were frequently affected by a condition which was known as erethism. They became quarrelsome, easily upset by even the mildest criticism, and liable to verbal and physical outbursts. One of the best descriptions of a patient with this syndrome is the Mad Hatter in 'Alice in Wonderland'! The fact that Lewis Carroll, who was a mathematics Don at Oxford, could describe the condition so well suggests that it was by no means uncommon in his day.

Psychotic signs may precede other signs in manganese poisoning, especially, it seems, in Chile, where manganese madness occurs relatively frequently amongst the miners. No cases have been reported in Britain this century. Cases of tetraethyl lead poisoning in this country are unheard of now, and cases reported from abroad have usually come about from the inappropriate use of leaded petrol as a solvent. In the USA, a number of cases of lead encephalopathy have been found in children sniffing petrol for kicks, some of whom have died as a result. The chlorinated naphthalenes are used as insecticides and do not produce toxic symptoms in normal working concentrations. Epileptic fits have been induced, however, in men who have been heavily exposed during the manufacture of these compounds.

In addition to causing mental changes, mercury, in its methylated form, may damage the cerebellum and the occipital cortex, resulting in disturbances of balance and defects of vision. Methyl mercury poisoning is rare in industry and most cases have resulted from environmental accidents of which the most notorious was the Minamata Bay disaster. This was caused by the discharge of industrial waste containing inorganic mercury into the sea where it was methylated by micro-organisms in the sea bed. The methyl mercury so formed entered the food chain and was concentrated by the fish which formed a substantial part of the diet of the population living around the bay. Other outbreaks of methyl mercury poisoning have occurred when seed grain dressed with the compound as a fungicide was eaten instead of sown. These episodes, particularly those which occurred in Iraq, are not so frequently commented on as that at Minamata Bay, but they are at least as serious, having affected many hundreds of people, large numbers of whom died.

The final effect on the CNS to which reference will be given here is Parkinsonism. This condition is similar in almost all respects to Parkinson's disease which is a common affliction in the elderly. The 'naturally' occurring form results from a depletion of the neurotransmitter dopamine in the basal ganglia, which are phylogenetically the oldest centres in the brain. Manganese is the most important of the toxic agents which cause Parkinson-like symptoms, but the means by which the disorder is induced is not clear. Since treatment with drugs which control the symptoms in the 'natural' variety are also effective in the toxic states, the underlying mechanism is presumably similar in both.

What remains unresolved is whether chronic low dose exposure to various organic solvents can cause organic psychosis. The 'Danish painters' syndrome' — much vaunted in the early 1980s — has not been corroborated in recent American or British studies. The best of these studies are, however, not without a measurable effect. It appears that some neurobehavioural tests of higher cerebral function do show a decremental change following long occupational exposure to organic solvents. The clinical and epidemiological significance of such results remain to be evaluated.

THE LIVER

Liver function is adversely affected by a relatively small number of organic solvents, prominent among which is carbon tetrachloride after liberation of a CCl_3 radical. Massive exposure to carbon tetrachloride results in the death of large numbers of liver cells and the patient becomes deeply jaundiced and may die. The capacity of the liver to regenerate itself is very great, however, and provided that the patient can be helped over the acute phase, and that any concomitant kidney damage does not prove fatal, a complete return to normal liver function is to be expected. Other industrial chemicals which can produce jaundice are derivatives of benzene (such as trinitrotoluene, dinitrophenol and toluene), yellow phosphorus and very large doses of DDT. An outbreak of jaundice in Epping which occurred in 1965 was traced to wholemeal flour contaminated with 4-4 diamino diphenyl methane, an aromatic amine, which had been spilt on the floor of the van in which the flour had been transported. All the affected patients recovered. Those handling this chemical at work have not shown liver damage at workplace concentrations or by inhalational routes.

The liver reaction which has received considerable notoriety in recent years is the development of angiosarcoma in men heavily exposed to vinyl chloride monomer. Angiosarcoma is a very rare, malignant tumour of the blood vessels and so the occurrence of several cases in one factory in the United States promptly alerted the occupational physician to the possibility that the cases were related to some exposure at work. Since the first report, about 50 cases have been reported, only a handful of which have come from Britain, and all in men exposed to very high concentrations of vinyl chloride monomer. It seems unlikely that new cases will arise in men with exposures to current low concentrations.

THE KIDNEY

The kidney is very vulnerable to damage from toxic materials because it has a rich blood supply in relation to its mass, and also because chemical compounds may be concentrated in its tissue when they are being excreted. Of the chemicals encountered in occupational practice, the two groups which are most likely to produce kidney damage are some of the heavy metals and the organic solvents. Damage to the kidney usually manifests itself by the appearance of substances in the urine which are normally held back by the intact renal tubules. In the cases of both mercury and cadmium, renal damage results in the appearance of protein in the urine. In some patients with mercury poisoning, the quantity of albumin in the urine may be so great as to interfere with normal fluid balance. This produces a condition known as the nephrotic syndrome which is characterized by albuminuria, hypoalbuminaemia and oedema. This condition is fully reversible once exposure is discontinued. Cadmium poisoning leads to the appearance in the urine of a low molecular weight protein, β_2 microglobulin.

Acute lead poisoning does not cause protein to appear in the urine but can give rise to the abnormal excretion of glucose, phosphate and amino acids, a combination referred to as Fanconi's syndrome. In lead poisoning, characteristic inclusion bodies are found in the nuclei of the cells of the proximal tubule. The significance of these inclusion bodies is obscure. Chronic exposure to lead may damage the kidney and induce structural deformation with impairment of the blood supply, which in turn may lead to the development of hypertension. In the early part of this century, lead workers were noted to be unduly likely to die from cerebrovascular disease secondary to hypertension, but this is no longer the case.

Carbon tetrachloride is the most dangerous solvent, so far as the kidney is concerned. Acute exposure can lead to the death of the renal tubules and complete cessation of kidney function. With the advent of renal dialysis, the outlook for this condition is no longer invariably hopeless, and if the patient can be supported over the acute phase, the tubular cells will regenerate and kidney function can be restored to normal.

Ethylene glycol, which is widely used in antifreeze solutions, is occasionally drunk by alcoholics when other forms of 'booze' are unavailable. It does them little good, however, since a substantial amount of the ethylene glycol is metabolized to oxalic acid. This deposits in the renal tissue in the form of calcium oxalate crystals which clog up the renal tubules and prevent them from carrying out their normal work.

THE CARDIOVASCULAR SYSTEM

Workplace hazards rarely have a direct effect on the cardiovascular system. However, certain organic solvents are thought to be capable of inducing cardiac arrhythmias and vinyl chloride can cause peripheral arterial spasm akin to the clinical features of hand–arm vibration syndrome. Methylene chloride is metabolized in part to carbon monoxide, and carbon disulphide appears to have a direct atherogenic potential.

These agents apart, most effects of workplace exposures on the cardiovascular system are secondary to target organ damage elsewhere. Examples include congestive heart disease from lung failure (cor pulmonale) and hypertensive heart disease from kidney failure.

THE BLOOD

There are only three chemicals which have an important effect on the blood of people at work: lead, benzene and arsine. Each produces an anaemia, but the mechanism whereby these materials achieve this common end differs markedly.

Lead. Lead is able to inhibit the activity of many of the enzymes in the body, especially those which contain active sulphydryl groups. A number of these enzymes are required for the synthesis of haem which, combined with the protein globin, forms haemoglobin, the pigmented complex that transports oxygen around the body in the red blood cells. The pathway through which haem is synthesized is outlined in Fig. 4.1 together with the steps inhibited by lead. The reserve capacity of the system is considerable, and exposure must be unduly great or prolonged to produce a serious degree of anaemia.

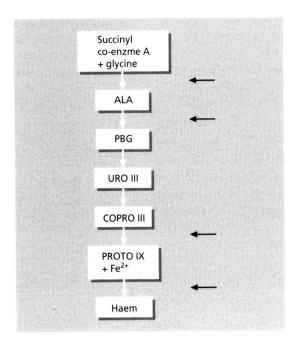

Fig. 4.1 Diagram showing the pathway of haem synthesis with the stages inhibited by lead (arrowed). ALA, δ-aminolaevulinic acid; PBG, porphobilinogen; URO III, uroporphyrinogen III; COPRO III, coproporphyrinogen III; PROTO IX, protoporphyrin IX.

Benzene. Benzene is unique amongst industrial poisons in having the capacity to depress bone marrow function. How it achieves this is not clear, although it is known to interfere with the synthesis of DNA. There may be several months or even several years between the onset (or cessation) of exposure and the development of anaemia. The severity of the anaemia depends upon the extent to which the bone marrow is damaged; in the worst cases, examination of the bone marrow may show that it is virtually acellular. This so-called aplastic anaemia has a poor prognosis although the patient can be kept alive for some time with regular blood transfusions. This disruption of bone marrow cell division can also lead to malignancy — in this case a form of leukemia.

Arsine. Arsine is a hydride gas of arsenic (AsH_3). The anaemia following exposure to arsine results from the destruction of circulating red blood cells, but details of how this state is reached are obscure. One consequence of the haemolysis of red cells is that the cellular sludge blocks the renal tubules, an event which will lead to the patient's certain death without artificial support. In the most severe cases of arsine poisoning, the patient may, literally, have no intact red cells, and the little oxygen which gets around the body is carried in solution in the plasma. Prompt transfusion and renal dialysis are usually effective in producing a recovery. Hydrides of phosphorus (phosphine) and antimony (stibine) can produce similar haemolysis of red cells to arsine.

FURTHER READING

Harrington, J.M. and Gill, F.S. (1992). *Occupational Health*, (3rd edn). Blackwell Scientific Publications, Oxford.

Levy, B.S. and Wegman, D.H. (1995). *Occupational Health*, (3rd edn). Little, Brown & Company, Boston.

The Health Effects of Some Physical Agents

J.M. Harrington and D. McBride

INTRODUCTION

In order to have an appropriate understanding of the agents which the hygienist is attempting to measure and control, he or she should know something of the health effects which may occur from exposure. This requires a knowledge of how the agent interacts with the body, and therefore what signs and symptoms may ensue. The health effects of chemical and biological agents are mainly covered in Chapter 4, with some further examples of dermatological effects in Chapter 2. The health effects of physical agents such as temperature, sound and pressure are dealt with here. The other chapters concerning physical agents are seen more from the engineer's viewpoint. For vibration, the reader is referred to Chapter 10 and for radiation to Chapters 13 and 14. More detailed accounts can be consulted by referring to the Further Reading list at the end of the chapter.

Of the three main classes of occupational hazard, chemical and biological agents tend to interact with the body in the same way, through a chemically mediated reaction, whilst physical agents interact by the transfer of energy. This energy can affect the body in a number of ways.

Some physical agents, such as temperature and pressure, are features of the normal environment, and cause harm by being in excess of that normally experienced. Some physical agents are stimuli for the senses and, if present in excess, may overwhelm the sensory organ. Physical agents can also transfer energy, the action of which is more akin to a chemical toxicity. An example is the possible action of an electromagnetic field in altering

electron spin states in cell surface receptors. Lastly, some physical agents have sufficient energy to cause direct damage to biomolecules, examples being the photochemical changes of ultraviolet light and damage to genetic material by ionizing radiation.

The body has defences to cope with all these challenges. Homeostatic mechanisms maintain the internal environment constant within a very wide range of external environmental conditions. Failure of these mechanisms eventually leads to the syndrome known as 'shock'. If the primary action of an agent is on a cell surface receptor, the target organ mechanism is important. If the agent is a mediator of a physical sense, the target is the sensory organ. DNA damage occurs naturally, and can be repaired by various mechanisms, but cancer may be induced if the process is imperfect.

TEMPERATURE

For the vast majority of workers, the temperature of their work place has importance only in terms of comfort zones, but for an important minority the temperature of the working environment varies greatly depending on the job done and where it is done (see also Chapter 12). It may be extremely hot for the foundry worker or very cold for cold storage operatives. Oil workers in an Alaskan winter (e.g. $-40°C$) experience markedly different temperatures from their colleagues undertaking similar work in the Arabian desert in summer (perhaps $+40°C$). At these extremes life can be threatened by temperatures which are at great variance with the normal body temperature of $37°C$. The normal thermoregulatory mechanisms are very efficient, and core body temperature is maintained at close to 37°C. Working raises the metabolic rate, and therefore the body temperature. Blood vessels in the skin dilate, carrying heat from the core to the surface where it is dissipated through convection, radiation and conduction, a process which is assisted by the evaporation of sweat. Discomfort due to the increased temperature gives a powerful stimulus to slow the rate of work. In cold climates, the opposite occurs. There is a stimulus to increase the metabolic rate, either through increased physical activity or shivering. Skin blood vessels constrict, helping to conserve core temperature, but causing cooling in the peripheries. Pre-existent circulatory disorders may therefore be exacerbated by the cold.

Effects of increased environmental temperatures

Most workers routinely exposed to heat will have been allowed to become adapted to their working environment over a period of time. During this time, the thermoregulatory mechanisms, for example the ability to sweat, will have been optimized. Those at risk of heat stress are those whose heat environment changes suddenly, for example the working of a new and deep seam in coal mining or the unexpected hot spell which overwhelms the ventilation system in a boiler room. Management should be aware of the possibility of such occurrences, and should ask for appropriate hygiene advice to determine if the working environment is acceptable. If work is performed under unsuitable conditions, particularly conditions of high humidity and low airflow, the core temperature of exposed workers may start to rise. The first signs of the resulting heat stress are discomfort and fatigue, and the natural reaction is to slow down the work rate or stop work, a protective mechanism which will allow cooling and recovery. Under certain circumstances, for example in rescue work and armed service, there may be powerful stimuli to exceed the limits of normal work capacity. Such workers should be trained to recognize this risk, and enforce a work/rest regime if necessary. They also need to be taught how to measure the thermal environment. This is made easier by the direct reading instruments which are now available, for example those which assess the WBGT (wet bulb globe temperature) index. In addition, those involved with work in high temperatures should be aware of the physiological changes which take place and the symptoms which occur on continued and uncontrolled exposure. There are nearly always premonitory symptoms, but if these are ignored, serious illness may develop with alarming rapidity.

Heat cramps

Sweating leads to the loss of large amounts of salt and fluid. Failure of adequate replacement, especially in the non-acclimatized worker, can result in painful, incapacitating and involuntary cramps, affecting the leg and abdominal muscles. Heat cramps are treated by rest and adequate fluid replacement, which should contain salt.

Heat exhaustion

Heat exhaustion occurs when the circulation fails to keep up with the extra demands placed upon it. Inadequate fluid replacement causes a fall in circulating blood volume, which is exacerbated by peripheral vasodilatation. Collapse occurs because of shock. The patient will look and feel ill, with all the typical signs of shock: a pale, clammy skin and extreme lethargy. Treatment is by rest, cooling and adequate fluid replacement.

Heat stroke

An impending failure of the sweating mechanism results in a rapid rise in core temperature, perhaps to above 40°C. The patient will usually have had signs of heat cramps or heat exhaustion. Collapse is accompanied by a hot dry skin. The condition is life threatening and unless urgent measures are taken to lower the temperature, convulsions and coma may ensue. Medical assistance will be necessary, but immersion in a cold bath and fluid replacement may be life saving — though cold water immersion has its inherent dangers as well.

Effects of decreased environmental temperatures

Cold injuries due to occupation are not common. Most workers exposed to extreme cold are well aware of the risks, and wear suitable protective clothing. Nevertheless, the health effects of decreased environmental temperatures are described here to increase awareness of the possible hazards involved in working under such conditions.

There are two main types of climate in which cold injuries may occur. In a cold, dry climate, snow and ice are usually present, and the temperature seldom rises above 0°C. A cold, wet climate is typical of winter in 'temperate' zones, where the temperature may vary from 10 to −12°C. In cold climates, the body maintains its temperature by decreasing the circulation to the periphery and by increasing the metabolic rate through an impulse to maintain physical activity, or by shivering where this is not possible. The effects of cold are first seen in the periphery.

Freezing injuries

Freezing injuries are most likely in a cold, dry climate in which the trunk is well protected by clothing, but the extremities are exposed, and may freeze. This takes place in stages. Rapid surface freezing produces a white spot on the skin known as 'frost nip'. Early recognition and rewarming prevents damage. Slower freezing in the deeper tissues produces frost bite. The skin is pale and solid, looking and feeling frozen. Ice crystals form in tissue fluid, and structural damage to cells always results. This damage is made worse by similar changes in blood vessels. On rewarming the damaged vessels leak, producing swelling which further compromises the circulation and adds to the tissue destruction. Some degree of tissue loss is inevitable. So long as infection and gangrene do not supervene, the extremity involved eventually mummifies and is sloughed or cast off.

Non-freezing injuries

Immersion or Trench foot results from poor circulation caused by the combination of cold, damp conditions and the pressure of standing in a relatively immobile position. Despite the epithet, the hands may be affected. The involved periphery becomes pale, swollen, macerated and numb. Although freezing does not take place, the circulatory changes may lead to tissue loss. There may also be damage to nerve tissue, and permanently altered sensation in the affected part.

Hypothermia

So long as warm clothing is worn and physical activity performed, core temperature can be maintained. Problems arise with exhaustion, hunger and when clothing becomes wet. Immersion in water is probably the most common cause of hypothermia, but cold, wet and windy conditions are also particularly treacherous. As the body temperature falls to 34°C, mental ability decreases with increasing fatigue, apathy and disorientation. Those who work outdoors in winter should be aware of these signs of apathy and unco-operation in others, and recognize feelings of fatigue and general numbness within themselves. If exposure develops, death occurs from coma and cardiac rhythm abnormalities as the temperature falls to below 30°C. The level of treatment depends on the length of exposure. If exposure is of short duration, for example immersion in water, rapid rewarming should be attempted. Hypothermia of longer duration is difficult to treat, as the body is lacking in oxygen, and cardiac arrest may occur. Slow, controlled rewarming under medical supervision is essential but difficult.

SOUND

The target organ for noise damage is the ear (see also Chapter 9). The pathway of sound reception is firstly mechanical transmission via the tympanic membrane and auditory ossicles. This mechanical energy is then transferred to the fluid in the inner ear. The inner ear is a membranous fluid-filled structure lying within the bone of the skull and consisting of the organ of hearing, the cochlea, and the organ of balance, the vestibular labyrinth. The sensory transducer of the cochlea is the organ of Corti, which lies on the basilar membrane of the cochlea. Within the organ of Corti lies the sensory apparatus, consisting of a highly specialized layer of 'hair cells'. The ionic composition of the fluids in the various membranous channels of the inner ear is such that depolarization occurs when the hair cells are displaced by the sound wave which travels along the basilar membrane. The resulting electrical impulse is transmitted to the brain via the auditory nerve. Disorders affecting this pathway before the cochlea cause what is known as a conductive deafness, whilst disorders of the cochlea or auditory nerve result in sensorineural or perceptive deafness.

Direct trauma to the ear occurs with impulses approaching explosive level, at around 35 kPa. Perforation of the eardrum and disruption of the auditory ossicles may occur, causing a conductive deafness. A tear in the basilar membrane is also possible, which results in severe (usually total) sensorineural deafness.

Two mechanisms are involved with lesser degrees of trauma. Firstly, minor damage may cause swelling of the hair cells in what is thought to be a biochemical disturbance. The resulting hearing loss is initially reversible, being a temporary threshold shift. The second mechanism is once again direct mechanical trauma, of a lesser degree than that which will cause disruption of the basilar membrane. Over a period of time, the hair cells become damaged, losing their sensory structures and characteristic shape. The transitional level between these two types of damage is not known. Indeed it may not exist, because it is thought that damage may persist if repeated often enough, and that a temporary threshold shift may eventually become permanent. The effect on hearing is of course deafness.

The range of hearing extends from 20 to 20 000 Hz. Noise affects the higher frequencies first, classically producing an increase in threshold at one frequency: the audiometric notch. The notch usually occurs at 4 kHz, but may lie between 2 and 6 kHz, and rarely occurs outside this range. The speech frequencies lie within the range of 500–2000 Hz, and because they are not at first affected, noise-induced hearing loss may initially pass unnoticed. The fine pitch discrimination necessary for the comprehension of speech is a complex and incompletely understood process which requires interaction between inner and outer hair cells, through neural feedback. As hair cells and neurones become depleted, the understanding of speech suffers because of this poor discrimination. Difficulty in conversation, especially with background noise, is the predominant symptom. In some cases amplification can make the situation worse, as the remaining neurones suddenly become 'saturated' with sound in a phenomenon known as 'recruitment'. The resulting distortion may be quite uncomfortable. The differential between achieving sufficient sound input for comprehension and the onset of recruitment may not be very great. As a result, it may be very difficult to communicate with someone who has recruitment: they cannot hear one minute, and accuse one of shouting the next! It is important to assess speech discrimination before recommending a hearing aid. It is obviously important to guard against this insidious onset of disability, and noise control levels are set by most Health and Safety legislatures. Even so, it is worthwhile bearing in mind that the sensitivity of hearing is subject to individual variability, and that a minority of workers may suffer hearing loss at levels at or below the legal limits for noise exposure.

PRESSURE

Humans are well adapted to live at atmospheric pressure. This adaptation is challenged by the increased pressures experienced in diving and the decreased pressures experienced in aviation. Problems may arise due to the rapid changes of pressure which may occur (barotrauma and decompression sickness), the changes of partial pressure of gases with depth (nitrogen narcosis and oxygen toxicity) and the rarefraction of atmosphere with altitude (altitude sickness).

Effects of increased pressure experienced by divers

Gas toxicity

Divers must have a breathing mixture containing oxygen which is supplied at the ambient pressure of the depth at which they are working.

The problem is that the main constituents of air, nitrogen and oxygen, are both toxic at depths greater than about 50 m. Oxygen is toxic to the central nervous system and lungs, whilst nitrogen has an anaesthetic effect resulting in decreased performance and euphoria. The oxygen in diving mixtures must therefore be diluted, the volume being made up with an inert gas, usually helium.

Barotrauma

During compression and decompression the air-containing spaces within the body must be allowed to equilibrate with the ambient pressure. Problems may arise in the upper respiratory tract or lungs. If the openings of the sinuses or the Eustachian tubes are blocked as a result of allergy or inflammation, pressure cannot equilibrate. A relative vacuum occurs on descent, and excess pressure on ascent. This causes mechanical stress on the tympanic membrane, which may perforate. Trapping of gas in the sinuses causes severe pain, whilst if the lungs are affected rupture of the alveoli and collapse of the lung (pneumothorax) may occur, causing chest pain and respiratory difficulty.

Decompression

During work under pressure, the gases used in the breathing mixture come to equilibrium in the tissues. The amount of gas dissolved depends on its partial pressure and solubility, and depends on the length of time worked. During decompression, dissolved gas must be allowed to escape from the tissues through the bloodstream and lungs. If decompression occurs too rapidly, the tissues may become supersaturated with gas. Irregularities, for example on blood vessel walls, may act as the nucleus for bubbles to form and decompression illness results.

Decompression illness

The symptoms occur when decompression has been too rapid. This occurs in accidental circumstances, such as running out of air, or when a diver has had an unpleasant or frightening experience, such as an encounter with a shark or conger eel. The resulting syndrome is complex. The symptoms are due to gas in the tissues, with some of the more life-threatening effects resulting from involvement of the nervous system. The primary symptoms are pain and discomfort, usually coming on within hours of decompression. There is a gradation in severity: from a creeping sensation under the skin (the 'creeps'), to severe limb, abdominal and chest pain (the 'bends' or 'chokes'). The neurological effects include paralysis of the limbs and epileptiform attacks, and permanent neurological damage may follow. The course of this acute illness is unpredictable. Seemingly minor symptoms may be followed by florid neurological signs. All symptoms of illness in divers should be treated seriously and managed with medical assistance, as urgent recompression and gradual decompression may be required at any stage. Previous attacks of decompression illness predispose divers to the condition occurring again. The effects may be apparent in the long bones, where bone death (dysbaric osteonecrosis) may be visible on X-ray.

Other conditions affecting divers

There are a number of features of the physical environment which also affect divers. Although sound travels faster in water, there is also greater attenuation, which may account for the fact that sensorineural hearing loss is not always shown in studies of divers' hearing. Visibility in water is often poor, because of turbidity in the water and poor light. The reduced sensory input which occurs because of these factors may be exacerbated by weightlessness, and cause acute disorientation.

Hypothermia may be a great problem, and the cold, wet and often cramped conditions experienced in diving provide an environment which is ideal for the spread of infection. In particular, maceration of the skin of the ear may allow bacterial infection with *Pseudomonas* or *Proteus* organisms, resulting in otitis externa, with severe pain and discharge. Dermatitis and bacterial skin infections also occur more commonly.

Aviation medicine

The most prominent physical hazards in aviation medicine are a direct converse of those in diving, and are due to pressure changes. Flying at altitude has the opposite effects on atmospheric gas constituents, in particular oxygen concentration is reduced. Hypoxia may occur at altitudes greater than 3000 m. This can result in mental changes, for example reduced reaction time and a decreased ability to concentrate. Anxiety and hypoxia also cause hyperventilation. Hyperventilation is ineffective in raising oxygen tension because of the shape of the oxygen dissociation curve, but it does lead to the washing-out of carbon dioxide. The resulting low carbon dioxide tension (hypocapnia) gives symptoms of light-headedness, flushing, tingling in the limbs and tunnel vision.

At altitudes of 8000 m or more, decompression symptoms may also occur. In commercial aircraft these effects are avoided by pressurization, whereby cabins are maintained at a pressure equivalent to around 2500 m. If cabin depressurization occurs in an emergency, decompression illness and barotrauma may result, along with the effects of hypoxia and extreme cold (−55°C at 10 000 m).

Most air passengers will have noticed the effects of mild barotrauma during descents from altitude. If Eustachian tube function is impaired, through nasal allergy or upper respiratory tract infection, air does not re-enter the middle ear and discomfort and conductive deafness occur. The prophylactic administration of boiled sweets is an attempt to open the Eustachian tube through the contraction of pharyngeal musculature.

Proprioception is of primary importance for flight control. Visual flights are carried out with the aid of instruments to navigate, but the horizon is used to maintain orientation. In instrument flight, navigation is carried out and orientation is maintained by reference to instruments. Problems may occur during transition from visual to instrument flight, especially if this occurs in other than straight and level flight, for example entering cloud whilst performing a descending turn in order to avoid it.

The vestibular organs are designed for a terrestrial environment, and may give unreliable information because of the rapidly changing forces in flight. Contradictory visual and equilibratory cues may be received and loss of control may result if the balance cues are relied upon rather than the instruments.

The effects of gravity are intensified in certain flying manoeuvres, although hopefully only in aerobatics and during military combat flying. 'Pulling positive G' occurs in loops where the head is orientated towards the centre of rotation, for example in pulling out of a dive. The effects on the limbs, head and neck make it difficult to carry out flight control movements. The effects on the circulation are to decrease the perfusion pressure to the brain, and temporary disorientation or a black-out may occur. 'Pushing negative G' occurs during the opposite manoeuvre, for example in outside loops. A 'red-out' is due to the increased perfusion pressure causing congestion and haemorrhage in the conjunctiva.

Working at altitude

Altitude sickness may be a problem in making the transition from living and working at sea level to working and living at altitude. Acclimatization occurs within 2–3 weeks, during which time the oxygen-carrying power of the blood is increased, because of an increase in haemoglobin concentration. During this period a worker is very easily fatigued, and will suffer the unpleasant symptoms of breathlessness (air hunger). Attempts to offset some of these effects in the unacclimatized person using pharmacological agents are not entirely successful and may carry adverse health effects of their own. Wherever possible, an otherwise fit worker should be allowed to acclimatize naturally before being expected to perform at full capacity.

FURTHER READING

Harding, R.M. and Mills, F.J. (1993). *Aviation Medicine*. BMJ Publishing, London.
Harrington, J.M. and Gill, F.S. (1992). *Occupational Health*. Blackwell Scientific Publications, Oxford.
Waldron, H.A. (ed.) (1989). *Occupational Health Practice*. Butterworth, London.

CHAPTER 6

The Nature and Properties of Workplace Airborne Contaminants

J.H. Vincent and L.M. Brosseau

INTRODUCTION

The science and practice of occupational hygiene are concerned with the interaction between humans and their working environments. Since much of this involves the local atmospheric environment, many agents which are potentially harmful are transported to the worker through the air. These are broadly classed as air pollutants, existing as matter (gases or aerosols), or energy (heat, sound, light and ionizing or non-ionizing radiation). This chapter is concerned with airborne pollutant matter.

The physical properties of matter are important in helping to understand how pollutant entities (gaseous or aerosol) are generated and dispersed in the workplace air, how they are transported to that part of the worker–environment interface where they are likely to be troublesome and how they might be monitored and controlled. This chapter aims to provide a basic framework of relevant physical ideas. It starts with a brief resumé of the general physical properties of matter, describing how the gaseous, liquid and solid phases are related to one another and how phase changes can take place. It then describes the properties of the air itself which transmits entities of pollutant matter, with particular emphasis on its important fluid properties. There follows a description of the nature and behaviour of aerosols and, finally, a description of the nature of the interaction between electromagnetic radiation and airborne pollutant matter, with emphasis on applications in monitoring methods. In view of the wide range of topics encompassed, the treatment throughout is necessarily of an introductory nature, and the reader is recommended to consult more specialized texts for in-depth coverage of specific areas. Some of these are listed at the end of the chapter.

PHYSICAL PROPERTIES OF MATTER

Matter is usually acknowledged to exist in three phases: solid; liquid; or gas. It consists of small particles called atoms, which in turn are made up of combinations of the fundamental particles of matter: protons; neutrons; and electrons. Each particular combination of these defines an element. Under certain conditions, atoms may combine together to form larger entities known as molecules. Whether or not atoms or molecules come together to form solids, liquids or gases depends on combinations of pressure, volume and temperature. The most familiar example is water which, over the ranges of familiar terrestrial conditions, can exist either as solid ice, liquid water or gaseous water vapour.

In the solid state, atoms are located in fixed positions which, for many stable materials, are arranged in regular and periodic patterns constituting the familiar stable crystallographic lattice structure. Amorphous (non-ordered) materials (e.g. glasses) are not strictly stable, and in time — sometimes a very long time — become crystalline. The atoms of a solid material are held together in this ordered way by inter-atomic forces, electrostatic in nature, which may be likened to a system of invisible springs by which each is connected to its neighbours. When people speak of atoms occupying fixed positions in the crystal lattice of a solid material, it should be understood that they are referring to their mean positions. In fact, for any temperature above absolute zero, 0 K, the atoms are in oscillatory motion about their mean locations and, as in any spring–mass system in motion, energy is continually being exchanged between the kinetic form (associated with velocity) and the potential form (associated with displacement). Averaged overall, energy is shared equally between the two energy forms.

If extra internal energy is given to a lump of solid matter in the form of heat, the atoms perform greater excursions about their mean locations. If enough energy is supplied, the solid melts and enters the liquid phase. At that point, bonds may be broken and remade, and individual atoms can move around in the lattice, changing places with one another. The state of the material has now become 'fluid'. It is of particular interest to occupational hygienists to consider what happens near the surface of a liquid. Atoms there are connected by their invisible 'springs' only with other atoms in the general direction of the body of the liquid; so, unlike atoms in the body of the liquid, they experience a net inward-seeking force. This accounts for the well-known phenomenon of surface tension. However, there is also a statistical probability that a given atom located instantaneously near the surface of the liquid may escape from the surface as a free entity and enter the gaseous vapour phase. This is the phenomenon of evaporation. Conversely, atoms or molecules in the vapour phase may enter the liquid through the surface, and so contribute to condensation. The magnitude and direction of the net flux of molecules across the surface are controlled by complex thermodynamic considerations.

If enough energy is supplied to a liquid, a temperature is eventually reached at which all the inter-atomic bonds can be broken permanently. All the atoms or molecules now become free to move at random, and the liquid becomes a gas in which all of the internal energy exists as kinetic energy.

The preceding scenario for the transition from the liquid to the gaseous or vapour phase applies in principle to all substances. For example, under extreme thermodynamic conditions (e.g. very low temperature), even a gas such as helium can become a liquid. In relation to occupational hygiene,

however, it is the convention to refer to gases as substances which, under workplace conditions, are always found in the free molecular phase (e.g. air). On the other hand, vapours are regarded as the free molecular phase of some other substances (e.g. organic solvents) which can, in the workplace, also be found in the liquid state.

PHYSICAL PROPERTIES OF THE WORKPLACE ATMOSPHERIC ENVIRONMENT

Basic properties

Occupational hygiene is concerned with the transport of pollutants of various kinds in the vicinity of human subjects, both through and by the workplace atmospheric air. Air is a mixture of gases, the main constituents being nitrogen (about 78% by volume) and oxygen (about 21% by volume), with a variety of other trace gases including argon, carbon dioxide and water vapour (which amount to about 1% by volume in total). It is a colourless, odourless gas of density $1.29 \, kg \, m^{-3}$ at a standard temperature of 293 K and pressure of $1.01 \times 10^5 \, Pa$ (STP, at sea-level).

Pollutants in the workplace air

In the widest sense, 'air pollution' defines the presence in the atmospheric air of entities of matter or energy, naturally occurring or synthetic, which have the potential to cause harm. In the context of occupational hygiene, this relates to the health and well-being of workers.

The universal unit of the concentration of any pollutant is its mass per unit volume of the atmosphere itself (e.g. μg of pollutant m^{-3} of air, or $mg \, m^{-3}$). However, gases and vapours are also commonly described in terms of the partial volume occupied (e.g. parts per million (ppm) or parts per billion (ppb)). For gases and vapours, the relationship between forms of expression is given (for STP conditions) by:

$$(mg \, m^{-3}) = \frac{(ppm) \times mol.wt \, (mass \, of \, gas \, or \, vapour \, in \, g \, mol^{-1})}{24.5 \, (l \, mol^{-1})} \quad (6.1)$$

For example, take the common gaseous air pollutant: sulphur dioxide. At a mass concentration of $0.3\,\text{mg m}^{-3}$ an exposed person would soon become aware of its presence. From Equation 6.1, this is equivalent to a partial volume of about 10^{-7} (or 0.1 ppm).

For aerosols, concentrations are usually expressed in terms of the mass per unit volume of air. However, depending on the measurement method used, aerosols may also be expressed in terms of the surface area of particulate per unit volume (e.g. as might be obtained using a light-scattering instrument) or the number of particles per unit volume (e.g. as might be obtained for asbestos fibres using an optical microscope).

Pollutant gases and vapours in air

Some of the above principles can be applied to materials which, while normally existing in the liquid phase, can also appear as vapours in air. This is a situation commonly encountered by occupational hygienists, since not all such materials are harmless.

Vapour pressure (VP) represents the pressure which would be exerted by vapour molecules in equilibrium with the same material in liquid form inside a closed container. For a material starting out as 100% liquid in a closed system, some of the molecules will evaporate into the vapour phase. For some materials, the attractive molecular forces between liquid molecules are relatively weak, so that the pressure exerted by the liquid in the closed container will be relatively high since a high proportion of the material will be present in the vapour phase. Conversely, for materials with stronger inter-molecular forces, relatively fewer molecules will be present in the vapour phase — so the vapour pressure will be correspondingly lower. Thus, it follows that materials with high vapour pressures are more likely to evaporate into the air than those with relatively lower vapour pressure. For example, hydrazine (N_2H_4, a colourless liquid) has a vapour pressure at STP (VP_{STP}) of 10 mmHg, while hexane ($CH_3(CH_2)_4CH_3$, another colourless liquid) has a vapour pressure of 124 mmHg. Thus the magnitude of vapour exposure is likely to be greater for hexane than for hydrazine.

This leads to a concept useful to occupational hygienists: the vapour hazard ratio (VHR) (see Chapter 17). For a given material, this is defined as:

$$VHR = \frac{SC}{OEL} \qquad (6.2)$$

where OEL is the relevant occupational exposure limit for the material (in parts per million by volume, ppm) and SC is the saturation concentration (also in ppm). SC is defined as:

$$SC = \frac{VP_{STP} \times 10^6}{BP} \qquad (6.3)$$

where barometric pressure (BP) is 760 mmHg. Applying this to hydrazine and hexane, we obtain the following:

hydrazine: SC = 13 158 ppm and OEL = 1 ppm, therefore VHR = 13 158,

hexane: SC = 163 158 ppm and OEL = 500 ppm, therefore VHR = 326.

From this we see that hydrazine is potentially much more hazardous to health than hexane, despite its lower vapour pressure and, hence, lower magnitude of exposure.

In some cases it is also important to consider the extent to which a material, when it is airborne, can exist as a vapour or an aerosol. To quantify this, SC (as defined in Equation 6.3) is first converted into a mass concentration (mg m^{-3}). This is then compared to the OEL (also expressed in mg m^{-3}). Thus we have the following possible scenarios:

1 if SC/OEL < 1, the airborne material will appear mostly as aerosol;

2 if 1 < SC/OEL < 100, the airborne material will contain some aerosol;

3 if SC/OEL > 100, the airborne material will appear as vapour.

For example, mercury has an OEL listed as $0.05\,\text{mg m}^{-3}$ under the assumption that the material is present as vapour and that there is no aerosol exposure. Mercury has a vapour pressure of 1.8×10^{-3} mmHg, giving it an SC of $19.6\,\text{mg m}^{-3}$. Therefore SC/OEL = 19.6/0.05 = 393. This confirms that the setting of an OEL for mercury based on the assumption of a vapour is correct.

Another physical property of pollutant gases and vapours in air of interest to occupational hygienists is their density. Significant differences in density in relation to that of the air itself can lead to stratification. For example, the density of carbon dioxide is $1.98\,kg\,m^{-3}$ (compared to $1.29\,kg\,m^{-3}$ for air), and in still atmospheres it can tend to accumulate near the floor. Although carbon dioxide is not toxic in itself, the fact that it displaces oxygen during this stratification can present a hazard in certain confined spaces. However this is not a problem in most industrial settings since there is usually sufficient mixing to prevent stratification.

Humidity

Water vapour is a normal and innocuous constituent of air and therefore is not a pollutant. However, it does not form a constant atmospheric constituent because the changes between phases for water (between solid ice, liquid water and gaseous water vapour) can all occur within the range of expected atmospheric conditions, even in workplaces.

The earlier description of how molecules of a liquid can enter the gaseous vapour phase may be enlarged upon to enable discussion of the important environmental question of humidity. This relates to the presence in the air of free water molecules. The mass of water vapour per unit volume of air is referred to as the absolute humidity. Its partial pressure cannot exceed the vapour pressure of water for a given temperature and atmospheric pressure. It reaches a pressure of 1 atmosphere ($1.01 \times 10^5\,Pa$) at the temperature at which water boils (393 K).

The water vapour in air is considered to be saturated when its partial pressure becomes equal to the vapour pressure. At lower pressures it is unsaturated, and relative humidity (RH, expressed as a percentage) is given by:

$$RH = \frac{\text{Partial pressure of water vapour}}{\begin{array}{c}\text{Vapour pressure of water at the}\\\text{same temperature}\end{array}} \times 100\% \quad (6.4)$$

For a given mass concentration of water vapour in the air, RH can be raised by lowering the temperature. Conversely, raising the temperature lowers RH. The temperature at which water vapour becomes saturated is known as the dew point. Below this, nucleation and condensation may take place, hence the appearance in the air of water droplets visible as mist or fog.

During evaporation, heat energy in the form of the kinetic energy of molecules is transferred from the liquid to the gas phase. Therefore, evaporation of water molecules from a moist body leads directly to a lowering in the temperature of the body, the rate of which depends on RH (being slowest when RH is highest). Thus we account for the familiar discomfort felt in warm air at high humidity, where the cooling of the skin by evaporation is inhibited (see Chapter 12).

AERODYNAMIC CONSIDERATIONS

The motion of air in workplaces is important in understanding how pollutant materials are conveyed to the worker. It is therefore important in each of the basic aspects of occupational hygiene: hazard recognition; evaluation; and control.

The starting point for describing the dynamic behaviour of a fluid (where, to a fluid dynamicist, air itself is a fluid) is Newton's second law, which states that the product of mass and acceleration of a 'body' is equal to the sum of all the forces acting on the body. For a fluid, this law is applied to each small elemental packet and the forces include body forces (e.g. buoyancy and gravity), pressure forces (associated with local gradients in static pressure) and shearing forces (associated with viscosity and local gradients in velocity). Applying this to each of the three available spatial dimensions, and including a fourth expression to ensure that continuity is maintained (so that the overall mass of fluid in the system under consideration does not change), yields the Navier–Stokes equations from which all else in fluid dynamics is derived. In general, these equations include the possibility that the fluid density may vary (i.e. the flow is compressible). However, as far as occupational hygiene is concerned, this feature may usually be neglected and flows may be treated as incompressible. This physical basis is deceptively simple. In practice, the resultant equations themselves are very complex when it comes to applying them to realistic systems, and analytical solutions for the behaviour of airflow systems are available only for the simplest cases. Fortunately, the advent of relatively inexpensive modern computers and appropriate software means that numerical solutions are now readily accessible. For present purposes, however, only a rudimentary qualitative picture is given.

Streamlines

One important set of solutions provided by the Navier–Stokes equations is the pattern of streamlines. It is this pattern which most graphically characterizes the flow. Described most simply, it is equivalent to the flow visualization that would be obtained by marking the fluid with a suitable visible tracer. To illustrate this Fig. 6.1 shows a typical flow system relevant to occupational hygiene. One feature in particular is worth noting: that there can be no transfer of fluid across streamlines. It therefore follows that the convergence of the streamlines represents an increase in fluid velocity (as the fluid is being 'squeezed' into a smaller volume); and conversely for diverging streamlines.

Boundary layers

A physical condition applicable to real fluids is that the velocity of the fluid must be zero at solid boundaries to the flow. This means that there must be a velocity gradient between the wall and the moving fluid outside, which in turn means that the fluid must be highly sheared. From the Navier–

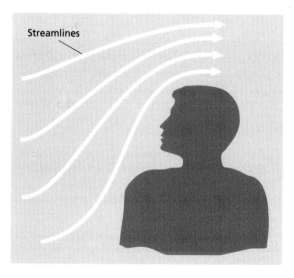

Fig. 6.1 A typical (simplified) streamline pattern relevant to occupational hygiene.

Stokes equations, this is where the effects of viscosity — the fundamental property of a fluid which reflects resistance to its motion — will be most strongly felt. It is from the effects of such boundary layers that, for aerosol particles and for other bodies immersed in fluids, the forces of drag and lift are derived. An important consequence of boundary layers which is important in all applications of fluid mechanics is the concept of dynamic similarity.

Similarity

It may be shown from the Navier–Stokes equations, as well as from dimensional arguments, that the dynamic nature of geometrically similar flows can be scaled between large- and small-scale systems provided that the dimensionless Reynolds number (Re) is kept constant. Re is defined as:

$$Re = \frac{D\,U\,\rho}{\eta} \qquad (6.5)$$

where D and U are characteristic dimensional and velocity scales for the system in question, and ρ and η are the fluid density and viscosity respectively. For example, for flow in a pipe, D would be the pipe internal diameter and U the mean velocity of the fluid flow in the pipe.

The Reynolds number concept is one of the most important ideas in fluid dynamics, originating from the work of Sir Osborne Reynolds in the 1880s. Physically, its meaning is strongly related to the boundary layer concept. It is, in effect, the ratio of the magnitude of inertial forces in the main body of the flow (e.g. near the axis of the pipe) to the magnitude of viscous forces close to the flow boundaries (e.g. near the pipe wall). For large Re (i.e. large U and D), it means that the boundary layer part of the flow has relatively small effect on the overall character of the flow system as a whole. On the other hand, for small Re (i.e. small U and D), the boundary layer flow and associated viscous effects dominate. Many properties of the flow (e.g. streamline pattern, drag force, etc.) vary quite sharply with changes in Re at small values of Re, but become much less sensitive to changes at large values.

Potential flow

For large enough *Re*, a given flow system may be treated for many purposes as if it were inviscid (i.e. having zero viscosity). Then the Navier–Stokes equations become much simpler and more amenable to mathematical treatment. In fact, they become equivalent to equations familiar to physicists and engineers working in other fields — for example, the flow of heat in a temperature field or the flow of electric charge in an electric field. Hence we refer to potential flow. Despite the idealized nature of its underlying assumptions, potential flow solutions have many practical applications relevant to occupational hygiene. For example, they have been widely and successfully used to describe the flow around aerosol sampling devices or into local exhaust ventilation systems.

Stagnation

An important property of a streamline is that, everywhere along its length, the sum of the local static pressure and the local dynamic pressure (i.e. that associated with the fluid velocity) is constant. This is Bernouilli's theorem. In the limiting case where the streamline intersects with the surface of a body, the fluid comes to rest at that point (Fig. 6.2). Here all the energy in the flow is converted into potential energy in the form of static pressure

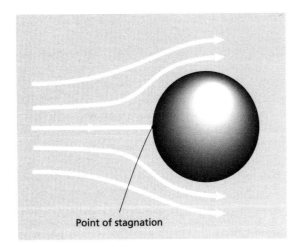

Point of stagnation

Fig. 6.2 Streamline pattern illustrating the phenomenon of stagnation.

and so the dynamic pressure falls to zero. The value of the static pressure therefore becomes a maximum, and the point where the streamline intersects with the surface is known as the stagnation point. To an occupational hygienist, this has two aspects of practical interest. The first is that stagnation points on surfaces often tend to be associated with increased aerosol deposition. The second is that it provides the principle of operation of the pitot-static tube, which is widely used in air velocity measurement (see Chapter 22).

Separation

Boundary layer separation is particularly important for flow about a body and is associated with the distribution of static pressure over the body surface. For frictionless inviscid flow, there is no net loss of energy along a streamline as it approaches the body, diverges to pass around it and then recovers on the downstream side. There is just the transformation of potential energy to kinetic energy (as the streamlines get closer together and, hence, the velocity increases) and back to potential energy again. However, for a streamline which passes close to the surface, and where there are friction losses, not all of the initial potential energy is recovered. The result is that the fluid in the boundary layer close to the surface of the body (on its downstream side) comes to rest prematurely. When and where this occurs, the flow breaks away from the body, enclosing a negative-pressure recirculating region which may or may not be turbulent (depending on the characteristic *Re* value for the flow, as discussed below). Some typical separated flows are illustrated in Fig. 6.3.

Turbulence

No discussion of fluid mechanics relevant to practical applications, no matter how rudimentary, would be complete without mention of the phenomenon of turbulence. This is relevant to many aspects of occupational hygiene.

The starting point for this discussion is the ideal, non-turbulent case known as laminar flow, in which the layers of the fluid (i.e. between the streamlines) slide smoothly over one another.

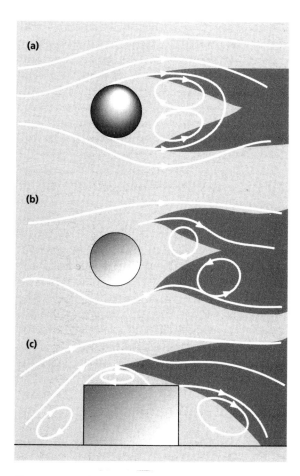

Fig. 6.3 Examples of some typical separated flows (darkly shaded areas indicate the presence of turbulence): (a) sphere (relatively stable wake region); (b) cylinder (vortex shedding in its wake); (c) surface-mounted prism (separation and re-attachment), relevant, for example, to flow around buildings.

However, from the Navier–Stokes equations it can be shown theoretically that, if inertial forces are large enough in relation to viscous forces (i.e. if Re for the flow is large enough, typically greater than about 2000), then a disturbance introduced into the flow can lead to overall instability. Such a disturbance might arise, for example, from the passage of the flow around some sort of flow blockage and the resultant flow separation. Amplification of the resultant triggering disturbance leads to a state of overall instability which appears as randomly fluctuating motions superimposed on the mean flow. Two of the consequences are: (1)

an apparent increase in the viscosity of the fluid (which, in the example of flow through a pipe, would appear as an increase in resistance to the flow); and (2) an accompanying sharp rise in its mixing properties. It is important to recognize that these consequences are associated with the properties of the turbulence and are not intrinsic properties of the fluid *per se*.

The origin of the turbulence has already been described as a small initial disturbance. But this in itself cannot provide the energy which drives the turbulent motions. This must derive from the mean flow itself. By the action of the mean flow, the initial, relatively large-scale fluctuating motions (i.e. eddies) created by the triggering disturbance are stretched and distorted, and so are broken down successively into smaller and smaller eddies. The energy from the mean flow which goes into the turbulence is therefore 'cascaded' down through the resultant range of eddy sizes until, eventually, the eddies become very small. At that point, when the Re values for the eddies themselves become very small, viscous forces take over inside the eddies and the energy is finally dissipated as heat. From this qualitative description, there emerges a physical picture of turbulence as a spectral phenomenon, characterized by a continuous distribution of eddy sizes and associated velocity fluctuations (superimposed on the mean flow). An important feature of this picture, arising from the second law of thermodynamics, is that the energy that goes from the mean flow into the turbulence cannot be recovered as useful kinetic energy and is irretrievably lost.

For many working purposes, this picture can be simplified so that turbulence may be described in terms of two 'bulk' properties: the characteristic intensity of the fluctuations (u', the root-mean-square value of the fluctuating velocity) and the characteristic mean length scale of those fluctuating motions (L). The degree of mixing increases with both, and a fair estimate of the diffusivity of a turbulent fluid (D_{ft}) may be obtained from:

$$D_{ft} \approx L\, u' \tag{6.6}$$

BASIC PHYSICAL PROPERTIES
OF AEROSOLS

What is an aerosol?

'Aerosol' is a scientific term which applies to any disperse system of liquid or solid particles suspended in a gas — usually air. It applies to a very wide range of particulate systems encountered terrestrially. Aerosols occur widely in workplace environments, arising from industrial processes and workplace activity, and so are of considerable interest to occupational hygienists. They take many different forms and a summary classification of a range of typical aerosols is given in Fig. 6.4. It contains not only examples of the workplace aerosols with which this book is primarily concerned but also, for the sake of comparison, some naturally-occurring and synthetic aerosols found in the outdoor atmospheric environment. Some aerosols of interest to occupational hygienists are listed below.

Dust   an aerosol consisting of solid particles made airborne by the mechanical disintegration of bulk solid material (e.g. during cutting, crushing, grinding, abrasion, transportation, etc.), with sizes ranging from as low as sub-micron to over 100 μm.

Spray   an aerosol of relatively large, liquid droplets produced by mechanical disruption of bulk liquid material, with sizes upwards of a few micrometres.

Mist   an aerosol of finer liquid droplets produced during condensation or atomization, with sizes up to a few micrometres.

Fume   an aerosol consisting of small, solid particles produced by the condensation of vapours or gaseous combustion products. Usually, such particles are aggregates of very small primary particles, with the individual units having dimensions of the order of a few nanometres and upwards.

Smoke   an aerosol of solid or liquid particles resulting from incomplete combustion, again usually in the form of aggregated, very small primary particles. The aggregates themselves

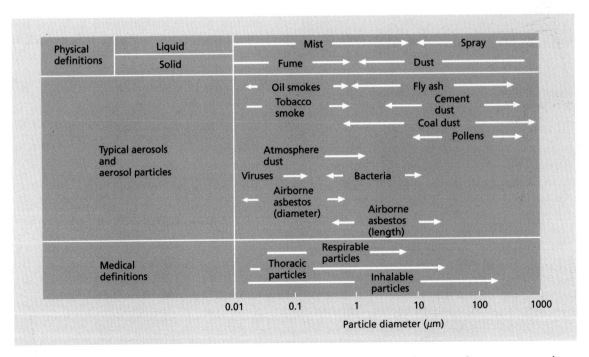

Fig. 6.4 Classification of typical aerosols ('medical' definitions refer to particle size fractions where exposure to the various parts of the human respiratory tract is possible).

have extremely complex shapes, frequently in the forms of networks or chains, having overall dimensions that can exceed 1 μm.

Bioaerosol an aerosol of solid or liquid particles consisting of, or containing, biologically viable organisms (viruses, bacteria, allergens, etc.), with sizes ranging from sub-micron to in excess of 100 μm.

Aerosol generation in workplaces

The majority of industrial processes generate aerosols in one form or another, usually as a side effect of the process itself and by a wide variety of physical and chemical means. These may include:

mechanical generation of dry aerosols: e.g. during mineral extraction, smelting and refining of metals, textiles manufacture, bulk chemical production and handling, woodworking, etc.;

mechanical generation of liquid droplet aerosols: e.g. during paint spraying, crop spraying, etc.;

formation by molecular processes: e.g. during combustion, chemical reactions, condensation, etc.;

and many others.

The evolution of aerosols

It cannot be assumed that an aerosol, once it has been dispersed, will remain in equilibrium and so retain the properties with which it began. Depending on the material in question, the initial generation process and the concentration of the aerosol, and other conditions in the surrounding air, a number of possibilities exist for evolutionary changes. These include:

growth by coagulation, agglomeration and coalescence: by the contact of particles with, and attachment to, one another, and in which the number concentration of particles decreases but the mass concentration stays the same;

disintegration: when a system of particles combined together to form a single particle is subjected to external forces such that the adhesive and cohesive bonds which hold the individual elements together are broken, and in which the number concentration increases but the mass concentration stays the same;

condensation: where particles are formed and grow by the condensation of molecules out of the vapour phase, and in which the mass concentration increases;

evaporation: where particles are decreased in size — or even disappear — by the transfer of molecules from the liquid to the vapour phase, and in which the mass concentration decreases.

These last two phenomena extend the earlier discussion about atmospheric water and other vapours to aerosols. From detailed consideration of the physics of phase transitions from liquid to vapour — and vice-versa — it may be shown that, in a system of droplets of a wide range of sizes, larger droplets can grow at the expense of smaller ones.

Particle shape

Particle shape can have a significant bearing on effects relevant to occupational hygiene: for example, on the way particles behave in the air, and how they behave after they have been deposited in the respiratory tract. Particle shape falls into a number of categories, some of which are shown schematically in Fig. 6.5. These include:

spherical particles (e.g. liquid mists, fogs and sprays, and some dry aerosols such as glassy spheres condensing out of some high-temperature processes);

compact or *isometric*, non-spherical, angular particles which have no preferred dimension or

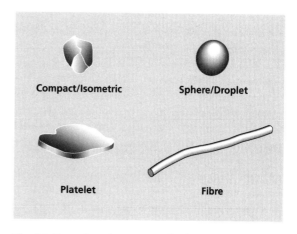

Fig. 6.5 Examples of some particle shapes found in occupational hygiene.

whose aspect ratio cannot be said to be substantially different from unity (e.g. most dusts,
including coal dust);

platelet particles (e.g. some dusts, such as mica);

fibrous or *acicular* particles which are long, thin,
needle-shaped particles (e.g. asbestos and synthetic mineral fibre dusts);

fractal particles, complex aggregates of much
finer primary particles (e.g. fumes and smokes).

Particle size

Particle size is a property which is extremely
important in virtually all aspects of aerosol behaviour. But it is a property whose definition is not
always as simple as might at first appear, and
can be somewhat elusive. Indices of particles size
include:

true geometric diameter (d) for a particle that is
perfectly spherical;

'effective' geometric diameter (d') for a non-
spherical particle, based on representative
widths; for example, dividing a two-dimensional
image of the particle into equal areas (Martin's
diameter) or contained within a pair of parallel
tangents to the particle perimeter (Feret's
diameter);

equivalent projected area diameter (d_p) is the
diameter of a sphere which, in two dimensions,
projects the same area as the particle in question;

equivalent surface area diameter (d_A) is the
diameter of a sphere which has the same surface
area;

equivalent volume diameter (d_v) is the diameter of
a sphere that has the same volume;

aerodynamic diameter (d_{ae}) is the diameter of a
sphere of water (density $10^3 \, \mathrm{kg \, m^{-3}}$) which has
the same falling speed in air as the particle in
question (see below).

Of these, perhaps the most important in the
occupational hygiene context is the latter — the
particle aerodynamic diameter. This governs the
airborne behaviour of most particles under most
conditions, and so is relevant to the inhalation of
particles by humans, deposition in the respiratory
tract, sampling and air cleaning.

For some particles, none of the above definitions
of particle size is truly appropriate, and further
considerations need to be invoked. This is the case
for fibres where both diameter and length need
to be defined. Complex aggregates such as those
formed during combustion (e.g. smokes) also pose
special problems. As already mentioned, these are
made up of large numbers of very small primary
particles and the degree of complexity is such as to
render difficult the definition of size in relation to
any of the measurable geometrical properties like
those described above. So, although aerodynamic
diameter can be usefully applied to describe aerodynamic behaviour, and a geometrical diameter
can be applied to describe aspects of visual appearance of individual particles or aerosols as a whole,
these do not always properly convey the full nature
of the particles. For many complex aggregated
particles the concepts of fractal geometry can
provide further information, leading to the concept
of a fractal dimension. These are derived from the
properties of some types of particle which reflect
the tendency to exhibit self-similar structure. That
is, observation under a microscope at increasing
magnification reveals a structure that continues to
repeat itself.

Elementary particle size statistics

Only rarely in practical situations — usually under
controlled laboratory conditions — do aerosols exist
that consist of particles all of one size. Such aerosols
are referred to as 'monodisperse'. More generally,
in workplaces and elsewhere aerosols consist of
populations of particles having wide ranges of
sizes, and so are termed 'polydisperse'. For these,
particle size within an aerosol needs to be thought
of in statistical terms.

Consider an ensemble of particles whose sizes
can be represented in terms of a single dimension
(d). The fraction of the total mass of particles with
dimension falling within the range d to $d + dd$ may
be expressed as:

$$dm = m(d) \, dd \qquad (6.7)$$

where

$$\int_0^\infty m(d) \, dd = 1 \qquad (6.8)$$

in which $m(d)$ is the mass frequency distribution

function. Alternatively, there are directly analogous expressions for the number frequency distribution function, $n(d)$.

It is often helpful in particle size statistics to plot distributions in the alternative cumulative form. For example, for the distribution of particle mass this is given in terms of the mass with dimension less than d, thus:

$$C_m(d) = \int_0^d m(d)\,\mathrm{d}d \qquad (6.9)$$

where C_m is the cumulative mass distribution, and similarly for mass. The fraction of mass with dimension less than d is given by:

$$\frac{\int_0^d m(d)\,\mathrm{d}d}{\int_0^\infty m(d)\,\mathrm{d}d} \qquad (6.10)$$

A typical mass distribution for a workplace aerosol is shown in Fig. 6.6, both in the frequency and cumulative forms. Note that the cumulative distribution describes the mass (e.g. in units of [mg]) contained in particles below the stated dimension. Since the cumulative distribution is obtained by integrating the frequency distribution, it follows conversely that the frequency distribution derives from differentiating the cumulative distribution. Thus, it is seen that the frequency distribution represents the mass fractions of particles contained within narrow size bands (and so may be expressed, for example, in units of [mg μm^{-1}]).

Figure 6.6 contains a number of important features. Firstly, the mass median particle diameter (d_m), at which 50% of the mass is contained within smaller particles and 50% is contained within larger ones, can be read off directly from the cumulative plot. Secondly, the frequency distribution shown exhibits a strong degree of asymmetry such

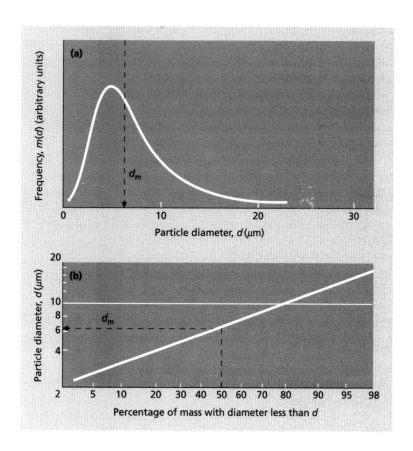

Fig. 6.6 Examples of aerosol size distributions: (a) frequency distribution; (b) cumulative distribution on log-probability axes.

that the peak lies at a value of d which is sub-stantially smaller than d_m, and there is a long tail in the distribution that extends out to relatively large particles. This characteristic is very common in practical polydisperse aerosol systems like those found in workplace environments. Very often, the overall distribution can be represented to a fair first approximation by the log-normal mathematical function:

$$m(d) = \frac{1}{d\sqrt{2\pi} \ln \sigma_g} \exp\left[-\frac{(\ln d - \ln d_m)^2}{2(\ln \sigma_g)^2}\right] \quad (6.11)$$

where σ_g is the geometric standard deviation, reflecting the width of the distribution. This is given by:

$$\sigma_g = \frac{d_{84\%}}{d_m} = \frac{d_m}{d_{16\%}} \quad (6.12)$$

For a perfectly monodisperse aerosol, $\sigma_g = 1$. More typically for aerosols found in the workplace environment, σ_g ranges from about 2 to 3. At this point, it is useful to note that, when the cumulative distribution is plotted on log-probability axes, it appears as a straight line if the distribution is log-normal (see Fig. 6.6(b)). Such log-normality (or even a reasonable approximation to it) provides some additional useful aspects. In particular, it enables conversions between relationships for distributions based on particle number, mass, surface area and any other aerosol property, using a set of equations (known as the Hatch–Choate equations) which have the form:

$$q\text{MD} = \text{NMD} \exp(q \ln^2 \sigma_g) \quad (6.13)$$

where NMD is the number median particle diameter and qMD is the median diameter weighted by d^q. For a given particle size d, in order to get from particle number to mass we need to multiply by d^3. Therefore it becomes obvious that $q = 3$ if we wish to use Equation 6.13 to convert distributions from number to mass.

The appearance of a log-normal particle size distribution is usually associated with a single aerosol generation process. In many workplaces, there may be more than one type of aerosol. In such cases, it is not unusual, for the aerosol as a whole, to find two or more particle size distributions superimposed. These are referred to as multimodal. A typical example is given in Fig. 6.7 for an aerosol in an underground mining situation where there is both relatively coarse dust (generated by the extraction process itself) and relatively fine diesel particulate (generated by underground transportation).

Electrical properties

In occupational hygiene applications and else-where, the electrical properties of aerosols have frequently been ignored, or — at best — occasionally invoked to provide qualitative explanations of un-expected, or otherwise implausible, observations. But in recent years, a growing body of experimental work has indicated that the state of static electri-fication (i.e. particle surface charge) in an aerosol may be of significant practical relevance in a num-ber of occupational hygiene areas. For example, it has now been established that it can affect the behaviour of particles in the lung after inhalation (leading to enhanced deposition in some cases), and can influence sampling and filtration.

Measurements of the electrical properties of workplace aerosols have shown that the following characteristics apply to a wide range of aerosol types.

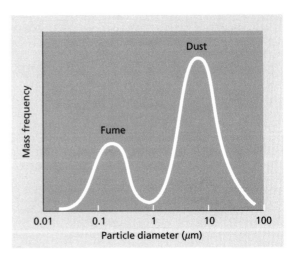

Fig. 6.7 Typical bimodal aerosol frequency distribution (from an underground mining situation, showing the dust and diesel fume components).

1 Each particle is charged either net positive or negative and, for the aerosol as a whole, the charges on individual particles are distributed almost symmetrically between positive and negative polarity.

2 The median magnitude of charge per particle for each given workplace aerosol ($|q_m|$) may be represented by the simple relation:

$$|q_m/e| = A\ d^n \qquad (6.14)$$

where n is a constant coefficient and, if particle diameter (d) is in [micrometres], A is the number of charges equivalent in magnitude to one electron ($|e|$) carried by a $1\,\mu m$ diameter particle. Typically it has been shown for workplace aerosols that A ranges from about 2 to 40 and n ranges from about 1 to 2.

THE MOTION OF AIRBORNE PARTICLES

The physical processes governing the motion of airborne particles are highly relevant to the transport and deposition of particles in ventilation ducts, deposition onto workplace surfaces, inhalation into and deposition inside the human respiratory tract, sampling and filtration, and so on. An elementary appreciation of the physics of particle motion is therefore important to occupational hygienists.

Drag force on a particle

When a particle of diameter d moves relative to the air, it experiences forces associated with the resistance (by the air) to its relative motion (as shown schematically in Fig. 6.8). For very slow, 'creeping' flow (at low Reynolds number) over the particle at velocity v, the drag force (F_D) is given by Stokes' law:

$$F_D = -3\ \pi\ d\ \eta\ v \qquad (6.15)$$

where the Reynolds number for the particle, defined as:

$$Re_p = \frac{d\ v\ \rho}{\eta} \qquad (6.16)$$

is very small ($Re_p < 1$) and where the minus sign indicates that the drag force is acting in the direction opposing the particle's motion. Strictly, this expression should be modified by three factors. The first is the Cunningham correction factor, which derives from the fact that, in reality, the air surrounding the particle is not continuous but is made up of individual gas molecules which are in random thermal motion (so particle motion — for small enough particles — takes the form of 'slip' between collisions with individual air molecules). The second factor concerns deviations from Stokes' law at Re_p values exceeding 1. The third relates to cases (the majority in practice) where particles are non-spherical. These corrections are described in

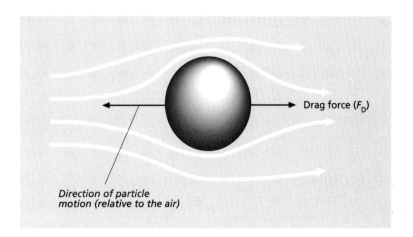

Fig. 6.8 Schematic to show the drag force on an aerosol particle.

detail in the aerosol science literature and should never be ignored. But in many occupational hygiene situations they may be quite small, so that — to a first approximation — Stokes' law may be a reasonable working assumption.

The starting point for all considerations of particle transport is the general equation of particle motion, again based on Newton's second law (mass × acceleration = net force acting). For the forces, the drag force describing the resistance of the fluid to the particle's motion has already been described. In addition, there may be an external force (e.g. gravity, electrical or some combination of forces), the effect of which is to generate and sustain particle motion. So long as the particle is in motion relative to the fluid, the drag force will remain finite. The proper relationship for describing the particle motion is a vector equation embodying the motion of the air and the particle, and the forces acting, each in all three available dimensions. It is not difficult, therefore, to envisage that the resultant set of equations which need to be solved for particle motion in specific cases can become quite complicated. However, the important principles involved can be illustrated by reference to one simple — but nonetheless extremely important — example.

Motion under the influence of gravity

The case of a particle falling under the influence of gravity in still air is shown schematically in Fig. 6.9. The equation of motion for a spherical Stokesian particle (i.e. a particle obeying Stokes' law) moving in the vertical (y) direction is given by:

$$m \, (dv_y/dt) = mg - 3 \pi \eta \, dv_y \quad (6.17)$$

where v_y is the particle's velocity in the y-direction, t is time, m is its mass and g the acceleration due to gravity. For a spherical particle, this expression may be re-organized to give:

$$dv_y/dt + (v_y/\tau) - g = 0 \quad (6.18)$$

where:

$$\tau = d^2 \, \gamma/18 \, \eta \quad (6.19)$$

in which γ is particle density. Closer inspection of Equation 6.19 reveals that τ has dimensions of

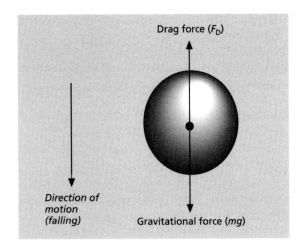

Fig. 6.9 Schematic to show the forces acting on a particle of mass m moving under the influence of gravity.

time, the significance of which we shall see shortly. Equation 6.18 is a simple first-order linear differential equation of the type familiar in many areas of science and engineering. In terms of the particle velocity at time t, it has the form:

$$v_y = g\tau[1 - \exp(- t/\tau)] \quad (6.20)$$

for the case where the particle starts from rest ($v_y = 0$) at time $t = 0$. This shows that particle velocity under the influence of gravity tends exponentially towards a terminal value: the sedimentation or falling speed, given by:

$$v_s = g \, \tau \quad (6.21)$$

Regardless of particle size (but under the broad, simplifying assumption that Stokes' law applies), particle velocity reaches $1/e$ of its final terminal value at $t = \tau$. The quantity τ is therefore referred to as the 'particle relaxation time'. Based on the above equations, we can estimate that for a 'fine' particle with the same density as water (i.e. $10^3 \, \text{kg m}^{-3}$) with $d = 1 \, \mu\text{m}$, $v_s \approx 30 \, \mu\text{m s}^{-1}$; for $d = 5 \, \mu\text{m}$, $v_s \approx 0.8 \, \text{mm s}^{-1}$; and for a 'coarse' particle with $d = 20 \, \mu\text{m}$, $v_s \approx 12 \, \text{mm s}^{-1}$; and so on. If we wished, we could then estimate the appropriate value for Re for each particle size and inspect the extent to which the assumption of Stokesian conditions is valid.

From the above, we could perform a simple

'back-of-the-envelope' calculation (always a good — and often revealing — first approach for an occupational hygienist) of the time it would take for particles of given type and size to sediment out completely in a room of given dimensions. For example, consider a cloud of monodisperse water droplets of diameter 20 µm, uniformly dispersed into a room of height 3 m. Under the most simple assumptions (no air movement or other deposition mechanisms), we may estimate that all particles will have settled to the floor of the room in a time $3 \text{ m} \div 12 \text{ mm s}^{-1}$; that is, in about 4 h.

Although the mechanism of gravitational settling is perhaps the most important in occupational hygiene, other relevant examples are those involving particle motion in electric fields or in thermal gradients. For these, the general physical approach is directly analogous to that for gravitational settling.

Motion without external forces

The concept of particle motion without the application of an external force is also important. For example, consider the simplest case where the air is stationary and a spherical particle is projected into it with finite initial velocity in the x-direction. Motion is described by the equation:

$$m \, (dv_x/dt) = -3 \, \pi \, \eta \, d \, v_x \qquad (6.22)$$

where now there is assumed to be no external force acting. This equation has the simple solution:

$$v_x = v_{x0} \exp \left(- t / \tau \right) \qquad (6.23)$$

where v_{x0} is the initial particle velocity relative to the fluid at time $t = 0$. This expression has particular relevance to moving air since it describes the fact that, although a particle injected into the flow with zero velocity at first lags behind the flow, it is progressively pulled along by the drag force exerted by the fluid until it eventually 'catches up' with it. At this point, the particle is then transported along at the same velocity as the air itself, and may thereafter be considered to be 'airborne'. This state of being airborne is therefore seen to stem directly from the particle drag force, and is obviously important in occupational hygiene.

Integration of Equation 6.23 yields a further important result, providing the distance travelled

by the particle relative to the air before it comes to rest, or — for the converse moving air case — catches up with it. Thus:

$$s = v_{x0} \, \tau \qquad (6.24)$$

where s is the stop distance. This concept is particularly important in considerations of how a particle behaves within moving air which is changing direction (i.e. in distorted flows, often encountered in the occupational hygiene context).

Similarity in particle motion

For particles moving in distorted air flows, we can examine the conditions under which their behaviour may be scaled. In this way it may be shown that, for systems which are geometrically alike, similar particle motion (i.e. in terms of relative trajectories) occurs, provided — in the first place — that:

$$St = \frac{d^2 \, \gamma \, U}{18 \, \eta \, D} \qquad (6.25)$$

is constant, where D and U are characteristic dimensional and velocity scales respectively. This dimensionless quantity is known as the Stokes' number. In addition, solutions for the motion of non-Stokesian particles will also depend on Re_p. However, as indicated before, Stokes' law is a fair working assumption for most workplace aerosols. Therefore the use of St alone for scaling purposes is usually adequate.

The physical significance of St becomes apparent for situations where the flow is distorted (i.e. divergent or convergent): for example, near a bluff obstacle in the workplace, inside a bent tube or duct (e.g. the lung airways or a ventilation duct) or in the vicinity of a sampler. Equation 6.25 with 6.19 gives:

$$St = \frac{\tau}{(D/U)} = \frac{\tau}{\tau_d} \qquad (6.26)$$

where, if D is the dimensional scale of the physical system which is responsible for the distortion, it is also equivalent to the dimensional scale of the distortion itself. It follows that D/U reflects the length of time (τ_d) for a packet of fluid to pass through the distorted flow region. St is therefore the ratio of the particle relaxation time to the time scale associated with the flow distortion, and so is a direct indication of how well the particle is able to respond to changes in the flow velocity and direction. Note, for example, that a very small particle with correspondingly small τ will yield a small value of St in many flow systems, indicating that the particle will tend to respond quickly to changes in the flow and so tend to 'follow' the airflow closely. A large particle, having large τ, and a correspondingly larger St, will tend to respond less effectively to the changing flow. A very large particle will therefore tend to continue along in the direction of its original motion, and not to 'see' the changes in flow direction and velocity.

The same concept can be viewed slightly differently. By combining Equations 6.24 and 6.25, we obtain another relationship:

$$St = \frac{s}{D} \qquad (6.27)$$

where St is now expressed as the ratio of particle stop distance (s) to the dimensional scale of the flow distortion. Similarly to the preceding argument, the particle will tend to follow the air flow when s is small compared to the flow distortion; and vice-versa when s is of the order of it, or larger.

From the preceding discussion, it is clear that St is an important measure of the ability of an airborne particle to respond to the movement of the air around it, and that particle trajectory patterns may differ to an extent dictated largely by the magnitude of St. The extremes are $St \ll 1$ and $St \gg 1$, with $St = 1$ representing some intermediate situation. Thus we have the concept of particle 'inertia', which is a function both of the particle itself and of the flow in which it is moving. It is illustrated in Fig. 6.10, and embodies one of the most important concepts in aerosol particle mechanics.

So far, we have assumed the absence of gravity. Of course, except in highly specialized working environments (e.g. space stations), gravity will always be present and so must be borne in mind. In some practical situations where the effects of gravity and inertia may both be important, dimensionless parameters in addition to St may have to be taken into account to compensate for the effects of gravity.

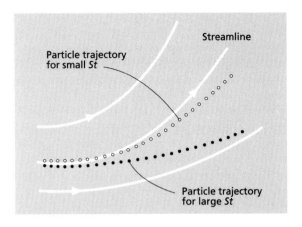

Fig. 6.10 Schematic to illustrate the concept of inertia.

Particle aerodynamic diameter

Two spherical particles having different diameters $(d_1$ and $d_2)$ and different densities $(\gamma_1$ and $\gamma_2)$ will have the same falling speeds in air provided, from Equations 6.19 and 6.21, that:

$$d_1^2\, \gamma_1 = d_2^2\, \gamma_2 \qquad (6.28)$$

where for simplicity, slip, Re_p and particle shape corrections have been neglected. Equation 6.28 leads directly to a new definition of particle size based on falling speed: namely, the particle aerodynamic diameter (d_{ae}) which was referred to earlier. Thus, for a given near-spherical particle:

$$d_{ae} = d\,(\gamma/\gamma^*)^{1/2} \qquad (6.29)$$

where d is the geometrical diameter of the particle and γ^* is the density of water $(10^3\,kg\,m^{-3})$. This does not apply to particles of extreme aspect ratio, notably long and thin fibres, for which separate equations have been developed and are described in the literature.

Impaction and interception

Consider what happens in a distorted aerosol flow, for example around a bend in a duct or about a bluff flow obstacle (Fig. 6.11). The air itself diverges to pass around the outside of the body. The flow of airborne 'inertialess' particles would do the same. However, as described above, real particles exhibit the features of inertial behaviour, in particular the tendency to continue to travel in the direction of

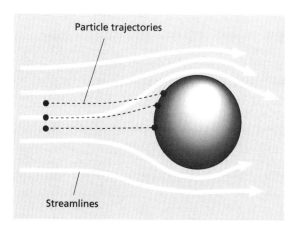

Fig. 6.11 Schematic to illustrate the phenomenon of impaction.

their original motion upstream of the body. This tendency is greater the more massive the particle, the greater its approach velocity and the more sharply the flow diverges. In the aerosol flow shown in Fig. 6.11, the result is that some particles will 'impact' onto the surface of the body. The effect is greatest for the heaviest particles approaching the body at the highest velocity. The efficiency of impaction (E) is defined as:

$$E = \frac{\text{Number of particles arriving by impaction}}{\text{Number of particles geometrically incident on the body}} \quad (6.30)$$

and is a strong function of the Stokes' number as described in Equation 6.25, where D is now the body dimension and U is the velocity of the approaching airflow. If all the particles that impact onto the body in the manner indicated actually stick and so are removed from the flow, then E is also equivalent to the collection efficiency. Therefore it is seen that impaction is important in aerosol collection in many situations, including during filtration and aerosol sampling.

This discussion can be extended to a particle whose trajectory, as traced by the motion of the particle's centre of gravity, passes by outside the body. If this trajectory passes close enough to the surface of the body and if the particle is geometrically large enough, it may be collected by interception, as illustrated in Fig. 6.12. Although for $d \ll D$ this effect on E is negligible, it becomes a significant influence if d becomes of the order of D, as for example it might in a filtration device made up of thin fibrous-collecting elements.

Elutriation

The term 'elutriation' is used to refer to another mode of particle deposition relevant to industrial hygiene: from a moving airstream under the influence of an externally applied force. Traditionally the term has been used to describe the gravitational separation of particles carried along by smooth laminar flow through a narrow horizontal channel

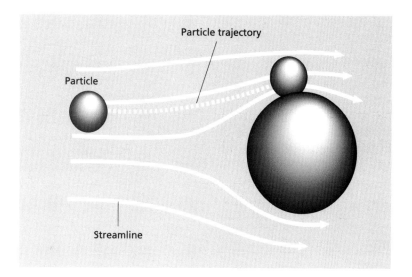

Fig. 6.12 Schematic to illustrate the phenomenon of interception.

where particles are deposited onto the floor of the channel. An extension of this idea is the gravitational elutriation that occurs during aerosol flow vertically upwards (e.g. through a vertical tube, or into an inverted sampling device). The general principle also applies if some other force (e.g. electrostatic) is the main agency of deposition. The process is relevant to aerosol behaviour, not only in sampling devices, but also in the airways of the lung after inhalation.

Aspiration

Aspiration is the process by which particles are withdrawn from ambient air through an opening in an otherwise enclosed body. It is therefore relevant to aerosol sampling systems. It is also relevant to the inhalation of aerosols by humans through the nose and/or mouth during breathing.

In order to identify the nature of the process of aspiration and to enable some generalizations, Fig. 6.13 shows schematically a body of arbitrary shape placed in a moving airstream. It has a single orifice located at arbitrary orientation with respect to the wind through which air is drawn at a fixed volumetric flow rate. There are two competing flow influences on particle transport: the external wind which diverges to pass around the outside of the body, and the convergent flow into the orifice. The interaction between these two gives rise to the complex, distorted overall flow pattern shown. It

may be thought of as having two parts, the external divergent part and the internal convergent part.

Particles moving in this flow system respond to the changes in flow velocity and direction in the ways described earlier. Generally in moving air, it is the wind that brings particles into the region of influence of the aspirating body, and it is inertial forces that provide the dominant influence on aerosol transport in that region. In fact, the system shown may be regarded as just a more complicated version of the impaction of particles onto a bluff body. This time, however, particles may be thought of as having to undergo two successive impaction processes: the first is, in effect, onto the surface of the body as governed by the external part of the flow; and the second is onto the plane of the orifice as governed by the internal part. Having established this picture, we may begin to construct a quantitative physical model for the efficiency with which particles are aspirated from the ambient air and into the body through the orifice.

Aspiration efficiency (A) may be defined for given particle aerodynamic diameter (d_{ae}), body geometry and dimensions (D), orifice geometry and dimensions (δ), orientation with respect to the wind direction (θ), external windspeed (U) and mean aspiration velocity (U_s) as:

$$A = \frac{\text{Concentration of particles in the air actually entering the orifice}}{\text{Concentration of particles in the undisturbed upstream air}} \quad (6.31)$$

provided that the airflow and aerosol upstream of the sampler are uniformly distributed in space. Aspiration efficiency defined in this way is the most basic description of performance for an aerosol aspirating system (such as an aerosol sampler). Starting with Equation 6.31, and from considerations of particle impaction from one region of the flow to another, a system of equations may be developed which can, in principle, provide estimates for A. For present purposes, it is sufficient to express some of the generalizations which arise. In the first instance:

$$A = f(St, U/U_s, \delta/D, \theta, B) \quad (6.32)$$

where St ($= d_{ae}^2 \gamma^* U/18nD$) is a characteristic Stokes' number for the aspiration system and B is

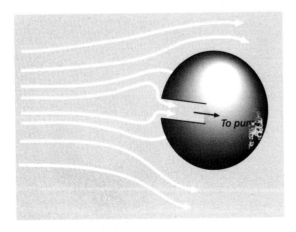

Fig. 6.13 Schematic to illustrate the concept of aspiration.

an aerodynamic shape ('bluffness' or 'bluntness') factor. Secondly:

$$A \rightarrow (U/U_s) \cos \theta \text{ as } St \rightarrow \infty \qquad (6.33)$$

indicating that A levels off for large particles approaching the body at high windspeeds. For very large particles and/or in environments with very little air movement, gravity may also play a role, and so an additional term, to reflect the effect of gravitational settling, may be required in Equation 6.32.

This forms the basis for understanding the performance characteristics of the simplest, and most widely researched, sampling system: the thin-walled tube. For many years this has formed the basis of aerosol sampling in stacks and ducts, under what have come to be known as isokinetic sampling conditions. With the thin-walled sampling tube aligned axially with the flow, and the sampling flow rate adjusted so that the velocity of the air entering the tube matches that in the duct (in the absence of the sampler), there is no distortion of the airstream and so particles of all sizes are aspirated with 100% efficiency (Fig. 6.14).

Diffusion

Particle motion has so far been assumed to be well ordered and, in theory at least, deterministic. In reality, however, even in apparently smooth airflows, aerosol particles exhibit random movement associated with their collisions with gas molecules,

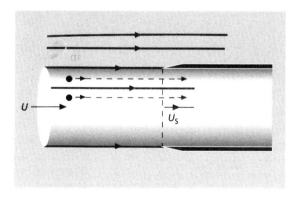

Fig. 6.14 Schematic to illustrate isokinetic sampling with a thin-walled sampling tube, where sampling velocity (U_s) is matched to the windspeed (U).

which themselves are in thermal motion (as described by the classical kinetic theory of gases). Such movement is independent of any convection associated with the air itself, and is known as 'molecular' (or 'Brownian') diffusion. As a result of this phenomenon, there is a net migration of particles from regions of high concentration to regions of low concentration. That is, although individual particles may diffuse in either direction, a greater number end up travelling down the concentration gradient. The resultant local net flux of particles by this process is described by Fick's law of classical diffusion, which for the simple one-dimensional case (for the x-direction) is:

$$\text{Local net flux} = -D_B \frac{dc}{dx} \qquad (6.34)$$

where c is the local concentration and D_B is the coefficient of Brownian diffusion. From classical kinetic theory for a small particle in the Stokes' regime, the latter is given by:

$$D_B = \frac{kT}{3 \pi \eta d_v} \qquad (6.35)$$

where T is the air temperature (in K) and k is the Boltzmann constant $(1.38 \times 10^{-23} \text{ J K}^{-1})$. The numerator represents the thermal energy of the gas molecules that is being transferred to the particles, and the denominator represents the loss of particle energy due to viscous effects. Therefore, D_B embodies the continual interchange of thermal energy between the gas molecules and particles, and vice-versa. Typically, for a particle of diameter 1 μm in air, D_B is very small: only of the order of $10^{-11} \text{ m}^2 \text{ s}^{-1}$.

Equation 6.34 leads directly to the general diffusion equation describing the local rate of change of concentration:

$$\frac{dc}{dt} = D_B \frac{d^2c}{dx^2} \qquad (6.36)$$

whose solution for the simple one-dimensional case of N_0 particles released initially at $x = 0$ at time $t = 0$, gives the Gaussian form:

$$c(x, t) = \frac{N_0}{(2 \pi D_B t)^{1/2}} \exp \left(\frac{-x^2}{4 D_B t} \right) \qquad (6.37)$$

for the concentration distribution along the x-direction at time t. The root mean square displacement of particles (in the one-dimensional case chosen) from their origin at time t is:

$$x' = (2D_B t)^{1/2} \qquad (6.38)$$

Aerosol diffusion in a flowing gas system is referred to as 'convective diffusion', and this aspect is perhaps the most relevant to occupational hygiene, especially in so far as deposition is concerned. In simple terms this may be envisaged by superimposing the possible excursion due to diffusion on the trajectories that would otherwise result in the absence of diffusion. The scaling parameter for this situation, analogous to the Stokes' number already described for inertial behaviour, is the Péclet number (Pe) which is given by:

$$Pe = \frac{U D}{D_B} \qquad (6.39)$$

where, as before, D and U are dimensional and velocity scales respectively. The smaller Pe is, the more pronounced the contribution due to diffusion.

The phenomenon of diffusion is important not only in how particles move from one point in an aerosol system to another, but also in how they move in relation to one another. It is responsible for collisions between particles which form a fundamental basis for the related phenomenon of coagulation (mentioned earlier).

Turbulent diffusion

Turbulent mixing of particles associated with the chaotic motions in a turbulent aerosol flow may be thought of as a form of diffusion over and above the molecular variety. In most cases, a fair approximation of the flux associated with turbulent diffusion may be described in terms of an expression which is directly analogous to Fick's law as given in Equation 6.34. The only difference is that the turbulent diffusivity of the particles, D_{pt}, replaces D_B.

An inertialess particle that is able to follow all of the fluid motions faithfully will have a turbulent diffusivity identical to that for the fluid itself. However, a relatively massive particle, of the type more representative of aerosols encountered in

reality, responds to each turbulent eddy as if it were a steady flow distortion of the type already described. Therefore, the particle's ability to respond to the turbulence must be related to an inertial parameter something like the Stokes' number already defined. This inertial parameter (K_{pt}) is given by:

$$K_{pt} = \frac{\tau u'}{L} \qquad (6.40)$$

where, as before, τ is the particle relaxation time and u' and L are the characteristic turbulence property values. This provides:

$$\frac{D_{pt}}{D_{ft}} = f(K_{pt}) \qquad (6.41)$$

where, as before, D_{ft} is the turbulent diffusivity for the fluid. As K_{pt} increases (i.e. larger particles, greater turbulence intensity, smaller length scale), the particle responds less and less well to the fluctuations and so its diffusivity falls. This trend is shown in Fig. 6.15. Eventually a stage is reached where the particle is so large, or the turbulence itself is such, that the particle does not 'see' the turbulence motions as it travels with the mean flow. In that limit, $D_{pt} \rightarrow 0$.

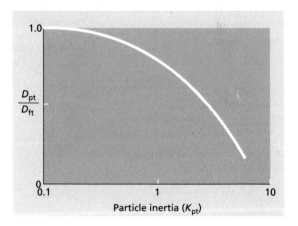

Fig. 6.15 Effect of particle inertia (represented by K_{pt}) on its ability to respond to the air motions in turbulent flow (as represented by D_{pt}/D_{ft}), showing that this ability falls as K_{pt} increases.

INTERACTIONS BETWEEN AEROSOLS AND ELECTROMAGNETIC RADIATION

Whereas most of the properties of aerosols outlined above can be directly linked, in one way or another, with health effects or environmental control, optical properties may appear to be somewhat peripheral. However, there are two aspects which are particularly relevant to occupational hygiene. The first concerns the visual appearance of a workplace aerosol. The fact that it is visible is usually an indication that worker exposure is high enough to demand attention. Furthermore, its visible intensity is a direct indication of the level of exposure. In addition, other qualitative features of the aerosol's appearance (e.g. colour) can provide some information about its physical nature. From such considerations, an occupational hygienist can learn a great deal from the visual appearance of a workplace aerosol. The second aspect is at the more quantitative level, where the optical properties of aerosols can form the basis of sophisticated aerosol instrumentation, for measuring not only aerosol concentration, but also particle size characteristics.

The physical basis of the optical properties of aerosols

The basic physical problem involved in the optical properties of aerosols concerns the interaction of electromagnetic radiation with individual suspended particles and with ensembles of such particles. If a particle has different dielectric properties to those of the surrounding medium, as reflected in their respective refractive indices, then it represents a dielectric inhomogeneity. As a result, interactions with incident light can be detected from outside. In general, the whole problem can be treated in terms of a plane electromagnetic wave incident on a particle whose geometric surface defines the boundaries of the inhomogeneity and whose dielectric properties are described by the refractive index for the particle medium. Mathematically, it is based on Maxwell's theory of electromagnetic radiation, the solutions of which explain the phenomena of reflection, diffraction, refraction and absorption. The first three of these constitute the phenomenon of light scattering. The latter concerns that part of the incident energy that goes into increasing the vibrational energy of the molecules in the ordered array inside the solid particle. Such absorbed energy appears in the form of heat, raising the temperature of the particle.

There is one further process that deserves mention: namely, the physical mechanism by which radiation incident at one wavelength can be scattered at another. This occurs by virtue of so-called 'inelastic' interactions involving the absorption and re-emission of radiation energy by the individual molecules of the particle. However, such interactions do not have much direct relevance to workplace aerosols. Therefore, attention here is focused on the simpler cases where the wavelengths of the incident and scattered radiation are the same. Such interactions are referred to as 'elastic'.

The first theory of light scattering was by Lord Rayleigh in the late 1800s, and applies to very small particles and molecules much smaller than the wavelength of the radiation λ. In effect, for visible light, this means particles with diameter less than about 0.05 μm. Under these conditions, the particles may be treated as 'point scatterers', and the resultant mathematical treatment is relatively simple. But the most significant advance, in terms of its relevance to aerosols, came in the early 1900s when G. Mie extended Rayleigh's theory to larger particles.

For a beam of light energy incident on a system of many suspended particles (e.g. an aerosol), the fraction of energy which interacts in the manner indicated is either scattered or absorbed. This energy is effectively removed, so that the beam itself may be regarded as having been attenuated or undergone extinction. The energy that remains in the beam is transmitted. From this picture, the interaction of light with an aerosol may be considered in one of two ways: either in terms of the extinction of the beam (or, conversely, its transmittance) or in terms of the scattered component.

The phenomenon of extinction is described by an important relationship: the Lambert—Beer law, which appears widely in science for describing the

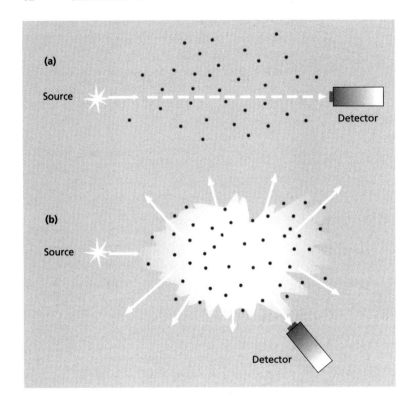

Fig. 6.16 Examples of practical scenarios involving the interaction of light with particles: (a) detection of transmitted light; (b) detection of scattered light.

effects of the interactions between energy (of all types) and matter. For the passage of light through an aerosol, it is written in the form:

$$\frac{I}{I_0} = \exp\left(-Q\,c\,t\right) \tag{6.42}$$

where I_0 and I are the light intensities before and after passing through the aerosol respectively, c is the aerosol concentration and t is the pathlength through the aerosol. The quantity Q is an extinction coefficient which embodies the physics of the interactions between the light and each individual particle.

Both light extinction and light scattering are relevant to occupational hygiene, in relation both to the visual appearance of aerosols and to aerosol monitoring instrumentation. Possible scenarios are summarized in Fig. 6.16.

INTERACTIONS BETWEEN GASES AND ELECTROMAGNETIC RADIATION

When electromagnetic radiation passes through a gaseous medium, energy may be removed from the beam if the wavelength of the radiation is such that energy can be absorbed by the gas molecules. Therefore, the phenomenon of extinction again applies, and the Lambert–Beer law re-appears, this time in the form:

$$\frac{I}{I_0} = \exp\left(-\,\alpha_\lambda\,c\,t\right) \tag{6.43}$$

where c is the concentration of the molecules with which the radiation is interacting, and I, I_0 and t are as defined before. In Equation 6.43, α_λ is an extinction coefficient embodying the physics of the interaction between the radiation and the gas through which it passes. It refers to the absorption spectrum of the gas and is strongly dependent on the wavelength (λ). In the ultraviolet region, from 0.25 to 0.40 µm, absorption takes place by electronic transitions in the gas molecules (e.g. excitation or ionization). In the visible region, from 0.40 to 0.70 µm, absorption is by vibrational–rotational excitation, although this is very weak in most gases and hence explains their invisibility to the human eye. The only common gas for which there is significant absorption in the visible region is nitrous oxide, which occurs as a visible brown gas. In the infrared region above 0.70 µm there are strong vibrational–rotational modes of excitation for most gases and vapours. This region is therefore particularly useful for application in detection systems for pollutant gases and is employed widely for instruments used in the occupational hygiene setting.

OVERVIEW

This chapter has given short outlines of various physical aspects of gases and aerosols relevant to the science and practice of occupational hygiene. These relate to the properties of airborne contaminant materials as they influence worker exposure: in particular their recognition, evaluation and control. This review underlines the point that occupational hygiene is first and foremost a scientific discipline. More in-depth background in any particular aspect described may be obtained by reference to the reading list given below and to the many other excellent sources now available.

FURTHER READING

Aerosol mechanics

Fuchs, N.A. (1964). *The Mechanics of Aerosols*. Pergamon Press, Oxford.
Hinds, W.C. (1982). *Aerosol Technology*. Wiley and Sons, New York.

Aerosol sampling

Vincent, J.H. (1989). *Aerosol Sampling: Science and Practice*. Wiley and Sons, Chichester.

Optical properties of aerosols

Hodkinson, J.R. (1966). The optical measurement of aerosols. In *Aerosol Science*, (ed. C.N. Davies), pp. 287–35. Academic Press, New York.

CHAPTER 7

The Sampling of Gases and Vapours: Principles and Methods*

R.H. Brown

INTRODUCTION

This chapter discusses the collection and analysis of gases and vapours found commonly in the industrial or workplace environment. It concentrates on descriptions of sampling methods for subsequent laboratory analysis and does not, therefore, include detailed discussions of direct-reading instruments, colorimetric indicators, tape samplers and other 'on-the-spot' testing devices. References to these are given at the end of the chapter.

THE NATURE OF INDUSTRIAL GASES AND VAPOURS

Materials hazardous to health may occur in the workplace atmosphere either as gases, vapours or aerosols. Gases are generally understood to be non-condensible at room temperature and vapours to be derived from volatile liquids. Therefore, under ordinary conditions, gases remain in the gaseous state even when present at high concentrations. Vapours, on the other hand, may condense at high concentrations and coexist in both gas and aerosol forms. However, unless an aerosol is deliberately produced, as in a spray operation, atmospheric concentrations of vapour pollutants rarely reach saturation conditions. Gases and vapours can therefore be considered similar and the same devices used to collect them. The sampling of aerosols is described in Chapter 8.

SAMPLING PROCEDURES

There are two basic methods for collecting gaseous samples. In one, called 'grab sampling', an actual sample of air is taken in a flask, bottle, bag or other suitable container. In the other, called 'continuous' or 'integrated sampling', gases or vapours are removed from the air and concentrated by passage through a solid or liquid sorbent medium.

Grab sampling usually involves the collection of instantaneous or short-term samples, usually within a few seconds or a few minutes, although similar methods can be used for sampling over longer periods. This type of sampling is acceptable when peak concentrations are sought, or when concentrations are relatively constant. This method is suitable for relatively inert gases, and vapours of liquids, but care should be taken in the choice of container to minimize adsorption on the container walls. The collection efficiency of grab sampling is normally 100%. However, sample decay may occur for various reasons, and collected samples are best analysed immediately.

Grab sampling is of questionable value when: (1) the contaminant or contaminant concentration varies with time; (2) the concentration of atmospheric contaminants is low; or (3) a time-weighted average exposure is required. In such circumstances, continuous or integrated sampling should be used. The gas or vapour in these cases is extracted from air and concentrated by: (1) solution in an absorbing liquid; (2) reaction with an absorbing solution (or reagent therein); or (3) collection onto a solid adsorbent. The collection efficiency of active sampling devices is frequently less than 100%;

therefore, individual efficiency percentages must be determined for each case. Later in this chapter another technique, 'diffusive' (or 'passive') sampling, is discussed.

SELECTION OF SAMPLING DEVICES

The first step in the selection of a sampling device and analytical procedure is to search the available literature. Primary sources are the compendia of methods recommended by the regulatory authorities, i.e. the UK Health and Safety Executive (HSE) or the US National Institute for Occupational Safety and Health (NIOSH) and the Occupational Safety and Health Administration (OSHA). Secondary sources are published literature references in, for example, *Annals of Occupational Hygiene*, *The American Industrial Hygiene Association Journal*, *Applied Occupational and Environmental Hygiene* or *Analytical Chemistry*, and books such as *The Intersociety Committee's Methods for Air Sampling and Analysis*.

If a published procedure is not available, one can be devised from theoretical considerations. However, its suitability must be established experimentally before application. Important criteria for selecting sampling devices are: solubility, volatility and reactivity of the contaminant; and the sensitivity of the analytical method.

Generally, non-reactive and non-adsorbing gaseous substances (i.e. substances which are chemically or electrically neutral, or of low polarity) may be collected as grab samples. Water-soluble gases and vapours, and those that react rapidly with absorbing solutions, can be collected in simple gas washing bottles. However, volatile and less soluble gaseous substances, and those that react slowly with absorbing solutions, require more liquid contact. For these substances, more elaborate sampling devices may be required, such as gas washing bottles of the spiral type or fritted bubblers. Insoluble and non-reactive gases and vapours are collected by adsorption onto activated charcoal, silica gel or other suitable adsorbent. Frequently, for a given contaminant, there will be a choice of sampling equipment.

Grab samplers

Evacuated flasks

These are containers of varying capacity and configurations. In each case, the internal pressure of the container is reduced. These containers are generally removed to a laboratory for analysis, although it is possible to achieve field readability if the proper equipment and direct-reading instrument are available. Some examples of evacuated flasks are heavy-walled containers, separation flasks and various commercial devices.

'Passivated' canisters

Stainless steel containers which have been specially treated to reduce adsorption effects have been used for collecting trace organic gases, especially the less reactive hydrocarbons and halocarbons. More recently, the Environmental Protection Agency (US-EPA) have used passivated canisters for ambient air analysis alongside adsorbent tubes.

Gas or liquid displacement containers

Any ordinary, sealable container can be used as a displacement sampler. Original air is replaced by test air by pumping or aspirating through the container with a double-acting rubber bulb aspirator or a battery or electrically operated vacuum pump. The volume of air swept out should be 10–15 times the container volume to achieve a sample collection efficiency of more than 99% (Fig. 7.1).

An alternative method for sampling with these containers is to fill them with water and allow the water to drain out slowly in the test area. The liquid becomes replaced by test air. Obviously, this procedure is not suitable for collecting water-soluble gases.

For soluble and reactive gases, an absorbent or reagent solution may be introduced into the gas displacement sampler. The usual procedure is to fill the sampler with test air and then add the absorbent. When dealing with partially or totally evacuated flasks, the reagent solution or absorbent is added before they are put under reduced pressure. In both cases, after the sample has been taken, the

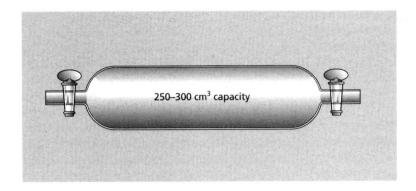

Fig. 7.1 Gas or liquid displacement type sampling bottle. Crown copyright. Reproduced with the permission of the Controller of Her Majesty's Stationery Office.

container is rotated to ensure an even distribution of the reagent on the inside surface of the sampler. This may take a few minutes or overnight, and so the equilibration time must be determined experimentally.

Flexible plastic containers

These bags are constructed from a number of plastic materials including polyester, polyvinylidene chloride, Teflon or other fluorocarbons. Plastic bags have the advantages of being light, non-breakable, inexpensive to ship and simple to use. However, they should be used with caution since storage stabilities for gases, memory effects from previous samples, permeability and precision and accuracy of sampling systems vary considerably.

Plastic bags should be tested before they are used. Some general recommendations are available in the published literature for the use of such bags for air sampling. A good review of specific applications up to 1967 is Schuette (1967). Posner and Woodfin (1986) made a useful systematic study of five bag types and six organic vapours. They concluded that Tedlar bags are best for short-term sampling while aluminized bags are better for long-term storage prior to analysis. Storage properties, decay curves and other factors will vary considerably from those reported for a given gas or vapour, since sampling conditions are rarely identical. Each bag, therefore, should be evaluated for the specific gas, or gas mixture, for which it will be used.

Continuous active samplers

Absorbers

The absorption theory of gases and vapours from air by solution, as developed by Elkins, Hobby and Fuller (1937) and verified by Gage (1960), assumes that gases and vapours behave like perfect gases and dissolve to give a perfect solution. The concentration of the vapour in solution is increased during air sampling until an equilibrium is established with the concentration of vapour in the air. Absorption is never complete, however, since the vapour pressure of the material is not reduced to zero but is only lowered by the solvent effect of the absorbing liquid. Some vapour will escape with continued sampling, but it is replaced. Continued sampling, however, will not increase the concentration of vapour in solution once equilibrium is established.

The efficiency of vapour collection depends on: (1) the volume of air sampled; (2) the volume of the absorbing liquid; and (3) the volatility of the contaminant being collected. Efficiency of collection, therefore, can be increased by: cooling the sampling solution (reducing the volatility of the contaminant); increasing the solution volume by adding two or more bubblers in series; or altering the design of the sampling device. Sampling rate and concentration of the vapour in air are not primary factors in determining collection efficiency.

Absorption of gases and vapours by chemical reaction depends on: the size of the air bubbles produced in the bubbler; the interaction of contaminant with reagent molecules; the rapidity of the reaction; and a sufficient excess of reagent solution. If the reaction is rapid and a sufficient excess of reagent is maintained in the liquid, complete retention of the contaminant is achieved regardless of the volume of air sampled. If the reaction is slow and the sampling rate is not low enough, collection efficiency will suffer.

A number of designs of bubblers and impingers are available: some are described in the Intersociety Committee book (Intersociety Committee, 1988). The function of different types is to provide sufficient contact between the contaminant in the air and the absorbing liquid, and although a sintered bubbler may have a higher collection efficiency than a bubbler, such devices tend to clog rapidly in field use. Both a midget Greenburg–Smith impinger (Fig. 7.2) and a 'Daco' non-spill impinger

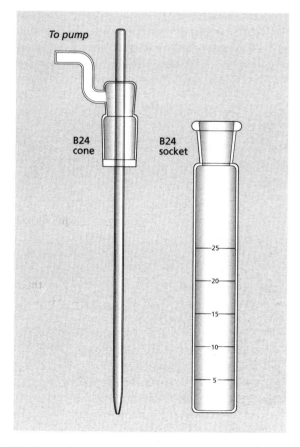

Fig. 7.2 Midget impinger. Crown copyright. Reproduced with the permission of the Controller of Her Majesty's Stationery Office.

have been found suitable for many applications. The flow rate to be used is a trade-off between being high enough to collect sufficient sample, and low enough to give good collection efficiency and minimize spray and evaporation losses.

Absorbers are suitable for collecting non-reactive gases and vapours that are highly soluble in the absorbing liquid, examples are: the absorption of methanol and butanol in water; esters in alcohol; and organic chlorides in butyl alcohol. They are also used for collecting gases and vapours that react rapidly with a reagent in the sampling media. For example, high collection efficiency is achieved when toluene diisocyanate is hydrolysed to toluene diamine in Marcali solution. Other examples include the reaction of hydrogen sulphide with cadmium sulphate, and ammonia neutralized by dilute sulphuric acid. Several methods for testing the efficiency of an absorbing device are available: (1) by series testing where enough samplers are arranged in series so that the last sampler does not recover any of the test gas or vapour; (2) by sampling from a dynamic standard atmosphere or from a gastight chamber or tank containing a known gas or vapour concentration; (3) by comparing results obtained with a device known to be accurate; and (4) by introducing a known amount of gas or vapour into a sampling train containing the absorber being tested.

Cold traps

Cold traps are used for collecting materials, in liquid or solid form, primarily for identification purposes. Vapour is separated from air by passing it through a coil immersed in a cooling system, i.e. dry ice and acetone, liquid air or liquid nitrogen. These devices are employed when it is difficult to collect samples efficiently by other techniques. Water is extracted along with organic materials, and two-phase systems result.

Plastic sampling bags

Plastic bags (as used for grab sampling) can also be used for collecting integrated air samples. Samples can be collected for 8 h, at specific times during the day, or over a period of several days. The bags may be mounted on workers as personal samplers or may be located in designated areas.

Solid adsorbents

Activated charcoal

Charcoal is an amorphous form of carbon formed by partially burning wood, nutshells, animal bones and other carbonaceous materials. A wide variety of charcoals are available; some are more suitable for liquid purification, some for decolorization and others for air purification and air sampling.

Ordinary charcoal becomes activated charcoal by heating it with steam to 800–900°C. During this treatment, a porous, submicroscopic internal structure is formed which gives it an extensive internal surface area (as large as 1000 m² per gram of charcoal) which greatly enhances its adsorption capacity.

Activated charcoal is an excellent adsorbent for most organic vapours. During the 1930s and 1940s, it was used in the then well-known activated charcoal apparatus for the collection and analysis of solvent vapour. The quantity of vapour in the air sample was determined by a gain in weight of the charcoal tube. However, its use was discouraged by the lack of specificity, accuracy and sensitivity of the analysis and the difficult task of equilibrating the charcoal tube.

Renewed interest in activated charcoal as an adsorbent for sampling organic vapours appeared in the 1960s. The ease with which carbon disulphide extracts organic vapours from activated charcoal, and the capability of microanalysis by gas chromatography, are the reasons for its current popularity. Today, air sampling procedures using activated charcoal are widely used by industrial hygienists and form the basis of the majority of the official analytical methods for organic materials recommended by the HSE, NIOSH or OSHA: i.e. the *Methods for the Determination of Hazardous Substances* series (MDHS) in the UK (Health and Safety Executive, 1981–94), or the *NIOSH Manual of Analytical Methods* (National Institute for Occupational Safety and Health, 1990) and the *OSHA Analytical Methods Manual* in the US (Occupational Safety and Health Administration, 1985).

Analytical information on selected charcoal procedures is provided in the MDHS series. A more extensive list can be compiled from NIOSH data and is given in Table 7.1. The NIOSH study showed that the charcoal tube method is generally adequate for hydrocarbons, chlorinated hydrocarbons, esters, ethers, alcohols, ketones and glycol ethers that are commonly used as industrial solvents. Compounds with low vapour pressure and reactive compounds (e.g. amines, phenols, nitrocompounds, aldehydes and anhydrides) generally have low desorption efficiencies from charcoal and require alternative sorbents such as silica gel, porous polymers or reagent systems for collection.

Inorganic compounds, such as ozone, nitrogen dioxide, chlorine, hydrogen sulphide and sulphur dioxide, react chemically with activated charcoal and cannot be collected for analysis by this method.

Even for substances recommended for sampling on charcoal, this sorbent may not always be ideal. Reference to Table 7.1 will indicate that carbon disulphide is the recommended desorption solvent for non-polar compounds, while a variety of desorption cocktails are required for the more polar compounds (e.g. alcohols, amines and nitrocompounds). Difficulties arise, therefore, when sampling mixtures of polar and non-polar compounds (e.g. mixtures of glycol ethers or of ketones) as each will give poor recoveries with the other's desorption solvent. As alternative, more universal solvents have not gained general recognition, it may be necessary to take two samples and desorb each one with a different solvent.

The volume of air that can be collected without loss of contaminant depends on the sampling rate, sample time, volatility of the contaminant and concentration of contaminant in the workroom air. For many organic vapours, a sample volume of 10 l (1.0 l min⁻¹) can be collected, without significant loss, in NIOSH-recommended tubes (Fig. 7.3). A breakthrough of more than 20% in the backup section indicates that some of the sample was lost. Optimum sample volumes are found in NIOSH procedures. The sample volume for gases and highly volatile solvents must necessarily be smaller. A 3% breakthrough was found to occur on NIOSH-recommended tubes at 0.2 l min⁻¹ for 15 min in an environment containing 5 ppm of vinyl chloride.

Table 7.1 Collection and analysis of gases and vapours (solvent desorption)

Method name	Test compounds	Sorbent*	Desorption solvent	NIOSH method no.
Alcohols I	t-Butyl alcohol Isopropyl alcohol Ethanol	C	99 : 1 CS_2 : 2-butanol	1400
Alcohols II	n-Butyl alcohol Isobutyl alcohol s-Butyl alcohol n-Propyl alcohol	C	99 : 1 CS_2 : 2-propanol	1401
Alcohols III	Allyl alcohol Isoamyl alcohol Methyl isobutyl carbinol Cyclohexanol Diacetone alcohol	C	99 : 5 CS_2 : 2-propanol	1402
Alcohols IV	2-Butoxyethanol 2-Ethoxyethanol 2-Methoxyethanol	C	95 : 5 CH_2Cl_2 : methanol	1403
Amines: aromatic	Aniline o-Toluidine 2,4-Xylidine N,N-Dimethyl-p-toluidine N,N-Dimethylaniline	S	95% ethanol	2002
Aminoethanol compounds	2-Aminoethanol 2-Dibutylaminoethanol 2-Diethylaminoethanol	S	80% ethanol	2007
Esters I	n-Amyl acetate n-Butyl acetate 2-Ethoxyethyl acetate Ethyl acrylate Methyl isoamyl acetate n-Propyl acetate, etc.	C	CS_2	1450
Hydrocarbons: BP 36−126°	Benzene, toluene Pentane through octane Cyclohexane Cyclohexene	C	CS_2	1500
Hydrocarbons: aromatic	Benzene Cumene Naphthalene, etc.	C	CS_2	1501
Hydrocarbons: halogenated	Chloroform Tetrachloroethylene p-Dichlorobenzene Bromoform, etc.	C	CS_2	1003
Ketones I	Acetone Cyclohexanone Diisobutyl ketone 2-Hexanone Methyl isobutyl ketone 2-Pentanone	C	CS_2	1300

Continued on p. 90

Table 7.1 (*continued*)

Method name	Test compounds	Sorbent*	Desorption solvent	NIOSH method no.
Ketones II	Camphor Ethyl butyl ketone Mesityl oxide 5-Methyl-3-heptanone Methyl *n*-amyl ketone	C	$99:1\ CS_2$: methanol	1301
Naphthas	Kerosene Petroleum ether Rubber solvent Stoddard solvent, etc.	C	CS_2	1550
Nitrobenzenes	Nitrobenzene Nitrotoluene 4-Chloronitrotoluene	S	Methanol	2005
Nitroglycerin and ethylene glycol dinitrate		T	Ethanol	2507
Pentachloroethane		R	Hexane	2517
Tetrabromoethane		S	Tetrahydrofuran	2003
Vinyl chloride		C	CS_2	1007

* C, charcoal; S, silica gel; T, Tenax; R, Porapak R.

Losses occurred before 5 l of the sample were collected in a 200 ppm vinyl chloride environment at a sampling rate of $0.05\,l\,min^{-1}$.

It is always best to refer to an established procedure for proper sampling rates and air sample volumes. In the absence of such information, breakthrough experiments must be performed before field sampling is attempted. The concentration of contaminant expected to be found in the field should be prepared in a sampling jar or fume chamber, and tests should be made on it. See MDHS 3 and 4 for the preparation of known concentrations.

Immediately before sampling, the ends of the charcoal tube are broken, rubber or Tygon tubing is connected to the backup end of the charcoal tube and air is drawn through the sampling train with a calibrated battery or electrically driven suction pump. A personal or area sample may be collected (see Chapter 17). The duration of the sampling may

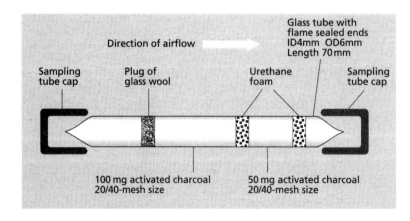

Fig. 7.3 Typical activated charcoal sampling tube. Dimensions in millimetres. Crown copyright. Reproduced with the permission of the Controller of Her Majesty's Stationery Office.

be several minutes or up to 8 h depending on the information desired. In all cases, airflow should be checked periodically with a flowmeter while the sampling is in progress. Afterwards, when sampling is completed, plastic caps or masking tape (but not rubber caps) are placed on the ends of the tube.

For each new batch of charcoal tubes, the analysis blank, the ageing, collection efficiency and recovery characteristics for a given contaminant must be determined. This may be achieved by introducing a known amount of the contaminant into a freshly opened charcoal tube, passing clean air through it to simulate sampling conditions and carrying through its analysis with the field samples. Another charcoal tube, not used to sample, is opened in the field and used as a field blank.

The first step in the analysis procedure is to remove the contaminant from the charcoal. The most frequently used liquid desorbant is carbon disulphide. Unfortunately, carbon disulphide does not always completely remove the sample from charcoal. Recovery varies for each contaminant and batch of charcoal used. The extent of individual recoveries must be determined experimentally and a correction for desorption efficiency applied to the analytical result. Over a narrow range of analyte concentrations, as used in the NIOSH validations, this desorption efficiency is essentially constant, but it may vary widely over larger concentration ranges, particularly for polar compounds. Desorption efficiency can also be affected by the presence of water vapour and of other contaminants. NIOSH recommends that methods should be used only where the desorption efficiency is greater than 75% and ideally it should be greater than 90%.

The practical desorption step in charcoal analysis is also critical since, upon the addition of carbon disulphide to charcoal, the initial heat of reaction may drive off the more volatile components of the sample. This can be minimized by adding charcoal slowly to pre-cooled carbon disulphide. Another technique is to transfer the charcoal sample to vials lined with Teflon septum caps and to introduce the carbon disulphide with an injection needle. The sealed vial will prevent the loss of any volatilized sample.

Several quality assurance schemes have been developed which apply to the charcoal tube method. One of these is the HSE Workplace Analysis Scheme for Proficiency (WASP). US schemes include the Proficiency Analytical Testing (PAT) Program and the Laboratory Accreditation Program of the American Industrial Hygiene Association (AIHA). Details of the WASP scheme may be obtained from the WASP Coordinator, Health and Safety Laboratory, Broad Lane, Sheffield, S3 7HQ, UK.

Silica gel

Silica gel is an amorphous form of silica, derived from the interaction of sodium silicate and sulphuric acid. It has several advantages over activated charcoal for sampling gases and vapours: (1) polar contaminants are more easily removed from the adsorbent by a variety of common solvents; (2) amines and some inorganic substances for which charcoal is unsuitable can be collected; and (3) the use of carbon disulphide is avoided.

One disadvantage of silica gel is that it will adsorb water. Silica gel is hydrophilic and polar substances are preferentially attracted to active sites on its surface. If enough moisture is present in the air, or if sampling is continued long enough, water will displace organic solvents, which are relatively non-polar in comparison, from the silica gel surface. With water vapour at the head of the list, compounds in descending order of polarizability are: alcohols; aldehydes; ketones; esters; aromatic hydrocarbons; alkenes; and paraffins.

Nevertheless, silica gel is an effective adsorbent for collecting many gases and vapours. Even under conditions of 90% humidity, relatively high concentrations of benzene, toluene and trichloroethylene are quantitatively adsorbed on 10 g of silica gel from air samples collected at the rate of $2.5 \, l \, min^{-1}$ for periods of at least 20 min or longer. Under normal conditions, hydrocarbon mixtures of two- to five-carbon paraffins, low molecular weight sulphur compounds (H_2S, SO_2, mercaptans) and alkenes concentrate on silica gel at dry ice−acetone temperature if the sample volume does not exceed 10 l. Significant losses of ethylene, methane, ethane and other light hydrocarbons occur if sampling volume is extended to 30 l.

More recent usage, however, has concentrated

on smaller tubes (in similar sizes to the NIOSH range of charcoal tubes) operated at room temperature. NIOSH recommends such tubes for a variety of more polar chemicals such as amines, phenols, amides and inorganic acids (see Table 7.1).

Much the same considerations apply to silica gel tubes as to the charcoal tubes. The sampling capacity and desorption efficiency for the compound of interest should be determined before use, or a reliable officially established method should be used. A variety of desorption solvents will be needed for desorbing specific compounds with high efficiency and polar desorption solvents, such as water or methanol, are commonly applied.

Thermal desorption

Because of the high toxicity and flammability of carbon disulphide, and the labour intensive nature of the solvent desorption procedure, a useful alternative is to desorb the collected analyte thermally. Except in a few cases, this is not practical with charcoal as adsorbent since the temperature needed for desorption (e.g. 300°C) would result in some decomposition of the analytes. Carbon molecular sieves or, more frequently, porous polymer adsorbents, in particular Tenax, Porapak Q and Chromosorb 106, are used instead. Thermal desorption has been adopted as a (non-exclusive) recommended method in the UK, Germany and the Netherlands, but it is less widely accepted in the USA.

The thermal desorption procedure typically uses larger tubes than the NIOSH method: usually 200–500 mg of sorbent are used, depending on type. Desorption can be made fully automatic, and analysis is usually carried out by gas chromatography. Some desorbers also allow automatic selection of sample tubes from a multiple-sample carousel. The whole sample can be transferred to the gas chromatograph, resulting in greatly increased sensitivity compared with the solvent desorption method. Alternatively, some desorbers allow the desorbed sample to be held in a reservoir from which aliquots are withdrawn for analysis, but then the concentrating advantage is reduced.

The main disadvantage of thermal desorption directly with an analyser is that it is essentially a 'one-shot' technique as, normally, the whole sample is analysed. This is why many such methods are linked to mass spectrometry. However, with capillary chromatography, it is usually possible to split the desorbed sample before analysis and, if desired, the vented split can be collected and re-analysed. Alternatively, the desorbate can be split between two capillary columns of differing polarity. Desorption efficiency is usually 100% for the majority of common solvents and similar compounds in a boiling range of approximately 50–250°C. Thus, the analysis of complex mixtures is easier than for charcoal or silica gel solvent desorption methods although, if a wide boiling range is to be covered, more than one sorbent may be required. For example, gasoline may be monitored by a Chromosorb 106 tube and carbon tube in series. Extensive lists of recommended sampling volumes and minimum desorption temperatures for Tenax and other sorbents are given in Brown and Purnell (1979) and the UK HSE method MDHS 72.

Relatively few quality assurance schemes have been developed which apply to the thermal desorption tube method. However, the HSE Workplace Analysis Scheme for Proficiency (WASP), noted above, includes tubes suitable for thermal desorption.

Coated sorbents

Many highly reactive compounds are unsuitable for sampling directly onto sorbents, either because they are unstable or cannot be recovered efficiently. In addition, some compounds may be analysed more easily, or with greater sensitivity, by derivatising them first. This can sometimes be achieved during the sampling stage. Methodologies have been developed, therefore, which use coated sorbents: either sorbent tubes or coated filters. Table 7.2 lists a number of such methods.

Wet chemistry and spectrophotometric methods

Several gases and vapours may be analysed by wet chemical methods or by ultraviolet spectrophotometry. There are two primary compendia of methods, issued by the Analytical Chemistry Committee of the AIHA (1965) and the Intersociety

Table 7.2 Collection and analysis of gases and vapours (coated sorbents)

Test compounds	Sorbent	Matrix*	Method no.
Acetaldehyde	2-(Hydroxymethyl)piperidine on Supelpak 20N	T	NIOSH 2538
Acrolein	2-(Hydroxymethyl)piperidine on Supelpak 20N	T	NIOSH 2501
Arsenic trioxide	Sodium carbonate	F	NIOSH 7901
Butylamine	Sulphuric acid	T	NIOSH S138
Diisocyanates	1-(2-Pyridyl)piperazine	F	OSHA 42
Formaldehyde	N-Benzylethanolamine on Supelpak 20F	T	NIOSH 2502
Isocyanate group	1-(2-Methoxyphenyl)piperazine	F	MDHS 25/2
Methylene dianiline	Sulphuric acid	F	NIOSH 5029

* T, sorbent tube; F, filter.

Committee (1988). Other useful sources are listed under Further Reading. Spectrophotometric methods have now been replaced largely by direct-reading instruments, detector tubes, high-performance liquid chromatography (HPLC) or other instrumental techniques.

CALCULATIONS

The collected sample is analysed, either directly if a gas phase or impinger sample or after desorption if collected on a solid sorbent, using appropriate gas or liquid standard solutions to calibrate the analytical instrument. Gas phase samples give a result directly in ppm (v/v), but other types of samples will give a mass of analyte per collected sample, or a concentration which can be converted to a mass by multiplying by the sample volume.

Mass concentration

The mass concentration of the analyte in the air sample is then calculated using the following equations.

1 Impinger:

$$C = \frac{m - m_{\text{blank}}}{\text{SE} \times V} \tag{7.1}$$

where C is the mass concentration of analyte in the air sample (mg m^{-3}), m is the mass of analyte in the sample (µg), m_{blank} is the mass of analyte in the blank (µg), SE is the sampling efficiency and V is the volume of air sampled (l).

2 Adsorbent tube:

$$C = \frac{m_1 + m_2 - m_{\text{blank}}}{\text{DE} \times V} \tag{7.2}$$

where m_1 is the mass of analyte on the first tube section (µg), m_2 is the mass of analyte on the backup tube section (if used) (µg) and DE is the desorption efficiency corresponding to m_1.

If it is desired to express concentrations reduced to specified conditions, e.g. 25°C and 101 kPa, then:

$$C_{\text{corr}} = C(101/P)(T/298) \tag{7.3}$$

where P is the actual pressure of air sampled (kPa) and T is the absolute temperature of air sampled (K).

Volume fraction

The volume fraction of the analyte in air, in ppm (v/v), is calculated by:

$$C' = C_{\text{corr}} (24.5/\text{mol.wt}) \tag{7.4}$$

where mol.wt is the molecular weight of the analyte of interest $(g\,mol^{-1})$.

DIFFUSIVE SAMPLERS

A diffusive sampler is a device which is capable of taking samples of gas or vapour pollutants from the atmosphere at a rate controlled by a physical process, such as diffusion through a static air layer or permeation through a membrane, but which does not involve the active movement of the air through the sampler. The adjective 'passive' is sometimes used to describe these samplers and should be regarded as synonymous with 'diffusive'.

This type of diffusive sampler should not be confused with the annular or aerosol denuders, which not only rely on diffusion to collect the gas or vapours, but also upon the air in question being simultaneously drawn through the annular inlet into the sampler. Aerosol particles have diffusion coefficients too low to be collected on the annular inlet and are trapped on a backup filter. Diffusive sampling in the occupational environment dates back at least to the 1930s when qualitative devices were described. The first serious attempt to apply science to quantitative diffusive sampling was in 1973 when Palmes described a tube-form sampler for sulphur dioxide. Since then, a wide variety of samplers have been described, some relying on diffusion through an air-gap, some relying on permeation through a membrane and some using both techniques, for the rate-controlling process in sampling. Many of these devices are commercially available.

The theoretical basis for diffusive sampling is now well established. Diffusion and permeation processes can both be described in derivations of Fick's first law of diffusion (see Equation 7.5). These result in expressions relating the mass uptake by the sampler to the concentration gradient, the duration of exposure and the sampler area exposed to the pollutant atmosphere. Expressions have also been derived for the application of Fick's law to diffusive sampling in the 'real' world, i.e. taking into account non steady-state sampling, the effects of fluctuating concentrations, sorbent saturation, wind velocity and turbulence at the sampler sur-

face, temperature, pressure, and so on. Except for sorbent saturation, which may lead to reduced (although sometimes predictable) uptake rates, these modifications to the basic Fick's law expression do not lead to significant errors for well-designed samplers. Such samplers may be regarded as truly integrating devices with accuracies similar to those of active samplers.

There are a variety of diffusive samplers, but only a selection of the major types manufactured can be described here. Diffusive equivalents to the more familiar pumped methods exist for nearly all types, the main exception being the direct collection of gas samples, where the nearest equivalent is an evacuated canister. Thus, the diffusive equivalent of an impinger is a liquid-filled badge such as the Pro-Tek™ inorganic monitor or the SKC badge; the diffusive equivalent of the charcoal tube is the charcoal badge such as the 3M OVM or the MSA VaporGard™ organic; and the diffusive equivalent of the thermal desorption method is the Perkin−Elmer tube or the SKC thermal desorption badge. There are also diffusive devices based on reagent impregnated solid supports. Two typical diffusive samplers are shown in Fig. 7.4.

In general, the regulatory authorities have been reluctant to accept diffusive monitoring methods, except in the UK and the Netherlands where several such methods have been adopted as non-exclusive recommended methods. However, the Luxembourg Symposium (Berlin, Brown and Saunders, 1987) came to the following conclusions.
1 The theoretical basis for diffusive sampling has been confirmed by laboratory and field trials.
2 Active and diffusive sampling are complementary approaches, having areas of applicability which may overlap. Each has its role in a strategy for monitoring worker exposure.
3 In general, there seems to be no significant difference between the accuracy and precision of diffusive sampling and those of other monitoring systems such as active pumped sampling.
4 It was agreed that, as a general principle, any method is acceptable by regulatory authorities and hygienists if used by experts within its defined limitations. This applies equally to diffusive samplers.

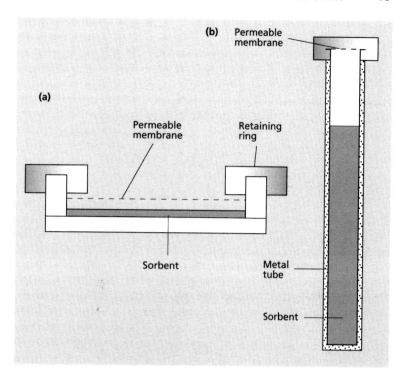

(a)

Permeable
membrane

Retaining
ring

Sorbent

(b) Permeable
membrane

Metal
tube

Sorbent

Fig. 7.4 Typical diffusive samplers:
(a) badge type sampler; (b) tube type
sampler. Crown copyright.
Reproduced with the permission of
the Controller of Her Majesty's
Stationery Office.

The symposium also concluded that validation of all sampling systems is essential both in the laboratory and in the field. It also recommended that an established evaluation protocol be followed such as the NIOSH (Kennedy *et al.*, 1987) or the Health and Safety Executive (1987) or that from Comité Européen de Normalisation (CEN) (1992).

Calibration

The basic expression of Fick's law is:

$$J = \frac{D\,(C_e - C_0)}{L} \quad (7.5)$$

and:

$$Q = \frac{(D\,A)\,t\,(C_e - C_0)}{L} \quad (7.6)$$

where J is the diffusive flux ($g\,cm^{-2}\,s^{-1}$), D is the coefficient of diffusion ($cm^2\,s^{-1}$), C_e is the external concentration being sampled ($g\,cm^{-3}$), C_0 is the concentration at the interface of the sorbent ($g\,cm^{-3}$), A is the cross-sectional area of the dif-

fusion path (cm^2), L is the length of the diffusion path (cm), Q is the mass uptake (g) and t is the sampling time (s).

It is apparent from inspection of these equations that the expression DA/L has units of $cm^3\,s^{-1}$ and therefore represents what can be considered as a 'sampling rate' of the diffusive sampler when compared to a pumped sampling system. This simple use of the sampling rate concept has been of considerable value to users of the devices and is often expressed in the dimensionally equivalent units of $ml\,min^{-1}$. Knowledge of the geometry of the sampler (which will be fixed for any given sampler type) permits the calculation of the sampling rate, provided the diffusion coefficient is known. A number of manufacturers have published tables of sampling rates calculated in this way, most of whom have used the same source of published diffusion coefficients. Diffusion coefficients that are not in this list can be calculated theoretically. Most manufacturers also publish lists of measured uptake rates, usually determined according to an established protocol, which are obviously more reliable than calculated values.

Environmental factors affecting monitor performance

Temperature and pressure

From Maxwell's equation, the diffusion coefficient (D) is a function of absolute temperature (T) and pressure (P):

$$D = f(T^{3/2}, P - 1) \qquad (7.7)$$

But from the general gas law:

$$PV = nRT \qquad (7.8)$$

and:

$$C = n/V = P/RT$$

where V is the volume, n is amount of gas (moles), R is the molar gas constant and C is the concentration.

Substituting Equations 7.7 and 7.8 in Equation 7.6, we get:

$$Q = f(P/T, \; T^{3/2}/P) = f(T)^{1/2} \qquad (7.9)$$

Thus Q, the mass uptake, is independent of pressure (P), but dependent on the square root of absolute temperature (T). In practice, the temperature dependence of the sampling rate of ambient temperature levels (about 0.2% per degree Celsius) may be ignored. However, temperature may affect the absorption or adsorption capacity of a sorbent adversely.

Humidity

High humidity can affect charcoal adsorption adversely, resulting in a reduction in saturation capacity for charcoal badges. If the sampler becomes saturated, C_0 in Equation 7.5 is no longer zero, and the sampling rate becomes non-linear. Porous polymers used for thermal desorption are relatively unaffected by humidity.

Transients

Simple derivations of Fick's law assume steady-state conditions, but in the practical use of such samplers, the ambient concentrations of pollutants are likely to vary widely. The question then arises whether a diffusive sampler will give a truly inte-grated response or will 'miss' short-lived transients before they have had a chance to diffuse into the sampler. This problem has been discussed theoreti-cally and practically. Generally, transients do not present a significant problem provided the total sampling time is well in excess of the time constant of the sampler, i.e. the time a molecule takes to diffuse into the sampler under steady-state con-ditions. The time constant of most commercial samplers is between 1 and 10 s.

Sorbent factors

All diffusive samplers rely on sorbents having a high affinity for the contaminant being sampled, i.e. C_0 equals zero in Equation 7.5, and uptake is linearly proportional to concentration and time of exposure. Useful checks on sorbent suitability are a back-diffusion test given in Bartley, Deye and Woebkenberg (1984) and the measurement of adsorption isotherms.

Face velocity

Diffusive samplers also rely on the external concen-tration, i.e. C_e in Equation 7.5, being maintained at the sampler surface. In the absence of sufficient air movement across the face of the sampler, transport of pollutant to the surface may itself be limited by diffusion, and the effective sampling rate will be reduced. At the other extreme, very high air velocities may induce turbulence within the sam-pler body if the draught shield is inadequate; the effective diffusion pathlength will be reduced and the sampling rate increased. The magnitude of these effects will vary with the geometry and design of particular samplers, although for the majority of modern samplers, sampling rates are reasonably constant within the range of air velocities likely to be encountered in workplace personal monitoring. Samplers with a large surface area ('badge' types) should not be used in 'static' positions where air velocities may be below their critical values for these types of samplers (about $0.2 \, \text{m s}^{-1}$).

Quality assurance

Relatively few quality assurance schemes have been developed which apply directly to diffusive methods. However, the NIOSH PAT (charcoal tube) and HSE WASP (thermal desorption tube) materials can be used instead; in the latter case, the same tube can be used in either pumped or diffusive mode, although the loadings may be different.

Calculations

The method of calculation of atmospheric concentrations is essentially the same as for pumped samplers, i.e. the collected sample is analysed and the total weight of analyte on the sampler determined. Then, as in Equation 7.2:

$$C = \frac{m_1 + m_2 - m_{\text{blank}}}{\text{DE} \times V}$$

(m_2 and DE are ignored for liquid sorbent badges). The total sample volume (V) is calculated from the effective sampling rate ($l\,min^{-1}$) and the time of exposure (min).

This calculation gives C in $mg\,m^{-3}$; strictly speaking, an appropriate sampling rate for the ambient temperature and pressure should be made as Equation 7.8 assumes C is in ppm. Alternatively, sampling rates can be expressed in units such as $ng\,ppm^{-1}\,min^{-1}$ (dimensionally equivalent to $cm^3\,min^{-1}$), when C' is calculated directly in ppm:

$$C' = \frac{m_1 + m_2 - m_{\text{blank}}}{(\text{DE} \times U \times t')} \times 100 \qquad (7.10)$$

where U is the sampling rate ($ng\,ppm^{-1}\,min^{-1}$) and t' is the sampling time (min). m_2 is relevant only to samplers with a backup section, and an additional multiplication factor may be needed to account for differing diffusion pathlengths to primary and backup sections.

Types of monitors

Diffusive samplers are available for both organic and inorganic species. Most organic monitors use activated charcoal as the collection medium. Both diffusion and permeation devices are available. As a general rule, organic badges can be used to monitor any compound that can be sampled by pumped charcoal tube methods. Each monitor has a unique design, so that sampling rates are not transferable from one type to another. The operational and other characteristics may also be different. Most

require gas chromatographic analysis for determination of the contaminant concentration.

Diffusion monitors for inorganic gases and vapours are more diverse in design and more chemi-specific than the more generally absorbing organic monitors. There are also many direct-reading, diffusive monitors for inorganic contaminants.

Accuracy of diffusive monitoring

The overall accuracy of diffusive monitors has been studied extensively. Most of the devices commercially available meet NIOSH, OSHA and CEN standards. NIOSH recommends that monitors produce results of ±25% for 95% of the samples tested in the range of 0.5–2.0 times the environmental standard. OSHA's accuracy requirement varies from ±25% to ±50%, depending on the concentration range. CEN's 'overall uncertainty' requirement varies from ±30% to ±50%, also depending on the concentration range.

Field and laboratory test results on several commercially available badges are found in the literature. Brown (1987), for example, examined the Perkin–Elmer tube for acrylonitrile, benzene, butadiene, carbon disulphide and styrene, and found the sampler to be at least as accurate as the equivalent pumped method. Laboratory precision was, on the average, 10% for the diffusive sampler. Field precision was 12% for the diffusive sampler and 13% for the pumped sampler. Kennedy, Cassinelli and Hull (1987) evaluated a range of inorganic samplers, including 3M, DuPont, MSA, REAL and SKC samplers, and found they generally met NIOSH criteria.

A European inter-laboratory comparison of the 3M badge exposed to butanol, pentanal, trichloroethane, octane, butyl acetate, 3-heptanone, xylene, α-pinene and decane generally displayed good agreement with the charcoal tube. Exceptions were butanol and pentanal, where the diffusive samplers read low. Again, excluding butanol and pentanal, overall laboratory precision varied between 9% (xylene) and 13% (heptanone). The contribution of inter-laboratory error was less than half of these values.

A study in which 78 pairs of side-by-side charcoal and 3M passive monitor samples were taken in the field and analysed for 22 organic chemicals indicated that the monitor assayed concentrations of 20 of these chemicals equally as well as charcoal tubes, on the basis of linear regression analysis.

Interpretation of results

The results of a measurement are only of value if they can be shown to be reliable and can be placed in context. Quality assurance schemes have been noted above, but Certified Reference Materials, internal quality assurance and external laboratory accreditation should also be taken into account. Measurements must also be interpreted in the context of a proper occupational hygiene assessment.

REFERENCES

Analytical Chemistry Committee (1965). *Analytical Abstracts.* American Industrial Hygiene Association, Akron, OH.

Bartley, D.L., Deye, G.J. and Woebkenberg, M.L. (1984). Diffusive Monitor Test: performance under transient conditions. *Applied Industrial Hygiene,* 2,(3), 119.

Berlin, A., Brown, R.H. and Saunders, K.J. (ed.) (1987). *Diffusive Sampling: an Alternative Approach to Workplace Air Monitoring.* CEC Pub. No. 10555EN. Commission of the European Communities, Brussels—Luxembourg.

Brown, R.H. (1987). Applications of the HSE diffusive sampler protocol. In *Diffusive Sampling: an Alternative Approach to Workplace Air Monitoring* (ed. A. Berlin, R.H. Brown and K.J. Saunders), pp. 189—95. CEC Pub. No. 10555EN. Commission of the European Communities, Brussels—Luxembourg.

Brown, R.H. and Purnell, C.J. (1979). Collection and analysis of trace organic vapour pollutants in ambient atmospheres. The performance of a Tenax-GC adsorbent tube. *Journal of Chromatography,* 178, 79—90.

Comité Européen de Normalisation (1992). *Workplace Atmospheres. Requirements and Test Methods for Diffusive Samplers for the Determination of Gases and Vapours.* PrEN 838.

Elkins, H.B., Hobby, A.K. and Fuller, J.E. (1937). The determination of atmospheric contamination; I: Organic halogen compounds. *Journal of Industrial Hygiene,* 19, 474—85.

Gage, J.C. (1960). The efficiency of absorbers in industrial hygiene air analysis. *Analyst,* 85, 196—203.

Health and Safety Executive (1981—94, in series). *Methods for the Determination of Hazardous Substances.* HSE Occupational Medicine and Hygiene Laboratory, Sheffield, UK.

Health and Safety Executive (1987). *Methods for the Determination of Hazardous Substances. Protocol for Assessing the Performance of a Diffusive Sampler.* MDHS 27. HSE Occupational Medicine and Hygiene Laboratory, Sheffield, UK.

Intersociety Committee (1988). *Methods of Air Sampling and Analysis,* (3rd edn). Lewis Publishers, Chelsea, MI.

Kennedy, E.R., Cassinelli, M.E. and Hull, R.D. (1987). Verification of passive monitor performance. Applications. In *Diffusive Sampling: an Alternative Approach to Workplace Air Monitoring,* (ed. A. Berlin, R.H. Brown and K.J. Saunders), pp. 203—8. CEC Pub. No. 10555EN. Commission of the European Communities, Brussels—Luxembourg.

Kennedy, E.R., Hull, R.D., Crable, J.V. and Teass, A.W. (1987). Protocol for the evaluation of passive monitors. In *Diffusive Sampling: an Alternative Approach to Workplace Air Monitoring,* (ed. A. Berlin, R.H. Brown and K.J. Saunders), pp. 190—202. CEC Pub. No. 10555EN. Commission of the European Communities, Brussels—Luxembourg.

National Institute for Occupational Safety and Health (1975). *NIOSH Manual of Analytical Methods,* (2nd edn). DHEW (NIOSH) Pub. No. 75—121.

National Institute for Occupational Safety and Health (1984). *NIOSH Manual of Analytical Methods,* (3rd edn). DHEW (NIOSH) Pub. No. 84—100.

Occupational Safety and Health Administration (1985). *OSHA Analytical Methods Manual.* OSHA Analytical Laboratories, Salt Lake City, UT.

Posner, J.C. and Woodfin, W.J. (1986). Sampling with gas bags; 1: Losses of analyte with time. *Applied Industrial Hygiene,* 1, 163—8.

Schuette, F.J. (1967). Plastic bags for collection of gas samples. *Atmospheric Environment,* 1, 515—19.

FURTHER READING

Arbetarskyddsverket (1987). Principer och methoder för provtagning och analys av ämnen upptagna på listan över hygieniska gränsvärden. Arbete och hälsa. *Vetenskaplig Skriftserie,* 1987, 17. Solna, Sweden.

Cohen, B.S. and Hering, S.V. (ed.) (1994). *American Conference of Governmental Industrial Hygienists: Air Sampling Instruments,* (8th edn). Chapters 18 (Detector tubes) and 19 (Direct reading instruments). ACGIH, Cincinnati, Ohio.

Deutsche Forschungsgemeinschaft (1985). *Analystische Methoden zur Prufung Gesundheitsschadlicher Arbeitsstoffe.* DFG. Verlag Chemie, Weinheim, FRG.

Nederlands Normalissatie-Instituut (1986—92, in series). *Methods in NVN Series (Luchtkwaliteit; Werkplekatmosfeer).* NNI, Delft, The Netherlands.

US Environmental Protection Agency (1984). *EPA Compendium of Methods for the Determination of Toxic Organic Compounds in Ambient Air.* EPA, Washington, DC.

The Sampling of Aerosols: Principles and Methods

D. Mark

INTRODUCTION

The term 'aerosol' is defined as a disperse system of solid or liquid particles suspended in a gas, most commonly air. In the workplace it applies to a wide range of particle clouds including: compact mineral and metallic particles produced in the process and manufacturing industries; agglomerated particles found in fumes during welding, metal smelting, etc.; fibrous particles such as asbestos and man-made-mineral fibres produced for insulation purposes; droplets from electroplating processes and cutting oils; and a number of bioaerosols produced in the agricultural, food and biotechnology industries.

Generally, as explained in Chapter 6, the aerodynamic behaviour of all aerosol particles is controlled by the same physical processes. It is the aerodynamic behaviour that governs whether the aerosol particle remains airborne, how far it travels from the source of production, whether it is captured by aerosol control systems and whether it reaches the human body. In the field of occupational hygiene, we are interested in controlling the levels of aerosol in the workplace air and thereby minimizing the risk to workers from adverse health effects due to exposure to the aerosol particles.

There are three main routes by which aerosol particles can reach the body and have the potential to cause harm. They are inhalation, skin deposition and the food chain. In the occupational field, exposure from particles depositing on food or drink is very rare, as meals are normally taken in specially provided areas away from the workplace. Skin

deposition is known to be a significant route of exposure for droplet aerosols and some metallic particles, but the most important route of exposure for aerosols is generally considered to be by inhalation.

This chapter concentrates on the sampling of aerosols for estimating the risk from inhalation. It starts by providing a scientific framework for the health-related sampling of aerosols by describing the sampling criteria and considering the sampling strategy to be employed. It then moves on to outline the basics of an aerosol sampling system and describes briefly the many systems that can be employed for the tasks specified. Sections describing procedures and errors involved in taking an aerosol sample follow, with special problems dealt with separately. With the current high international activity on standards for aerosol sampling (in Europe and the USA), and improvements in detector technology, it must be emphasized that this chapter describes the current state of affairs. A final section is included, therefore, that deals with future developments and how they may affect the occupational hygienist measuring aerosol concentrations in the workplace.

HEALTH-RELATED AEROSOL SAMPLING CRITERIA

It has long been realized that different aerosol-related health effects may be linked to different sizes of aerosol. Until recently, two sizes were considered to be important for health effects. Coarse particles, which could be deposited in the upper regions of the respiratory tract, were thought to be associated with toxic effects, whilst the finer particles, which could penetrate into the gas exchange region of the lung, were implicated as the cause of pneumoconioses, such as that found in coalminers.

The sampling of coarse particles for health-related purposes was based, in the past, on the use of samplers for so-called 'total' aerosol. Whilst the implicit assumption in their use was that they collected a sample of all sizes of airborne particles with 100% efficiency, in practice, early samplers were not designed with regard to their sampling efficiencies and measurements of 'total' aerosol would have varied greatly, dependent upon the instrument used. More recently, a form of standardization based on a physical rationale has been achieved by specifying a fixed mean air velocity entering the sampler of $1.25\,\mathrm{m\,s^{-1}}$.

The sampling of fine aerosols has historically borne more relevance to those particles that are thought to be responsible for disease in the deep lung, such as pneumoconiosis. In the late 1950s and 1960s a number of definitions were proposed for the so-called *respirable* fraction, representing particles that penetrated to the gas exchange region of the lung. Shown in Fig. 8.1, they were the British Medical Research Council (BMRC) curve (Orenstein, 1960), the US Atomic Energy Commission (AEC) curve (Lippmann and Harris, 1962) and the American Conference of Governmental Industrial Hygienists (ACGIH) curve (American Conference

of Governmental Industrial Hygienists, 1968). They were pragmatic curves, because not only did they fit the available deposition data reasonably well, but they were also matched by suitable samplers. However, they were different and therefore measurements made according to one criterion could not necessarily be compared with those made by the other.

Over the last 10 to 15 years, considerable progress has been made on the provision of internationally acceptable definitions for health-related aerosol fractions in workplace atmospheres. Collaboration between members of committees of the International Organization for Standardization (ISO), the Comité Européen de Normalisation (CEN) and the ACGIH has produced a set of agreed definitions for health-related aerosol fractions in both workplace and ambient atmospheres. The workplace set has been published by CEN as EN 481 (Comité Européen de Normalisation, 1993a) and is currently available from the British Standards Institution as BS 6069, EN 481. It is expected to be officially published in the USA by the end of 1994. The three main fractions are provided for occupational hygiene use: inhalable, thoracic and respirable, and they are shown in Fig. 8.2.

The inhalable fraction (E_I) is defined as the mass fraction of total airborne particles which is inhaled through the nose and/or mouth. It was derived from wind tunnel measurements of the sampling efficiency of full-size tailor's mannequins and replaces the very-loosely defined 'total' aerosol fraction used previously. For industrial workplaces it is given by:

$$E_\mathrm{I} = 50\,[1 + \exp\,(-0.06D)] \qquad (8.1)$$

where D is the particle aerodynamic diameter.

The thoracic fraction (E_T) is defined as the mass fraction of inhaled particles penetrating the respiratory system beyond the larynx. It is given by a cumulative log-normal curve, with a median aerodynamic diameter of $11.64\,\mu\mathrm{m}$ and geometric standard deviation of 1.5.

The respirable fraction (E_R) is defined as the mass fraction of inhaled particles which penetrates to the unciliated airways of the lung (the alveolar region). It is given by a cumulative log-normal curve with a median aerodynamic diameter of

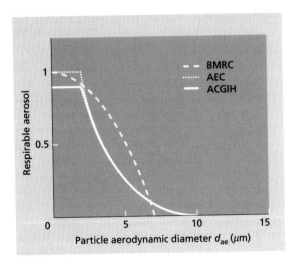

Fig. 8.1 Some historically important definitions for respirable aerosol.

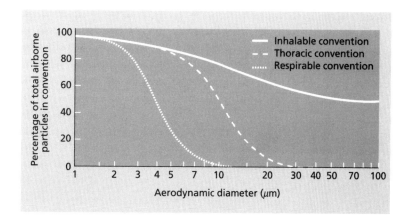

Fig. 8.2 ISO/CEN/ACGIH sampling conventions for health-related aerosols.

4.25 μm and a geometric standard deviation of 1.5.

These sampling conventions comprise the target specifications for the design of sampling instruments for the health-related sampling of aerosols in the workplace. However, these conventions cannot be consistently applied without an agreed testing protocol. This is the subject of continuing work by the CEN/TC137/WG3, who were instrumental in producing the CEN sampling conventions. A draft pre-standard has been produced (Comité Européen de Normalisation, 1993b) which is currently (1994) undergoing evaluation in a pilot study on the performance of personal inhalable aerosol samplers. It is expected that the full standard will be published in 1996. In the protocol, assessment of the suitability of samplers is based upon the overall inaccuracy (bias and precision) by which the sampler measures the mass of a chosen aerosol fraction from a wide range of occupationally-occurring size distributions. Early indications show that some of the currently-used sampling instrumentation may be able to meet the requirements of the new conventions and the test protocol.

The agreements reached in these new conventions have given renewed impetus to the move towards a new set of standards based on the three fractions (inhalable, thoracic and respirable) replacing the old 'total' and respirable aerosol combination. To see which aerosol types fall into which categories, it is necessary to reconsider the types of health effects associated with the deposition of particles of various types at the various parts of the respiratory tract. For example, the deposition of some biologically-active particles (e.g. bacteria, fungi, allergens) in the extrathoracic airways of the head may lead to inflammation of sensitive membranes in that region, such as symptoms of 'hay fever' (e.g. rhinitis). Other types of particle (e.g. nickel, radioactive material, wood dust) depositing in the same region may lead to more serious local conditions, such as ulceration or nasal cancer. For the health-related measurement of all such aerosols, it is appropriate to sample according to a criterion based on the inhalable fraction.

The next class of aerosols comprises particles which may provoke local responses in the tracheo-bronchial region of the lung, leading to such effects as bronchoconstriction, chronic bronchitis, bronchial carcinoma, etc. For the health-related measurement of all such aerosols, it is appropriate to sample the thoracic fraction.

The third class of aerosols contains particles which deposit in the alveolar region, leading to pneumoconiosis, emphysema, alveolitis and pulmonary carcinoma, etc. It also contains asbestos fibres, which may cause mesothelioma in the nearby pleural cavity. In relation to these, respirable aerosol continues to provide the most appropriate sampling criterion.

Finally, as a general rule, for aerosol substances that are soluble and are known to be associated with systemic effects (where toxic material can enter the blood after deposition in any part of the respiratory tract and be transported to other organs), standards should be specified in terms of the inhalable fraction.

Fibrous aerosols

Fibrous aerosol particles — those with long aspect ratio such as asbestos and man-made mineral fibres — have, historically, been considered separately by the scientific community. The definition of what is 'respirable' for such particles is based not only on the aerodynamic factors that govern the deposition of fibres in the lung after inhalation, but also on their known dimension-associated health risks. For example, in the case of asbestos, long, thin fibres are thought to be more hazardous to health than short, fat ones. This is because they are capable of penetrating deep into the alveolar region of the lung, and the normal lung defence mechanisms are less able to eliminate long particles than isometric ones of similar aerodynamic diameter. Selection of the respirable fraction of the airborne fibres is therefore carried out, after they have been collected on filters, by sizing and counting under the microscope. Unlike for isometric particles, it is the number, not the mass, of particles that is measured.

The internationally agreed criteria for respirable asbestos fibres is that they should have an aspect ratio of $3:1$, length $>5\,\mu m$ and diameter $<3\,\mu m$. This was agreed in 1979 by the Asbestos International Association (AIA, 1979) and is still widely used today. Both sampling and microscopy procedures are prescribed in this document, many versions of which have been proposed in different countries. Whilst this prescriptive approach should lead to consistency in fibre measurements, it is not consistent with the more general conventions described above which specify instrument performance and not particular instrument designs.

Biological aerosols

There are currently no internationally agreed definitions for the sampling of biological aerosols (bioaerosols), and work is in progress in a number of countries to resolve the situation. However, although not explicitly stated in the document EN 481 (Comité Européen de Normalisation, 1993a), bioaerosols that are harmful to the various regions of the body should be sampled using instruments that select particles according to the health-related sampling conventions described in EN 481.

The additional problems posed by bioaerosols are that some of the particles only cause problems to the human body when alive. These particles (bacteria, viruses, moulds, etc.) are detected by culturing them on media such as agar, and so they must be kept alive and unharmed during the sampling process. For these particles it is the number rather than the mass concentration that is determined. This area is changing rapidly and it is hoped that agreed conventions and methodology will be available soon. The samplers currently available will be described later in this chapter.

SAMPLING STRATEGY

A detailed discussion of sampling strategy is given in Chapter 17. Nevertheless, it is an essential part of the sampling process and therefore will be briefly discussed here.

The most important question to ask before setting out to develop a sampling strategy is 'Is it necessary to sample?'. In the UK, the Control of Substances Hazardous to Health (COSHH) Regulations state clearly that an assessment of the likely risk to health at the workplace should be carried out first. Only if the estimated risk may be significant is it recommended that a sampling programme be instigated. There are then a whole number of questions (outlined in Chapter 17) that need to be answered before a reliable sampling strategy can be achieved.

If sampling is to be carried out to assess the true exposures of individual workers (or of groups of workers), one of the most important questions is whether a personal or static sampling strategy should be used (or a combination of both). In static (or area) measurements, the chosen instrument is located in the workplace atmosphere, and provides a measurement of aerosol concentration which is (hopefully) relevant to the workforce as a whole. For the case of personal measurements, the chosen instrument is mounted on the body of the exposed subject and moves around with him (or her) at all times.

When choosing one or other of these, some important considerations need to be taken into account. For a few workplaces (e.g. some working groups in longwall mining), it has been shown that reasonably good comparison may be obtained using suitably placed static instruments and personal samplers. More generally, however, static samplers have been found to perform less well, tending to give aerosol concentrations which are consistently low compared to those obtained using personal samplers. One advantage with static samplers is that a relatively small number of instruments may be used to survey a whole workforce. If this can be shown to provide valid and representative results, it is a simple and cost-effective alternative. Furthermore, the high flow rates that are available for static samplers mean that, even at very low aerosol concentrations, a relatively large sample mass can be collected in a short sampling period. The use of personal samplers is more labour intensive. More instruments are deployed and this leads to greater effort in setting them up and in recovering and analysing the samples afterwards. By definition, personal sampling involves the direct co-operation of the workers themselves. Also, for such samplers, it is inevitable that the capacities of the pumps used will be limited by their portability. So flow rates will usually be low (rarely $> 4\,l\,min^{-1}$). However, personal aerosol sampling is the only reliable means of assessing the true aerosol exposures of individual workers, so that it is by far the most common method of aerosol measurement in workplaces.

A combination of both static and personal measurements should provide the most cost-effective and comprehensive sampling strategy. Personal samplers can be used to provide the detailed individual exposure information for regulatory purposes, for example, on one shift every month, whilst coverage of the other shifts may be achieved by using a strategically placed static monitor providing continuous assessment. Provided that the work process is relatively stable, an alarm monitor may be employed, set to trigger when the level is reached at which personal exposure is expected to exceed the occupational exposure limit. This system would require calibration with personal sampling to set the appropriate trigger level.

THE BASICS OF AN AEROSOL SAMPLING SYSTEM

An aerosol sampling instrument (or sampler) always comprises a number of components which contrib-

ute to the overall accuracy with which a sample is taken. These components are: the sampling head; the transmission section; the particle size selector (which is not always present); the collecting or sensing medium; calibrated flow monitoring and control; and the pump. A simple schematic diagram of these essential components is given in Fig. 8.3.

The sampling head

Many occupational hygienists have, in the past, overlooked the choice of sampling head. Instead they have concentrated on the performance of the pump, the choice of filter and the analytical technique to be employed, and have used any filter holder of suitable size, without knowing its particle sampling efficiency. This approach may lead to large errors in the mass concentration measured. For example, currently there is a wide range of different personal sampling heads used for the measurement of so-called 'total aerosol'. Recent

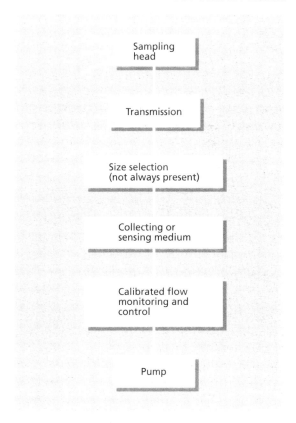

Fig. 8.3 The basic components of an aerosol sampling system.

wind tunnel tests (Vincent and Mark, 1990) have shown that these samplers exhibit widely differing sampling efficiencies under typical workplace conditions and therefore would not be expected to give the same mass concentration values. However, this situation will soon be improved because, with the recent approval of the new inhalable aerosol convention described above, instrument manufacturers will, and users must, demonstrate that their equipment meets the new convention if the result is to be used for regulatory purposes. Work is currently underway within Europe and the USA to provide a test protocol to demonstrate compliance of samplers to the new conventions.

For the thoracic and the respirable fractions, the performance of the sampler entry, although not as important as for the inhalable fraction, should nevertheless be taken into account. The most suitable approach for a sampler for the thoracic or respirable fraction (and one that mimics the way that particles from the ambient arrive at their site of deposition) is to use an inhalable aerosol entry followed by a suitable size selector. Suitable entries are available for both personal and static samplers.

The transmission section

This concerns the transport of particles that have entered the sampler entry, to the collecting or sensing region. Particle inertia and sedimentation forces can result in considerable deposition onto the internal walls of the transmission section, especially when the sampling head is remote from the sensing region and particles are conducted down narrow pipework and bends. This results in a loss of particles reaching the sensing region and is dependent on both the aerodynamic diameter of the particles and their composition. Droplets and soft, sticky particles will stick to the walls once deposited, whilst hard, granular particles may bounce off the walls and become re-entrained into the airflow. Electrostatic forces may also be important when the particles are highly charged and the sampler is made from non-conducting material. In addition, therefore, the humidity of the sampled air may play a role in both increasing the conductivity of the surface and reducing particle bounce.

For personal samplers, these wall losses can

introduce a significant error into the measurement. Losses of up to 100% have been reported for some non-conducting 'total' aerosol samplers, and these losses cannot be easily accounted for as they depend upon the roughness of handling of the particle-laden sampling head. For static samplers similar problems occur, and are especially evident in continuous particle counters and particle size analysers.

Size selectors

For the thoracic and respirable fractions, some form of particle size selector is used to select the relevant portion of the sampled aerosol. Particles are generally selected by aerodynamic means using physical processes similar to those involved in the deposition of particles in the respiratory system. Gravitational sedimentation processes are used to select particles in horizontal and vertical elutriators; centrifugal sedimentation is used in cyclones; inertial forces are used in impactors; whilst porous foams employ a combination of both sedimentation and inertial forces.

Owing to their size, and the requirement to be accurately horizontal or vertical for correct operation, elutriators are only used in static samplers. Cyclones, impactors and foams, however, can be used in either personal or static samplers.

Filters

A filter is the most common means of collecting the aerosol sample in a form suitable for assessment. Assessment might include gravimetric weighing on an analytical balance before and after sampling to obtain the sampled mass. It might also include visual assessment using an optical or electron microscope, and/or a range of analytical and chemical techniques.

The choice of filter type for a given application greatly depends on how it is proposed to analyse the collected sample. Many different filter materials are now available, with markedly different physical and chemical properties. These include fibrous (e.g. glass), membrane (e.g. cellulose nitrate) and sintered (e.g. silver) filters. Membrane filters have the advantage that they can retain particles effectively on their surface (which is good for microscopy), whereas fibrous filters have the advantage of providing in-depth particle collection, and hence a high load-carrying capacity (which is good for gravimetric assessment).

Filters are available in a range of dimensions (e.g. 25–100 mm diameter) and pore sizes (e.g. 0.1–10 μm). Collection efficiency is usually close to 100% for particles in most size ranges of interest. However, sometimes reduction in efficiency might be traded against the lower pressure drop requirements of a filter with greater pore size. For some types of filter, electrostatic charge can present aerosol collection and handling problems – in which case, the use of a static eliminator may (but not always) provide a solution. For other types, weight variations due to moisture absorption can cause difficulty, especially when being used for the gravimetric assessment of low masses. It is therefore recommended that the stabilization of filters overnight in the laboratory be carried out before each weighing, together with the use of blank 'control' filters to establish the level of variability. It is preferable that temperature and humidity be controlled in the balance room, especially when collected particle weights are low.

The chemical requirements of filters depend on the nature of the analysis which is proposed. As already mentioned, weight stability is important for gravimetric assessment. If particle counting by optical microscopy is required, then the filters used must be capable of being rendered transparent (i.e. cleared). Direct on-filter measurements of mineralogical composition (e.g. by infrared spectrophotometry, X-ray diffraction, scanning electron microscope and energy-dispersive X-ray analyses, X-ray fluorescence, etc.) are often required. For these, filters must allow good transmission of the radiation used, with low background scatter. Collected samples may also be extracted from the filter prior to analysis, using a range of wet chemical methods, ultrasonication, ashing, etc., each of which imposes a range of specific filter requirements.

Pumps

Most samplers require a source of air movement so that particulate-laden air can be aspirated into the instrument. For personal and static (or area) sampling, the main difference in terms of pump requirements is the flow rate, which tends to be low for personal sampling (usually from 1 to $4 \, l \, min^{-1}$), and larger (up to $100 \, l \, min^{-1}$ and even higher) for static sampling. The main limiting factor for a personal sampling pump is its weight, since it must be light enough to be worn on the body (usually on a belt) without inconvenience to the wearer.

A wide range of lightweight, battery-powered pumps is available for personal sampling (and also static sampling, if desired). These instruments are based on diaphragm, piston and rotary pumping principles. Those in practical use are equipped with damping devices to reduce the effects of flow pulsations. The actual volumetric flow rate will depend first on sampling considerations (e.g. entry conditions to provide the desired performance), and then the amount of material to be collected for accurate assessment, analytical requirements, etc. Internal flowmeters, usually of the rotameter type or digital counters, are incorporated into most pumps, but these must always be calibrated against a primary flow rate standard (e.g. a spirometer). It should also be noted that the flow rate may vary with the resistance imposed by the filter and its collected aerosol mass. For this reason, flow rates should be checked periodically during sampling and adjusted if necessary. However, flow-controlled pumps are now available which eliminate the need for such regular attention during sampling. Finally, for sampling in potentially explosive atmospheres (e.g. coalmines, chemical plants), intrinsically safe or flame-proof pumps should be used. Performance requirements for personal sampling pumps are specified in a new draft European Prestandard (prEN 1232) (Comité Européen de Normalisation, 1993c).

PRACTICAL SAMPLERS FOR COARSE AEROSOL

Static (or area) samplers

Over many years, static samplers have been developed for the sampling of coarse aerosol in workplace atmospheres. The simplest are open-filter arrangements mounted on the box which contains the

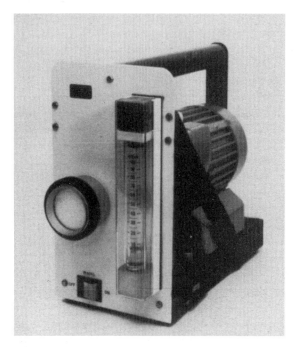

Fig. 8.4 Typical pump-mounted static sampler for coarse aerosols. Photograph courtesy of Bird & Tole Ltd., High Wycombe, UK.

inside the head. This capsule also houses the filter, and the whole capsule assembly (tare weight of the order of a few grams) is weighed before and after sampling to provide the full mass of aspirated aerosol. This system eliminates the possibility of errors associated with internal wall losses. When the capsule is mounted in the sampling head, the entry itself projects about 2 mm out from the surface of the head, creating a 'lip' around the orifice itself. This has the effect of preventing the secondary aspiration of any aerosol particles which strike the outside surface of the head and fail to be retained. The performance of this sampler, shown in Fig. 8.5(b), is in good agreement with the inhalability curve for particles with aerodynamic diameter up to about 100 μm. At present this is the only static sampler designed specifically for the inhalable fraction which is available commercially.

Personal samplers

For reasons outlined above, personal sampling is generally the preferred approach for workplace aerosols. Here, a large number of different devices have been used for coarse aerosol, again historically originating for the purpose of sampling for 'total' aerosol. The simplest is the open-filter arrangement, the one shown in Fig. 8.6 being the 25 mm open-filter. Other personal samplers for total aerosol that are at present widely used by occupational hygienists in Britain are the single (4 mm) hole sampler recommended by the Health and Safety Executive (HSE) for lead aerosol and the modified seven-hole version recommended for general coarse aerosol sampling (Health and Safety Executive, 1989). These too are shown in Fig. 8.6. Both of these closed-face samplers also employ 25 mm filters, and all three samplers are intended for use at the sampling flow rate of $2 \, l \, min^{-1}$.

pump (Fig. 8.4), or systems in which the same open-filter holder is mounted independently. The sampler shown is widely used in a number of industries in Britain (e.g. nuclear and cotton). Similar devices have been used elsewhere, both in workplace and in ambient air sampling. However, their sampling performances have very rarely been tested, and the few experiments that have been carried out reveal that none of the samplers come close to matching the inhalability criterion.

In the light of such data, new generations of aerosol sampler are beginning to emerge, this time designed from the outset to match the inhalability criterion. One designed for use in workplaces is the $3 \, l \, min^{-1}$ Institute of Occupational Medicine (IOM) static inhalable aerosol sampler (Mark et al., 1985), shown in Fig. 8.5(a). It incorporates a number of novel features. The sampler contains a single sampling orifice located in a head which is mounted on top of the housing containing the pump, drive and battery pack and rotates slowly about a vertical axis. The entry orifice forms an integral part of an aerosol collecting capsule which is located mainly

Experiments have been conducted to compare the peformances of these samplers with the inhalability curve (Mark and Vincent, 1986). It is particularly important to note here, that as well as for the other personal samplers discussed below, only data obtained with each sampler tested whilst mounted on a life-sized torso (e.g. of a mannequin) are considered useful in this context. It should not be assumed that, if such samplers were tested

(a)

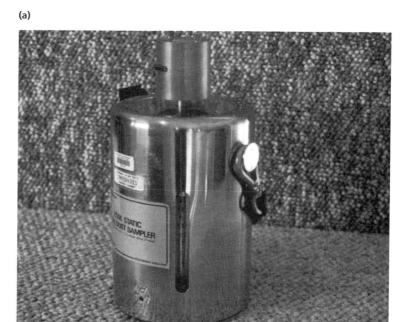

(b)

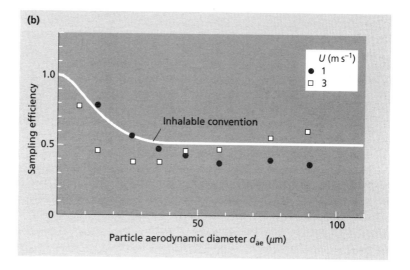

Fig. 8.5 IOM static inhalable aerosol sampler (from Mark *et al.,* 1985): (a) instrument shown complete; (b) performance of IOM static inhalable aerosol sampler.

independently, they would necessarily provide the same results, because the aerodynamic conditions governing the airflow around the sampler would be quite different. It follows, therefore, that devices designed as personal samplers should not be used in the static mode. Unfortunately, this common-sense guideline is widely ignored.

The results for the three samplers in Fig. 8.7 indicate that they all match the inhalability criterion quite well for particles with particle aerodynamic diameter up to about 15 μm, and for windspeeds of 1 m s^{-1} and below. But for conditions outside these ranges, yet typical of those found in many work-places (especially outdoor workplaces), the perform-ances are less satisfactory, with strong windspeed dependency (especially for the single-hole and seven-hole samplers) and with a tendency towards under-sampling. Interestingly, it was found that

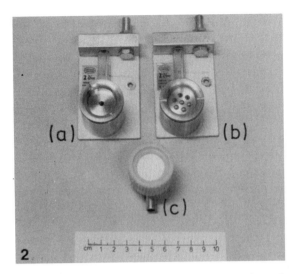

Fig. 8.6 Three personal samplers for coarse aerosols used in the UK: (a) single-hole sampler (Health and Safety Executive, 1981); (b) seven-hole sampler (Health and Safety Executive, 1989); (c) open-faced filter holder. From Mark and Vincent (1986).

the performances of these, and other personal samplers, are not strongly dependent on where the device is mounted on the torso.

The physical design features of these three samplers are, in one way or another, representative of those exhibited by most of the many other samplers which have been designed and used over the years in many countries. One is the 37 mm plastic cassette which is employed widely — either open-faced or closed-faced — by occupational hygienists in the USA (Fig. 8.8). Test results for this sampler are limited in number and range of particle sizes covered, but are sufficient to show that this sampler too provides an inadequate measure of the inhalable fraction (except, for fine particles), again tending to under-sample with respect to the inhalable fraction.

In the light of the generally poor performances of many existing 'total' aerosol samplers with respect to the inhalability criterion, a new personal sampler has been proposed. This is the $2 l\,min^{-1}$ IOM personal inhalable aerosol sampler (Mark and Vincent, 1986) shown in Fig. 8.9(a). It features a 15 mm diameter circular entry which faces directly outwards when the sampler is worn on the torso. Like the IOM static inhalable aerosol sampler in Fig. 8.5,

the entry is incorporated into an aerosol-collecting capsule which, during sampling, is located behind the face-plate. Use of this capsule ensures that the overall aspirated aerosol is always assessed. In addition, as for the static sampler, the lips of the entry protrude outwards slightly from the face-plate in order to prevent over-sampling associated with particle blow-off from the external sampler surfaces. Experimental data for this instrument are shown in Fig. 8.9(b), and show a good match with the inhalability curve. Once again, this instrument is the only one presently available commercially which adequately matches the inhalability criterion.

It should be noted that whilst writing this chapter, the author is involved (with many others) in a major project, funded by the EU (European Union) Measurement and Testing Programme and the UK Health and Safety Executive, to study the suitability of a protocol proposed by CEN/TC137/WG3 for testing the performance of health-related aerosol samplers in relation to the new sampling conventions. Personal samplers for coarse aerosols are being used as the vehicles for the evaluation which involves testing eight types of sampler in a large wind tunnel. The samplers are mounted on the torso of a life-size tailor's mannequin and exposed to nine aerosol sizes in the range $6-100\,\mu m$ in three windspeeds: 0.5, 1 and $4\,m\,s^{-1}$. This will provide a comprehensive set of data on the performance of most of the personal samplers used for sampling coarse aerosols worldwide. Early results confirm the notion that the design of personal sampling heads affects their performances, and are consistent with the evaluations described above.

PRACTICAL SAMPLERS FOR RESPIRABLE AEROSOL

The history of sampling fine aerosols in workplaces began with the respirable fraction, in particular with the emergence in the 1950s of the BMRC respirable aerosol criterion. A number of types of sampling device have since been developed. Most have in common the fact that they first aspirate a particle fraction which is assumed to be representative of the total workplace aerosol, from which the desired fine fraction is then aerodynamically separated inside the instrument, using an arrangement

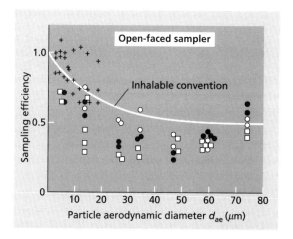

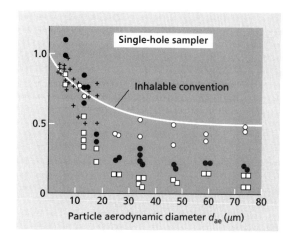

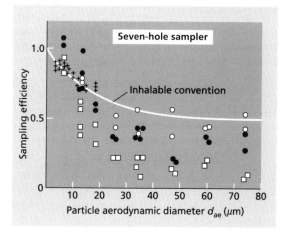

Fig. 8.7 Performance of the three personal samplers for coarse aerosols shown in Fig. 8.6. Sampling efficiency (A_{app}) is given as a function of particle aerodynamic diameter for samplers mounted on a torso. From Vincent (1989).

whose particle size-dependent penetration characteristics match the desired criterion. It is the fraction which remains uncollected inside the selector and passes through to collect onto a filter (or some other collecting medium) which is the fine fraction of interest.

Static samplers

A variety of static samplers for respirable aerosol have been built and successfully used in practical occupational hygiene. Some achieve particle size selection by the mechanism of horizontal gravitational elutriation. One example is the British $2.5 \, l \, min^{-1}$ MRE Type 113A sampler shown in Fig.

8.10; another is the similar, but higher flow rate, $100 \, l \, min^{-1}$ Hexhlet. The penetration characteristics of such devices can be easily tailored, using the elutriator theory developed by Henry Walton (1954), to closely match the BMRC respirable aerosol curve (itself originally derived from elutriator theory). However, recent wind tunnel studies (Mark, Lyons and Upton, 1993) have shown that the overall sampling efficiency (inlet and size selection) is affected by varying windspeed as shown in Fig. 8.11.

Other static respirable aerosol samplers have been designed to operate on the principles of cyclone selection. One example is the German $50 \, l \, min^{-1}$ TBF50 sampler (Stuke and Emmerichs,

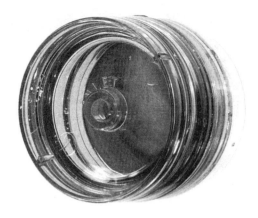

Fig. 8.8 37 mm plastic cassette personal sampler, shown in the closed-face mode.

1973); another is the French $50 \, l \, min^{-1}$ CPM3 (Fabries and Wrobel, 1987). Although such cyclones can be designed having well-defined penetration characteristics, prediction of performance from theory is more complicated than for horizontal elutriators.

Personal samplers

Horizontal gravitational elutriators are satisfactory for static respirable aerosol sampling, but are inevitably rather bulky and not conducive to miniaturization. Therefore, horizontal gravitational elutriation is not an option for personal respirable aerosol samplers. On the other hand, cyclones are ideally suited for such purposes, and have found wide application. Well-known examples are the British $1.9 \, l \, min^{-1}$ cyclone known as SIMPEDS and shown in Fig. 8.12; and the American $1.7–2.1 \, l \, min^{-1}$ 10 mm cyclone, whose selection characteristics have been shown to be in good agreement with the BMRC and ACGIH curves respectively.

One further device has some interesting and unusual features and so deserves special mention. This is the French CIP10 shown in Fig. 8.13. Although this instrument is aimed primarily at collecting a finer (respirable) aerosol fraction, it is capable of also providing the concentration of the inhalable and thoracic fractions by the inclusion of special inserts in place of the size-selecting foam. It is particularly interesting because the instrument incorporates its own built-in pumping unit, consisting of a battery-driven, rapidly rotating polyester

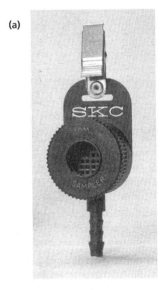

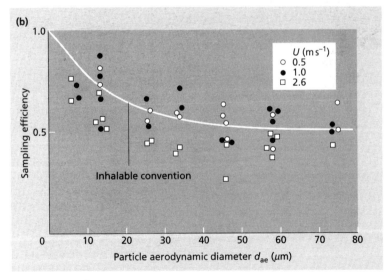

Fig. 8.9 IOM personal inhalable aerosol sampler: (a) conducting plastic version sold by SKC Ltd., Blandford Forum, Dorset, UK; (b) performance (aspiration efficiency, A) of the original prototype version mounted on torso.

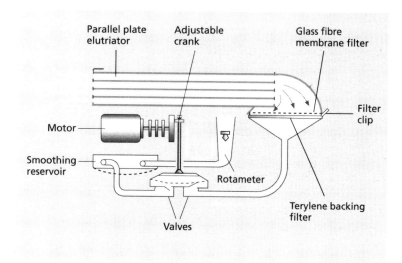

Fig. 8.10 MRE 113A static respirable aerosol sampler.

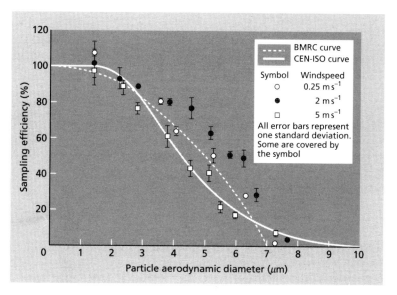

Fig. 8.11 Performance of MRE 113A static respirable aerosol sampler in comparison with respirable conventions.

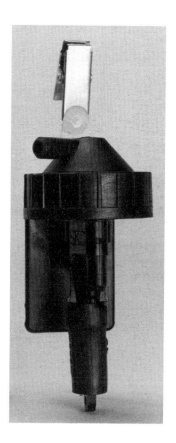

Fig. 8.12 SIMPEDS personal respirable aerosol sampler.

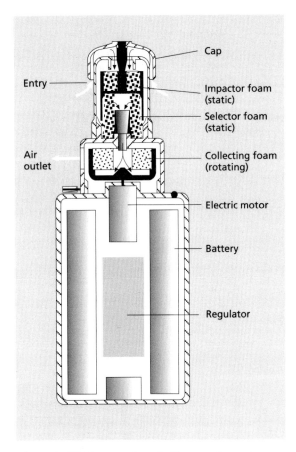

Fig. 8.13 CIP10 personal respirable aerosol sampler.

foam plug. The aerosol is aspirated through a downwards-facing annular entry and is progressively selected by a combination of mainly gravitational and inertial forces in two static, coarse-grade foam plugs located inside the entry as well as on the finer-grade rotating one. As a result of the low-pressure drop characteristics of such foam filtration media, a very high flow rate — by personal sampler standards — can be achieved: up to $10\,l\,min^{-1}$.

PRACTICAL SAMPLERS FOR THORACIC AEROSOL

Static samplers

Methodology for the sampling of thoracic aerosol in the occupational context was not widely considered prior to the establishment of the ISO and ACGIH criteria. For workplaces, the only aerosol standard that approaches the thoracic fraction is in the US cotton industry where a criterion was established in 1975 by the US National Institute of Occupational Safety and Health, based on a selection curve which falls to 50% at $15\,\mu m$ (compared with $11.64\,\mu m$ in the new CEN/ISO/ACGIH thoracic fraction). This implies recognition of the role of particle deposition in the large airways of the upper respiratory tract in cotton workers' byssinosis. The recommended static sampling method employs the concept of vertical elutriation, and an example of the sampler is shown in Fig. 8.14.

Personal samplers

The MSP personal environmental monitor, shown in Fig. 8.15, uses a single-stage impactor designed to select the thoracic fraction according to the

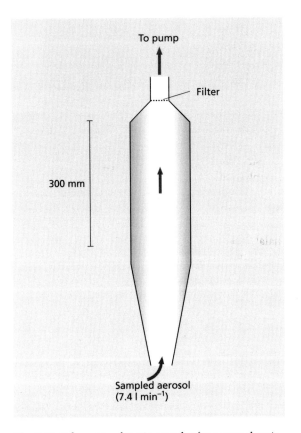

Fig. 8.14 Schematic of static sampler for cotton dust in the USA.

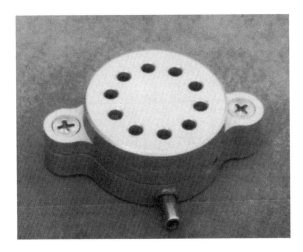

Fig. 8.15 MSP personal sampler for the PM10 definition of the thoracic fraction. Photograph courtesy of MSP Corporation, Minneapolis, USA.

earlier American PM10 definition. With a flow rate of $41\,\text{min}^{-1}$, it has a very sharp sampling curve which excludes some of the large particles allowed in the ISO/CEN/ACGIH thoracic convention. This sampler has been widely used in the USA for monitoring personal exposures in non-occupational situations, such as homes and public places, and has formed part of a major study to investigate aerosol exposures both indoors and outdoors.

There are a number of other samplers currently under development for the thoracic fraction. One is a modification of the CIP10 respirable aerosol sampler (described above) in which the foam size selector has been replaced by an inertial particle selection device. The other prototype sampler uses a porous foam size selector behind the IOM inhalable aerosol entry. These samplers should soon be commercially available.

INVESTIGATIONAL INSTRUMENTS

In all of the instruments described above, the sampled aerosol is collected on a filter or some other substrate which may be assessed separately after sampling has been completed. Such instrumentation is suitable when time-averaged measurement can be justified. However, there are occasions where short-term (or even real-time) measurement is required: for example, when investigating the major sources of aerosol emission from

an industrial process and the subsequent efficiency of control procedures introduced to minimize that emission. They may also form the basis of an alarm monitoring system of the type described above.

Optical techniques, based on the principles of light extinction and scattering, provide an effective means by which aerosol can be assessed in real time. They provide the great advantage that measurement can be made without disturbing the aerosol — provided of course that the particles can be introduced into the sensing zone of the instrument without loss or change. Their disadvantage is that interactions between light and airborne particles are strongly dependent on particle size and type, and so results are frequently difficult to interpret.

In workplaces, aerosol concentrations are usually too low to provide significant attenuation and so optical instruments operating on the basis of the detection of the scattered light are more widely used. There are many possibilities (e.g. optical geometry, scattering angle, etc.) on which to base an instrument, and a correspondingly wide range of instruments has appeared on the market. The most successful have been those designed for the monitoring of aerosol fractions within specific particle size ranges — in particular, the respirable fraction. They include the British safety in mines scattered light instrument (SIMSLIN) which is based on the horizontal elutriator system of the MRE Type 113A gravimetric respirable dust sampler described earlier, but with the elutriated aerosol entering an optical sensing zone in which scattered infrared light from a diode laser is collected within the angles 12° to 20° from the forward direction and focused onto a photodiode (Fig. 8.16). SIMSLIN has been shown to provide a response that is approximately proportional to the instantaneous respirable mass concentration of mine dusts. A more recent version is the optical scattering instantaneous respirable dust indication system (OSIRIS), in which the data can be telemetered to a central monitoring station. In the American respirable aerosol monitor (RAM), the aspirated aerosol is passed through a cyclone which allows the respirable fraction to penetrate to the sensing zone, where infrared light scattered in the near-forward direction is detected by a photodiode. A somewhat different approach is adopted in the German TM-digital, where the

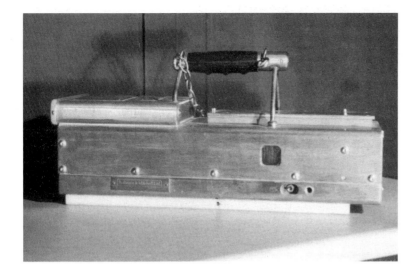

Fig. 8.16 SIMSLIN static scattered light instrument for respirable aerosol.

aerosol enters the sensing region by direct convection without the aid of a pump (Fig. 8.17). In the sensing region, scattered infrared light is detected at an angle of 70° to the forward-facing photodiode. This instrument also has been shown to respond directly to the respirable dust mass concentration in mine environments. An important extension of the RAM is a personal device — the MINIRAM — which, like the TM-digital, is an essentially 'passive' device, having no pump (Fig. 8.18). Similar principles are used in the hand-held wand-type instruments such as the AMS950 produced by Casella (London) Ltd. (Fig. 8.19). These are widely used in walk-through surveys of workplaces to determine which processes are the major dust sources, and for this purpose the variation in response of the instrument with particle size and refractive index must not be forgotten.

The second type of instrument is based on the interaction between a focused light beam and each individual single particle. Such instruments are referred to as 'optical particle counters'. From light-scattering principles, if an individual particle can be detected and registered electronically, it can be not only counted but also sized (i.e. placed into a given size band or 'channel' based on the magnitude of signal arising from the scattered light). By such means, instruments can be designed which are capable either of counting particles within specified size ranges or of providing an overall particle size

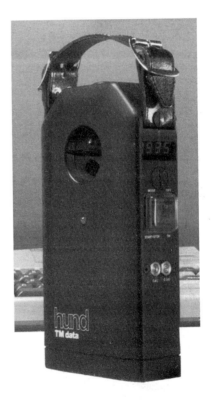

Fig. 8.17 Hund Corporation version of the TM-digital respirable aerosol monitor.

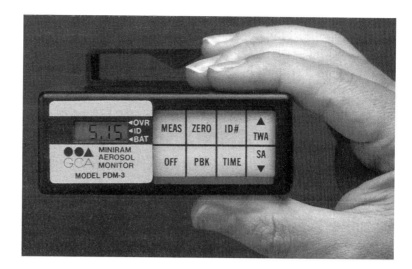

Fig. 8.18 MINIRAM miniature real time aerosol monitor. Photograph courtesy of GCA Corporation, Bedford, UK.

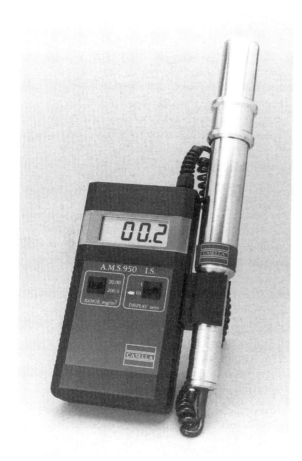

Fig. 8.19 Casella AMS950 hand-held aerosol monitor. Photograph courtesy of Casella London Ltd., Bedford, UK.

distribution. As with aerosol photometers, many practical instruments have evolved within this category, and have been widely used in research both in laboratories and in workplaces. The fibrous aerosol monitor (FAM) is a version that sets out to provide counts of fibrous particles conforming to the 'respirable' fibre definition (as discussed earlier), even in the presence of non-fibrous particles.

A wide range of other types of direct-reading instruments is available. One is based on the beta-attenuation concept, where the mass of particulate material deposited on a filter, or some other surface, is determined from the reduction in intensity of beta-particles passing through the accumulated layer. In such instruments, the change in attenuation reflects the rate at which particles are collecting on the filter and hence on the concentration of the sampled aerosol. One advantage of this approach over optical instruments is that the attenuation of beta-particles is directly dependent on particulate mass, and is almost independent of aerosol type or particle size distribution.

Another class of devices is what might be referred to as 'vibrational mass balances'. The frequency of mechanical oscillation of a piezoelectric crystal (e.g. quartz) is directly proportional to the mass of the crystal. Change in effective mass of the crystal, such as that due to the deposition of particles on its surface, is reflected in the change in its mechanical resonant frequency. The piezobalance, manufactured by TSI Inc., St Paul, Minnesota, USA, is one example of an instrument of this sort. A recent development of this principle (TEOM: tapered element oscillator microbalance) involves the use of a tapered glass tube which is fixed at the large end and supports a filter at the narrow end. The tube and filter are oscillated, and again the deposition of particles on the filter causes a change in the resonant frequency of the tube (the principles of this method are given in Fig. 8.20).

An interesting, and potentially very useful, development has been the combination of direct-reading instruments and video recording of the operation. In this procedure the operator wears a direct-reading personal monitor, and the contaminant levels are superimposed on the video film of the operational process. Although mostly used for the sampling of gases and vapours, some success has been obtained using the MINIRAM light scattering device as the monitor. It has proved to be a very useful tool in demonstrating to operators ways in which they can reduce their personal exposures.

ERRORS INVOLVED IN TAKING AN AEROSOL SAMPLE

As with any measurement process, there are errors associated with that measurement. Aerosol sampling comprises a number of different stages, each one with its own error which contributes to the overall inaccuracy of the measurement of aerosol concentration. There are systematic errors, which we can control, such as:
● bias in concentration due to inadequate performance of the sampling head;
● errors in setting and maintaining the required flow rate;
● analytical errors: gravimetric and chemical.
There are also random errors over which we have little control, except in the design of the sampling strategy. These errors are associated with:
● choice of who to sample and where;
● variation in day-to-day aerosol concentration.
These errors all combine to give an overall error or uncertainty in the measurement of aerosol concentration.

Performance of the sampling head

As mentioned above, it is essential that the sampling head be chosen specifically for the aerosol fraction of interest (i.e. inhalable, thoracic or respirable). Recent experiments have shown that there are wide variations in the sampling efficiencies of sampling heads previously used to collect so-called 'total' aerosol. Studies in a range of different industries have shown that aerosol concentration comparisons of two types of personal sampler for coarse particles can have ratios ranging from 1:1 to 3:1. Similar problems can be found for samplers for the respirable fraction.

It is therefore essential (and soon to be required in Europe) that, if sampling for health-related purposes, suitable samplers should be chosen that have been shown to meet the requirements of the relevant sampling convention specified in European Standard EN 481.

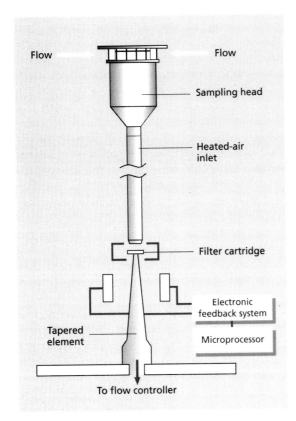

Fig. 8.20 Principle of operation of the tapered element oscillating microbalance (TEOM).

Flow rate setting and control

Errors in the flow rate through samplers can have significant effects on the mass concentration measured. Both the entry efficiency and the selection efficiency of the size selector (if present) can be affected by incorrect flow rate setting and control.

The flow rate through most modern sampling pumps is easily adjusted by means of a single screw and, once set, is maintained by in-built flow control systems which compensate for build-up of particles on the filter. However, despite the fact that some pumps have inbuilt rotameter flowmeters, it is still necessary to check the flow rate entering the sampler using a primary standard, such as a bubble flowmeter. This is because the rotameters are either fixed in series in the flow line, or on the pump exhaust, where flow rate measurement is unreliable. The flowmeter is fixed to the sampler entry so that the true flow rate through the sampler is measured. This process has been speeded up dramatically in recent years by the introduction of automatic bubble flowmeters, such as the Gilibrator manufactured by Gilian Inc., New Jersey, USA.

Analytical errors: gravimetric

The majority of aerosol samples taken in the workplace are analysed gravimetrically. Whilst this may seem to be a simple process, in order to obtain reliable results a number of precautions are necessary.

Ideally, all weighing should be carried out in a temperature and humidity controlled room set aside specially for the purpose. If full environmental control is not available, then care should be taken to ensure that the room is not subject to large changes in temperature due to, for example, solar gain and time-controlled central heating. The room should be big enough to contain a solid bench upon which the balance is sited and a set of shelves for storing filters and cassettes for conditioning prior to weighing. This conditioning should be allowed before each weighing (i.e. before and after aerosol exposure) and preferably for a period of at least 12 h — overnight is a useful time. Conditioning in a desiccator, which is sometimes used, is not rec-

ommended as the filter rapidly gains weight when transferred to the balance and is therefore very difficult to weigh. For some membrane filters made from cellulose esters, PVC, PTFE and polycarbonate, excess surface electrical charge must be neutralized, either with a radioactive source or a high electric field, before accurate weighing can be achieved. Finally, even with all these precautions it is essential that a small number of filters (about 10% of the batch) be kept unexposed to aerosol to serve as blank controls, so that residual changes in filter weight due to moisture uptake and changes in balance performance can be allowed for.

Provided that the above precautions are taken and a suitable balance is used, a weighing accuracy of ± 0.03 mg is easily achievable.

Analytical errors: chemical

Many aerosol samples taken in workplaces contain a variety of different compounds. If measurement of a specific compound within the mixture, such as lead, nickel, cadmium, etc. is required, then the collected sample must be analysed by atomic absorption spectrometry or other methods to determine the concentration of that compound. For solid aerosol particles the main difficulty in the analysis process is ensuring that all the collected particles are removed from the filter. Digestion of the filters by acid washing or low-temperature ashing are methods generally employed for this purpose.

Random errors: variability of exposure

Most operations in workplaces lead to short-term fluctuations in pollutant emissions. If the substance is acutely toxic it is important to measure the peak concentrations, to set short-term occupational exposure limits (STELs) and to instigate control procedures to protect the worker. For most substances, we are interested in the longer-term integrated exposure, and full-shift sampling is required. However, even when sampling for a longer period, significant errors in assessing the actual exposure of a worker to aerosols can arise. Day-to-day exposure levels for a given worker can be very variable, as can exposure levels between workers doing the same job, and between workers doing different jobs. This variability is random in nature and there is some evidence to suggest that exposure measurements follow a log-normal distribution pattern. Variations in full-shift exposure levels of up to 1000 : 1 have been observed — large enough to dwarf the instrumental errors described above!

To ensure that a sampling campaign gives realistic estimates of individual exposure, it is essential that the above variability is taken into account when deciding the duration and frequency of sampling and who and where to sample. This topic is the subject of much guidance from the regulatory authorities such as the UK Health and Safety Executive and the US National Institute of Occupational Safety and Health, and a draft CEN standard is soon to be approved by the European Union. It is considered in more detail in Chapter 17.

SPECIAL PROBLEMS

Fibrous aerosol particles

Fibrous aerosols can pose extreme risks to health and so are of special interest. Because of their unusual morphological properties, and the role of these properties in the aetiology of lung disease, fibres are specifically excluded from the ISO, CEN and ACGIH conventions. Instead, there is a separate rationale for particle size-selective measurement, based on an appreciation of both the nature of particle motion which governs fibre deposition in the deep lung, and the biological effects that influence the fate of the particles after deposition. Thus it has been a widespread convention since the 1960s to assess 'respirable' fibres in terms of the airborne number concentration, rather than mass concentration used for all other particles. Furthermore, these respirable fibres are not selected by aerodynamic means, but are defined when examined by optical microscopy under phase contrast conditions as those particles having a length-to-diameter ratio greater than 3, length greater than 5 μm and diameter less than 3 μm.

The practical criteria that have emerged for fibres are based not only on the properties of the particle which can bear directly on possible health effects,

but also on the technical means readily available for assessing them. Optical microscopy is relatively cost-effective and straightforward. However, to set an upper limit for fibre diameter smaller than 3 μm (which might be justified in the light of some of the biological evidence) could result in counting problems since a higher proportion would lie beyond the physical limits of detection by optical means. Therefore, the criteria currently in use for routine analysis are based on pragmatic as well as scientific considerations.

As already indicated, the definition of a 'respirable' fibre is based on purely geometric criteria so that selection is best carried out not aerodynamically but visually under the microscope. This means that, in practical sampling, the main priority is to achieve deposition onto a suitable surface (e.g. a membrane filter) which can then be 'cleared' and mounted for subsequent visual analysis. It follows that actual physical sampling can be very simple, and usually involves the collection of particles directly onto an open filter contained within a downwards-pointing filter holder. The filter holder is generally fitted with a cowl or some other baffle to protect the filter from large airborne material as well as from curious fingers. An example of such a sampler, as recommended for use in the UK (MDHS 39), is given in Fig. 8.21. The filters used are normally membranes made from mixed cellulose esters, which are easily made transparent (cleared) with acetone vapour from commercially available acetone boilers. The samplers are used routinely in both the static mode to monitor asbestos clearance sites, and the personal mode to estimate individual exposure.

Bioaerosols

The term 'bioaerosols' includes a wide range of airborne particles which are derived from living matter. They include micro-organisms ranging in size from sub-micron viruses to fungal spores which may exceed 200 μm. Between these extremes there is a wide variety of bacteria, fungi (including both yeasts and moulds) and spores, and non-viable fragments of micro-organisms. Some viruses and bacteria are pathogenic (e.g. anthrax) and must be alive to cause harm, whilst allergic responses such as

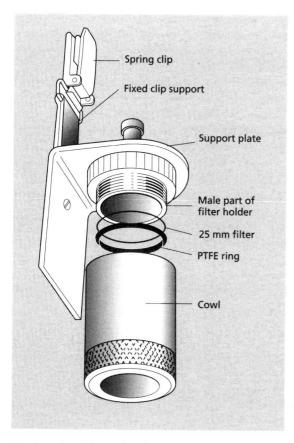

Fig. 8.21 Cowled sampling head for asbestos and other fibres.

Labels on figure:
Spring clip
Fixed clip support
Support plate
Male part of filter holder
25 mm filter
PTFE ring
Cowl

asthma and hay fever, etc., may be caused by fragments of cells as well as the live organism. Examples of all these types of particles can occur at the workplace, which includes farming situations as well as the indoor workplaces usually considered.

The principles of sampling are similar to those described above, but, as well as meeting the sampling criteria for inorganic aerosols, samplers for some bioaerosols must also collect the particles with minimal shear forces and static electricity forces, and must retain the particles in a moist atmosphere. This is because some micro-organisms (such as viruses, etc.) are fragile and are easily killed, thereby rendering them harmless to humans. Despite the wide-ranging occurrence of bioaerosols and the increased understanding of their role in many diseases, there are no approved guide-lines describing standard methods for the sampling of bioaerosols in most environments. A large number of reviews concerning sampling methods used to assess bioaerosols have been published. These include reviews covering all applications such as those by Burge and Solomon (1987), Chatigny *et al.* (1989) and Griffiths and DeCosemo (1994).

The most commonly used samplers for bio-aerosols in workplaces are the Andersen microbial sampler (AMS) shown in Fig. 8.22 and the all-glass impinger (AGI) shown in Fig. 8.23. These are both static instruments which are designed to keep the collected particles alive. The AMS achieves this by collection onto a nutrient agar medium, whilst the AGI relies on particle collection into a liquid reservoir. Other devices designed specifically for collecting bioaerosols which have been used in workplaces include: the Casella slit sampler, the surface air sampler and the Biotest RCS sampler, all of which use agar for particle collection and retention; and cyclones with inlet spray-wetters such as the aerojet general liquid scrubber air sampler (Decker *et al.*, 1969). In these latter devices, collection fluid is continuously injected at the sampler inlet via a hypodermic syringe so that bioaerosol particles deposited on internal walls of the sampler are continuously swept into the collection reservoir.

Although all the samplers described above have been designed to keep the bioaerosol particles alive (and we do not yet know how well this has been achieved), no attempt has been made to control the physical sampling efficiencies of the samplers. Some recent work on the AMS and the AGI has shown that their physical sampling efficiencies are dependent on both windspeed and particle size in a manner that does not conform to the ISO/CEN health-related sampling conventions. To obtain a reliable estimate of the health-related concentration of micro-organisms, measurements of the particle size distribution and windspeed should be made at each sampling location. Major studies are currently being carried out in both the USA and Europe to fully characterize the performances of samplers currently used for sampling bioaerosols. It is expected that improved methods should result.

Two main methods of assessment are carried out for bioaerosols. Viable particles are assessed by

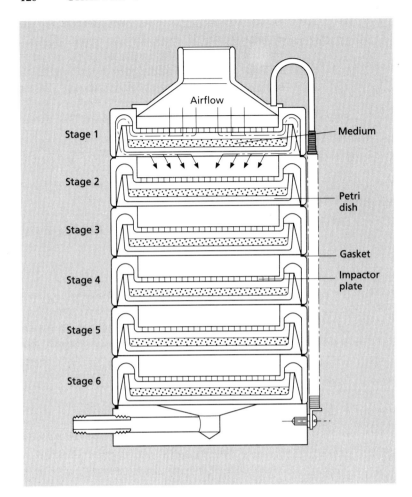

Fig. 8.22 Andersen microbial sampler (AMS), Graesby Anderson Ltd., Orpington, UK.

counting the number of colony-forming units (CFUs) visible after culturing on a suitable growth medium such as agar. The total number of all bioaerosol particles sampled (both viable and non-viable) are determined by microscopy methods, such as epifluorescence microscopy, and (more recently) immunoassay methods, such as ELISA (enzyme-linked immunosorbent assay).

Two-phase compounds

Some compounds such as arsenic, aromatic carboxylic acid anhydrides, isocyanates, etc. can occur both as aerosols and vapours under certain conditions in workplaces. For the first two compounds, the particles are sampled with a normal sampling head (seven-hole sampler in the UK) and are collected on a filter. The vapour penetrating is then collected either on a second, treated filter or on an absorbent tube. For isocyanates however, midget impingers are used, with both aerosol and vapour being collected in the liquid.

These methods are applicable when the two phases are analysed together. However, it is likely that the aerosol and vapour phases will deposit in different regions of the respiratory tract, and so it may be important to determine the concentrations of the two phases separately. For this purpose it is essential that they remain in their original airborne state once collected to ensure that there is not cross-contamination between phases. This situation is very difficult to achieve, as air passing through

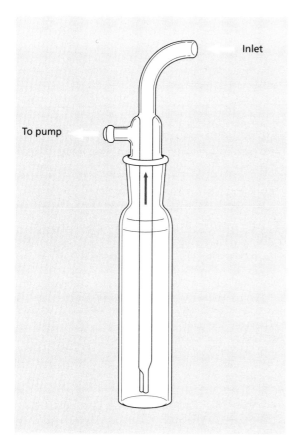

Fig. 8.23 All-glass impinger (AGI) for bioaerosols.

collected particles may cause off-gassing, whilst there may also be back diffusion from the absorbent stage once the sampling pump has been switched off.

A method proposed by Soderholm (1993) involves the simultaneous sampling of the aerosol and the vapour phase separately. This is achieved by using a diffusive sampler to collect the vapour phase, and an inhalable aerosol sampler fitted with a filter for the particles followed by an adsorbent stage to collect the airborne vapour and the vapour released from the collected particles.

FUTURE DEVELOPMENTS

The sampling of aerosols in all environments, including occupational, is going through a period of great change, with the emphasis in all measure-ments being on international standardization. For aerosols, international agreement has recently been reached for a set of health-related sampling conventions. The next step, which is currently under way, is the establishment of an agreed test protocol by which the performance of aerosol samplers can be tested for compliance with the health-related conventions. This work, which was mentioned earlier, will involve the classification of samplers according to the range of conditions in which they will give reliable results. Once this has been achieved, and provided that an agreed sampling strategy is followed, there is no reason why reliable, valid measurements of occupational exposures cannot be achieved. These will have the added benefit of being internationally comparable.

Currently, continuously recording instruments are used as investigational tools to determine major aerosol sources, and as educational tools to reduce aerosol exposure by altering work practices. It is expected that this will continue, but with an additional use as alarm monitors in an overall sampling strategy employing both periodic personal sampling supported by continuous monitoring of all work shifts.

With an increasing incidence of allergenic diseases, such as asthma, which are thought to be caused by inhaling bioaerosols, and the increasing production of process micro-organisms, there is a desperate need for standardized guidance on the sampling of bioaerosols. Research work is currently being carried out in laboratories worldwide to develop practical, reliable and standard methods. It is expected that there will not be one universally applicable method but possibly two: one for micro-organisms that must be kept viable, using samplers that both treat the micro-organisms gently and keep them wet; and one where viability is not important and existing methodology for inorganic aerosols can be used.

REFERENCES

American Conference of Governmental Industrial Hygienists (1968). *Threshold Limit Values of Airborne Contaminants*. ACGIH, Cincinnati, Ohio.

Asbestos International Association (1979). *Recommended Technical Method No. 1: Reference Method for the Determination of Airborne Asbestos Fibre Concen-*

trations at Workplaces by Light Microscopy (Membrane Filter Method). AIA Health and Safety Publication, London.

Burge, H.A. and Solomon, W.R. (1987). Sampling and analysis of biological aerosols. *Atmospheric Environment*, **21**,(2), 451–4.

Chatigny, M.A., Macher, J.M., Burge, H.A. and Solomon, W.A. (1989). Sampling airborne microorganisms and aeroallergens. In *Air Sampling Instruments for Evaluation of Atmospheric Contaminants*, (7th edn), (ed. S.V. Hering). American Conference of Governmental Industrial Hygienists, Cincinnati, Ohio.

Chung, K.Y.K., Ogden, T.L. and Vaughan, N.P. (1987). Wind effects on personal dust samplers. *Journal of Aerosol Science*, **18**, 159–74.

Comité Européen de Normalisation (1993a). *Workplace Atmospheres. Size Fraction Definitions for Measurement of Airborne Particles*. CEN Standard EN 481.

Comité Européen de Normalisation (1993b). *Workplace Atmospheres. Assessment of Performance of Instruments for Measurement of Airborne Particles*. Draft CEN Prestandard.

Comité Européen de Normalisation (1993c). *Workplace Atmospheres. Requirements and Test Methods for Pumps used for Personal Sampling of Chemical Agents in the Workplace*. CEN Prestandard prEN 1232.

Decker, H.M., Buchanan, L.M. and Frisque, D.E. (1969). Advances in large volume air sampling. *Contamination Control*, **8**, 13–17.

Fabries, J-F. and Wrobel, R. (1987). A compact high flowrate respirable dust sampler. *Annals of Occupational Hygiene*, **31**, 195–209.

Griffiths, W.D. and DeCosemo, G.A.L. (1994). The assessment of bioaerosols: a critical review. *Journal of Aerosol Science*, **25**, 1425–58.

Health and Safety Executive (1981). *Control of Lead: Air Sampling Techniques and Strategies*. Guidance Note EH 28. HSE, London.

Health and Safety Executive (1989). *General Methods for the Gravimetric Determination of Respirable and Total Inhalable Dust*. MDHS 14. HSE, London.

Hering, S.V. (ed.) (1989). *Air Sampling Instruments for Evaluation of Atmospheric Contaminants*, (7th edn). American Conference of Governmental Industrial Hygienists, Cincinnati, Ohio.

Lippmann, M. and Harris, W.B. (1962). Size-selective samplers for estimating 'respirable' dust concentrations. *Health Physics*, **8**, 155–63.

Mark, D. and Vincent, J.H. (1986). A new personal sampler for airborne total dust in workplaces. *Annals of Occupational Hygiene*, **30**, 89–102.

Mark, D., Vincent, J.H. and Gibson, H. (1985). A new static sampler for airborne total dust in workplaces. *American Industrial Hygiene Association Journal*, **46**, 127–33.

Mark, D., Lyons, C.P. and Upton, S.L. (1993). Performance testing of the respirable dust sampler used in British coal mines. *Applied Occupational and Environmental Hygiene*, **8**,(4), 370–80.

Orenstein, A.J. (1960). Recommendations adopted by the Pneumoconiosis Conference. In *Proceedings of the Pneumoconiosis Conference*, pp. 619–21. Churchill, London.

Soderholm, S.C. (1993). Measuring the particle/vapour distribution of an air contaminant. Paper presented at the *American Industrial Hygiene Conference and Exposition, New Orleans, May 1993*.

Stuke, J. and Emmerichs, M. (1973). Das gravimetrische Staubprobenahmegerat TBF50. *Silikosebericht Nordrhein-Westfalen*, **9**, 47–51.

Vincent, J.H. and Mark, D. (1990). Entry characteristics of practical workplace aerosol samplers in relation to the ISO recommendations. *Annals of Occupational Hygiene*, **34**, 249–62.

Walton, W.H. (1954). Theory of size classification of airborne dust clouds by elutriation. *British Journal of Applied Physics*, **5** (Supplement): S29–40.

CHAPTER 9

Noise

K. Gardiner

INTRODUCTION

This chapter aims to describe the basic physical properties of sound, the parameters by which it is measured and the means by which it can be controlled. Vibration is dealt with in Chapter 10.

NOISE

Basic acoustics

Sound is the form of energy which is detected by the hearing mechanism. This sensation is produced when the eardrum is vibrated by a minute, fluctuating pressure change in the air inside the ear canal. This fluctuation has, in turn, been caused by a disturbance such as the vibrating cone of a loudspeaker or turbulent jet, by a vibrating machine panel or the vocal cords. Sound is propagated through materials by the longitudinal oscillation of individual molecules and interaction with adjacent molecules (hence it cannot pass through a vacuum).

The simplest form of vibration that a source can exhibit is known as simple harmonic motion (SHM). This motion is exhibited by the molecules of the propagating materials at a rate determined by the bulk modulus (κ) and density (ρ) of the material. It may be shown that the velocity of sound (c) in a material is given by:

$$c = \sqrt{\frac{\kappa}{\rho}} \qquad (9.1)$$

When sound passes through air, the vibration of air particles causes a minute fluctuating pressure

known as the acoustic pressure, which is superimposed on the existing atmospheric pressure (about $101\,325\,\mathrm{N\,m^{-2}}$); the smallest detectable acoustic pressure is in the order of $2 \times 10^{-5}\,\mathrm{N\,m^{-2}}$. This is much smaller than diurnal atmospheric pressure changes and the Eustachian tube ensures that the air pressure in the middle ear and ear canal are equalized so that the eardrum is free to respond to small acoustic pressures.

For the simplest sounds, the acoustic pressure (p) (Fig. 9.1) may be described by a sinusoidal function:

$$p = A \frac{\sin}{\cos} \omega t \qquad (9.2)$$

where A is the amplitude (i.e. the maximum value) ($\mathrm{N\,m^{-2}}$), t is time (s) and ω is angular frequency ($\mathrm{rad\,s^{-1}}$). This equation is cyclic over a periodic time of $T = 2\pi/\omega$, i.e. has the same value at times

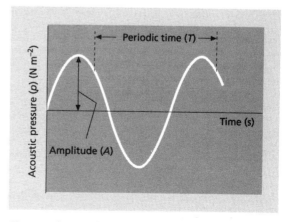

Fig. 9.1 Change of acoustic pressure with time for a pure tone.

$t = t_0$ and $t = t_0 + 2\pi/\omega$. It is more convenient to express the periodicity in terms of its frequency (f): the number of cycles produced in 1 s, where $f = 1/T$ (s^{-1} or hertz (Hz)). The audible frequency range is about 15 Hz to 18 kHz, although acoustic pressures do exist at lower (infrasonic) and higher frequencies (ultrasonic).

Because of the finite value of sound velocity, points along the path of propagation exhibit phase differences. In Fig. 9.2, points 'a' and 'b' are separated by a distance X (m). The time taken for the sound to travel from 'a' to 'b' is X/c seconds. Hence the phase at 'b' is delayed by X/c on 'a' so that if:

$$p = A \frac{\sin}{\cos} \omega t, \text{ at 'a'} \qquad (9.3)$$

then

$$p = A \frac{\sin}{\cos} \omega \left(t - \frac{X}{c} \right) \text{ at 'b'}$$

and

$$p = A \frac{\sin}{\cos} (\omega t - kX)$$

where k is ω/c (a wave constant). Where X has a value such that $X = 2\pi, 4\pi, 6\pi$, etc., 'a' and 'b' are said to be in phase.

Two adjacent points which are in phase are separated by a distance known as the wavelength (λ). Hence:

$$k\lambda = 2\pi$$

therefore

$$\lambda = Tc \qquad (9.4)$$

(i.e. the time taken for the sound to travel through a distance equal to λ is T). It follows that $f\lambda = c$, so that the wavelength of sounds of different frequencies may be calculated.

Since the velocity of sound in air is approximately $340 \, \text{m s}^{-1}$ at ground level, the wavelengths of audible sounds will range from 23 m (15 Hz) to 19 mm (18 kHz). The physical dimensions of objects encountered in buildings are also of this range and so the behaviour of sound in factories, for example, is greatly dependent on its frequency. In general, propagation of high-frequency sound is very directional: when high-frequency sounds meet a barrier, reflection occurs. Low-frequency sounds tend to diffract around barriers and to be generally non-directional.

Sound quantities

The rate at which sound energy leaves its source is known as 'sound power' (W) (measured in watts). A source of sound approximating to a point will produce a spherical sound field, so that the sound power is dissipated over an ever-increasing area. Thus the quantity of sound entering the ear depends on the sound power and its distance from the source (r). The average amount of energy passing through a unit area in unit time is known as the 'sound intensity' (I) (W m^{-2}). From Fig. 9.3:

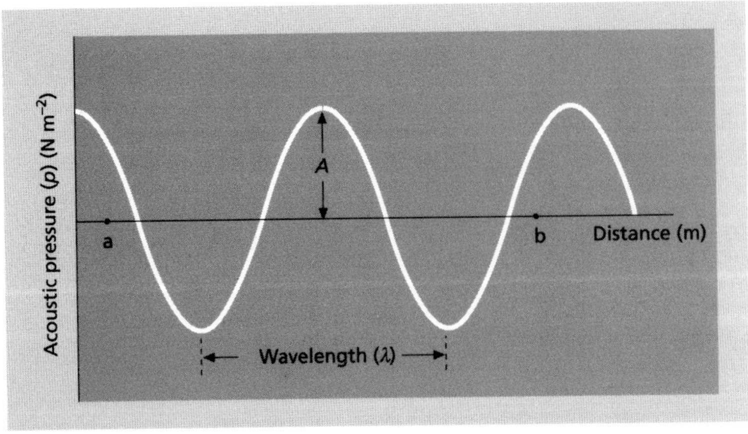

Fig. 9.2 Change of acoustic pressure with distance for a pure tone.

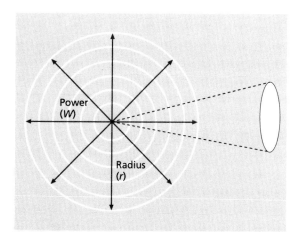

Fig. 9.3 Distribution of sound propagated from a point source.

$$I = \frac{\text{Sound power}}{\text{Surface area of sphere}} = \frac{W}{4\pi r^2}$$

hence

$$I \propto \frac{1}{r^2} \text{ (an inverse square law)} \qquad (9.5)$$

If a plane reflecting barrier is placed immediately behind the source, a hemispherical field is produced, so that the surface area is halved and the intensity doubled. If the field is further modified by reflection, the intensity will also change. In general:

$$I = \frac{QW}{4\pi r^2} \qquad (9.6)$$

where Q is the directivity factor. ($Q = 2$ for a hemispherical field and 4 for a quarter-spherical field, etc.)

The value of acoustic pressure corresponding to the energy content of the sound wave is not the amplitude, since this value is never maintained by the wave, but is the average in time of the square of the pressure. This may be shown to be the root-mean-square (rms) value (p_{rms}), which is $A/\sqrt{2}$ for a sinusoidal function (Fig. 9.4). Furthermore:

$$I_{av} = \frac{p_{rms}^2}{\rho c} \qquad (9.7)$$

where ρc is termed the characteristic impedance of the medium (for air $\rho c = 1.2 \times 340 \simeq 400$ rayls). This relationship shows that an average intensity of $10^{-12}\,\text{W}\,\text{m}^{-2}$ produces an rms acoustic pressure of $2 \times 10^{-5}\,\text{N}\,\text{m}^{-2}$ in air.

Bel scales

The Weber–Fechner law states that the change in a physiological response at a stimulus is proportional to the relative change in the stimulus, i.e.:

$$\delta R \propto \frac{\delta S}{S} \qquad (9.8)$$

where δR is the change in response and S is the stimulus (e.g. sound intensity). The response to a stimulus change from S_1 to S_2 may be found by integrating the above expression:

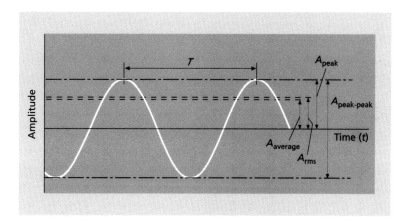

Fig. 9.4 Relationship between root-mean-square (rms), peak and average values for a sinusoidal signal. From Waldron (1989).

$$R_2 - R_1 = K \ln \frac{S_2}{S_1} \qquad (9.9)$$

where K is the constant of proportionality.

The unit of response is chosen so that the constant of proportionality becomes unity when logarithms to the base 10 are used. These units are bels:

$$\text{Response (in bels)} = \log_{10} \frac{S_2}{S_1} \qquad (9.10)$$

This logarithmic scale has the property of 'compressing' the very wide stimulus range encountered in acoustics ($10^{-12}\,\text{W}\,\text{m}^{-2}$ up to $1\,\text{W}\,\text{m}^{-2}$) into more manageable figures. However, the bel is a rather large unit and decibels (dB) are more practicable. Hence:

$$\text{Change in dB} = 10 \log_{10} \frac{S_2}{S_1} \qquad (9.11)$$

It is important to realize that the decibel scale is a scale of comparison and can compare sound levels on either side of a wall, each end of a 'silencer' or a worker's hearing, with an accepted norm.

In noise measurement, S_1 is often given an agreed reference value so that noise level scales are produced. The most commonly encountered scales are listed below.

1 *Sound intensity level scale*:

$$\text{Reference intensity} = 10^{-12}\,\text{W}\,\text{m}^{-2}$$

$$\text{Sound intensity level} = 10 \log_{10} \left(\frac{I}{10^{-12}} \right) \quad (9.12)$$

where I is the intensity of interest ($\text{W}\,\text{m}^{-2}$).

2 *Sound power level scale*:

$$\text{Reference intensity} = 10^{-12}\,\text{W}$$

$$\text{Sound power level} = 10 \log_{10} \left(\frac{W}{10^{-12}} \right) \quad (9.13)$$

where W is the power of interest (W).

3 *Sound pressure level scale*. Since it is the square of the sound pressure of a wave that is proportional to its intensity, the sound pressure level (SPL) is defined as:

$$\text{SPL} = 10 \log_{10} \frac{p_{\text{rms}}^2}{p_{\text{ref}}^2} \qquad (9.14)$$

where p_{rms} is the sound pressure of interest. The reference pressure (p_{ref}) is chosen to correspond, in air, with the reference sound intensity (I_{ref}) of $10^{-12}\,\text{W}\,\text{m}^{-2}$ and ρc of 400 rayls, i.e.:

$$I_{\text{ref}} = \frac{p_{\text{ref}}^2}{400} \qquad (9.15)$$

therefore

$$p_{\text{ref}} = 2 \times 10^{-5}\,\text{N}\,\text{m}^{-2}$$

and

$$\text{SPL (dB)} = 20 \log_{10} \left(\frac{p_{\text{rms}}}{2 \times 10^{-5}} \right)$$

For sounds in air, the intensity level and sound pressure level are numerically equal.

Properties of the decibel scale

When more than one source of sound is encountered, combined sound level may be calculated by finding the total amount of sound intensity occurring, and calculating the new sound intensity level from that.

Equal source levels

Example: find the combined sound intensity level when two similar sources of 40 dB each are heard together:

$$40\,\text{dB} = 4\,\text{bels} = \log_{10} \left(\frac{I}{10^{-12}} \right) \quad (9.16)$$

where I is the sound intensity of each source.

$$\text{Total combined intensity} = 2I$$

therefore

$$\text{Combined intensity level} = 10 \log_{10} \left(\frac{2I}{10^{-12}} \right)$$

$$= 10 \log_{10} \left(\frac{2 \times 10^{-8}}{10^{-12}} \right)$$

$$= 10 \log_{10} 2 + 10 \log_{10} 10^4$$

$$= 3 + 40 = 43\,\text{dB}$$

This doubling of intensity will always give an extra 3 dB. If three similar sources are combined, the combined level will be almost 5 dB (i.e. $10 \log_{10} 3$) above the individual levels; four sources give an increase of 6 dB.

As a normal ear cannot distinguish a change of < 1 dB, even under ideal listening conditions, fractions of decibels are rarely used in practice.

Unequal source levels

The contribution of the lower level is quite small and so the increase will be < 3 dB.

Example: find the combined level when similar sounds of 60 dB and 70 dB are heard together:

$$60\,dB = 6 \text{ bels} \qquad 70\,dB = 7 \text{ bels}$$

$$= 10 \log_{10} \left(\frac{I_1}{10^{-12}} \right) \qquad = 10 \log_{10} \left(\frac{I_2}{10^{-12}} \right)$$

therefore

$$\frac{I_1}{10^{-12}} = 10^6 \text{ and } \frac{I_2}{10^{-12}} = 10^7 \qquad (9.17)$$

(NB: I_1 is only 10% of I_2)

$$\text{Combined intensity level} = 10 \log_{10} \left(\frac{I_1 + I_2}{10^{-12}} \right)$$

$$= 10 \log (10^6 + 10^7)$$
$$= 10 \log_{10} (10^7 \times 1.1)$$
$$= 70 + 0.4$$
$$= 70\,dB$$

(i.e. no increase on the higher level)

(This approximation is justified since the normal variation of even supposedly steady noise is always > 1 dB).

Since levels separated by 10 dB (or more) produce no significant increase on the higher level when combined, and identical levels give a 3 dB increase when combined, estimation of the combined levels of sounds separated by < 10 dB may be made mentally.

Example: find the combined level when similar sounds of 54 dB and 47 dB are heard together:

Over-estimate: 54 dB and 54 dB combine $\Rightarrow$ 57 dB
Under-estimate: 54 dB and 44 dB combine $\Rightarrow$ 54 dB
Combined level must be between 54 and 57 dB, say 55 dB (actually 54.8 dB).

Background noise

The total noise level existing in any location is made up of noise from many different sources. In a factory, for example, there will be a certain noise level when the plant is turned off. If this background noise level is > 10 dB below the plant noise level, the measured level will be that due to the plant. If the background noise level and plant noise levels are equal, the total level measured will be 3 dB greater. Since the background noise cannot be removed, the true level of the plant noise must be calculated from measurements of the background noise alone (i.e. with plant turned off) and the total level (i.e. with plant turned on).

Example: background noise alone $= 75$ dB and total level of plant and background $= 80$ dB:

$$75\,dB = 10 \log_{10} \left(\frac{I_b}{10^{-12}} \right)$$

$$\text{and } 80\,dB = 10 \log_{10} \left(\frac{I_b + I_p}{10^{-12}} \right) \qquad (9.18)$$

therefore

$$\frac{I_b}{10^{-12}} = 10^{7.5} \text{ and } \frac{I_b}{10^{-12}} + \frac{I_p}{10^{-12}} = 10^8$$

$$\text{Level of plant alone} = 10 \log_{10} \left(\frac{I_p}{10^{-12}} \right)$$

$$= 10 \log_{10} (10^8 - 10^{7.5})$$
$$= 78\,dB$$

where I_b is the intensity of background noise alone and I_p is the intensity of plant noise alone.

Loudness

The frequency response of the ear is not linear, the ear being the most sensitive to sounds in the $1-5$ kHz frequency range and particularly insensitive at low frequencies. Loudness is the subjective assessment of sound quantity and has a complex relationship with the sound pressure level actually presented to the ear. When the sound pressure levels of pure tones of different frequencies which are judged to be equal in loudness are plotted, these 'equal loudness curves' (Fig. 9.5) exhibit 'dips' at

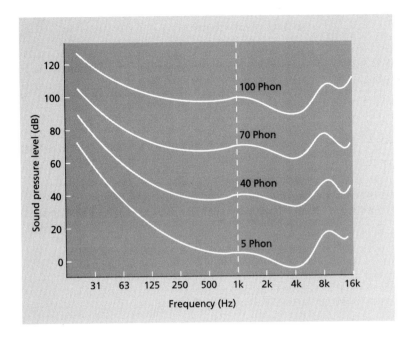

Fig. 9.5 Equal loudness curves for pure tones.

around 4 kHz and 12 kHz which are due to one-quarter and three-quarter wave resonance in the ear canal. Furthermore, these equal loudness curves are not parallel, the ear's response becoming more linear as the level increases. Since loudness level depends on frequency and sound pressure level, a new scale was introduced to facilitate comparisons of loudness level. Sounds which are equal in loudness level are assigned the same numerical value of phons. Hence, all points on any one curve bear the same value in phons taken as numerically equal to the number of decibels the curve possesses at 1 kHz. A doubling of loudness occurs when the loudness level increases by 10 phon.

Frequency analysis

Since the perception of sounds depends on level and frequency, a full investigation of noise must include the measurement of the sound pressure level of each frequency present. This would be an arduous task if the total frequency range were to be covered. Since the ear is fairly insensitive to low and very high frequencies, a reduced range is acceptable in nearly all cases (a range of 45 Hz to 11 200 Hz is most common).

Even in this reduced range, single frequency measurements would be time-consuming and so

this range is divided into eight frequency groups (or bands), and the total number of decibels in each group is measured. Each band is one octave wide, the upper frequency of the octave band being twice the lower frequency, and the geometric mean frequency being taken as the octave band's 'label'. This can be shown as: $f_2 = 2f_1$, where f_1 and f_2 are the lower and upper band limits and $(f_0)^2 = (f_1 \times f_2)$ for the centre or mean frequency. International agreements have produced 'preferred octave bands' which have mean frequencies of 63, 125, 250, 500, 1k, 2k, 4k and 8k Hz.

Octave band analysis is useful in gaining a quick guide to the frequency distribution of the noise, but, as Fig. 9.6 demonstrates, much detail is lost, and the lower levels contribute little to the total level in each band (because of the properties of the logarithmic scale). Less detail is lost if one-third-octave bands are used (upper frequency = $2\frac{1}{3} \times$ lower frequency), and $\frac{1}{3}$-octave band levels combine to give the octave band level. Therefore $\frac{1}{3}$-octave band levels are always less than the octave band level. Figure 9.7 shows the improved detail given by $\frac{1}{3}$-octave band analysis.

INSTRUMENTATION

A wide variety of sound level meters are avail-

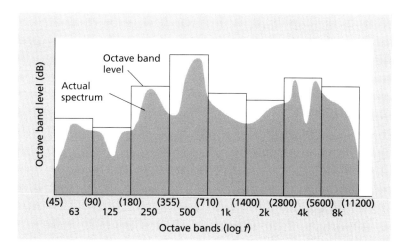

Fig. 9.6 Frequency analysis of a noise, showing octave band levels.

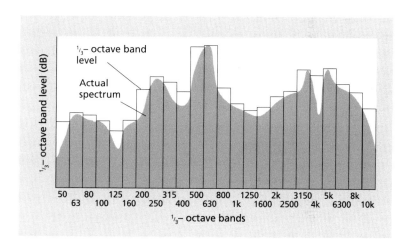

Fig. 9.7 Comparison of octave and $\frac{1}{3}$-octave band analysis.

able which have different facilities and levels of accuracy and precision. In the UK, four grades of intergrating sound level meters are specified in BS 6698 (IEC 804). Clearly the equipment selected should be suitable and sufficient to enable the assessment of interest to be successfully completed. The characteristics of the four types of meter are given in Table 9.1.

Early attempts to give the sound level meter a similar frequency response to that of the ear resulted in the weighting networks A, B and C. These were based on the ear's response at 40, 70 and 100 phon. Their relative response is shown in Fig. 9.8. When the A, B and C networks are used, the meter readings are quoted as dB(A), dB(B) and dB(C) respectively. This extra complication was

found unhelpful and the B and C weighting networks have fallen from general use. The dB(A) scale has been shown to have certain unexpected advantages when assessing the nuisance value of a noise, and remains in common use (see Table 9.2). Additional weighting networks D and E have been added: D is used for aircraft noise only and E is another attempt at a loudness level measurement.

Estimation of dB(A) level from octave band levels

The corrections given in Table 9.3 are applied to the respective octave band levels, and the total level in dB(A) is found by combining the eight corrected band levels.

Table 9.1 Characteristics of meter types

BS/IEC grade	Typical use	Amplitude range on a single setting	Typical overall accuracy	Comment
0	Lab reference	70 dB	±0.5 dB	
1	Lab and field	60 dB	±1.0 dB	
2	General field	50 dB	±1.5 dB	Lacks accuracy if significant component of noise above 10 kHz
3	Field survey	50 dB	±3.0 dB	Lacks accuracy if significant component of noise above 6 kHz

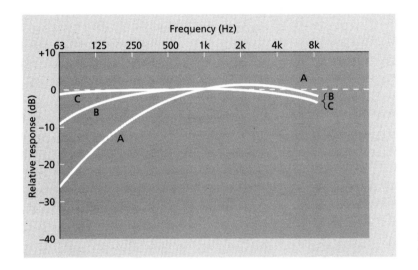

Fig. 9.8 Relative responses of the weighting networks.

Table 9.2 Typical levels in dB(A) of a range of common noise

Type of noise	Typical level in dB(A)
Jet at 30 m	140
Riveting, grinding metals at 1 m	120
Pop group	110
Machine shop with heavy plant	90
City traffic	80
Typing pool	55
Quiet office	40
Countryside at night	20

Measurement of fluctuating levels

Because noises are rarely steady or regularly fluctuating, methods of assigning numerical values to them have been devised and are being constantly reviewed.

Equivalent continuous sound level (L_{eq})

This is the notional steady level that would have emitted the same 'A' weighted sound energy over the same time as the actual noise, i.e.:

Table 9.3 Octave band corrections for 'A' weighting

Octave band mid-frequency	63	125	250	500	1k	2k	4k	8k	Hz
Correction	−26	−16	−9	−3	0	+1	+1	−1	dB

$$L_{eq} = 10 \log_{10} \frac{1}{T} \int_0^T \left(\frac{p_A}{2 \times 10^{-5}} \right)^2 dt \quad (9.19)$$

where T is measurement time and p_A is the instantaneous 'A' weighted acoustic pressure in pascals in the undisturbed field in air at atmospheric pressure.

Since a doubling of sound energy increases the level by 3 dB, and a tenfold increase raises the level by 10 dB, noise which is nominally 90 dB(A) for 4 h and 70 dB(A) for 4 h will not produce an L_{eq} of 80 dB(A). In this case:

$$\text{Average energy} = \left[\frac{(4 \times 100\text{-fold}) + (4 \times 1)}{8} \right]$$
$$= \frac{404}{8} \quad (9.20)$$

therefore giving a 50.5-fold increase on an energy content of 70 dB(A), which is equivalent to 87 dB(A). Thus the L_{eq} is more dependent on the higher levels occurring in the measurement period.

When the duration of work and measurement T (see Equation 9.19) are 8 h (28 800 s), in the UK the L_{eq} is called the 'daily personal noise exposure' ($L_{EP,d}$). It is this measure of noise exposure that is required for comparison with the first two action levels of 85 and 90 dB(A). Where more sophisticated equipment is not available, it is possible to calculate an $L_{EP,d}$ by use of the following formulae:

$$f = \frac{t}{8} \text{ antilog } [0.1 (L-90)] \quad (9.21)$$

and

$$L_{EP,d} = \frac{\log f_{tot}}{0.1} + 90 \text{ dB(A)}$$

where t is the exposure to sound level L (in hours) and f_{tot} is the total value of fractional exposure f over the working day. However, a more simple means is by the use of a nomogram (Fig. 9.9), as is highlighted by the two following examples. When there is only one significant level of noise during the day the value of $L_{EP,d}$ can be obtained from the nomogram in Fig. 9.9. By drawing a straight line connecting the measured level on the L scale with the exposure duration on the t scale, $L_{EP,d}$ can be read at the point of intersection with the centre scale.

Example: a person is exposed to a sound level of 102 dB(A) for $2\frac{1}{4}$ h per day. During the rest of the day the level is below 75 dB(A) which may be ignored. From Fig. 9.9, $L_{EP,d} = 96$ dB(A) (rounded to the next higher decibel).

When periods of exposure at more than one level are significant, the exposure at each level can be converted to a value of 'fractional exposure' (f) using the nomogram in Fig. 9.9. The values of 'f' received during one day should be added together, and the total value of f converted to $L_{EP,d}$ using the centre scale of the nomogram.

Example: a person is exposed to the pattern of sound in the first two columns of the table below. The third column shows the corresponding values of f which are added together and converted to $L_{EP,d}$.

Sound level dB(A)	Duration of exposure	f (from Fig. 9.9)
114	10 min	5.2
105	45 min	3.0
92	10 h	2.0
	Total:	10.0

From Fig. 9.9, $L_{EP,d} = 100$ dB(A) (to the nearest decibel).

Weekly average noise exposure

The weekly average of an employee's daily personal noise exposure ($L_{EP,w}$) can be calculated from the following formula and is expressed in dB(A):

$$L_{EP,w} = 10 \log_{10} \left[\frac{1}{5} \sum_{k=1}^{k=m} 10^{0.1 \, (L_{EP,d})_k} \right] \quad (9.22)$$

where $(L_{EP,d})_k$ is the $L_{EP,d}$ value for each of m working days of the week.

Single event noise exposure level (L_{AX})

At present this is used for single, short events and is also based on energy. The L_{AX} is the level which, if it lasted for 1 s, would have emitted the same energy as the actual event. In practice, the time of

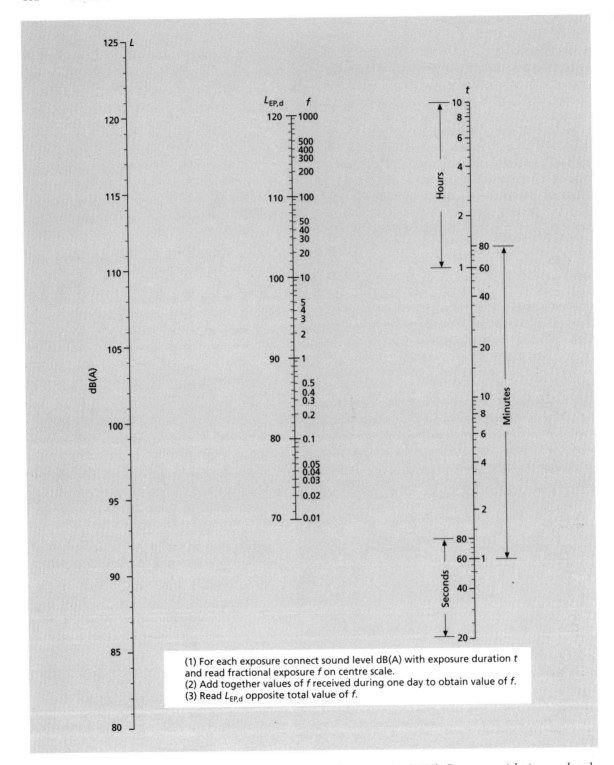

Fig. 9.9 Nomogram for calculation of $L_{EP,d}$. From Health and Safety Executive (1990). Crown copyright is reproduced with the permission of the Controller of HMSO.

the actual event is taken as the time for which the level is within 10 dB of its maximum.

$$L_{AX} = 10 \log_{10} \int_{t_1}^{t_2} \left(\frac{p_{(A)}}{2 \times 10^{-5}} \right)^2 dt \quad (9.23)$$

where t_1 and t_2 define the time interval (in seconds) in which the level remains within 10 dB of its maximum.

Since L_{eq} and L_{AX} use the same concept over different times, they may be related:

$$L_{eq} = 10 \log_{10} \frac{1}{T} \sum_{i=1}^{N} 10 \left(L_{AXi}/10 \right) \quad (9.24)$$

where N is the number of events in time T.

Statistical levels (L_n)

Statistical levels are used to assess the variation of level with time. Consider the noise 'history' shown in Fig. 9.10. It can be seen that 70 dB(A) was exceeded on two occasions during the 20 s of the measurement: firstly for $\frac{1}{2}$ s; secondly for $1\frac{1}{2}$ s, i.e. 70 dB(A) was exceeded for $(\frac{1}{2} + 1\frac{1}{2})/20$ of the time, i.e. 10%. For this noise history 70 dB(A) is the 'ten per cent level' (L_{10}): the level exceeded for 10% of the time. The L_{10} is a useful measure as it provides a well-defined 'near peak' evaluation of a varying noise level. Other percentages can also be used, such as the L_{90} which is a well-defined 'near background' level (45 dB(A) in Fig. 9.10).

In 1969, the USA became the first country in the western world to introduce industrial noise regu-lations, setting a limit of 90 dB(A), but measured with a simple sound level meter (slow response), for an 8 h daily exposure. In 1971, this limit was incorporated with the Occupational Health and Safety Act, and defined as '100% Noise Dose'. In 1972, the Department of Employment in the UK settled on a limit of 90 dB(A) for an 8 h daily ex-posure and published the 'Code of Practice for Reducing the Exposure of Employed Persons to Noise'. This has subsequently been updated by the Noise at Work Regulations 1989, in which the three action levels of 85 and 90 dB(A) (as $L_{EP,d}$ values) and 200 pascals (140 dB or 20 µPa) (as a peak sound pressure) have been set.

The British approach to the problem of noise fluctuation was to employ the equal energy con-cept of the L_{eq} of either 85 or 90 dB(A) for 8 h per day, subject to a maximum level of 140 dB (fast response) for unprotected ears. By contrast, the Occupational Safety and Health Act (OSHA) of the USA allows an increase of 5 dB for a halving expo-sure duration up to a maximum of 115 dB(A). This relationship makes an allowance for the recovery of temporary threshold shift (TTS) during the periods of less intense noise when exposure time has been reduced.

Noise dose may be defined for both countries as:

$$\text{Noise dose} = 100 \int_{0}^{T/8} \left(\frac{p_{(t)}}{0.632} \right)^n dt \; \% \quad (9.25)$$

where $p_{(t)}$ is the A weighted varying sound pressure (N m^{-2}), 0.632 N m^{-2} corresponds to 90 dB(A), T is

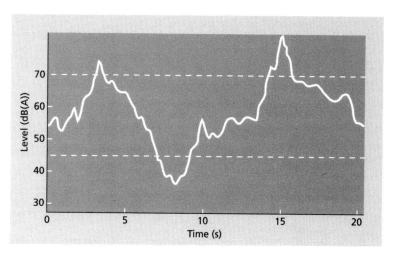

Fig. 9.10 History of a fluctuating noise.

the measurement duration (in hours) and n takes the value 2 in the UK (and most of Europe) and 1.2 in the USA. Comparison of 100% dose for different exposures is given in Table 9.4.

Noise dosemeter (dosimeter)

If workers experience many different levels during their shifts, their noise dose calculations can only be achieved accurately by means of an instrument capable of measuring the L_{eq} over the whole shift. Personal noise dosemeters are convenient as they fit into the worker's pocket, and the read-out (depending on type) is directly in percentage dose, L_{eq}, max peak, $Pa^2 h$, etc.

Guidance for the UK Noise at Work Regulations recommends that measurement should be made in the 'undisturbed field', however, results are unlikely to be significantly affected by reflections if the microphone is kept at least 4 cm away from the operator and most dosemeter microphones are provided with a clip to hold them onto the brim of a safety helmet or overall lapel (Fig. 9.11). The microphone should also be placed on the side of the subject likely to receive most noise. Thus the microphone receives the same sound pressure as the worker's ear, which the dosemeter 'A weights' and then, after squaring (or in the USA raising to 1.2th power), totals over the measurement period, and displays as the noise dose.

The advantage in using the concept of noise dose is that the 'usual rules' of arithmetic apply, the

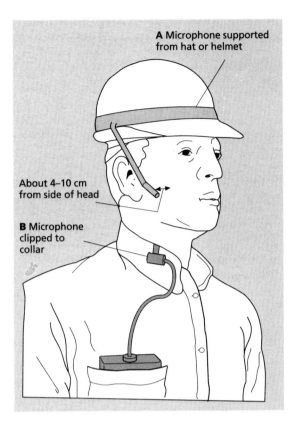

Fig. 9.11 Location of microphone for dosemeters. A, head-mounted microphone; B, collar- or shoulder-mounted microphone. From Health and Safety Executive (1990). Crown copyright is reproduced with the permission of the Controller of HMSO.

maximum permitted in one shift being always 100%. For example, if a worker receives 60% of the dose in the first 2 h, he/she may only receive 40% during the remaining 6 h. He/she must therefore be moved to a location with a lower L_{eq}. This may be calculated as follows:

$$40\% \text{ in } 6\,h = \frac{40}{6}\,\% \text{ per h}$$

$$= \left(\frac{40}{6} \times 8\right)\% \text{ in } 8\,h \quad (9.26)$$

$$= 53\tfrac{1}{3} \simeq 50\%$$

Thus, the new L_{eq} (to give a noise dose of 50% in 8 h):

$$= 87\,dB(A) \text{ in the UK}$$
$$(85\,dB(A) \text{ in the USA})$$

Table 9.4 Comparison of duration and levels in the UK and USA for 100% dose at 90 dB(A) over 8 h

Exposure permitted (h day^{-1})	UK L_{eq} (dB(A))	OSHA dB(A) (slow)	
8	90	90	
4	93	95	
2	96	100	
1	99	105	
$\frac{1}{2}$	102	110	
$\frac{1}{4}$	105	115	
$\frac{1}{8}$	108	115	
$\frac{1}{16}$	111	115	max
$\frac{1}{32}$	114	115	
$\frac{1}{64}$	117	115	

Such a relocation of a worker would call upon good industrial relations within the organization.

Aural comfort

Various criteria have evolved to provide guidance on acceptable maximum background noise levels in different situations. In general, the quieter the activity, the lower the acceptable background level. Low-frequency sounds are less well heard and so their acceptable levels are greater than higher frequency sounds which the ear detects readily.

Noise criteria curves (NC)

In the 1950s, research in the USA determined the maximum levels in the eight octave bands (63 Hz–8 kHz) that caused minimal interference with two women conversing on the telephone. As a result, curves numbered from 15 to 70 (the octave band sound level at 1 kHz) were produced for use in the office environment. These were known as noise criteria (NC) curves (Fig. 9.12). The background noise in an environment is measured in decibels (linear) and the intensities at each octave band plotted on the graph. The NC rating for that environment is taken as the number of the curve above the highest value.

A number of different environments have been assigned NC values and these are given below. For example, the NC for a typing pool is 45 and therefore background noise levels measured in the office of interest in excess of this value are too noisy.

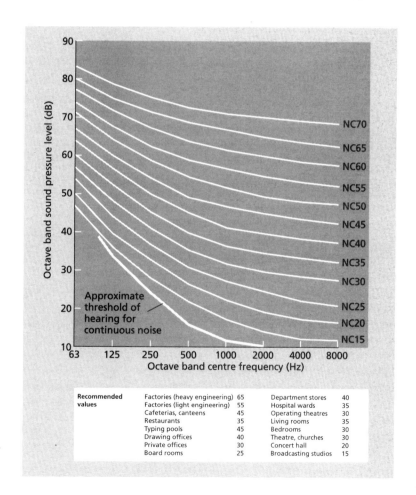

Fig. 9.12 Noise criteria (NC) curves and recommended values showing NC 30 for a private office.

Recommended values				
	Factories (heavy engineering)	65	Department stores	40
	Factories (light engineering)	55	Hospital wards	35
	Cafeterias, canteens	45	Operating theatres	30
	Restaurants	35	Living rooms	35
	Typing pools	45	Bedrooms	30
	Drawing offices	40	Theatre, churches	30
	Private offices	30	Concert hall	20
	Board rooms	25	Broadcasting studios	15

Noise rating curves (NR)

This method uses the same concept as the NC system, but the curves are based on the results of a large-scale survey of the reaction of the community to noise and as a result have a much wider range (0–135) than the NC curves. The rating of rooms in dwellings involves the corrections shown in the table of Fig. 9.13. For example, a living room (NR 30) in a residential urban area (+5) suffering an impulsive noise (−5) for 6% of the time (+10) would be assessed at NR (30 + 5 − 5 + 10) = NR (40), i.e. the background noise may rise to NR 40 when the impulsive noise is present without conditions becoming unacceptable. Existing background noises may be assigned NR values as with NC curves.

The main advantage of using criteria which utilize data from octave band analysis, such as these two (NR and NC), is that by comparison with these curves the frequencies of most concern are easily identified. A dB(A) value, on the other hand, has incorporated this frequency.

Noise and materials

Materials reflect, absorb and transmit sound, the proportions depending on the material and the frequency of the sound (Fig. 9.14).

The *absorption coefficient* (α) is defined as:

$$\frac{\text{Intensity of sound reflected by material}}{\text{Intensity of sound incident on same area of material}}$$

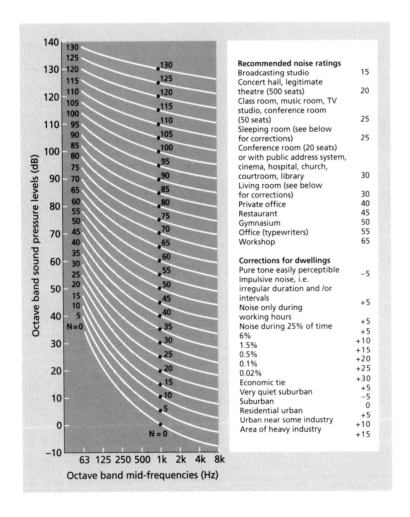

Recommended noise ratings

Broadcasting studio	15
Concert hall, legitimate theatre (500 seats)	20
Class room, music room, TV studio, conference room (50 seats)	25
Sleeping room (see below for corrections)	25
Conference room (20 seats) or with public address system, cinema, hospital, church, courtroom, library	30
Living room (see below for corrections)	30
Private office	40
Restaurant	45
Gymnasium	50
Office (typewriters)	55
Workshop	65

Corrections for dwellings

Pure tone easily perceptible	−5
Impulsive noise, i.e. irregular duration and /or intervals	+5
Noise only during working hours	+5
Noise during 25% of time	+5
6%	+10
1.5%	+15
0.5%	+20
0.1%	+25
0.02%	+30
Economic tie	+5
Very quiet suburban	−5
Suburban	0
Residential urban	+5
Urban near some industry	+10
Area of heavy industry	+15

Fig. 9.13 Noise rating curves and recommended values.

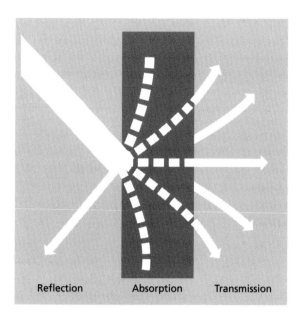

Fig. 9.14 Diagrammatic representation of reflection, absorption and transmission.

The *reflection coefficient* (r) is defined as:

$$\frac{\text{Intensity of sound absorbed by material}}{\text{Intensity of sound incident on same area of material}}$$

The *transmission coefficient* (τ) is defined as:

$$\frac{\text{Intensity of sound transmitted by material}}{\text{Intensity of sound incident on same area of material}}$$

It follows that $r + \alpha + \tau = 1$.

For many materials in practical use τ is very much smaller than α or r, and so in some situations it is convenient to take $\alpha + r = 1$. Such a situation is met in the consideration of the growth and decay of sound in an enclosure where the very small amount transmitted through the walls has an insignificant effect.

Absorption coefficient

Absorption is really the conversion of sound into other forms of energy. Materials which absorb sound may be classified into three categories.
1 Porous materials: sound enters the pores and the viscous forces so generated lead to heat production.

2 Non-porous panels: sound energy is converted into vibrational (i.e. mechanical) energy.
3 Perforated materials: the perforations act as cavity resonators, absorbing narrow bands of frequency.
An idealized summary of the behaviour of these materials is given in Fig. 9.15.

Though in theory α can never exceed unity, standard measurement methods can arrive at values in excess of 1. These procedures calculated α on a projected surface area, and should the material be made up into a non-plane shape its active area will be greater than that used in the calculation, giving α a value greater than unity.

Transmission coefficient

The transmission coefficient depends on the material's density and thickness and the frequency of the sound being transmitted. Mention has already been made of the small value of τ usually encountered ($\tau \approx 0.0001$ at 500 Hz for a brick wall). It is more convenient to express transmission quantities in terms of a transmission loss (TL), defined as:

$$TL = 10 \log_{10} \frac{1}{\tau} \text{ dB} \qquad (9.27)$$

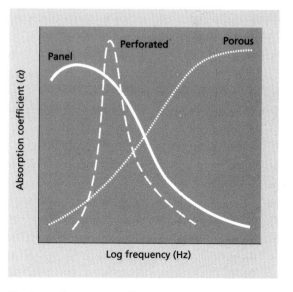

Fig. 9.15 Absorption coefficient variation with frequency.

So, for the brick wall:

$$TL = 10 \log_{10} \frac{1}{0.0001}$$

$$= 40\,dB$$

Sound insulation

Figure 9.16 shows the general behaviour of partitions used in buildings. For the lowest frequencies, the behaviour of the partition depends mainly on its edge fixing and stiffness; the TL falls as the frequency increases. For the highest frequencies, the behaviour depends on wavelengths, there being certain frequencies where the wavelength in air corresponds exactly with the wavelength of the bending wave set up in the flexing wall. When such coincidences occur there is little energy lost and so the TL is low. Above and below these critical frequencies the TL remains high.

In the intermediate frequency range, the mass per unit area of the partition is the controlling quantity, the behaviour of the partition obeying the Mass law as a first approximation. This states:

$$TL = 20 \log_{10} mf - 43\,dB \qquad (9.28)$$

where m is the mass per unit area of wall (= density × thickness) and f is the frequency of the sound. Actual partitions vary greatly from this general picture. It is imperative that measurements made on 'real' partitions should cover the required frequency range (usually 100–3150 Hz) in some detail (at least $\frac{1}{3}$-octave bands). Trade literature often quotes single, averaged, figures for the TL of a product. This should be used only as a guide because of the large variations occurring over the frequency range.

Composite partitions

Where more than one material is used in a wall, the average transmission loss for the composite partition may be found by calculating the area-weighted average transmission coefficient (τ_{av}):

$$\tau_{av} = \frac{\sum\limits_{i=1}^{N} \tau_i S_i}{\sum\limits_{i=1}^{N} S_i} \qquad (9.29)$$

where S_i is the area of the ith material in the partition.

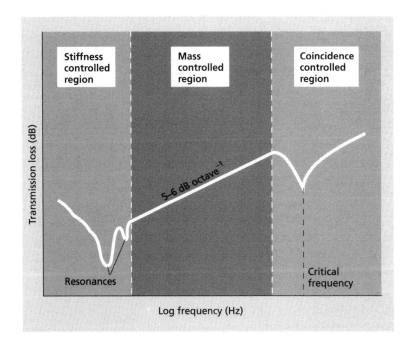

Fig. 9.16 Generalized variation of transmission loss of a typical building partition with frequency.

Thence:

$$TL_{av} = 10 \log_{10} \frac{1}{\tau_{av}} \qquad (9.30)$$

This method gives a good estimate when the sound fields on each side of the partition are diffuse. Air gaps are classed as a material making up the partition having a TL equal to 0 dB (i.e. $\tau = 1$). Their effect on TL_{av} is marked, a small air gap reducing the insulation value of a wall considerably.

Sound in enclosed spaces

The total sound field produced in an enclosed space has two components (Fig. 9.17).

1 The direct sound field: which travels from source to listener by the shortest route without encountering any room surface.

2 The reverberant sound field: which reaches the listener after at least one reflection from a room surface.

The size of the direct field depends on the acoustic power of the source, the distance between the source and the listener and the position of the source in the space (which affects the directionality of the source). The size of the reverberant component depends on the amount of sound reflected at each reflecting surface and the number of reflections that each individual sound wave undergoes before reaching the listener. This is found to depend on the area-weighted average absorption coefficient $(\bar{\alpha})$ and the room's surface area (S):

$$\bar{\alpha} = \frac{\sum\limits_{i=1}^{N} S_i \alpha_i}{\sum\limits_{i=1}^{N} S_i} \qquad (9.31)$$

where S_i is the surface area of the ith material and α_i is the respective absorption coefficient.

The reverberant component does not vary greatly over a given room, whereas the direct sound component for a point source varies inversely with the square of the distance from the source. Therefore, near the source, where the direct component dominates, the total sound field falls rapidly as the distance increases, becoming constant in the far field where the field is predominantly reverberant (Fig. 9.18).

It may be shown that the sound pressure level (SPL) at a point in a room is related to the acoustic power of the source by the following expression:

$$SPL = L_w + 10 \log_{10} \left(\frac{Q}{4\pi d^2} + \frac{4(1 - \bar{\alpha})}{S\bar{\alpha}} \right) \qquad (9.32)$$

where L_w is acoustic power (W), Q is a directivity factor, d is the distance from the source (m), S is the total surface area of the room and $\bar{\alpha}$ is an area-

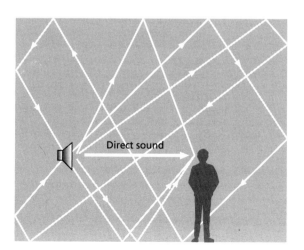

Fig. 9.17 Distribution of sound in an enclosed space.

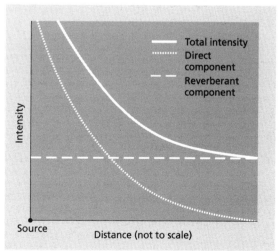

Fig. 9.18 Contribution of direct and reverberant sound to total field.

weighted average absorption coefficient. Readings of sound pressure levels taken near the source greatly depend on the position of the microphone. It is good practice to make these measurements at least 1 m from the source where the variation in level is not so large.

Reverberation time

Since the velocity of sound is finite, reverberation components arrive at different times, following the direct component. Thus, the total sound field does not start and stop but grows and decays. The time taken for a total sound decay of 60 dB is known as the reverberation time, and is a useful guide to the acoustic quality of a room (Fig. 9.19).

Work by Sabine has shown that the reverberation time (RT) of a room of moderate absorption is given by:

$$RT = \frac{0.16\,V}{A} \text{ seconds} \qquad (9.33)$$

and

$$A = \sum_{i=1}^{N} S_i \alpha_i$$

where V is the room volume (m^3). Since the absorption coefficients vary with frequency, the rever-

beration time also varies across the frequency range.

Sabine's formula may be used to estimate the reverberation times of a planned room and to calculate the change in absorption necessary to comply with the recommended optimal values. The optimum reverberation time depends on the volume of the room and the activity taking place. Such values are based on subjective judgements and are available in chart or tabular form.

Doubling the absorption in a room will halve its reverberation time, and the reverberant component of the total field. Therefore the noise level in a room will fall by about 3 dB in the far field if the room absorption is doubled.

Measurement of hearing

The most commonly used assessment of hearing is the determination of the threshold of audibility. This is the level of sound required to be just audible. It is not absolutely fixed for the individual but seems to vary over a range of 2−6 dB from day to day, and from determination to determination. In practice it is necessary to take the threshold as the level which is just heard 50% of the times for which it is presented.

In addition, further variations occur if the test sounds are presented from above or below the

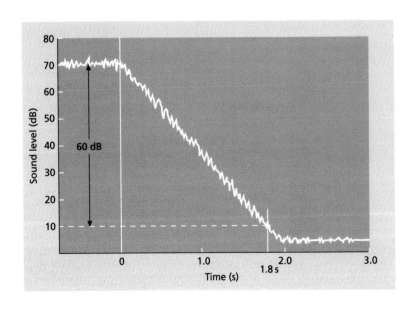

Fig. 9.19 Reverberation time. From Waldron (1989).

threshold range. The 'descending threshold' is found by presenting the higher levels first; the 'ascending threshold' is reached by beginning with levels below the threshold range and increasing them until the sounds are just heard. Because of these variations, 5 dB steps of level are used in practical audiometry, the likely variation being smaller than the step.

Standard hearing

In 1952, two groups of workers (at the National Physical Laboratory and the Central Medical Establishment, RAF) tested a total of 1200 subjects, aged from 18 to 23 years. The subjects were screened for good general health and no otological history. Although the techniques employed in the threshold tests were slightly different, comparable results were obtained and became adopted in the 1954 British Standard. Two interesting facts emerged. Firstly, the spread of hearing threshold for these young, carefully screened volunteers was quite large, the standard deviation being at least 6 dB at all audiometric frequencies. Secondly, comparison with the US Standard (based on small samples) showed that the US Standard underestimated hearing acuity by some 10 dB.

Further investigations in other countries confirmed the British findings and in 1964 the ISO published 'Standard Reference Zeros for Pure Tone Audiometers' (ISO 389). In this Standard, standard hearing is assigned 0 dB hearing level (HL), and is referred to as the level generated by a headphone of agreed construction into an artificial ear (a 6 cm^3 cavity). This level has different values across the frequency range, but standard hearing is 0 dBHL at every frequency.

The pure tone audiometer

Pure tone signals are generated (usually 125, 250, 500, 1k, 2k, 3k, 4k, 6k and 8k Hz) which, after amplification, are passed to the headphone. With the hearing level control at 0 dBHL, the level of the signal is automatically adjusted at each frequency to be that required by the ISO standard reference zero. When the hearing level control is set to 50 dBHL, for example, 50 dB more than the reference zero emerges from the headphones at each frequency. Thus, the audiometer makes no attempt to present signals of equal loudness to the subject, as equal loudness increments are not identical at different frequencies.

The subject to be tested is comfortably seated and ears checked for absence of wax. The headphones are fitted, ensuring that the earphone orifice coincides with the ear canal. The subject is asked to indicate, by raising a finger or operating a signal lamp, when sounds are heard (no matter how faintly). Verbal communication should be discouraged once testing has begun. A general assessment of hearing will have already been made from casual conversation before the test, and a sufficiently high signal at 1 kHz for about 1 s is presented so that a confident response is made. This level is reduced in steps until the subject no longer responds. The threshold is then crossed by raising the signal until a response is made. Threshold is taken when the same level is just heard on three occasions.

The other frequencies are then tested and 1 kHz repeated as a check. If there is significant difference, the subject should be retested. The other ear is then tested. Results are conveniently recorded on an audiogram (Fig. 9.20). An experienced audiometrician will complete the test in about 15 min.

The demand for large-scale screening and monitoring by industry has greatly increased the use of the automatic audiometer. In this instrument the frequency is changed, and the hearing level control motor driven, automatically. The hearing level value is traced by a pen onto an audiogram. The subject is instructed to press a switch when they can hear the signal (which steadily reduces the signal) and to release the switch when the signal is no longer audible (which steadily increases the signal). In this way the threshold crossings are drawn out (Fig. 9.21). Simultaneous supervision of up to three machines is possible.

Test conditions

Careful listening is essential for these tests and so the subject must be placed in a very quiet environment. The headphones give some attenuation at middle and high frequencies which can be increased by the provision of hemispherical shells fitting

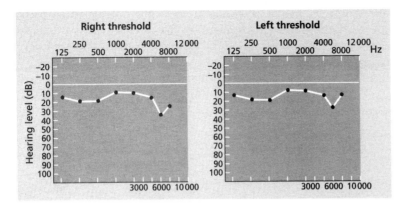

Fig. 9.20 Pure tone audiogram.

over each earphone. Better protection is given by purpose-built test booths (or carefully designed rooms). Such quiet conditions are essential as many of those screened will have normal hearing. In order to test to −10 dBHL with an error not exceeding 2 dB, the background level at the ear should not exceed the octave band levels given in Table 9.5.

Limitations of audiometry

The primary objective of legislation specific to noise is that it should prevent or reduce the incidence of noise-induced hearing loss (NIHL) rather than the simple reduction of noise exposure *per se*. It is therefore implicit that employers should

assess the hearing levels of their workforce in order to identify those that require additional protection. Audiometry should be able to accurately measure the hearing of an industrial population from 16 to at least 65 years old and to be able to reliably detect small changes over time.

The 'audiometric zero' is set at the mode hearing level of young, non-noise-exposed, otologically normal people at each frequency (see earlier section 'standard hearing'). It therefore follows that a number of the younger population will have hearing levels markedly better than audiometric zero. Individuals with the most sensitive hearing (in the top 5% of the population) will have hearing levels ranging between −8 dB at 500 Hz and 1 kHz to

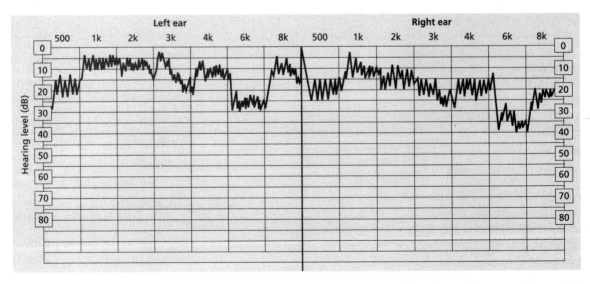

Fig. 9.21 Audiogram from an automatic (self-recording) audiometer. The threshold is taken as the mean of the peaks' average and valleys' average.

Table 9.5 Maximum allowable noise levels for audiometry: (a) at ear, for measurements down to −10 dBHL with error not exceeding 2 dB (no headphones); (b) in booth if MX41/AR cushions are used with audiometer headphones

(a)									
Octave band mid-frequency	63	125	250	500	1k	2k	4k	8k	Hz
Maximum noise at ear	61	46	31	7	1	4	6	9	dB
(b)									
Octave band mid-frequency	63	125	250	500	1k	2k	4k	8k	Hz
Maximum noise in booth	62	48	36	14	16	29	37	32	dB

−14 dB at 8 kHz (manual audiometer), with the data about 3 dB better if conducted on an automatic selfrecording audiometer. In addition, the audiogram will range by about 5 dB above and below the mean level. As it is desirable for the audiometer to present inaudible sounds to each individual, it should range down to −20 dB at 500 Hz and 1 kHz to −25 dB at 8 kHz.

In the main, audiometry only measures hearing levels down to −5 dB (as it is assumed that these are 'normal people'), however, if an individual with a true hearing level of −15 dB was tested it would simply be recorded as −5 dB. If that individual was exposed to noise, conventional audiometry would only facilitate the identification of hearing loss when it had degraded to worse than 0 dB. This would appear as a degradation of 5 dB but in reality would be ≥ 15 dB, thereby failing to identify a susceptible individual. Improvements in audiometers would also necessitate that the facilities in which these tests are carried out would have to be at least 10 dB quieter than is currently recommended.

It has been reported that the 10% of the population most susceptible to NIHL, when exposed to $L_{EP,d}$ of 90 dB(A), could be expected to exhibit hearing level changes at 4 kHz of 13 dB over a five year period (Robinson, 1987). It would therefore not be unreasonable if audiometry were to be able to detect a change in hearing half this value − a suggested objective is to be reliably able to detect a 5 dB change. However, to be able to detect a 5 dB change over time the resolution of each audiogram must be to less than 2.5 dB. Conventional audiometry is only able to resolve to '5 dB at best' (Department of Health and Social Security, 1982).

The accuracy of audiometry can be affected by three main factors: technical limitations; the

'learning' effect; and fit of the headphones. There are two characteristics of self-recording audiometers which could affect resolution, these being step width and the calculation of the mean hearing levels at each frequency. Step widths are usually 2.5 dB, but to achieve this with any resolution step widths should not exceed 1−1.5 dB and many audiometers have computers which indicate mean hearing level at each frequency but round-off to the nearest 2.5 dB!

The learning effect is where the examinee becomes more proficient over the period of the test, with the result that the ear first tested is worse than the second. Some audiometers re-test the first ear and significant differences between the first and second test of the same ear are indicative of this effect. The magnitude of this effect could be as much as 2.5 dB.

Audiometry is known not to be very repeatable (the very criteria you need and want) (Department of Health and Social Security, 1982) and this may be partly due to headphone location. It has been recommended that at least two tests are conducted (without removal of the headphones) until the difference between tests is ≤ 2 dB.

Further tests

Headphone stimulation tests the complete auditory pathway, from canal to brain, and malfunction in any part of the pathway will give an elevated hearing level indicating a hearing loss. Such losses are classified into:

1 conductive losses, due to malfunction in the outer and middle ear; and

2 sensorineural losses, due to malfunction in the inner ear and auditory nerve.

To isolate the loss caused by sensorineural deafness, the cochlea is stimulated by vibrating the skull with a small electromagnetic vibrator applied to the mastoid area. The pure tone audiometer is calibrated so that the thresholds obtained for a normally hearing subject are numerically equal for both headphone and vibrator tests. A difference between hearing levels for headphone (air-conduction) and vibrator (bone-conduction) tests indicates a conductive loss.

One important complication is that the inter-aural attenuation by vibration stimulation is almost 9 dB — stimulating one ear also stimulates the other. The non-test ear must be sufficiently occupied with masking noise from a headphone so that the pure tone threshold determination of the test ear may be accomplished. Interaural attenuation for air-conducted sound is around 40 dB and so the masking noise does not interfere with the test ear unless it is too great. The correct amount to be used may be found by increasing the masking level in 10 dB steps until the test ear threshold is identical for three successive determinations. This need for masking has delayed the introduction of an automatic bone-conduction audiometer.

Pure tone manual and automatic audiometric tests are subjective in that they rely on the co-operation of the subject. If the subject is unable or unwilling to co-operate, objective tests are now available in some of the larger hospitals. One such method detects the electrical activity of the cortex (using small surface electrodes) at levels very near threshold even when the subject is asleep. This method has been used where there have been disputes over the amount of hearing present in a subject.

NOISE EXPOSURE AND HEALTH

The effects of excessive exposure to noise are discussed in detail in Chapter 5.

Noise immission level

A UK government-sponsored investigation using 1000 subjects has suggested that the amounts of threshold shift are related to the total noise exposure (dependent on the noise level and its duration). The actual shift in threshold, corrected for natural loss of acuity with age, was found to correlate well with the noise immission level (NIL), defined as:

$$NIL = L_A + 10 \log_{10} t \qquad (9.33)$$

where L_A is the level of noise in dB(A) (L_{eq} if noise fluctuates) and t is the number of years' duration.

Although industrial noises have many different spectra, the UK investigation found this to have no significant effect on the threshold shifts of those tested. The precise amount of shift varied considerably from subject to subject. The likely effect of various NILs on hearing is shown in Fig. 9.22. It will be noted that the maximum threshold shift occurs at 4 kHz, which is a characteristic of this noise-induced hearing loss (although some people exhibit their maximum shifts at 6 kHz). In the early stages of exposure the threshold shift diminishes after a few hours' rest. Increased exposure leads to increased shifts of which only part is recoverable with rest. The amount remaining after 40 h is termed a 'permanent threshold shift' (PTS), the recovered shift being termed a 'temporary threshold shift' (TTS). TTS recovery exhibits a 'bounce effect', shown in Fig. 9.23, being rapidly reduced in the first minute, and increasing in the second minute, of rest. Subsequent recovery tends to follow a logarithmic relationship with time. For consistency, TTSs are measured after 2 min of rest have elapsed (TTS_2).

Over many years of noise exposure the total loss increases and a greater proportion of it becomes permanent. Standard agreed amounts of presbycousis (see Chapter 5), based on large-scale tests, can be deducted from audiometric test results to estimate the amount of noise-induced hearing loss present.

Hearing conservation

The greatest noise level received by many in the course of their occupation are the levels encountered whilst travelling to and from work, rather than at work. For many people, the amount of NIHL accrued will depend on their leisure activities. However, very high noise levels are associated with many industries, and if the hearing of those employed there is to be conserved, exposure to

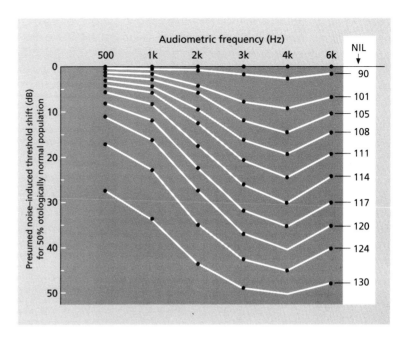

Fig. 9.22 Likely effects of noise immission levels (NILs) on hearing.

such noise must be controlled. It is necessary to decide upon a level of exposure which affords sufficient reduction for hearing conservation and, at the same time, is realistic. Too low a level at work does not prevent loss due to leisure activities, etc., and would cause grave engineering and economic problems.

NIHL affects those frequencies which are required for good speech reception (the information content of speech depending on the consonants which are high frequency). Small losses at these frequencies affect speech intelligibility insignificantly, and so a limited amount of NIHL at the end of a working life may be tolerated. If these amounts are restricted to < 15 dB at 4000 Hz, between 10 and 15 dB at 3000 Hz and < 10 dB at 500, 1000 and 2000 Hz, then it has been found that a NIL over 50 years of 105 dB will just meet this criterion for the majority of the working population. For a few individuals the losses will be greater with this exposure.

It is unlikely that the same conditions will occur for 50 years, and a NIL of 104 dB over 40 years will more adequately meet this criterion for most of the working population. A 40-year NIL of 104 dB implies an L_{eq} of 88 dBA, at home and at work. If levels at work are controlled to be < 88 dBA, then the conversation criterion will not be exceeded there. If a duration of 30 years is taken, a NIL of 105 is obtained with an L_{eq} of 90 dB(A). Such an increase has an insignificant effect on hearing conservation but a dramatic effect on noise control problems (a 2 dB change implies a sound intensity increase of 60%).

Control of noise exposure levels

As with the control of any overexposure in the work environment one must attempt to prevent rather than control exposure and if prevention or elimination is not possible then to descend

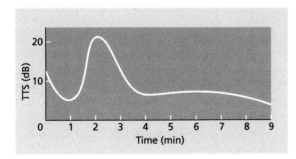

Fig. 9.23 The 'bounce effect'.

down the hierarchy of acceptable/effective control measures (see Chapter 21). Control of noise exposure provides the classic example of viewing the work environment in three distinct sections: source; transmission path; and receiver (Fig. 9.24).

Noise reduction at source

Since movement causes vibration which is passed on to the air particles and perceived as sound, minimization of movement in any process will achieve a measure of noise control at source. A number of methods of preventing noise generation are given below.

1 Substitution of a quieter process, i.e. welding not riveting.

2 Avoiding or cushioning of impacts.

3 Introduce or increase the amount of damping.

4 Reduction of turbulence of air exhausts and jets by silencers, either of the 'absorption' type where the attenuation (insertion loss) is achieved by a lining of absorbent material, or the 'expansion chamber' type where the insertion loss is achieved by acoustic mismatch between the volume of the chamber and inlet/outlet pipe (a number are now a hybrid of these two types).

5 Introduction of low-noise air nozzles and pneumatic ejectors.

6 Matching the pressure of the supplied air to the needs of the air-powered equipment.

7 Avoiding 'chapping' airstreams by rotating components.

8 Improved design of fans, fan casings, compressors etc.

9 Dynamic balancing of rotating parts.

10 The use of better quality control in design and manufacturing procedures to obviate the need for *post hoc* rectification.

11 Better machine maintenance.

12 Limit the duration for which a noisy machine or part of a machine is used.

Control of the transmission path

Having made every effort to control the noise exposure at the source, the next most appropriate course of action is to minimize the progress of the energy from the source to the receiver. A number of examples are given below.

1 Use of correctly chosen reflecting and absorbent barriers for the direct component.

2 Use of correctly chosen absorbent material on surrounding surfaces to minimize the reflected component.

3 Use of anti-vibration mountings under machines.

4 Enclosure of the source.

5 Provision of a noise refuge.

6 Increasing the distance between source and receiver:

  (a) segregation of noisy processes;

  (b) use of remote control;

  (c) use of flexible exhaust hoses to ensure the exhaust is discharged away from the operator(s).

7 Active noise control: where the addition of a second source with the same amplitude but with reversed phase causes destructive superposition.

Control of noise exposure for the receiver

Reduction of the time for which a worker is exposed

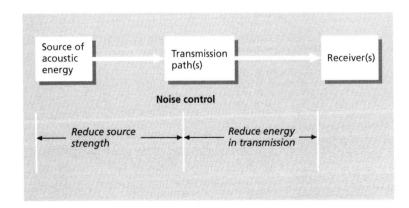

Fig. 9.24 Energy flow diagram.

to high levels of noise will achieve a lowering of their noise dose. However, a short period in a high level will increase the dose markedly, and no amount of time spent at lower levels can reduce this dose already received. Job rotation within shifts will also allow reduction in time spent in the higher level.

Work study of a task may show that the presence of a worker at their machine is unnecessary throughout the shift — machines may be minded as long as visual contact is maintained. The worker may mind their machine from within an acoustic enclosure possessing a viewing window. When they are required at the machine they may leave this refuge, wearing personal protection for these comparatively short periods.

Ear protection

Ear protection is rarely comfortable when worn for long periods. The isolation, perspiration and enclosed feeling experienced encourage its removal. Once removed, even for the shortest period, the majority of protection it affords is lost since the dose received from the higher level will be large.

Ear protection is, therefore, to be regarded as a last resort measure, emphasis being placed on the reduction of noise at its source and its transmission. There are a number of different types of personal protectors, a brief description of which are given below.

Earmuffs

These usually consist of hard plastic cups which surround the ears. A seal is made with the head by cushions filled with soft foam or a viscous liquid. A headband is used to retain the two cups in the correct position with the appropriate pressure.

Some earmuffs are designed to: emphasize the attenuation of certain frequencies; passively attenuate loud noises more than quiet sounds ('amplitude sensitive'); actively attenuate at certain intensities or frequencies by the use of electronics incorporated within the cup; detect the noise out-side the cup and then to generate (as far as possible) the same noise inside the cup but exactly out of phase which thereby cancels the incident noise.

Earplugs

Earplugs are designed to fit into the ear canal and are generally of three types: permanent, disposable and reusable. The permanent types are available in a variety of sizes and therefore care is needed in selection — if these are required then 'custom moulded' are better than 'universal fitting'. Disposable plugs are made from various compressible materials and if correctly fitted will fit most people. Reusable plugs require regular cleaning and replacement due to the degradation of the material over time.

Attenuation of earmuffs and earplugs

As the working population differs in terms of head size and shape, ear size and shape, etc. manufacturers quote a mean attenuation and, to provide a degree of uncertainty, its standard deviation. These data are generated by determining the level of hearing in each octave band of a group of subjects both with and without the protection. As it is better to 'fail-safe', a level of 'assumed protection' is calculated by subtraction of one standard deviation away from the mean in that octave band. However, this still may leave a proportion of the population under-protected and therefore it may be prudent to subtract two standard deviations (see Chapter 23).

Calculation of received noise level when ear protection is worn

The 'assumed protection' is subtracted from an octave band spectrum of the offending noise, 'A' weighted corrections are made in each band and the total 'A' weighted level calculated.

Example: a plant room containing a large compressor yields the following octave band analysis near the ear of the attendant:

Mid-frequency	63	125	250	500	1k	2k	4k	8k	Hz
SPL	104	98	95	87	84	80	78	72	dB

The total level in dB(A) may be found by correcting this spectrum using Table 9.3 and summation of the different intensities by use of Fig. 9.25 (see also section 'Properties of the decibel scale').

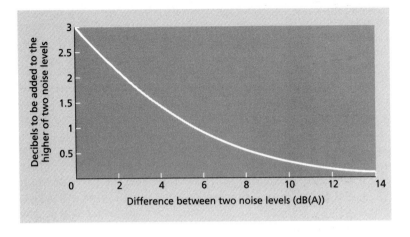

Fig. 9.25 Noise level addition chart.

Mid-frequency	63	125	250	500	1k	2k	4k	8k	Hz
SPL	104	98	95	87	84	80	78	72	dB
Correction	−26	−16	−9	−3	0	+1	+1	−1	dB
Corrected level	78	82	86	84	84	81	79	71	dB

```
        83          88          85          80
           89              86
              90 dB(A)
```

∴ Estimated level = 90 dB(A).

Tests on the earmuff to be worn give the following results:

Mid-frequency	63	125	250	500	1k	2k	4k	8k	Hz
Mean attenuation	—	15	19	25	28	39	46	43	dB
Standard deviation	—	1.5	2	2.1	1.7	1.7	1.5	2.6	dB
Assumed protection	0	13.5	17	22.9	26.3	37.3	44.5	40.4	dB

Therefore, received 'A' weighted levels with earmuff are:

Mid-frequency	63	125	250	500	1k	2k	4k	8k	Hz
Corrected level	78	82	86	84	84	81	79	71	dB
Assumed protection	0	13.5	17	22.9	26.3	37.3	44.5	40.4	dB
Received level	78	68.5	69	61.1	57.7	43.7	34.5	30.6	dB

```
        78          69          57.7        36
           78              58
              78 dB(A)
```

∴ Estimated received level with earmuffs = 78 dB(A).

Noise Survey Report

Name and Address of Premises ....

Date of Survey ....   Survey Conducted by ....

Equipment Used ....   Date of Last Calibration ....

Description of Workplace ....

Location	Number of Persons Exposed	Noise level (Leq)	Duration of Exposure	$L_{EP, d}$	Peak Pressure	Comments

Octave Band Data dB

Location	63 Hz	125 Hz	250 Hz	500 Hz	1 kHz	2 kHz	4 kHz	8 kHz

Sketch of Workplace

Signature ....

Date ....

Fig. 9.26 Sample noise survey report.

It will be noted that, as the calculations have been performed approximately, the results can only be estimates for a given individual.

Other tests on ear protection

Some countries have developed standard methods of testing the physical properties of ear protection: their behaviour in extremes of temperature, reaction to prolonged vibration and consistency of springiness of the headband of an earmuff. Such tests try to simulate the conditions that the device will encounter in the workplace, and indicate the likelihood of the ear protection retaining its initial fit and attenuation.

Survey report

As with all occupational hygiene survey work, the accurate documentation of sampling strategy issues (see Chapter 17) such as when, where, what was happening, etc., along with the actual results, should always be made at the time of the survey. This can be facilitated by the use of a record sheet. Although no single means of recording data would be suitable and sufficient for all situations, an example is given in Fig. 9.26.

Usually of great importance in noise surveys is the location of the person or process of interest relative to walls, other machines, etc. and the number of machines operative and inoperative at the time. This information should all be recorded. It is also hoped that the 'sketch of the workplace'

section of the record sheet will be used to undertake noise mapping. This is where sound measurements around a machine or process are taken and lines drawn between the points of equal intensity. These noise contours assist in the identification of areas likely to give rise to excessive exposure and where personal hearing protectors may be necessary. If a number of these are completed for different situations (i.e. a different number of machines operative or variations in production rate) in the same locality, the magnitude of the effect of each is very apparent.

REFERENCES

Department of Health and Social Security (1982). *Report of the Industrial Injuries Advisory Council*. HMSO, London.

Health and Safety Executive (1990). *Noise at Work — Noise Assessment, Information and Control*. Noise Guides 3 to 8. HMSO, London.

Waldron, H.A. (ed.) (1989). *Occupational Health Practice*, (3rd edn). Butterworths, Sevenoaks.

FURTHER READING

Robinson, D.W. (1987). *Noise Exposure and Hearing — A New Look at the Experimental Data*. HSE Contract Report No. 1. HSE, Bootle.

Sharland, I. (1979). *Woods Practical Guide to Noise Control*. Woods, London.

Sound Research Laboratories Ltd. (1991). *Noise Control in Industry*. Spon, London.

CHAPTER 10
Vibration

M.J. Griffin

INTRODUCTION

Vibration is oscillatory motion. The human body is exposed to vibration in many occupations. The effects may be variously described as pleasant or unpleasant, insignificant or interesting, beneficial or harmful. This chapter defines methods of evaluating occupational exposures to vibration, introduces the various human responses and lists possible preventative procedures. Detailed guidance on the application of alternative evaluation procedures will be found in the relevant guides and standards and other texts (e.g. Griffin, 1990).

Hand-transmitted vibration. This is the vibration that enters the body through the hands. It is caused by various processes in industry, agriculture, mining and construction where vibrating tools or workpieces are grasped or pushed by the hands or fingers. Exposure to hand-transmitted vibration can lead to the development of several disorders.

Whole-body vibration. This occurs when the body is supported on a surface which is vibrating (e.g. sitting on a seat which vibrates, standing on a vibrating floor or lying on a vibrating surface). Whole-body vibration occurs in all forms of transport and when working near some machinery.

CHARACTERISTICS OF VIBRATION

Vibration magnitude

During the oscillatory displacements of an object it has alternately a velocity in one direction and then a velocity in the opposite direction. This change of velocity means that the object is constantly accelerating, first in one direction and then in the opposite direction. Figure 10.1 shows the displacement waveform, the velocity waveform and acceleration waveform for a movement occurring at a single frequency (i.e. a sinusoidal oscillation). A vibration can be quantified by either its displacement, its velocity or its acceleration. For practical convenience, the magnitude of vibration is now usually expressed in terms of the acceleration and measured using accelerometers. The units of acceleration are metres per second per second (i.e. $m\,s^{-2}$). The acceleration due to gravity on Earth is approximately $9.81\,m\,s^{-2}$.

The magnitude of an oscillation could be expressed as the difference between the extremities reached by the motion (i.e. the peak-to-peak acceleration) or the maximum deviation from some central point (i.e. the peak acceleration). The magnitude of vibration is now most commonly expressed in terms of an average measure of the acceleration of the oscillatory motion, usually the root-mean-square value (i.e. $m\,s^{-2}$ rms). For a sinusoidal motion, the rms value is the peak value divided by $\sqrt{2}$ (see Fig. 9.4 in Chapter 9).

When observing vibration it is sometimes possible to estimate the displacement caused by the motion. For a sinusoidal motion the acceleration (A) can be calculated from the frequency (f), in Hz, and the displacement (D):

$$A = (2\pi f)^2\, D \qquad (10.1)$$

For example, a sinusoidal motion with a frequency of 1 Hz and a peak-to-peak displacement of 0.1 m

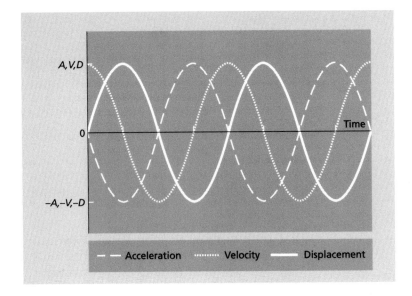

Fig. 10.1 Displacement, velocity and acceleration waveforms for a sinusoidal vibration. If the vibration is of frequency f and peak displacement D, the peak velocity $V = 2\pi fD$ and the peak acceleration $A = (2\pi f)^2 D$.

will have an acceleration of $3.95\,\mathrm{m\,s^{-2}}$ peak–peak, $1.97\,\mathrm{m\,s^{-2}}$ peak and $1.40\,\mathrm{m\,s^{-2}}$ rms. The above expression may be used to convert acceleration measurements to corresponding displacements. However, the conversion is only accurate when the motion occurs at a single frequency (i.e. it has a sinusoidal waveform as shown in Fig. 10.1).

Logarithmic scales for quantifying vibration magnitudes in decibels are sometimes used. When using the reference level in ISO 1683 (International Organization for Standardization, 1983), the acceleration level L_a is expressed by:

$$L_a = 20 \log_{10}\left(\frac{a}{a_0}\right) \qquad (10.2)$$

where a is the measured acceleration (in $\mathrm{m\,s^{-2}}$) and a_0 is the reference level of $10^{-6}\,\mathrm{m\,s^{-2}}$. With this reference, an acceleration of $1\,\mathrm{m\,s^{-2}}$ corresponds to $120\,\mathrm{dB}$ and an acceleration of $10\,\mathrm{m\,s^{-2}}$ corresponds to $140\,\mathrm{dB}$. Other reference levels are used in some countries.

Vibration frequency

The frequency of vibration is expressed in cycles per second using the SI unit, hertz (Hz). The frequency of vibration influences the extent to which vibration is transmitted to the surface of the body (e.g. through seating), the extent to which it is transmitted through the body and the response to vibration within the body. From above it will be seen that the relationship between the displacement and the acceleration of a motion is also dependent on the frequency of oscillation: a displacement of 1 mm will correspond to a low acceleration at low frequencies but a very high acceleration at high frequencies. Consequently, the vibration visible to the human eye does not provide a good indication of vibration acceleration.

Oscillations at frequencies below about 0.5 Hz can cause motion sickness. The frequencies of greatest significance to whole-body vibration are usually at the lower end of the range from 0.5 to 100 Hz. For hand-transmitted vibration, frequencies as high as 1000 Hz or more may have detrimental effects.

Vibration direction

The responses of the body differ according to the direction of the motion. Vibration is usually measured at the interfaces between the body and the vibrating surfaces in each of three orthogonal directions. Figure 10.2 shows a co-ordinate system used when measuring vibration in contact with a hand holding a tool. The axes may differ at the second handle on the same tool; a diagram is often necessary to define the axes of measurement.

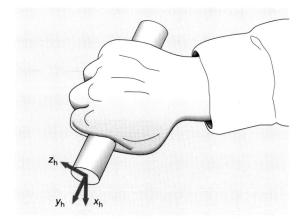

Fig. 10.2 Axes of vibration used to measure hand-transmitted vibration.

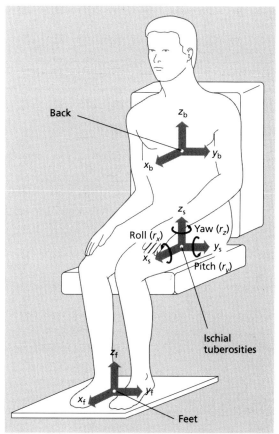

Fig. 10.3 Axes of vibration used to measure whole-body vibration.

The three principal directions for seated and standing persons are: fore-and-aft (x-axis), lateral (y-axis) and vertical (z-axis). The vibration is measured at the interface between the body and the surface supporting the body (i.e. between the seat and the ischial tuberosities for a seated person; beneath the feet for a standing person). Figure 10.3 illustrates the translational and rotational axes for an origin at the ischial tuberosities of a seated person. A similar set of axes is used for describing the directions of vibration at the back and feet of seated persons. The vibration of a control held in the hand, or a display viewed by the eyes, can also be important.

Vibration duration

Some effects of vibration depend on the total duration of vibration exposure. Additionally, the duration of measurement may affect the measured magnitude of the vibration. The rms acceleration may not provide a good indication of vibration severity if the vibration is intermittent, contains shocks or otherwise varies in magnitude from time to time (see below).

HAND-TRANSMITTED VIBRATION

Prolonged and regular exposure of the fingers or the hands to vibration or repeated shock can give rise to various signs and symptoms of disorder. The precise extent and interrelationship between the signs and symptoms are not fully understood but five types of disorder may be identified (Table 10.1). The various disorders may be interconnected: more than one disorder can affect a person at the same time and it is possible that the presence of one disorder facilitates the appearance of another. The onset of each disorder is dependent on several variables, such as the vibration characteristics, the dynamic response of the fingers or hand, individual susceptibility to damage and other aspects of the environment. The terms 'vibration syndrome', or 'hand−arm vibration syndrome' (HAVS), are sometimes used to refer to one or more of the effects listed in Table 10.1.

Table 10.1 Five types of disorder associated with hand-transmitted vibration exposures. Some combination of these disorders is sometimes referred to as the 'hand–arm vibration syndrome' (HAVS). From Griffin (1990)

Type	Disorder
Type A	Circulatory disorders
Type B	Bone and joint disorders
Type C	Neurological disorders
Type D	Muscle disorders
Type E	Other general disorders (e.g. of the central nervous system)

Vascular effects (vibration-induced white finger)

The first published cases of the condition now most commonly known as 'vibration-induced white finger' (VWF) are acknowledged to be those reported in Italy by Loriga (1911). A few years later, cases were documented at limestone quarries in Indiana. VWF has subsequently been reported to occur in many other widely varied occupations in which there is exposure of the fingers to vibration (see Griffin, 1990).

Signs and symptoms

VWF is characterized by intermittent blanching of the fingers. The finger tips are usually the first to blanch but the affected area may extend to all of one or more fingers with continued vibration exposure. Attacks of blanching are precipitated by cold and therefore usually occur in cold conditions or when handling cold objects. The blanching lasts until the fingers are rewarmed and vasodilation allows the return of the blood circulation.

Many years of vibration exposure often occur before the first attack of blanching is noticed. Affected persons often have other signs and symptoms, such as numbness and tingling. Cyanosis and, rarely, gangrene, have also been reported. It is not yet clear to what extent these other signs and symptoms are causes of, caused by, or unrelated to, attacks of 'white finger'.

Diagnosis

There are other conditions that can cause similar signs and symptoms to those associated with VWF.

VWF cannot be assumed to be present merely because there are attacks of blanching. It will be necessary to exclude other known causes of similar symptoms (by medical examination) and also to exclude primary Raynaud's disease (also called 'constitutional white finger'). This exclusion cannot yet be achieved with complete confidence. However, if there is no family history of the symptoms, if the symptoms did not occur before the first significant exposure to vibration and if the symptoms and signs are confined to areas in contact with the vibration (e.g. the fingers but not the ears etc.), they will often be assumed to indicate VWF.

Diagnostic tests for VWF can be useful but, at present, they are not infallible indicators of the disease. The measurement of finger systolic blood pressure during finger cooling, and the measurement of finger rewarming times following cooling, can be useful, but many other tests are in use.

The severity of the effects of vibration are sometimes recorded by reference to the 'stage' of the disorder. The staging of VWF is based on verbal statements made by the affected person. In the Taylor–Pelmear system, the stage of VWF was determined by the presence of numbness and tingling, the areas affected by blanching, the frequency of blanching, the time of year when blanching occurred and the extent of interference with work and leisure activities. A more simple procedure, the Stockholm Workshop staging system, was subsequently evolved (Table 10.2). In this system, the staging compounds the frequency of attacks of blanching with the areas of the digits affected by blanching.

A numerical procedure for recording the areas of the digits affected by blanching is known as the 'scoring system' (Fig. 10.4). The blanching scores for the hands shown in Fig. 10.4 are 01300_{right}, 01366_{left}. The scores correspond to areas of blanching on the digits commencing with the thumb. On the fingers a score of 1 is given for blanching on the distal phalanx, a score of 2 for blanching on the middle phalanx and a score of 3 for blanching on the proximal phalanx. On the thumbs, the scores are 4 for the distal phalanx and 5 for the proximal phalanx. The blanching score may be based on statements from the affected person or on the visual observations of a designated observer (e.g. a nurse).

Table 10.2 Stockholm Workshop scale for the classification of vibration-induced white finger . From Gemne *et al.* (1987)

Stage	Grade	Description
0		No attacks
1	Mild	Occasional attacks affecting only the tips of one or more fingers
2	Moderate	Occasional attacks affecting distal and middle (rarely also proximal) phalanges of one or more fingers
3	Severe	Frequent attacks affecting all phalanges of most fingers
4	Very severe	As in stage 3, with trophic skin changes in the finger tips

* If a person has stage 2 in two fingers of the left hand and stage 1 in a finger on the right hand the condition may be reported as 2L(2)/1R(1). There is no defined means of reporting the condition of digits when this varies between digits on the same hand. The scoring system is more helpful when the extent of blanching is to be recorded.

Neurological effects

Neurological effects of hand-transmitted vibration (e.g. numbness, tingling, elevated sensory thresholds for touch, vibration, temperature and pain, and reduced nerve conduction velocity) are now recognized as separate effects of vibration and not merely as symptoms of VWF (see Griffin, 1990). A method of reporting the extent of vibration-induced neurological effects of vibration has been proposed (Table 10.3). This staging system is not currently related to the results of any specific objective test: the 'sensorineural stage' is a subjective impression of a physician, based on the statements of the

Table 10.3 Proposed 'sensorineural stages' of the effects of hand-transmitted vibration. From Brammer, Taylor and Lundborg (1987)

Stage	Symptoms
0_{SN}	Exposed to vibration but no symptoms
1_{SN}	Intermittent numbness with or without tingling
2_{SN}	Intermittent or persistent numbness, reduced sensory perception
3_{SN}	Intermittent or persistent numbness, reduced tactile discrimination and/or manipulative dexterity

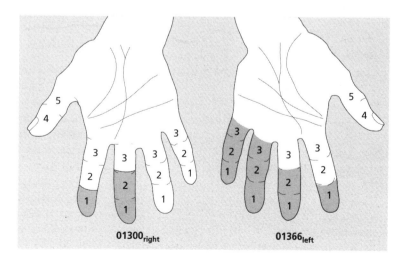

Fig. 10.4 Method of scoring the areas of the digits affected by blanching. From Griffin (1990).

affected person or the results of any available clinical or scientific testing.

Muscular effects

The research literature includes several reports of muscle atrophy among users of vibrating tools. More commonly, workers exposed to hand-transmitted vibration report difficulty with their grip, including reduced dexterity, reduced grip strength and locked grip. Many of the reports are derived from symptoms reported by exposed persons rather than signs detected by physicians, and could be a reflection of neurological problems. Measurements of muscle function have rarely been obtained using repeatable tests.

Muscle activity may be of great importance to tool users since a secure grip can be essential to the performance of the job and safe control of the tool. The presence of vibration on a handle may encourage the adoption of a tighter grip than would otherwise occur and a tight grip may increase the transmission of vibration to the hand. If the chronic effects of vibration result in reduced grip this may help to protect operators from further effects of vibration, but interfere with both work and leisure activities.

Articular effects

Many surveys of the users of hand-held tools have found evidence of bone and joint problems: most often among men operating percussive tools, such as those used in metalworking jobs, mining and quarrying. It is speculated that some characteristic of such tools, possibly the low-frequency shocks, is responsible. Some of the reported injuries relate to specific bones and suggest the existence of cysts, vacuoles, decalcification or other osteolysis, degeneration or deformity of the carpal, metacarpal or phalangeal bones. Osteoarthrosis and olecranon spurs at the elbow, and other problems at the wrist and shoulder, are also documented (see Griffin, 1990).

Notwithstanding the evidence of many research publications, there is not universal acceptance that vibration is the cause of articular problems and there is currently no dose–effect relationship which predicts their occurrence. In the absence of specific information, it seems that adherence to current guidance for the prevention of vibration-induced white finger may provide reasonable protection.

Other effects

Effects of hand-transmitted vibration may not be confined to the fingers, hands and arms: many studies have found a high incidence of problems such as headaches and sleeplessness among tool users and have concluded that these symptoms are caused by hand-transmitted vibration. Although these are real problems to those affected, they are 'subjective' effects which are not accepted as real by all researchers. Some current research is seeking a physiological basis for such symptoms. At present it would appear that caution is appropriate, but it is reasonable to assume that the adoption of the modern guidance to prevent vibration-induced white finger will also provide some protection from any other effects of hand-transmitted vibration within, or distant from, the hand.

Tools and processes causing hand-transmitted vibration

The vibration of tools varies greatly, depending on tool design and method of use, so it is not possible to categorize individual tool types as 'safe' or 'dangerous'. However, Table 10.4 lists tools and processes which are sometimes a cause for concern.

Preventative measures for hand-transmitted vibration

Protection from the effects of hand-transmitted vibration requires action from management, tool manufacturers, technicians and physicians at the workplace and from tool users. Table 10.5 summarizes some of the actions which may be appropriate.

When there is reason to suspect that hand-transmitted vibration may cause injury, the vibration at tool–hand interfaces should be measured. It will then be possible to predict whether the tool or process is likely to cause injury and whether any other tool or process could give a lower vibration severity.

Table 10.4 Tools and processes potentially associated with vibration injuries. After Griffin (1990), Chapter 14

Type of tool	Examples of tool type
Percussive metalworking tools	Riveting tools Caulking tools Chipping tools Chipping hammers Fettling tools Hammer drills Clinching and flanging tools Impact wrenches Swaging Needle guns
Grinders and other rotary tools	Pedestal grinders Hand-held grinders Hand-held sanders Hand-held polishers Flex-driven grinders/polishers Rotary burring tools
Percussive hammers and drills used in mining, demolition and road construction	Hammers Rock drills Road drills, etc.
Forest and garden machinery	Chain-saws Anti-vibration chain-saws Brush saws Mowers and shears Barking machines
Other processes and tools	Nut runners Shoe-pounding-up machines Concrete vibro-thickeners Concrete levelling vibro-tables Motorcycle handlebars

The duration of exposure to vibration should also be quantified. Reduction of exposure time may include the provision of exposure breaks during the day and, if possible, prolonged periods away from vibration exposure. For any tool or process having a vibration magnitude sufficient to cause injury, there should be a system to quantify and control the maximum daily duration of exposure of any individual.

Gloves are sometimes recommended as a means of reducing the adverse effects of vibration on the hands. When using the frequency weightings in current standards, commonly available gloves do *not* normally provide effective attenuation of the vibration on most tools. Gloves and 'cushioned'

handles may reduce the transmission of high frequencies of vibration but current standards imply that these are not usually the primary cause of disorders. Gloves may protect the hand from other forms of mechanical injury (e.g. cuts and scratches) and protect the fingers from temperature extremes. Warm hands are less likely to suffer an attack of finger blanching and some consider that maintaining warm hands while exposed to vibration may also lessen the damage caused by the vibration.

Workers who are exposed to vibration magnitudes sufficient to cause injury should be warned of the possibility of vibration injuries and educated on the ways of reducing the severity of their vibration exposures. They should be advised of the symptoms to look out for and told to seek medical attention if the symptoms appear.

There should be pre-employment medical screening wherever a subsequent exposure to hand-transmitted vibration may reasonably be expected to cause vibration injury. Medical supervision of each exposed person should continue throughout employment at suitable intervals, possibly annually. There is no single test which will diagnose the existence or extent of all possible effects of hand-transmitted vibration (see above). Tests in common use include direct and indirect measures of finger blood flow, the measurement of finger systolic blood pressure, the determination of various tactile thresholds and more extensive neurological investigations. Although these and other investigations may assist the diagnosis of specific disorders, their sensitivities and specificities are currently unknown (Faculty of Occupational Medicine of the Royal College of Physicians, Working Party on Hand-transmitted Vibration, 1993a and b).

National and International Standards

ISO 5349 (International Organization for Standardization, 1986) and BS 6842 (British Standards Institution, 1987a) use the same frequency weighting (called W_h in BS 6842) to quantify the severity of hand-transmitted vibration over the frequency range 8–1000 Hz. This weighting is applied to measurements of vibration acceleration in each of the three axes of vibration at the point of entry of vibration to the hand.

Table 10.5 Some preventative measures to consider when persons are exposed to hand-transmitted vibration. After Griffin (1990), Chapter 19

Group	Action
Management	Seek technical advice
	Seek medical advice
	Warn exposed persons
	Train exposed persons
	Review exposure times
	Policy on removal from work
Tool manufacturers	Measure tool vibration
	Design tools to minimize vibration
	Ergonomic design to reduce grip force, etc.
	Design to keep hands warm
	Provide guidance on tool maintenance
	Provide warning of dangerous vibration
Technical at workplace	Measure vibration exposure
	Provide appropriate tools
	Maintain tools
	Inform management
Medical	Pre-employment screening
	Routine medical checks
	Record all signs and reported symptoms
	Warn workers with predisposition
	Advise on consequences of exposure
	Inform management
Tool user	Use tool properly
	Avoid unnecessary vibration exposure
	Minimize grip and push forces
	Check condition of tool
	Inform supervisor of tool problems
	Keep warm
	Wear gloves when safe to do so
	Minimize smoking
	Seek medical advice if symptoms appear
	Inform employer of relevant disorders

Care is required to obtain representative measurements of tool vibration with appropriate operating conditions. There can be difficulties in obtaining valid measurements using some commercial instrumentation (especially when there are high shock levels). It is wise to determine acceleration spectra and inspect the acceleration time-histories before accepting the validity of any measurements.

The frequency-weighted acceleration on different tools may be compared. The standards imply that if two tools expose the hand to vibration for the same period of time, the tool having the lowest frequency-weighted acceleration will be least likely to cause injury or disease.

Occupational exposures to hand-transmitted vibration can have widely varying daily exposure durations — from a few seconds to many hours. Often, exposures are intermittent. To enable a daily exposure to be reported simply, the standards refer to an equivalent 4 h (ISO 5349) or an equivalent 8 h (BS 6842) exposure.

Table 10.6 shows a relationship between years of vibration exposure, 4 h energy-equivalent frequency-weighted acceleration and the prevalence of finger blanching as proposed in an Annex to ISO

Table 10.6 Number of years before blanching develops in 10–50% of vibration-exposed persons according to ISO 5349 (International Organization for Standardization, 1986)

Weighted acceleration, $a_{hw(eq, 4 h)}$ (m s^{-2} rms)	Percentage of population affected by finger blanching				
	10%	20%	30%	40%	50%
2	15	23	> 25	> 25	> 25
5	6	9	11	12	14
10	3	4	5	6	7
20	1	2	2	3	3
50	< 1	< 1	< 1	1	1

5349. These relationships are illustrated graphically in Fig. 10.5. The values in Fig. 10.5 and Table 10.6 refer to frequency-weighted acceleration referenced to the frequency range 8–16 Hz. Figure 10.6 shows how the magnitudes required for a predicted prevalence of 10% vibration-induced white finger after 8 years depend on vibration frequency from 8 to 1000 Hz for exposure durations from 1 min to 8 h per day.

The percentage of affected persons in any group of exposed persons will not always closely match the values shown in Table 10.6 or Figs 10.5 and 10.6. The frequency-weighting, the time-dependency and the dose–effect information are based on less than complete information and they have been simplified for practical convenience. Additionally,

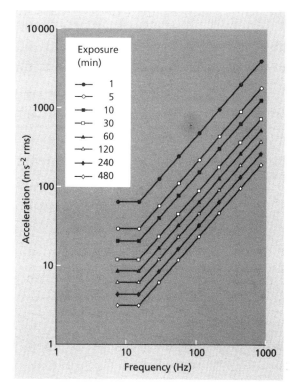

Fig. 10.6 Acceleration magnitudes predicted to give 10% prevalence of vibration-induced white finger after 8 years for daily exposure durations from 1 min to 8 h, according to ISO 5349 (International Organization for Standardization, 1986).

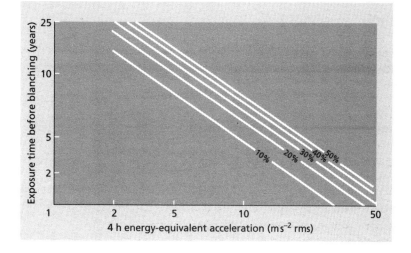

Fig. 10.5 Years of exposure to 4 h energy-equivalent frequency-weighted hand-transmitted vibration required for finger blanching in 10–50% of exposed persons, according to ISO 5349 (International Organization for Standardization, 1986).

the number of persons affected by vibration will depend on the rate at which persons enter and leave the exposed group. Neither the average exposure time nor the 'mean latency' (i.e. the average period of vibration exposure before those with symptoms of VWF develop the condition) are appropriate measures of the exposure period for this calculation.

An Annex to BS 6842 summarizes current knowledge and the assumptions concerning dose–effect data for VWF but does not include the detailed table of prevalence rates given in the International Standard. It states that vascular symptoms do not normally occur if the frequency-weighted acceleration is below $1 \, \text{m s}^{-2}$ rms.

The Machinery Safety Directive of the European Community (89/392/EEC) states that machinery must be designed and constructed so that hazards resulting from vibration produced by the machinery are reduced to the lowest practicable level, taking into account technical progress and the availability of means of reducing vibration. It is proposed that the instruction handbooks for hand-held and hand-guided machinery should specify the equivalent acceleration to which the hands or arms are subjected where this exceeds some stated value (currently proposed as a frequency-weighted acceleration of $2.5 \, \text{m s}^{-2}$ rms). The relevance of any such value will depend on the test conditions to be specified in other standards. Very many hand-held vibrating tools can exceed this value. The specified tests will not encompass all realistic exposures and so may not represent the exposures received in some jobs. Additionally, the different exposure durations involved in different jobs will carry different degrees of risk.

Standards defining test conditions for the measurement of vibration on chipping and riveting hammers, rotary hammers and rock drills, grinding machines, pavement breakers and a range of garden and forestry equipment (including chain-saws) are in preparation (see ISO 8662-1 (International Organization for Standardization, 1988).

Current standards for evaluating hand-transmitted vibration provide guidance which cannot be ignored. However, those concerned with the design or evaluation of situations involving hand-transmitted vibration should anticipate that further understanding of the relevant pathology, physiology and biodynamics may yield improvements to the methods of assessing the safety of exposures to hand-transmitted vibration.

WHOLE-BODY VIBRATION

Vibration of the whole body is produced by various types of industrial machinery and by all forms of transport. The vibration may affect health, comfort and the performance of activities. The comments of persons exposed to vibration mostly derive from the sensations produced by vibration rather than a knowledge that the vibration is causing harm or interfering with their activities.

Effects on comfort

The relative subjective reaction (e.g. discomfort) expected for different oscillatory motions can usually be predicted from measurements of the vibration. For very low magnitude motions it is possible to estimate the percentage of persons who will be able to feel vibration and the percentage who will not be able to feel the vibration. For higher vibration magnitudes, an approximate indication of the extent of subjective reactions is available in a semantic scale of discomfort (e.g. BS 6841) (British Standards Institution, 1987b).

Limits to prevent vibration discomfort must vary between different environments (e.g. between buildings and transport), between different types of transport (e.g. between cars and trucks) and within types of vehicle (e.g. between sports cars and limousines). The design limit depends on external factors (e.g. cost and speed) and the comfort in alternative environments (e.g. competitive vehicles).

Effects of vibration magnitude

The absolute threshold for the perception of vertical whole-body vibration in the frequency range 1 to 100 Hz is approximately $0.01 \, \text{m s}^{-2}$ rms. A magnitude of $0.1 \, \text{m s}^{-2}$ will be easily noticeable, magnitudes around $1 \, \text{m s}^{-2}$ rms are usually considered uncomfortable and magnitudes of $10 \, \text{m s}^{-2}$ rms are usually dangerous. The precise values depend on vibration frequency and exposure duration and they are different for other axes of vibration (see BS 6841 and Griffin, 1990).

A doubling of vibration magnitude (expressed in $m\,s^{-2}$) produces an approximate doubling of discomfort. A halving of vibration magnitude can therefore produce a considerable improvement in comfort.

Effects of vibration frequency and direction

The dynamic responses of the body, and the relevant physiological and psychological processes, dictate that subjective reactions to vibration depend on vibration frequency and vibration direction. Frequency weightings are given in BS 6841: this is currently the most up-to-date published standard giving guidance concerned with vibration discomfort.

Effects of vibration duration

Vibration discomfort tends to increase with increasing duration of exposure to vibration. The precise rate of increase may depend on many factors but a simple 'fourth power' time dependency is sometimes used to approximate how discomfort varies with exposure duration, from the shortest possible shock to a full day of vibration exposure (i.e. (acceleration)^4 × duration = constant). This time dependency is more consistent with available information and expectations than either an 'energy time dependence' or the ISO 2631 (International Organization for Standardization, 1974) time dependence (see below).

Vibration in buildings

Acceptable magnitudes of vibration in buildings are close to vibration perception thresholds. The effects of vibration in buildings are assumed to depend on the use of the building, in addition to the vibration frequency, direction and duration. Guidance is given in various standards (e.g. ISO 2631-2) (International Organization for Standardization, 1989). BS 6472 (British Standards Institution, 1992) defines a procedure which combines the assessment of vibration and shock in buildings by using the 'vibration dose value' (see below).

Effects on health

Epidemiological studies have reported disorders among persons exposed to vibration from occupational, sport and leisure activities. The studies do not all agree on either the type or the extent of disorders, and rarely have the findings been related to measurements of the vibration exposures. However, it is widely believed that disorders of the back (back pain, displacement of intervertebral discs, degeneration of spinal vertebrae, osteoarthritis, etc.) may be associated with vibration exposure (see Chapter 5 and Appendix 5 of Griffin, 1990). There may be several alternative causes of an increase in disorders of the back among persons exposed to vibration (e.g. poor sitting postures, heavy lifting). It is not always possible to conclude confidently that a back disorder is solely, or primarily, caused by vibration.

Other disorders which have been claimed to be due to occupational exposures to whole-body vibration include abdominal pain, digestive disorders, urinary frequency, prostatitis, haemorrhoids, balance and visual disorders, headaches and sleeplessness. Further research is required to confirm whether these signs and symptoms are causally related to exposure to vibration.

Method of vibration evaluation

Epidemiological data alone are not sufficient to define how to evaluate whole-body vibration so as to predict the relative risks to health from the different types of vibration exposure. A consideration of such data in combination with an understanding of biodynamic responses and subjective responses is used to provide current guidance. The manner in which the health effects of oscillatory motions depend upon the frequency, direction and duration of motion is currently assumed to be similar to that for vibration discomfort. However, it is assumed that the 'total' exposure, rather than the 'average' exposure, is important and so a 'dose' measure is used.

ISO 2631 (International Organization for Standardization, 1974 and 1985) defined exposure limits (Fig. 10.7) which were '... set at approximately half the level considered to be the threshold of pain

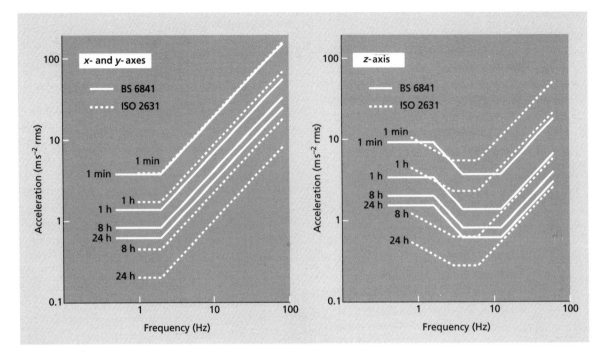

Fig. 10.7 Comparison of ISO 2631 (International Organization for Standardization, 1985) exposure limits with an 'action level' based on a vibration dose value (VDV) of $15 \, \mathrm{m \, s^{-1.75}}$ from BS 6841 (British Standards Institution, 1987). When seated: x-axis = fore-and-aft; y-axis = lateral; z-axis = vertical. From Griffin (1990).

(or limit of voluntary tolerance) for healthy human subjects ...'. Although the latest version of ISO 2631 was published in 1985, it is similar to the 1974 version which was based on research conducted before 1970. BS 6841 (British Standards Institution, 1987b) is more up-to-date and broadly consistent (though not identical) with a draft revision of the International Standard. Figure 10.7 also shows an 'action level' for vertical vibration derived from BS 6841.

The 'vibration dose value' (VDV) can be considered to be the magnitude of a 1 s duration of vibration which will be equally severe to the measured vibration. The vibration dose value uses a 'fourth power' time dependency to accumulate vibration severity over the exposure period from the shortest possible shock to a full day of vibration (see BS 6841):

$$\mathrm{VDV} = \left[\int_{t=0}^{t=T} a(t)^4 \, \mathrm{d}t \right]^{1/4} \qquad (10.3)$$

where $a(t)$ is the frequency-weighted acceleration. If the exposure duration (t, seconds) and the frequency-weighted rms acceleration (a_{rms}, m s^{-2} rms) are known, the 'estimated vibration dose value' (eVDV) can be calculated:

$$\mathrm{eVDV} = 1.4 \, a_{\mathrm{rms}} t^{1/4} \qquad (10.4)$$

An action level based on the vibration dose value is applicable over a wider range of duration than the exposure limit in ISO 2631 and can be used to evaluate the severity of repetitive shocks. This 'fourth power' time dependency is also considerably simpler to use than the time dependency in ISO 2631 (see below).

Effects on performance

Vibration may interfere with the acquisition of information (e.g. by the eyes), the output of information (e.g. by hand or foot movements) or the complex central processes that relate input to output (e.g. learning, memory, decision making). Effects of oscillatory motion on human performance may impair safety.

The greatest effects of whole-body vibration are on input processes (mainly vision) and output processes (mainly continuous hand control). In both cases there may be disturbance occurring entirely outside the body (e.g. vibration of a viewed display or vibration of a hand-held control), disturbance at the input or output (e.g. movement of the eye or hand) and disturbance affecting the peripheral nervous system (i.e. afferent or efferent system). Central processes may also be affected by vibration, but understanding is currently too limited to make confident generalized statements.

The effects of vibration on vision and manual control are primarily caused by the movement of the affected part of the body (i.e. the eye or hand). The effects may be decreased by reducing the transmission of vibration to the eye or to the hand, or by making the task less susceptible to disturbance (e.g. increasing the size of a display or reducing the sensitivity of a control). Often, the effects of vibration on vision and manual control can be much reduced by redesign of the task.

Simple cognitive tasks (e.g. simple reaction time) appear to be unaffected by vibration, other than by changes in arousal or motivation or by direct effects on input and output processes. This may also be true for some complex cognitive tasks. However, the sparsity and diversity of experimental studies allow the possibility of real and significant cognitive effects of vibration. Vibration may influence 'fatigue', but there is little relevant scientific evidence and none which supports the complex form of the so-called 'fatigue-decreased proficiency limit' offered in ISO 2631.

Control of whole-body vibration

Wherever possible, reduction of vibration at source is to be preferred. This may involve reducing the undulations of the terrain or reducing the speed of travel of vehicles.

Methods of reducing the transmission of vibration to operators require an understanding of the characteristics of the vibration environment and the route for the transmission of vibration to the body. For example, the magnitude of vibration often varies with location: lower magnitudes will be experienced in some areas. Table 10.7 lists some preventative measures which may be considered.

Seats can be designed to attenuate vibration. However, most seats exhibit a resonance at low frequencies which results in higher magnitudes of vertical vibration occurring on the seat than on the floor! At high frequencies there is usually attenuation of vibration. In use, the resonance frequencies of common seats are in the region of 4 Hz. The amplification at resonance is partially determined by the 'damping' in the seat. Increases in the damping of the seat cushioning tend to reduce the amplification at resonance but increase the transmissibility at high frequencies. There are large variations in transmissibility between seats and these result in significant differences in the vibration experienced by people.

A simple numerical indication of the isolation efficiency of a seat for a specific application is provided by the 'seat effective amplitude transmissibility' (SEAT) (see Griffin, 1990). A SEAT value greater than 100% indicates that, overall, the vibration on the seat is 'worse' than the vibration on the floor. Values below 100% indicate that the seat has provided some useful attenuation. Seats should be designed to have the lowest SEAT value compatible with other constraints.

A separate suspension mechanism is provided beneath the seat pan in 'suspension seats'. These seats, used in some off-road vehicles, trucks and coaches, have low resonance frequencies (around 2 Hz) and so can attenuate vibration at frequencies above about 3 Hz. The transmissibilities of these seats are usually determined by the seat manufacturer, but their isolation efficiencies vary with operating conditions.

National and International Standards for evaluating whole-body vibration

No precise limit can be offered to prevent disorders caused by whole-body vibration, but standards define useful methods of quantifying vibration sev-

Table 10.7 Summary of preventative measures to consider when persons are exposed to whole-body vibration. After Griffin (1990), Chapter 5

Group	Action
Management	Seek technical advice
	Seek medical advice
	Warn exposed persons
	Train exposed persons
	Review exposure times
	Policy on removal from work
Machine manufacturers	Measure vibration
	Design to minimize whole-body vibration
	Optimize suspension design
	Optimize seating dynamics
	Ergonomic design to provide good posture, etc.
	Provide guidance on machine maintenance
	Provide guidance on seat maintenance
	Provide warning of dangerous vibration
Technical at workplace	Measure vibration exposure
	Provide appropriate machines
	Select seats with good attenuation
	Maintain machines
	Inform management
Medical	Pre-employment screening
	Routine medical checks
	Record all signs and reported symptoms
	Warn workers with predisposition
	Advise on consequences of exposure
	Inform management
Exposed persons	Use machine properly
	Avoid unnecessary vibration exposure
	Check seat is properly adjusted
	Adopt good sitting posture
	Check condition of machine
	Inform supervisor of vibration problems
	Seek medical advice if symptoms appear
	Inform employer of relevant disorders

erity. BS 6841 (British Standards Institution, 1987b) offers the following guidance.

High vibration dose values will cause severe discomfort, pain and injury. Vibration dose values also indicate, in a general way, the severity of the vibration exposures which caused them. However there is currently no consensus of opinion on the precise relation between vibration dose values and the risk of injury. It is known that vibration magnitudes and durations which produce vibration dose values in the region of $15\,\mathrm{m\,s^{-1.75}}$ will usually cause severe discomfort. It is reasonable to assume that increased exposure to vibration will be accompanied by increased risk of injury.

At high vibration dose values, prior consideration of the fitness of the exposed persons and the design of adequate safety precautions may be required. The need for regular checks on the health of routinely exposed persons may also be considered.

A vibration dose value of $15\,\mathrm{m\,s^{-1.75}}$ has been called a 'tentative action level'. It may be appropriate for organizations to limit vibration or repeated shock exposures to higher or lower values depending on the situation. The vibration dose value provides a robust measure by which highly variable and complex exposures can be compared. The tentative action level merely serves to indicate the approximate values which might be excessive. Figure 10.8 illustrates the root-mean-square accelerations corresponding to a vibration dose value of $15 \, m \, s^{-1.75}$ for exposures between 1 s and 24 h.

Unlike the 'exposure limit' in the old ISO 2631, the vibration dose value 'action level' does not allow very high magnitudes at short durations or require very low magnitudes for long-duration exposures. Any exposure to continuous vibration, or intermittent vibration, or repeated shock may be compared with the action level by calculating the vibration dose value. It would be unwise to exceed the action level without consideration of the possible health effects of an exposure to vibration or shock.

The Machinery Safety Directive of the European Community (89/392/EEC) states that machinery must be designed and constructed so that hazards resulting from vibration produced by the machinery are reduced to the lowest practicable level, taking into account technical progress and the availability of means of reducing vibration. The Machinery Safety Directive encourages the reduction of vibration by means additional to reduction at source (e.g. good seating).

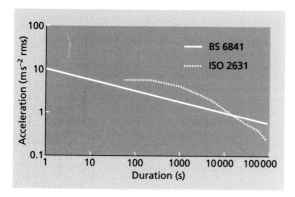

Fig. 10.8 Action level corresponding to a vibration dose value (VDV) of $15 \, m \, s^{-1.75}$ (see BS 6841 (British Standards Institution, 1987)) compared with exposure limit from ISO 2631 (International Organization for Standardization, 1974 and 1985).

CONCLUSIONS

Mechanical oscillation of the human body can produce discomfort, interfere with the performance of activities and cause pathological and physiological changes in the body. Those responsible for the health of workers should be aware of the relevant standards for evaluating the effects of vibration. These standards provide valuable information and should not be ignored. Nevertheless, the complexity of the interactions between oscillatory motion (i.e. vibration and shock) and the functions of the body are great. It is helpful to be aware of the uneven scientific support for some of the information in the current standards: reading may be beneficially extended into the scientific literature.

REFERENCES

Brammer, A.J., Taylor, W. and Lundborg, G. (1987). Sensorineural stages of the hand−arm vibration syndrome. *Scandinavian Journal of Work, Environment and Health*, **13**, (4), 279−83.

British Standards Institution (1987a). *Measurement and Evaluation of Human Exposure to Vibration Transmitted to the Hand*. British Standards Institution BS 6842.

British Standards Institution (1987b). *Measurement and Evaluation of Human Exposure to Whole-body Mechanical Vibration and Repeated Shock*. British Standards Institution BS 6841.

British Standards Institution (1992). *Evaluation of Human Exposure to Vibration in Buildings (1 Hz to 80 Hz)*. British Standards Institution BS 6472.

Council of the European Communities (Brussels) (1989). On the approximation of the laws of the member states relating to machinery Council Directive (89/392/EEC). *Official Journal of the European Communities*, **June**, 9−32.

Faculty of Occupational Medicine of the Royal College of Physicians, Working Party on Hand-transmitted Vibration (1993). *Hand-transmitted Vibration: Clinical Effects and Pathophysiology, Part 1*. Report of a working party. The Royal College of Physicians of London.

Faculty of Occupational Medicine of the Royal College of Physicians, Working Party on Hand-transmitted Vibration (1993). *Hand-transmitted Vibration: Clinical Effects and Pathophysiology. Part 2*. Background papers to the working party report. The Royal College of Physicians of London.

Gemne, G., Pyykko, L., Taylor, W. and Pelmear, P. (1987). The Stockholm Workshop scale for the classification of cold-induced Raynaud's phenomenon in the hand−arm vibration syndrome (revision of the Taylor−Pelmear scale). *Scandinavian Journal of Work, Environment and Health*, **13**, (4), 275–8.

Griffin, M.J. (1990). *Handbook of Human Vibration*. Academic Press, London.

International Organization for Standardization (1974). *Guide for the Evaluation of Human Exposure to Whole-body Vibration*. International Standard ISO 2631.

International Organization for Standardization (1983). *Acoustics — Preferred Reference Quantities for Acoustic Levels*. International Standard ISO 1683.

International Organization for Standardization (1985). *Evaluation of Human Exposure to Whole-body Vibration — Part 1: General Requirements*. International Standard ISO 2631-1.

International Organization for Standardization (1986). *Mechanical Vibration — Guidelines for the Measure-ment and the Assessment of Human Exposure to Hand-transmitted Vibration*. International Standard ISO 5349.

International Organization for Standardization (1988). *Hand-held Portable Tools — Measurement of Vibration at the Handle — Part 1: General*. International Standard ISO 8662-1.

International Organization for Standardization (1989). *Evaluation of Human Exposure to Whole-body Vibration — Part 2: Continuous and Shock-induced Vibration in Buildings*. International Standard ISO 2631-2.

Loriga, G. (1911). Il lavoro con i martelli pneumatici. The use of pneumatic hammers. *Bollettino Ispett. Lavoro*, **2**, 35–60.

CHAPTER 11
Light and Lighting

N.A. Smith

INTRODUCTION

Light is a natural phenomenon required to enable everyday activities to be carried out. It is essential to our basic existence, yet ironically it is very often taken for granted. Modern lifestyles are such that humans have become less dependent upon natural light since the introduction of artificial light sources.

The role of light and lighting in the field of occupational hygiene has become progressively more important and the necessity to overcome problems associated with ill-conceived lighting installations is more readily apparent.

This chapter gives the practising occupational hygienist an insight into the basic concepts of light and lighting with the underlying emphasis on its application to the workplace. It is not the purpose of the chapter to introduce the reader to in-depth detail of the science of illumination; this can be found in specialist reference texts.

FUNDAMENTALS

The electromagnetic spectrum, visible radiation and light

Light is a form of energy. This form of energy is known as 'radiation' and is electromagnetic in character. This means that the radiation has both an electric and a magnetic field, both of which vary sinusoidally with time. All electromagnetic radiation propogates with a velocity of $3 \times 10^8\,\mathrm{m\,s^{-1}}$.

The electromagnetic spectrum is shown in Fig. 11.1 and it can be seen that visible radiation (i.e.

radiation which is detected by the human eye) occupies the approximate wavelength range between 380 and 760 nm.

In essence, radiation is the cause and light the effect, with changes in wavelength within the visible spectrum producing changes in the colour of the light output.

Infrared and ultraviolet radiation

At wavelengths at the extremities of the visible part of the electromagnetic spectrum, the radiation becomes progressively infrared (IR) at the long wavelength end and ultraviolet (UV) at the short wavelength end. Both IR and UV radiation have been sub-divided into three groups A, B and C, with corresponding limiting wavelengths as shown in Table 11.1. Excessive or prolonged exposure to IR or UV radiation may lead to human tissue damage.

Rectilinear propagation of light

An observer can only see an object when light from the object enters the eye. Since it is impossible to see around obstacles, then it is clear that light travels in straight lines — a phenomenon referred to as 'rectilinear propagation of light'. Light is therefore represented by straight lines called 'rays'. A collection of rays is termed a 'beam' or a 'pencil'.

Terms and definitions

There are many terms and definitions associated with lighting. A comprehensive list is given in

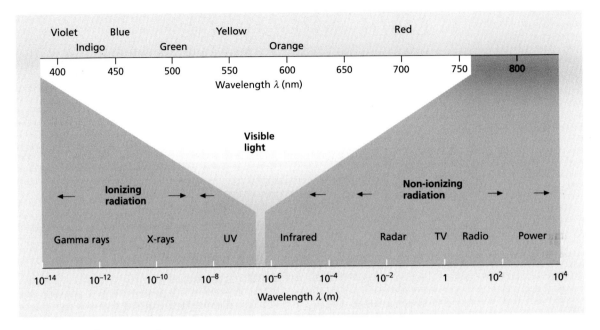

Fig. 11.1 The electromagnetic spectrum.

Smith (1991). An abridged schedule is provided here.

Candela   The SI unit of luminous intensity.

Colour appearance   The appearance of a surface under a given light.

Colour rendering index   A measure of how colours under a particular light compare with a standardized set of conditions.

Daylight factor   The ratio of illuminance due to daylight at a particular point in a building to the simultaneous horizontal external illuminance from an unobstructed sky, expressed as a percentage. Sunlight is excluded.

Flux, luminous   The light emitted by a source or received by a surface.

Table 11.1 Sub-division of infrared and ultraviolet radiation groups

| Sub-division | Wavelength range (nm) | |
	Infrared	Ultraviolet
A	780–1400	315–400
B	1400–3000	280–315
C	3000–1 000 000	200–280

Glare index   A measure of the degree of discomfort glare.

Illuminance   The amount of light falling on a surface divided by the area upon which it is falling. Measured in lumen m^{-2} or lux.

Light loss factor (or Maintenance factor)   A factor which takes into account the reduction in output from a luminaire due, *inter alia*, to: (1) depreciation in output from a lamp due to ageing; and (2) cleanliness of luminaire optical system.

Lumen   The SI unit of luminous flux.

Luminaire   The apparatus which controls the distribution of light and contains all the components for fixing, protecting and connecting the lamp.

Luminance   The flow of light in a given direction (measured in candela m^{-2}) from a surface element.

Luminance contrast   A measure of contrast as a ratio of luminance difference (task to background) to luminance of background.

Luminous efficacy   The ratio (luminous flux)/ (electrical power) = (output)/(input) measured in lumen W^{-1}.

Luminous intensity   A measure of the luminous flux emitted within a small conical angle in the direction of a surface. Measured in candela (SI unit).

Lux   The SI unit of illuminance.

Reflectance   A term given to the ratio (reflected flux)/(incident flux).

Spacing-to-height ratio   The ratio of spacing between centres of adjacent luminaires to the mounting height above the working plane.

Utilization factor   The ratio of the amount of luminous flux falling on the working plane to the total flux emitted by the luminaires.

Working plane   The horizontal, vertical or inclined plane on which the task lies. Normally assumed to be a horizontal plane 0.85 m above floor level, unless specified otherwise.

Colour

Figure 11.1 shows that within the visible spectrum, light of varying wavelengths produce corresponding changes in colour. The colours range from violet at the high-frequency (low-wavelength) end of the spectrum to red at the low-frequency (high-wavelength) end.

In considering colour, it is important to make a clear distinction between lights and pigments. If two coloured lights are superimposed, the resultant colour is not the same as that produced by mixing pigments of the same two colours. This difference is due to:

1 pigment colours being impure whilst coloured lights are pure; and

2 the resultant colour from coloured lights being the sum of the constituent colours, i.e. an additive process, whereas the resultant colour from pigments is a subtractive process.

Figure 11.2 illustrates the effects produced.

Colour appearance and colour rendering

Any coloured object has the ability to reflect certain parts of the visible spectrum of incident light falling upon it better than others. Its colour appearance will therefore depend upon the spectral emission of the incident light. The ability of a light source to reveal the true colours of objects seen in its light is known as 'colour rendering'.

A shopper buying an article of clothing may take

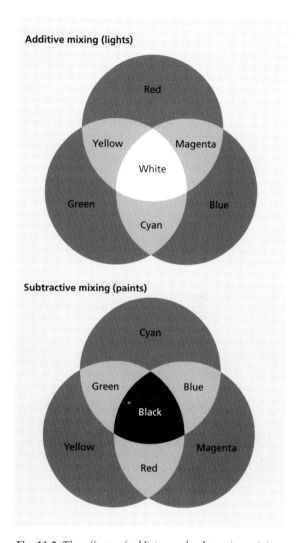

Fig. 11.2 The effects of additive and subtractive mixing.

it to a nearby window so as to gain an accurate indication of its colour since daylight does not distort surface colour. At the other extreme most objects viewed when lit by a low-pressure sodium lamp will give an almost totally false impression of their surface colour.

A colour rendering index (CRI) value ranging from 0 to 100 gives a numerical indication of the colour rendering properties of light sources: 0 indicates total distortion of colours and 100 indicates *no* distortion of colours. The CRI values of a selection of light sources together with details of the corresponding CRI group are shown in Table 11.2.

Table 11.2 Typical colour rendering index (CRI) values of lamps together with corresponding CRI groups

Lamp type	CRI group	CRI index	Comment
		100	
GLS Tungsten halogen	1A		Accurate colour discrimination is essential e.g. colour printing
Fluorescent (Northlight, artificial, daylight)		90	Good colour rendering is necessary for reasons of appearance, e.g. merchandising
Fluorescent (White, warm white), CSI, MBI	1B	80	
Fluorescent (Warm white, natural)	2	70	Moderate colour rendering is required
High-pressure sodium de-luxe		60	
High-pressure mercury Mercury blended	3	50	Poor colour quality is acceptable
		40	
High-pressure sodium SON, SON-TD	4	30	Very poor colour quality. Colour rendering is of lesser significance. Some distortion is acceptable
		20	
Low-pressure sodium		10	Total colour distortion sets in. Efficacy increases to a maximum value
		0	

Basic laws of lighting

The cosine law

A vertical plane ABCD is located at 90° to the flow of light as shown in Fig. 11.3. If the plane is rotated through an angle of $\theta°$ (shown by the inclined plane EFGH) then the illuminance on the inclined plane is reduced by the ratio $\cos \theta°:1$.

The inverse square law

Consider a point source of light at S as shown in Fig. 11.4. The flux reaching plane A, B and C is constant. If the distance SB = 2 × SA then the area of plane B is four times the area of plane A. There-fore, the illuminance on plane B is one quarter of the illuminance on plane A. Similarly if the distance SC = 3 × SA then the area of plane C is nine times the area of plane A and the illuminance on plane C is one ninth of the illuminance on plane A.

In general, illuminance varies inversely as the square of the distance from the point source. Thus:

$$\text{Illuminance } (E) \propto \frac{1}{(\text{Distance})^2} \qquad (11.1)$$
$$\text{(lux)}$$

THE EYE AND VISION

Construction of the eye

The eye, a cross-section of which is shown in Fig.

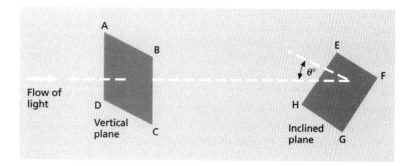

Fig. 11.3 The cosine law.

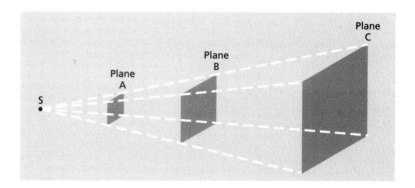

Fig. 11.4 The inverse square law.

11.5, is effectively an instrument which collects light rays and subsequently focuses them into an image on its rear surface.

Initially, light enters the eye through the cornea, which by virtue of its rounded shape behaves like a convex lens. Behind the cornea is the iris — a

coloured annular structure — which opens and closes, analogous to the diaphragm of a camera, in order to control the amount of light entering the eye. Within the centre of the iris is the pupil. Light having passed through the cornea passes through the iris and then into a transparent body called the

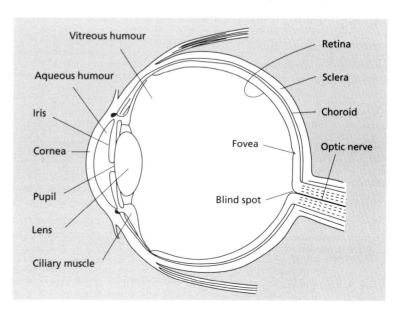

Fig. 11.5 Cross-section through the eye.

lens. The shape of this lens is variable and can be changed by the ciliary muscle.

The ciliary muscle controls the lens in order to focus the light entering the eye accurately on the retina. The retina is a light-sensitive layer at the back of the eye. Photosensitive cells within the retina convert the light falling on the retina into signals, which are carried via the optic nerve to the brain. The photosensitive cells are sub-divided into cones and rods.

The cones are active at high levels of illuminance and allow us to see detailed colour in daylight. This type of vision is referred to as 'photopic'. At lower illuminance levels, as might be typified under road lighting, the cones become progressively less sensitive, with a simultaneous lessening in appreciation of colours. Such vision is referred to as 'mesopic'. At even lower levels of illuminance, typified by approaching darkness, the cones become insensitive and only the rods operate leading to a 'grey' vision often referred to as 'scotopic' vision.

Essentially there are three types of cone, sensitive to red, blue and green light respectively. The signals generated in the cones are subsequently transmitted, via the optic nerves, to the brain which interprets the signals. Any variation in either the spectral distribution of the light source, or the colour-sensitive elements of the eye, will influence the final sensation of colour. In the centre of the retina is a small dimple termed the fovea which contains only cones. This concentration of cones makes the fovea the centre of the eye's sharpest vision.

The aqueous humour is a water-like fluid which washes the front of the eye in the space between the cornea and the lens. The vitreous humour is a transparent jelly-like fluid, which occupies the interior of the eye and helps the eye to keep its shape.

Sensitivity of the eye

The sensitivity of the eye is not constant over all wavelengths within the visible spectrum. The sensitivity, for the light-adapted eye, is greatest at a wavelength of 555 nm and diminishes at the extremes of the visible spectrum as shown in Fig. 11.6. If lights of different colours but of the same

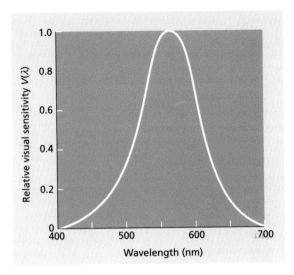

Fig. 11.6 Sensitivity of the eye.

intensity are directed into the eyes of an observer, the colours at the middle of the visible spectrum will appear brighter than those at the extremes. Thus light sources whose output is within the yellow–orange region of the spectrum (e.g. low-pressure sodium lamps — monochromatic output at 589 nm) will have a greater efficacy than light sources whose output is more biased towards the red or blue ends of the visible spectrum.

When the eye is dark-adapted, i.e. is operating in darkened environments, the sensitivity of the eye shifts. This shift is known as 'Purkinje's shift'.

Retinal fatigue

If the eye concentrates for a short time on an intense source of red light and then the gaze is transferred very quickly to a sheet of white paper, the observer perceives a blue/green image of the original source. On looking at the white background the complementary colour of the original source will be detected. The nerves of the retina which detected the original red source of light have become 'fatigued'. When the observer transfers their gaze to the white paper, all the nerves of the retina are excited, but since in that part of the retina where the image of the red source fell those nerves are fatigued, then this area of the retina will record a peacock-blue colour.

Visual perception

Visual perception can be thought of as a sequence of processes:

1 the emission of light from a source, or alternatively the reflection of light from an object;

2 the radiant energy reaching the eye (which is effectively an interface between the outside world and the brain) and subsequently being absorbed by the retina;

3 the transfer of radiant energy in the retina into electrochemical signals for onward transmission to the brain;

4 the creation in the brain, following receipt of the incoming signals, of an image which is a facsimile of the scene originally viewed.

Memory has a significant role to play in the process of interpretation. The information received on the retina is compared with similar recalled experiences. Comparison with previous similar visual experiences, and their confirmation using evidence of other senses, leads to the brain linking the information received on the retina with the real world.

Characteristics of vision

There are three highly significant factors which influence the eye's ability to see: accommodation, adaption and acuity.

Accommodation

Accommodation is the ability of the eye to focus on an object; a process which involves two separate and automatic operations, i.e.:

1 the adjustment of the lens so that the image subsequently formed on the retina is sharp;

3 the convergence of the signal from each eye so that there is one 'real image' in the brain.

Figure 11.7 represents the two operations.

Adaption

The eye will function over a brightness range of one million to one, but it is only capable of coping with brightness ranges of typically one thousand to one simultaneously. The eye responds to the brightness range by varying its sensitivity to the brightness of the object being viewed. This change in the eye's sensitivity is termed adaption. It does not occur instantaneously. In changing from a low

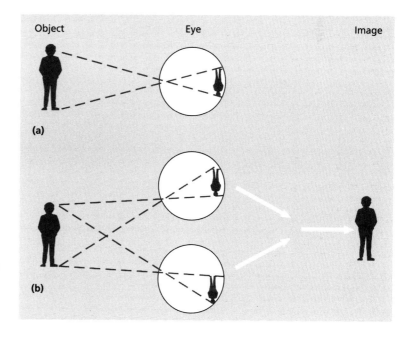

Fig. 11.7 Accommodation: (a) the lens adjusts so as to focus on the object being viewed; (b) the message signal from both eyes is brought together to form one image in the brain whilst simultaneously being inverted.

brightness to a high brightness the adaption typically takes place in seconds, whereas in traversing from a high brightness to a low brightness the change may take several minutes.

Two processes are involved in the eye's changing sensitivity.

1 The iris opens and closes quickly in response to variations in brightness. This process only provides a limited amount of control.

2 The retina changes in sensitivity but this tends to be a relatively slow process.

As a consequence the iris compensates for small changes in brightness whilst the retina responds to large brightness changes. As these processes use energy, visual fatigue can result.

Under normal daylight conditions, the sensitivity of the eye peaks at a wavelength of 555 nm. When the eye is adapted to darkened conditions the sensitivity of the eye peaks at a wavelength of 505 nm. The relationship between relative sensitivity and wavelength for both the light- and dark-adapted eye is shown in Fig. 11.8.

Acuity

Visual acuity is the ability to discern detail. It is influenced by the luminance of the object being viewed. The Snellen chart, named after the Dutchman Herman Snellen, is used by optometrists and enables visual acuity to be determined using a combination of letter size and distance between

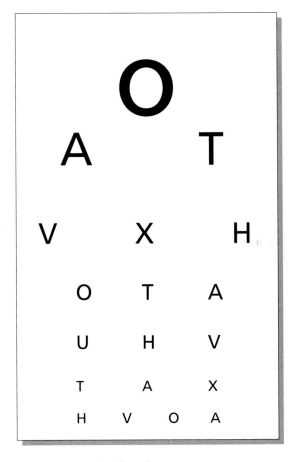

Fig. 11.9 Typical Snellen chart.

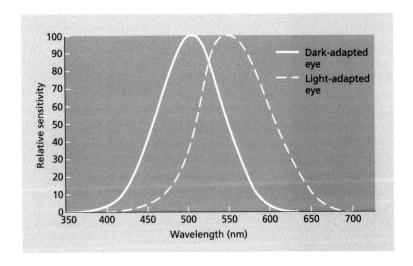

Fig. 11.8 Variation in spectral sensitivity of the human eye.

the chart and the observer. Figure 11.9 represents a typical Snellen chart.

Visual acuity can also be determined from the expression:

$$\text{Visual acuity} = \frac{1}{\text{(Angle subtended at the eye)}} \qquad (11.2)$$

where the angle is measured in minutes of arc. Figure 11.10 shows the mathematical processes involved in calculating visual acuity using Equation 11.2.

Example: consider the letter 'C' included in the wording of a warning sign displayed in a factory. Calculate the distance (L) at which an observer with a visual acuity of 1.0 will just be able to distinguish the gap in the letter C if the height of the gap is 30 mm.

If visual acuity is 1.0, then from Equation 11.2 the angle subtended at the eye is also 1.0 (minute of arc). Figure 11.11 shows the trigonometry used in the calculation.

$$1 \text{ minute of arc} = \left(\frac{1}{60}\right)^{\circ}$$

$$\theta = \left(\frac{1}{60}\right)^{\circ}$$

$$\frac{\theta}{2} = \left(\frac{1}{120}\right)^{\circ}$$

$$= 0.00833^{\circ}$$

From Fig. 11.11

$$\tan\left(\frac{\theta}{2}\right)^{\circ} = \frac{15\,\text{mm}}{L}$$

$$1.4538 \times 10^{-4} = \frac{0.015\,\text{m}}{L}$$

$$L = 103.18\,\text{m}$$

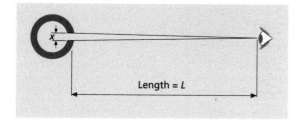

Fig. 11.10 Method of calculating visual acuity.

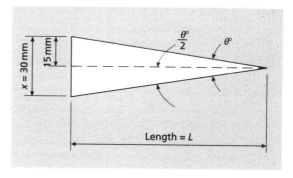

Fig. 11.11 Trigonometry used in example.

If the variation in acuity with task illuminance is plotted graphically, it will be shown that acuity initially increases rapidly, the initial rate of change decreasing, until a point is reached where the characteristic levels off. Figure 11.12 is a typical curve, relating to a particular task. If the task is a relatively simple one, then maximum performance (the point where the characteristic levels off) will be achieved with a relatively low level of illuminance.

By definition acuity tends to be an academic indicator of the eye's ability to discern detail. When a visual task is under consideration it is necessary to determine not only whether the task can be undertaken but also the ability of the eye to carry

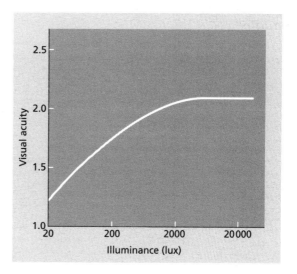

Fig. 11.12 Typical relationship between visual acuity and prevailing illuminance.

out the task with speed and accuracy, a combination referred to as visual performance.

There is a link between accuracy and speed and it can be shown that the plot of performance against illuminance is very similar to the plot of acuity against illuminance. Whilst there will be variation from task to task, these characteristics tend to level off at the point where the individual obtains maximum accuracy corresponding to the point where manual dexterity will not allow work at a faster rate. Figure 11.13 shows typical characteristics of accuracy and speed against illuminance. Figure 11.14 gives typical acuity curves for three tasks having low, medium and good contrast. It will be evident that the low-contrast task requires a much greater illuminance in order for it to be performed adequately. Figure 11.15 shows the relationship between typical relative illuminance required for reading print on paper, as an example of a visual task, against the age of the individual reading the print.

Visual fatigue

The causes of visual fatigue can be conveniently divided into three categories.

1 *Constitutional*: where the overall state of the health of the individual is important.

2 *Ocular*: where the effects of deteriorating vision and/or the effects of ageing are significant.

3 *Environmental*: where the levels of illuminance and the general characteristics of the immediate vicinity are influential. The environmental causes of visual fatigue can be categorized into:

(a) those which are influenced by the visual task itself, and

(b) those which are influenced by the visual environment in which the task is carried out.

The visual task

When the light signal detected by the eyes is of low level, the brain attempts to amplify the signal by feedback to the eye. This process subsequently produces strain when the feedback becomes continuous. Characteristics of the visual task which subsequently lead to eyestrain include:
* minute detail;
* excessively low contrast task/background;
* movement of task;
* surface finish of task.

The visual environment

Characteristics of the visual environment which, either singularly or in combination, subsequently lead to eyestrain include:
* inadequate illuminance;
* excessively high contrast (task/background);
* presence of glare;

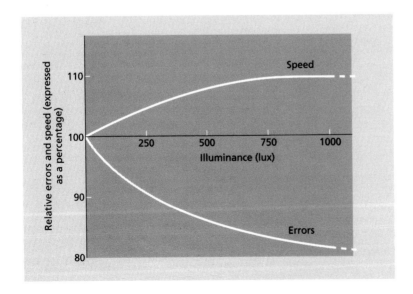

Fig. 11.13 Typical relationship between speed and errors, and prevailing illuminance.

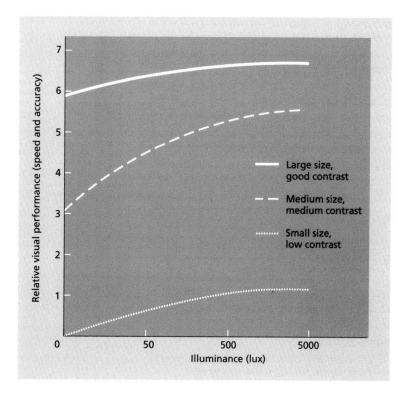

Fig. 11.14 Typical relative visual performance versus illuminance for different tasks and contrast levels.

- flicker from fluorescent sources;
- general feeling of lack of well-being within an environment.

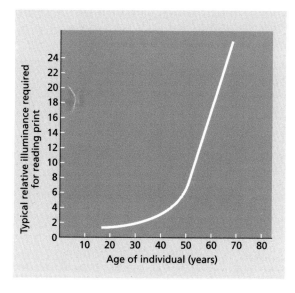

Fig. 11.15 Typical relative illuminance required for reading print versus age of individual.

Glare

Many definitions of the term 'glare' have been put forward. The term is synonymous with the effect perceived when viewing the headlights of an oncoming vehicle, being more pronounced on a dark, wet night. In reality, glare is any situation where contrast within the field of view is excessive. The two main forms of glare are 'disability glare' and 'discomfort glare'.

Disability glare, as the name would imply, prevents or disables an individual from seeing a particular task. The earlier reference to the headlights of an oncoming vehicle is an example of disability glare. In such situations it is almost impossible to discern the scene immediately surrounding the headlights. The disabling effect within the eye is due in part to a veil of scattered light in the optic media within the eye and is likely to be more prevalent in elderly people. Disability glare is proportional to the intensity of the offending source.

Discomfort glare, which is more likely to occur in interiors, may not disable an individual from performing a particular visual task, but prolonged exposure to such an environment will cause discomfort. It may be that such discomfort will take several hours to materialize, often developing as a headache. Discomfort glare can be produced as a result of a badly designed lighting installation. Almost invariably, glare is an unwanted phenomenon, but occasionally it is possible to use glare to advantage. One such advantage is the use of high-powered lamps mounted on security checkpoints at factory entrances. In such circumstances would-be intruders cannot see if the checkpoint is manned.

Glare index

It is possible to assign a numerical value to the magnitude of discomfort glare. This value is known as the 'glare index'. Such values are then compared with limiting values of indices for typical interiors as specified in the *Code for Interior Lighting* (Chartered Institution of Building Services Engineers, 1994).

The procedure for calculating glare index is a two-stage process. Initially, an uncorrected index value is read from published tables where the length and width of the interior being considered are quoted in terms of the mounting height (H). H is taken as the distance between the eyes of a seated individual and the horizontal centre line of the luminaires. The eye level of a seated observer is taken as 1.2 m above ground level. Account is taken, in the published tables, of variation in fabric reflectances of the interior being considered.

The final glare index value, which is the value used when making the comparison with given limiting values, is calculated by applying conversion factors to the uncorrected index value depending upon:
1 the luminous flux of the luminaire;
2 variation in the mounting height from the seated eye level value of 1.2 m.

In order to avoid the presence of discomfort glare, the final or corrected value should not exceed the limiting index value quoted in the *Code of Interior Lighting* (Chartered Institution of Building Services Engineers, 1994) for the interior under consideration. Calculation of glare index values must be made in both axial and transverse directions relative to the layout of the interior. Further

details of the calculation of glare index values are given in Smith (1991). Figure 11.16 shows methods of reducing glare from windows.

LAMPS AND LUMINAIRES

Lamps can be divided into two types: filament lamps and discharge lamps.

Filament lamps

These lamps rely on the principle of incandescence for the production of light. Essentially, a metallic filament is heated by means of an electric current until it incandesces, giving off visible radiation. The domestic lamp (GLS lamp) is an everyday example of the filament lamp.

A progression from the GLS lamp is the tungsten halogen lamp. Quartz glass is used for the envelope and the addition of a trace of one of the halogen elements, e.g. iodine, allows the iodine to combine with the tungsten, which has evaporated from the filament, to form tungsten iodine. The tungsten iodine vapour is then carried back to the filament by convection currents where it separates out, the tungsten being redeposited on the original filament. The iodine is subsequently released and the cycle is repeated. The envelope of a tungsten halogen lamp should never be touched by human skin, since the greases and acids contained within the skin will attack the quartz glass and subsequently produce weak spots which may ultimately lead to premature failure.

Discharge lamps

In discharge lamps there is no direct electrical connection within the lamp as is the case with filament lamps. A discharge lamp consists of a glass tube containing a gas or vapour.

When a voltage is applied to the lamp, energy is imparted to atoms resulting in the displacement of electrons to higher energy levels. The electrons subsequently fall back to their original levels, thereby releasing energy in the form of electromagnetic photons. The nature of the gas or vapour will determine the wavelength and thereby the colour of the output from the lamp.

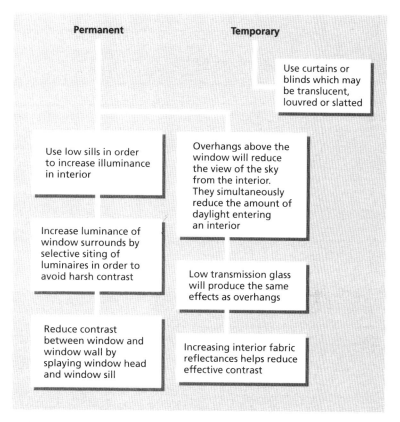

Fig. 11.16 Methods of reducing glare from windows.

Discharge lamps can be further sub-divided into low-pressure and high-pressure lamps. Low-pressure lamps include fluorescent lamps and low-pressure sodium (SOX) lamps. The latter emit monochromatic light at a wavelength of approximately 589 nm. These lamps have the advantage of almost instantaneous restrike in the event of momentary loss of electrical supply. The monochromatic output of the SOX lamp is at a wavelength close to that of the maximum sensitivity of the eye and therefore the lamp has a very high efficacy value. A further advantage is that SOX lamps are extremely useful in foggy conditions since the monochromatic light cannot be split up into constituent wavelengths by the water droplets in suspension in the atmosphere.

However, a major disadvantage of the SOX lamp is that its colour rendering index value is almost zero. Objects seen in the light from a SOX lamp will have their surface colours severely distorted, unless the surface colour wavelength is matched to the output from the lamp.

Fluorescent lamps are used extensively in interiors. Electronic circuitry involving high-frequency supplies allows regulation of the light output which, if used in sympathy with levels of prevailing daylight, can be used in energy-saving installations. The light output from fluorescent lamps is influenced by the ambient temperature.

High-pressure lamps include mercury vapour, metal halide and high-pressure sodium lamps. Such lamps are used extensively for road lighting, lighting for civic and amenity areas together with floodlighting for car parks, railway sidings and building sites.

Mercury vapour and metal halide lamps, if broken, emit potentially dangerous ultraviolet radiation. Disposal of broken and spent lamps needs to be carefully controlled. Details of acceptable methods of control are given in *Disposal of Discharge Lamps* (Health and Safety Executive, 1989).

Table 11.3 gives typical characteristics and applications of lamp types.

Table 11.3 Characteristics and applications of lamp types

Lamp type (and symbol)	Typical lamp efficacy (lumens per watt)	Typical lamp life (h)	Typical applications
Tungsten filament (GLS)	8–18	1000–2000	Domestic, display
Tungsten halogen (TH)	18–24	2000–4000	Display, traffic signals, overhead projectors (OHP)
Mercury vapour (MB)	40–60	5000–10 000	Industrial, road lighting
Metal halide (MBI)	65–85	5000–10 000	Floodlighting, area and amenity lighting
Fluorescent (MCF)	50–100	5000–10 000	General, domestic, commercial
Low-pressure sodium (SOX)	100–175	6000–12 000	Road lighting
High-pressure sodium (SON)	65–120	6000–20 000	Industrial, road lighting, civic and amenity lighting

Luminaires

Formerly known as the 'light fitting', the luminaire supports the lamp and provides the necessary electrical connections. Luminaires control the flow of light, direct it towards the working plane and control the brightness of the output of the luminaire visible to the occupants within the interior. Additionally, the luminaire provides the means of fixing the lamp to the building fabric, together with providing a housing for the lamp control gear.

Luminaires have to operate in a variety of environments, including dusty, wet, corrosive and the generally hostile. Luminaire construction is defined in BS 4533 (British Standards Institution, 1990) and BS EN 60598-1 (British Standards Institution, 1993). The Ingress Protection (IP) system for specifying the degree of protection which is provided by an enclosure also includes luminaires. The degree of protection is designated by a two-digit reference number. The first digit (0–6 inclusive) describes the degree of protection from the ingress of solid foreign objects. The second digit (0–8 inclusive) describes the degree of protection against the ingress of water.

DAYLIGHT FACTOR AND DAYLIGHT

Daylight factor

This is the relationship connecting values of internal illuminance and external illuminance, both values being restricted to daylight as a source:

$$\text{Daylight factor} = \frac{\text{Daylight illuminance at a point within a room}}{\begin{array}{c}\text{Simultaneous illuminance} \\ \text{on a horizontal plane outside} \\ \text{the building from a} \\ \text{completely unobstructed sky} \\ \text{(excluding sunlight)}\end{array}} \times 100\%$$

(11.3)

The daylight factor is essentially a geometrical characteristic of an interior/window combination. Its value is not influenced by changes in external illuminance and at any point in an interior its numerical value is constant.

The daylight factor comprises three separate components as shown in Fig. 11.17. The components are: (1) the sky component, which is due to light received directly from the sky; (2) the

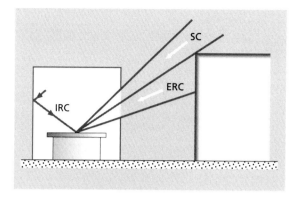

Fig. 11.17 The three components of daylight factor: SC, sky component; ERC, externally reflected component; IRC, internally reflected component. Daylight factor = Σ (SC + ERC + IRC).

externally reflected component, which is due to light reflected from external obstructions, e.g. adjoining buildings; and (3) the internally reflected components, which are due to light reflected from internal surfaces in the building, e.g. walls, floor, ceiling.

Daylight

In the UK, the exterior illuminance due to daylight typically reaches 35 000 lux at noon during July, whilst at noon in December the exterior illuminance typically reaches 8000 lux. When the exterior illuminance falls below 5000 lux, daylighting is generally accepted as being too weak to provide adequate lighting within an interior.

The above values are exterior values. The interior illuminance due to daylight is significantly lower, with typically only 10% of the exterior illuminance filtering through to interiors. Furthermore this figure is variable and is influenced by, for example, distance from windows.

The daylight factor calculation, referred to previously, is relative to an individual point within an interior. Clearly, in order to develop a more meaningful pattern of the effects of daylight within an interior it would be necessary to develop a grid of such values throughout the building. The concept of an average daylight factor overcomes the necessity to perform multiple calculations from point to point. The average daylight factor is given by:

$$\text{Average daylight factor (\%)} = \frac{T\,W\,\theta\,M}{A\,(1 - R^2)} \qquad (11.4)$$

where T is the diffuse transmittance of glazing (clear single glazing = 0.85 and double glazing = 0.75), W is the nett area of glazing (m^2), θ is the angle subtended in the vertical plane by sky visible from the geometric centre of the window (in degrees), A is the total area of interior wall surface, including floor, ceiling, walls and windows (m^2), R is the average reflectance value of the internal surface (weighted according to surface areas) and M is a maintenance factor which takes into account dirt on lamps and luminaires and deterioration of light output.

It is generally accepted that when the average daylight factor is greater than typically 5%, the building interior will give the appearance of being lit cheerfully by daylight. Conversely, if the average daylight factor drops below typically 2%, natural daylight will rarely be satisfactory and artificial lighting is likely to be required constantly.

LIGHTING SYSTEMS AND LIGHTING DESIGN

Lighting systems

Systems used in commercial and industrial interiors can be divided into three major groups: general lighting, localized lighting and local lighting. General lighting installations aim to provide, as far as is practical, an approximately uniform illuminance over the whole of the working plane. Near uniform illuminance is often achieved using the Lumen method of design (see below). Localized lighting is a system designed to provide the required illuminance on the work areas, together with a reduced level of illuminance in adjacent areas. Local lighting is lighting for a small area surrounding the task, typically provided by small fluorescent luminaires. Figure 11.18 shows the essential differences between the three systems.

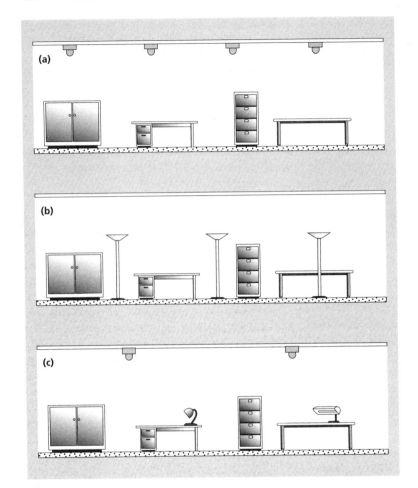

Fig. 11.18 Types of lighting systems: (a) general lighting; (b) localized lighting; (c) local lighting.

Lighting in offices

Many office occupations involve the reading of typed information. The visual task is therefore influenced by the size of the type used, together with type clarity and also the reflectance values of both type and paper.

Offices are often illuminated with ceiling-mounted luminaires arranged to provide an average level of illuminance on the working plane. It is usually the case that such lighting schemes have been designed with little regard for the type of visual tasks likely to be carried out within the office. Many offices can be lit using daylight for a substantial part of the working year. However, the levels of indoor illuminance from daylight may not necessarily be sufficient to allow many tasks to be carried out.

Windows not only admit light but maintain a link for the room occupants with the outside world. There is therefore a clear advantage in using light sources capable of producing an output which approaches that of natural daylight. For this reason fluorescent lamps are preferred extensively for office lighting. *CIBSE LG7* (Chartered Institution of Building Services Engineers, 1993) refers to office lighting.

Visual task lighting

When analysing particular tasks an assessment should be made of the adaption and accommodation involved in the task at hand, together with a further assessment of the frequency at which the task is being performed. Determining the objects that require viewing, and establishing under what conditions viewing needs to take place, together with a detailed survey of the existing lighting outlining any deficiencies, will be highly beneficial in forming an overall view of task lighting requirements.

Many methods of design for lighting systems aim to achieve a relatively uniform distribution of illuminance at the working plane level. Unfortunately, this often simultaneously produces unacceptable visual task lighting. When visual task lighting is considered, and good task lighting conditions ultimately achieved, it is likely that a more acceptable working environment will be established which avoids the effects of visual distraction and/or visual fatigue. Relatively bright reflections within the task will limit its visibility and may subsequently lead to discomfort.

The human eye acknowledges details within a visual task by discriminating between the darker and lighter parts of the task. The variation in 'brightness' of a visual task is determined from the luminance contrast. Luminance contrast (C) is given by:

$$C = \left| \frac{L_t - L_b}{L_b} \right| \qquad (11.5)$$

where L_t is the luminance of the task and L_b is the luminance of the background. Both quantities are expressed in candela m^{-2}. The vertical (modulus) lines indicate that all values of luminance contrast are to be considered as positive.

The contrast of a visual task will be influenced by the reflectance properties of the task itself. If the task material has a matt finish, then incident light upon the task will be reflected equally in all directions. This infers that the direction of the incident light will be insignificant.

It is more often the case, however, that the task has a non-matt or specular finish (mirror-like). In such cases, defocussed images of high-luminance sources, e.g. luminaires, will be seen reflected in the task. Such images produce 'veiling reflections', a form of indirect glare. 'Veiling reflections' are so termed because they produce a veil of light in front of the task.

Reflecting glare fools the eye into thinking that the environment is brighter than it is. This results in the eye failing to adapt correctly to the value of illuminance required for the visual task and leads to visual fatigue. In such cases the direction of the incident light is highly significant.

There is a link between contrast and reflectance. Consider black ink — with a typical reflectance value of say 5% — on a piece of white paper — with the paper having a typical reflectance value of say 85%. The ink is usually perceived by the contrast, or difference, in luminance between the black ink and the white paper. The luminous contrast, as has been shown, can be calculated from Equation 11.5. Alternatively, it can be calculated from the reflectances of the ink and the paper, providing that both the ink and the paper are illuminated uniformly. Thus:

$$C = \left| \frac{R_{paper} - R_{ink}}{R_{paper}} \right| \times 100\% \qquad (11.6)$$

where R_{paper} is the reflectance of the paper and R_{ink} is the reflectance of the ink.

Using Equation 11.6, luminous contrast for the black ink on the white paper is calculated as:

$$C = \left| \frac{85 - 5}{85} \right| \times 100\%$$
$$= 94.1\%$$

Lumen method of design

The main aim of the Lumen method of design is to achieve a uniform general level of illuminance on a working plane within an interior. This method takes no cognizance of the task likely to be performed in the interior.

With the Lumen method, the illuminance (E) (lux) is found from:

$$E = \frac{n \times LDL \times LLF \times UF}{Area} \qquad (11.7)$$

where n is the number of lamps, LDL is the lighting design lumens per lamp (i.e. the lamp output, after an initial period of operation), LLF is the light loss factor (which takes into account the depreciation of light output due to lamp ageing, dirt on luminaire, etc.) and UF is the utilization factor (which is found from the luminaire manufacturer's literature).

Example: an office 8 m × 6 m is to be lit to a

general level of 500 lux on the working plane, using fluorescent lamps each having an output of 4500 lumen. If the light loss factor is 0.82 and the utilization factor is 0.44 calculate the number of lamps required:

$$E = \frac{n \times LDL \times LLF \times UF}{Area}$$

therefore

$$n = \frac{E \times Area}{LDL \times LLF \times UF}$$

$$= \frac{500 \times 48}{4500 \times 0.82 \times 0.44}$$

$$= 14.78$$

i.e. 15 lamps, possibly in a 5×3 array.

Inspection lighting

The purpose of inspection lighting is to highlight inconsistencies in a product so that it can be rejected if the defect is considered unacceptable. The techniques used are shown in Table 11.4.

Emergency lighting

The purpose of emergency lighting is to enable people to move in relative safety to an escape route, and subsequently to vacate the premises in the event of an interruption of supply to the main lighting system. Emergency lighting may be in use at all times, known as a 'maintained system', or it may come into operation only in the event of the failure of the main electrical supply. Such a system is referred to as 'non-maintained'. A further subdivision of emergency lighting defines: (1) 'escape lighting' which is that part of emergency lighting relative to escape routes; and (2) 'standby lighting' which is designed to allow normal activities to continue in the event of a loss of the main electrical supply.

In accordance with BS 5266 (British Standards Institution, 1988), emergency lighting should be operative within 5 s of the supply interruption. In situations where the occupants within an interior are familiar with the layout and escape routes then

Table 11.4 Inspection lighting techniques

Inspection	Technique
Scratches on polished or glossy surfaces	Directional light applied to surface. Reflections from irregularities appear light on dark background
Surface flatness	Monochromatic light (typically from SOX lamps) used in conjunction with optical flats, creates optical fringes revealing defects
Defects in transparent materials, e.g. glass, plastics	Output from lamp is deliberately polarized, transmitted through the product being inspected and then analysed using a second polarizer. Defects will produce variations in the pattern of transmitted light
Surface finishes	Ultraviolet radiation causes some materials to fluoresce. Products to be inspected are coated with fluorescent material which will reveal darkened areas where there are irregularities or discontinuities in the surface finish
Rotating components	Rotating components appear stationary using the stroboscopic effect
Colour matching*	Special fluorescent lamps in accordance with BS 950 (British Standards Institution, 1967)

* Care should be taken to avoid confusion with 'metamerism', i.e. where the colours of two articles appear identical under one light source but appear different under another source of light.

the time interval can be extended up to a maximum of 15 s with the approval of the enforcing authority.

Exterior lighting

It is essential to appreciate that exterior lighting and interior lighting present different problems. Such differences include reflectance, size and mounting height.

Reflectances: these are critical when considering interior lighting but with exterior lighting there is an almost total absence of reflectances;

Size: interiors are relatively small compared with the size of exteriors to be lit;

Mounting height: mounting heights in interiors tend to be small compared with exteriors, where often poles or towers are used.

The lighting of exteriors typically involves providing illumination for a small number of persons, often occupied in carrying out work of little visual difficulty. Such installations require a lower level of illuminance than is required for interior lighting. Typical examples of exterior lighting installations include: building and civil engineering sites; car parks; factory yards; railway yards and sidings; loading bays; gantry and crane yards; and storage areas.

For railway yards, sidings, factory yards and car parks, it is usual to use high-powered lamps at high mounting heights. On building and civil engineering sites, lighting is often required 24 h per day. On these sites it is usual to use portable lighting equipment which can be relocated as the site work progresses. When siting luminaires in loading bays, it is necessary to take cognizance of the likely positions of vehicles during loading, in order to avoid the vehicles becoming obstructions and creating unwanted shadows. Storage areas can cause special problems. For areas free from obstruction it is more advantageous to use multiple luminaires on a single support. Increasing the mounting height can reduce unwanted shadows caused by obstructions. However, it will then be necessary to use higher-rated lamps. For gantry and crane yards, structural members supporting the gantries can be used for the mounting of luminaires. Attention must be paid to the possibility of shadows being created by the working movement of the equipment.

Hazardous-area lighting

Explosive atmospheres

BS 5345 (British Standards Institution, 1989) categorizes hazardous areas into three zones. Zone 0 refers to an area where an explosive gas/air mixture is present continuously. Zone 1 refers to an area where an explosive gas/air mixture is likely to occur in normal operation. Zone 2 refers to an area where an ignitable concentration is not likely to occur during normal operation.

Mains-powered lighting is not permitted in a Zone 0 atmosphere. Betalights are, however, allowed in Zone 0 atmospheres. Typically these are sealed borosilicate glass capsules coated internally with phosphor and filled with tritium gas.

Grouping of apparatus

BS 5345 (British Standards Institution, 1989) classifies luminaires to be used in hazardous atmospheres into: (1) Group I for application in the coal-mining industry; and (2) Group II for application in other industries. Group II luminaires are further divided into sub-groups, depending upon their suitability for use with gases and vapours, thus: Group IIA is the propane group; Group IIB is the ethylene group; and Group IIC is the hydrogen group. Full details of the protection afforded by electrical equipment against explosion are given in Part I of BS 5435.

Ignition temperature

'Ignition temperature' is defined as the lowest temperature, determined by a standardized method, at which the most explosive mixture of a given substance and air will just ignite at a heated surface.

LIGHTING FOR AREAS CONTAINING VISUAL DISPLAY UNITS

In order to exercise control over the working environment in which visual display units (VDUs) are used, legislation has been introduced which affects both employed and self-employed workers who habitually use VDUs for a significant part of their normal work. The Health and Safety (Display Screen Equipment) Regulations (Health and Safety Executive, 1992) came into force on 1 January 1993. The regulations implement a European directive (European Community, 1990) on minimum safety and health requirements for work with display screen equipment. Employers have a requirement to ensure that VDU workstations comply with the regulations.

General lighting requirements. In accordance with the Schedule to the regulations, any room lighting or task lighting provided shall ensure satisfactory lighting conditions and produce an appropriate contrast between the VDU screen and the background environment, taking into account the nature of the work and the visual requirements of the operator or user. Any possible disturbing glare and reflections on the VDU screen, or other equipment, shall be prevented by co-ordinating workplace and workstation layout with the location and technical characteristics of the artificial light sources.

Reflections and glare. In accordance with the Schedule to the regulations, workstations shall be designed so that sources of light such as windows and transparent or translucent walls cause no direct glare and no distracting reflections on the screen. Windows shall be fitted with a suitable system of adjustable covering so as to attenuate the daylight that falls on the workstation.

Luminaires for VDU areas

In the UK, *CIBSE LG3* (Chartered Institution of Building Services Engineers, 1989) gives recommendations about luminaires for use in areas where there are VDUs. These recommendations were introduced into the UK before the EC display screen directive (European Community, 1990) and the Health and Safety Regulations (Health and Safety Executive, 1992). The UK Health and Safety Executive recommends that employers should grade visual display tasks, according to the degree of severity and intensity, into one of three categories. In each category the luminance above a specified cut-off angle is limited to 200 candela m^{-2}.

Figure 11.19 shows the cut-off angles for each of the three categories described.

Category 1. Used in areas where VDU screens are constantly in use, where there is a high density of screens and where errors in discerning the information displayed on the screen are likely to have

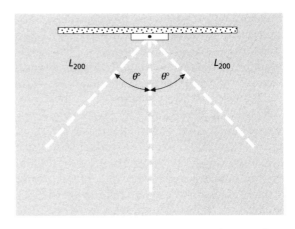

Fig. 11.19 Classification of luminaires used in visual display unit (VDU) areas. $\theta° =$ cut-off angle. L_{200} represents a luminance limit of 200 candela m^{-2} above the cut-off angle. Category 1, $\theta = 55°$; Category 2, $\theta = 65°$; Category 3, $\theta = 75°$.

serious consequences, e.g. in air traffic control rooms.

Category 2. Used in areas where VDU screens are used intermittently or where a lesser number of screens are in constant use and where the accuracy of the information displayed on the screen is considered to be important.

Category 3. Used in areas where VDU screens are used occasionally, where there is a low density of screens and where the information displayed on the screen is considered to be of lesser importance, e.g. routine office tasks.

Use of uplighters

Uplighters, producing a form of indirect lighting, are often used in areas containing VDUs. Essentially, the light is directed onto the ceiling from where it is then reflected downwards. This method of illuminating an area overcomes the problem of direct vision of the light source itself and thereby the effects of glare on display screens are almost totally eliminated. Unfortunately, in order to prevent adverse lighting conditions, the use of uplighters places certain restrictions on the finish and colour of the room fabrics. In extreme cases it is possible to inadvertently create a large luminous ceiling which amplifies the oscillations in light output produced by the alternating electrical supply to the lamps used. This will create an unwanted effect which may lead to visual fatigue when subjected to prolonged exposure.

Methods of avoiding problems encountered with VDUs are listed in Fig. 11.20.

LIGHTING SURVEYS

A full lighting survey will give details of any defects in the lighting systems and enable remedial action to be taken.

Survey techniques

Preliminaries

Scale drawings should be produced, giving details of all principal working surfaces, windows, luminaires and other structural and/or decor features. Where confusion is likely to develop, sectional views will be beneficial.

Preliminary report sheet

Figure 11.21 shows a typical preliminary report sheet.

Determination of the minimum number of measuring points

For the results of a lighting survey to be meaningful there must be a minimum number of measuring points within the interior being surveyed. The number of points will be influenced by the geometry of the interior. One method of determining the minimum number of measuring points is to calculate the room index (RI) of the interior and then calculate the corresponding minimum number of measuring points. RI is calculated by:

$$RI = \frac{Length \times Width}{MH\,(Length + Width)} \tag{11.8}$$

where MH is the mounting height above the working plane. The minimum number of measuring points is subsequently found by:

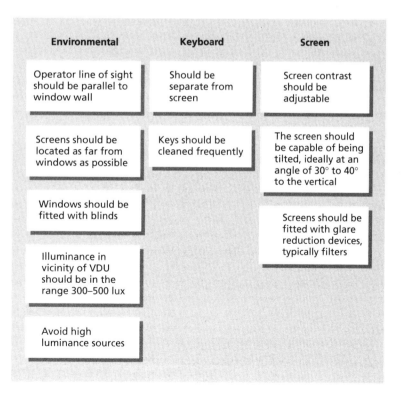

Fig. 11.20 Methods of avoiding problems encountered with visual display units (VDUs).

Environmental	Keyboard	Screen
Operator line of sight should be parallel to window wall	Should be separate from screen	Screen contrast should be adjustable
Screens should be located as far from windows as possible	Keys should be cleaned frequently	The screen should be capable of being tilted, ideally at an angle of 30° to 40° to the vertical
Windows should be fitted with blinds		Screens should be fitted with glare reduction devices, typically filters
Illuminance in vicinity of VDU should be in the range 300–500 lux		
Avoid high luminance sources		

Lighting survey sheet

Date .... Time ....

Location Address ....

Survey Person ....

Reason for Survey ....

Room Dimensions:　　L = ...．　　W = ...．　　　　　H = ...．

Window Dimensions:　H = ...．　　W = ...．

Daylight Availability:　Side Glazing ....　Roof Glazing ....

Artificial Lighting:　Luminaires/Lamps ....

Luminaire Type ....

Lamp Type ....

Lamp Rating ....

Date of Lamp Change ....

Condition of Equipment and Room Fabrics:

Ceiling ....

Walls ....

Floor ....

Windows ....

Luminaires ....

Principal Visual Tasks ....

Principal Planes of Interest ....

CIBSE Recommended Illuminance Values ....

Fig. 11.21 Typical preliminary report sheet.

$$\text{Minimum number of measuring points} = (X + 2)^2 \quad (11.9)$$

where X is a parameter whose value is dependent upon the RI. For all values of RI less than 3.0, the value of X is taken as the next highest integer. For all values of RI equal to or greater than 3.0, the value of X is fixed at 4.0. Table 11.5 gives examples of the relationship between RI, X and the minimum number of measuring points. A typical layout of measuring points is shown in Fig. 11.22.

This procedure describes the minimum number of measuring points. However, it may be considered beneficial to select a higher number of measuring points if the room geometry so dictates.

Table 11.5 Relationship between room index, parameter X and minimum number of measuring points

Room index	Parameter X	Minimum number of measuring points
0.9	1	9
1.9	2	16
2.0	3	25
3.0	4	36
3.4	4	36
5.1	4	36

Measuring equipment

Illuminance meters

The spectral response of the cells used in the instruments differs from the response of the human visual system. The response is typically corrected by the use of filters and when filters are incor-

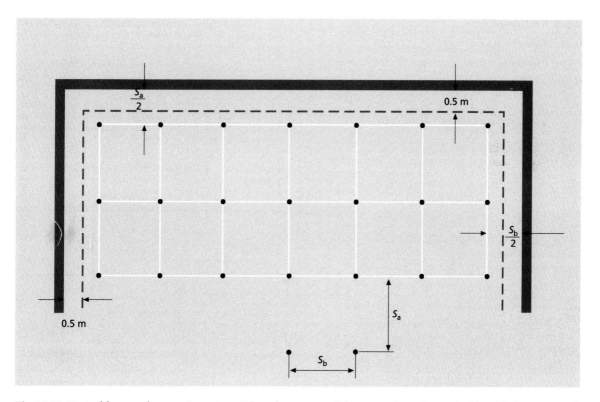

Fig. 11.22 Typical layout of measuring points. When the centres of the measuring points coincide with the centres of the lighting points within an interior then the use of more than the minimum number of lighting points is recommended in order to minimize errors. Measurements should ideally be taken on a horizontal plane, typically 0.8 m above floor level. Measuring points within 0.5 m of boundary walls are not considered appropriate.

porated the instrument is referred to as 'colour corrected'.

A further correction is applied to take into account the direction of incident light falling upon the detector cell. Instruments which are capable of accurately measuring illuminance from differing directions of incident light are said to be 'cosine corrected'.

Luminance meters

Luminance meters use photovoltaic cells similar to those used in illuminance meters. Such instruments also have to be colour corrected.

Daylight factor meters

Instruments are available which measure the value of the daylight factor directly.

Interpretation of data

Levels of illuminance should be compared with CIBSE requirements for the type of interior under consideration. 'Patchy' lighting should be avoided wherever possible. To this end the uniformity ratio is a useful indicator:

Table 11.6 Typical illuminance levels

Location or event	Typical illuminance levels (lux)
Starlight	0.2
Moonlight	2.0
Side road or estate road lighting	5.0–10.0
Domestic interior lighting	100–300
Workshop benches	400–500
General offices	500–750
Drawing offices	500–750
'Bad light' stops play at cricket	1000
Sports ground lighting for colour TV transmission	1500–2000
Operating theatres	10 000–50 000
Bright sunlight	50 000–100 000

NB: CIBSE *Code for Interior Lighting* (Chartered Institution of Building Services Engineers, 1994) gives details of recommended illuminance levels for domestic, commercial and industrial applications.

$$\text{Uniformity ratio} = \frac{\text{Minimum illuminance}}{\text{Mean illuminance}} \quad (11.10)$$

The minimum acceptable value of the uniformity ratio is 0.8.

Typical lighting levels

Typical illuminance levels relative to everyday events are listed in Table 11.6.

REFERENCES

British Standards Institution (1967). *Specification for Artificial Daylight for the Assessment of Colour.* British Standards Institution BS 950 Part 1.

British Standards Institution (1988). *Code of Practice for the Emergency Lighting of Premises Other Than Cinemas and Certain Other Specified Premises Used for Entertainment.* British Standards Institution BS 5266 Part 1.

British Standards Institution (1989). *Code of Practice for Selection, Installation and Maintenance of Electrical Apparatus for use in Potentially Explosive Atmospheres (other than Mining Applications or Explosive Processing and Manufacture).* British Standards Institution BS 5345 Part 1.

British Standards Institution (1990). *Electric Luminaires.* British Standards Institution BS 4533 Part 101.

British Standards Institution (1993). *Luminaires. General Requirements and Tests.* British Standards Institution BS EN 60598-1.

Chartered Institution of Building Services Engineers (1989). *Areas for Visual Display Terminals.* CIBSE Lighting Guide No. 3.

Chartered Institution of Building Services Engineers (1993). *Lighting for Offices.* CIBSE Lighting Guide No. 7.

Chartered Institution of Building Services Engineers (1994). *Code for Interior Lighting.*

European Community (1990). *Directive on the Minimum Safety and Health Requirements for Work with Display Screen Equipment.* EC Directive 90/270/EEC.

Health and Safety Executive (1989). *Disposal of Discharge Lamps.* HELA Data Sheet. HSA 253/3/100/8.

Health and Safety Executive (1992). *Health and Safety (Display Screen Equipment). Regulations.*

Smith, N.A. (1991). *Lighting for Occupational Hygienists.* H and H Scientific Consultants Ltd., Leeds.

CHAPTER 12

The Thermal Environment

A. Youle

INTRODUCTION

Humans are warm-blooded animals; the body core temperature (i.e. the temperature deep in the body tissues) must normally be regulated to remain within a narrow range, typically $37.0 \pm 0.5°C$ $(98.4 \pm 1°F)$. This process, termed 'heat home-ostasis', is required because many of the bio-chemical and cellular processes on which bodily functions depend, take place efficiently and cor-rectly only within this narrow range. External conditions which permit the narrow control con-ditions to be maintained are termed thermally 'neutral' or in the 'neutral zone'. Outside this zone the environment can be considered to be applying either heat or cold 'stress' to the body, with poten-tial thermal 'strain' effects. The usual maximum deviation of core temperature that can be tolerated in fit people is approximately $\pm 2°C$, but with potential strain effects. In the extreme, if the core temperature drops to about 31°C, strain is manifest by loss of consciousness and death can ensue rapidly; above 43°C the thermoregulation mech-anism can fail, again with potentially fatal conse-quences (see Chapter 5).

The body generates heat continuously, by the conversion of food to energy via the metabolic system, and using the energy in the form of work done. The majority of energy is converted to heat, which contributes to maintaining the body tem-perature, but may cause overheating. There must be an appropriate balance between the heat gener-ated and the heat lost to, or gained from, the environment to maintain heat homeostasis.

THERMAL BALANCE

Whenever a temperature difference occurs between an object and its surroundings, heat transfer processes will occur to reduce this difference. The processes available, depending on the physical circumstances prevailing, are: conduction, convec-tion, radiation and phase changes (e.g. evaporation). This transfer will apply to any such circumstances in occupations, e.g. heating effects of furnaces, solar heat gains through glazing in buildings, chill-ing from a cold wind or heat distribution from a heating system.

In particular, heat exchange mechanisms are continuously functioning between the human body and its surroundings. Under normal circumstances, there is a net loss from the body to its surroundings for the body's core temperature to remain constant, i.e. there is an equilibrium between internal heat production and heat loss from the surface (Fig. 12.1). This thermal balance can be expressed in the form of the equation:

$$M = \pm K \pm C \pm R - E \qquad (12.1)$$

where M is the rate of metabolic heat production; K, C and R are the loss or gain of heat by conduction, convection and radiation respectively; and E is the heat loss from the skin and respiratory tract due to the evaporation of moisture. Other factors which may affect the balance are the external work (w) performed by or on the body (affecting M) and the rate of change in the store of heat (S) in the body.

The value of metabolic heat production in the basal state, i.e. with complete physical and mental

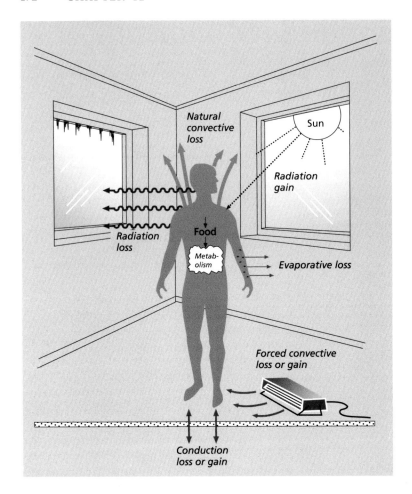

Fig. 12.1 Heat balance mechanisms for the human body.

rest, is about 45 W m^{-2} (i.e. per m^2 of body surface area) for a 30 year-old male. With the surface area of a typical male being 1.8 m^2, this amounts to ~80 W for the whole body. As activity or physical work increases, the metabolic rate also increases. Typical values of M for differing activities are given in Table 12.1. Maximum values are obtained during severe muscular work and may be as high as 900 W m^{-2} for brief periods. Such a high rate can seldom be maintained and performance at 400–500 W m^{-2} is very heavy exercise but an overall rate that may be continued for about 1 h. Metabolic heat is largely determined by muscle activity during physical work but may be increased at rest in the cold by the involuntary muscle contractions involved in shivering.

The metabolic rate figures quoted can be related to energy consumed by the body through the breakdown of food, or work done due to activity. The energy content of food is usually quoted (e.g. on packaging) in units of 'Cals' which correspond to kilocalories (kcal). A physically active male adult typically consumes, in one day, food of energy content 3000 Cals (kcal), i.e. 12.6 MJ. Averaged over a 24 h period this would correspond to a metabolic rate of approximately 145 W (i.e. corresponding to an activity of standing to light work, see Table 12.1). If a balance is not maintained between energy consumed and work done, then body weight is either lost or gained. Activity over 24 h at the basal state (75 W) is equivalent to a consumption of approximately 1500 kcal, whilst in the extreme case for long duration, heavy exercise, consumptions of 6000–9000 kcal can occur, corresponding to continuous exercise of 300–450 W.

Taking work done (w) into account in the heat balance equation given above, $M - w$ is the actual heat gain by the body during work, or $M + w$ when

Table 12.1 Metabolic rates for differing activities

Activity	Typical rate per person (W)	Rate per m² of body surface (W)
Sleeping	75	43
Resting	90	47
Sitting	105	60
Standing	125	70
Light work	160	90
Strolling	200	107
Walking	280	154
Heavy work	450	250
Running (typical)	1000	600
Intense athletic activity (5–10 min)	1600	900
Shivering	1000	600

NB: a typical male adult has a body area of $1.8\,m^2$. Surface area can be determined from the du Bois equation, knowing the weight and height:

$$A = W^{0.425} \times H^{0.725} \times 71.84$$

where A is the surface area in square centimetres, W is the weight in kilograms and H is the height in centimetres.

negative work is performed. In positive work, some of the metabolic energy appears as external work so that the actual heat production in the body is less than the metabolic energy produced. With negative work, e.g. 'braking' while walking downstairs, the active muscle is stretched instead of shortened, so that work is done by the external environment on the muscles and appears as heat energy. Thus the total heat liberated in the body during negative work is greater than the metabolic energy produced.

Conduction

Heat is conducted between the body and static solids or fluids with which it is in contact. The rate at which heat is transferred by conduction depends on the temperature difference between the body and the surrounding medium, the thermal conductivity of the material (k) and the area of contact. For steady state conditions this can be expressed by:

$$K = k\,(t_1 - t_2)/d \qquad (12.2)$$

where K is the heat loss in watts per surface area of the body $(W\,m^{-2})$, t_1 and t_2 are the temperatures of the body and material respectively (°C), k is

a constant, i.e. the thermal conductivity (in $W\,m^{-1}\,°C^{-1}$) of the material involved and d (m) is the thickness of material across which the temperature difference occurs.

In normal circumstances, conduction transfer from the body direct to objects is voluntarily minimized as sensations of discomfort arise, as for instance when resting a bare arm onto a good conductor (e.g. metal). The value for K in the heat balance equation is thus often ignored. However, immersion in cold water is an example where conduction losses are very significant and can quickly lower the body temperature to dangerous levels.

Conduction is an important consideration in relation to providing a protective layer to the body to reduce the effective external surface temperature and reduce losses by other means (particularly in cold conditions), or in extreme circumstances to protect the body from high heat gains (e.g. in furnace repair work). In considering conduction of heat at the body surface through clothing, it is usually more appropriate to refer to resistivity, the reciprocal of k, which is expressed as resistance (or insulation) to heat flow across a given thickness of material, in units of $m^2\,°C\,W^{-1}$.

An arbitrary unit of insulation, the 'clo', is used for expressing the insulation value of clothing. By definition 1.0 clo is the insulation provided by clothing sufficient to allow a person to be comfortable when sitting in still air at a uniform temperature of 21°C. 1.0 clo is equivalent to a clothing resistance (insulation) value of $0.155\,m^2\,°C\,W^{-1}$. Examples of clo values are given in Table 12.2.

Convection

Normally, the surface temperature (i.e. of the skin or external layer of clothing) of a person is higher than that of the surrounding air. Therefore, air close to the body becomes warmer and will rise by natural convection, with cooler air taking its place. Heat exchange by convection is dependent on the temperature difference between the surface and the air and a factor known as the 'convective heat transfer coefficient'. The transfer can be expressed by the equation:

$$C = h_c\,(t_1 - t_2) \qquad (12.3)$$

Table 12.2 Typical values for the insulation of clothing (in clo units)

Clothing assembly	Clo
Naked	0
Shorts	0.1
Light summer clothing	0.5
Typical indoor clothing	1.0
Heavy suit and underclothes	1.5
Polar clothing	3–4
Practical maximum	5

where C is the convection loss per unit area $(\mathrm{W\,m}^{-2})$, h_c is the convective heat transfer coefficient (in units of $\mathrm{W\,m}^{-2}\,{}^{\circ}\mathrm{C}^{-1}$) and t_1 and t_2 are the temperature (°C) of the body surface and the adjacent air, respectively.

The value of h_c depends on various factors, including the nature of the fluid medium, the geometry and surface texture of the object and the temperature differences prevailing. Typically for still air (i.e. air velocity $< 0.1\,\mathrm{m\,s}^{-1}$) the value lies in the range 1.5–4.3, and the process is termed 'natural' or 'free' convection. For the body, the transfer coefficient depends principally on the temperature difference between clothing (t_{cl}) and air (t_a) (in °C) and is given by the approximate relationship:

$$h_c = 2.38\,(t_{cl} - t_a)^{0.25} \qquad (12.4)$$

Air velocity (v), due to the body moving through the air (with some parts, e.g. arms and legs, having a higher relative velocity to the air than the rest of the body) or air moving across the body, will significantly increase the convection loss via an increase in h_c. This is termed 'forced convection', with the heat transfer coefficient now strongly dependent on air velocity, rising typically to 9 at an air speed of $1\,\mathrm{m\,s}^{-1}$ to 25 at $5\,\mathrm{m\,s}^{-1}$ and to 50 at $10\,\mathrm{m\,s}^{-1}$. The value is approximately dependent on $v^{\frac{1}{2}}$. There are a variety of expressions for this dependence in the literature, some examples being:

$$h_c = 5.8 + 4.1\,v \qquad \text{for} \qquad v < 5\,\mathrm{m\,s}^{-1} \qquad (12.5)$$

$$h_c = 7.8\,v^{0.8} \qquad \text{for} \qquad v > 5\,\mathrm{m\,s}^{-1} \qquad (12.6)$$

Radiation

Radiant heat emission from a surface depends on the absolute temperature T (in kelvin, K, i.e. °C + 273) of the surface to the fourth power, i.e. proportional to T^4. Radiation transfer R (in $\mathrm{W\,m}^{-2}$) between similar objects 1 and 2 can then be given by the expression:

$$R = \sigma\varepsilon\,(T_1^4 - T_2^4) \qquad (12.7)$$

where σ is the Stefan–Boltzmann constant ($5.67 \times 10^{-8}\,\mathrm{W\,m}^{-2}\,\mathrm{K}^{-4}$) and ε is the emissivity of the objects.

Because of the T^4 relationship, radiation exchange is particularly relevant when dealing with objects of high surface temperature. Examples are: energy from the sun (surface temperature approximately 6000 K) and molten or 'red-hot' steel ($\sim$1000–1500 K). Similarly if significant heating effect by radiation is required from a small source (for heating purposes) then it must be at a high temperature (e.g. a bar electric fire).

For many indoor situations, the surrounding surfaces are at a fairly uniform temperature and the radiant environment can be described by the mean radiant temperature (MRT). The radiant heat exchange between the body surface area (clothed) and surrounding surfaces (in $\mathrm{W\,m}^{-2}$) can then be given by:

$$R = \sigma\varepsilon\,f_{\text{eff}}\,f_{cl}\,[(t_{cl} + 273)^4 - (t_r + 273)^4] \qquad (12.8)$$

where ε is the emissivity of the outer surface of the clothed body, f_{eff} is the effective radiation area factor (i.e. the ratio of the effective radiation area of the clothed body to the total surface area of the clothed body), f_{cl} is the clothing area factor (i.e. the ratio of the surface area of the clothed body to the surface area of the nude body), t_{cl} is the clothing surface temperature (°C) and t_r is the MRT (°C). MRT is defined as the temperature of uniform surrounding surfaces which will result in the same heat exchange by radiation from an object (e.g. a person) as in the actual environment. MRT can be estimated from the temperature of the surrounding surfaces, weighted according to their relative influence on a person, by the angle between the person and the radiating surface. t_r is therefore dependent on both a person's posture and their location in a room. The MRT (t_r) can alternatively be obtained by measurement (see section on 'Surveying the thermal environment').

The value of f_{eff} is typically 0.70 for seated persons and 0.73 for standing persons. The emissivity for human skin is close to 1.0 and most types of clothing have an emissivity of about 0.95. These values are influenced by colour for short wave thermal radiation such as solar radiation (i.e. as emitted from very hot objects).

An approximation can be made when small temperature differences prevail, where the rate of heat transfer by radiation between surfaces is related to the first power of the temperature difference. The expression is then in the same form as that for heat transfer by convection, namely:

$$R = h_r (t_1 - t_2) \qquad (12.9)$$

where R is the radiant heat transfer per unit area (W m^{-2}), h_r is the radiant heat transfer coefficient $(\text{W m}^{-2} \, ^\circ\text{C}^{-1})$ and t_1 and t_2 are the temperatures of the two surfaces (in °C). h_r depends on the nature of the two surfaces, their temperature difference and the geometrical relationship between them. Typically its value is 5.5 for transfer from a person seated in comfortable conditions. This form of equation for radiation transfer is used in many of the simple rational thermal models of comfort and stress.

It is to be noted that the simplified expression for radiation transfer is of similar form to the convection loss expression. The relative loss of heat from the body by the two mechanisms is thus directly related to the relative values of the transfer coefficients, demonstrating that typically the loss by radiation is twice that by natural convection.

Evaporation

At rest in a comfortable ambient temperature, an individual loses moisture by evaporation of water diffusing through the skin (cutaneous loss) and from the respiratory passages. Total water loss in these conditions is approximately $30 \, \text{g h}^{-1}$, with a corresponding heat loss due to evaporation. Such heat loss is known as 'insensible' (or 'latent') loss, with a corresponding insensible water loss. This term refers to heat loss without an associated

temperature change, in contrast to 'sensible' heat loss (or gain) where heat transfer (by conduction, convection or radiation) causes temperature changes which are detectable by the 'senses'. Typically, at rest in comfort, total body heat loss is made up from 70% sensible loss and 30% insensible, i.e. latent, loss.

The latent heat of vaporization of water is $2453 \, \text{kJ kg}^{-1}$ at 20°C and this skin loss results in a heat loss equal to approximately $10 \, \text{W m}^{-2}$. This loss is increased by the process of sweating. For example, a high sweat rate, e.g. of $1 \, \text{l h}^{-1}$, will dissipate about 680 W over the whole body, corresponding to the metabolic rate for high activity (see Table 12.1). This value of heat loss is only obtained if all the sweat is evaporated from the body surface; sweat that drips or is removed from the body is not providing effective cooling.

Evaporation transfer is expressed in terms of the latent heat taken up by the environment as the result of evaporative loss and the vapour pressure difference which constitutes the driving force for diffusion. This can be expressed as:

$$E = h_e (p_{sk} - p_a) \qquad (12.10)$$

where E is the rate of heat loss by evaporation per unit area of body surface (W m^{-2}), h_e is the mean evaporation coefficient (approximately $3 \times 10^{-3} \, \text{W m}^{-2} \, \text{Pa}^{-1}$) and p_{sk} and p_a are the partial pressures of water vapour at the skin surface and in the ambient air (in pascals, Pa). The values of p_a can be obtained from psychrometric data (see later). As an example, for a skin condition of 32°C and 100% relative humidity and an air condition of 23°C and 50% relative humidity, the values of p_{sk} and p_a are 4800 and 1400 Pa respectively, and E is therefore approximately $10 \, \text{W m}^{-2}$.

If the actual rate of evaporation (E_1) is less than the theoretical maximum rate possible (E_{max}), in the prevailing conditions, the ratio E_1/E_{max} can be used as a measure known as 'skin wettedness'. The skin surface may be considered as a mosaic of wet and dry areas. With a wettedness value of 0.5 the rate of evaporation achieved would be equivalent to half the skin surface being covered with a film of water, the other half being dry. For insensible cutaneous water loss the value is about 0.06 and the maximum value is 1.0 when the skin is fully wet. This concept is of importance in some of the rational heat stress indices.

Heat storage

The specific heat of the human body is 3500 J kg^{-1} °C^{-1} (compared to water at 4200 J kg^{-1} °C^{-1}). If a 65 kg individual has a change in mean body temperature of 1°C over a period of 1 h, the rate of heat storage is approximately 230 kJ h^{-1}, or 63 W, i.e. comparable with the basal metabolic rate. In the equation for thermal balance, S can be either positive or negative, but in determining storage the difficulty is to assess the true change in mean body temperature. A simple measured change alone is not sufficient because of the different weightings contributed by the core and shell. Typical formulae combining measurements of skin and core temperature to give a mean body temperature are:

$$0.90\ t_{core} + 0.10\ t_{skin} \quad \text{in hot conditions} \quad (12.11)$$

and

$$0.67\ t_{core} + 0.33\ t_{skin} \quad \text{in cold conditions} (12.12)$$

The weighting coefficients change because the volume of the warm core effectively reduces during vasoconstriction in cold surroundings.

Overall balance

Under normal temperature conditions providing comfort for sedentary activity, i.e. with a metabolic rate of typically 100–120 W and light to medium clothing, the relative losses by the four heat transfer mechanisms are:

conduction	0%
convection	25%
radiation	45%
evaporation	30%.

The precise relative values will depend on the exact conditions prevailing.

As the ambient conditions increase in temperature, the loss mechanisms by convection and radiation decrease, as the temperature difference between the body surface and the surroundings decreases. Hence to maintain balance, the evaporative loss increases by sweating. When the temperature difference reaches zero, or is reversed, convection and radiation losses cease and become gains and the only loss mechanism is evaporation. Thermal balance may not then be maintained, leading to a rise in core temperature and associated physiological effects.

Conversely, as temperatures fall below comfort values, convection and radiation losses increase. In the extreme the balance is lost and the core temperature will fall. These effects are summarized in Fig. 12.2.

Four of the thermal parameters affecting the heat transfer mechanisms are related to the environment: air temperature, mean radiant temperature, humidity conditions and air velocity, and two are related to the individual: activity and clothing. The time exposed to the prevailing conditions is of

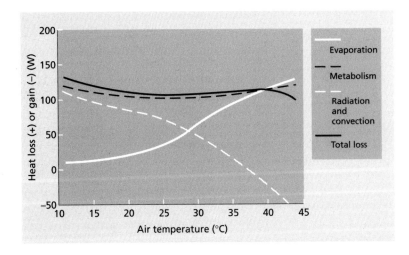

Fig. 12.2 Relative rates of heat transfer from the body with ambient conditions (air temperature).

importance when balance is not maintained, as this will affect the magnitude of the change in body temperature and the resulting health risks.

Many of the rational thermal models or indices quantify the loss/gain mechanisms via the simple equations previously quoted (or more complex versions), based on prevailing conditions of the surroundings and assumptions on activity and clothing. In this way assessments of heat balance and trends in the core temperature can be made and quantified within the index and related to recommended exposure times to the particular environment.

EVALUATION OF AN ENVIRONMENT

Thermal indices

The thermal environment can be assessed in either subjective terms or by objective measurements. In the former case individuals are asked to give an opinion on the thermal environment which they are experiencing. This is usually undertaken by the use of a standard subjective scale with which they are provided (e.g. Fig. 12.3). This is particularly relevant in assessing thermal comfort in, for instance, office-type environments where a large number of people may be experiencing a similar objective environment. However, in extreme environments such an approach would yield little useful or reliable data except perhaps to warn that a problem is imminent.

An alternative approach is to quantify the objective parameters making up the environment, i.e. air temperature, radiant temperature, humidity and air velocity, together with activity and clothing. However, specification of these six parameters to define the thermal environment is both cumbersome and of little use to all except the experienced worker in the field. Thus, much effort has been put into developing 'thermal indices' which summarize the prevailing conditions by a single number which can then be related to criterion for the index to indicate the severity of the environment in question.

The purpose of an index is to 'sum-up' the inter-relation of the six objective parameters in a single figure in relation to the thermal performance (or heat balance) of the human body. The various parameters may change, but in such a way as not to affect the thermal balance, and hence the value of the index itself would not change. For instance, a rise in air temperature may be compensated for by a fall in radiant temperature or a rise in air velocity (or visa versa); an increase in activity may be balanced by a reduction in clothing or in air/radiant temperature. In such cases the index value would remain constant although the separate parameters are changing. Alternatively, where a change in parameters (whether one or all six) causes a change in the thermal balance, then this would be reflected in a change in the single parameter, i.e. the index.

Indices do not necessarily take into account all six parameters. For simplicity, they may consist of a dominant factor only (e.g. wet bulb) as a simple assessment of heat stress for a given type of activity (e.g. mining). Alternatively, some of the parameters may be assumed to be fixed or constant (e.g. activity and clothing), thus simplifying the interrelation of the remaining four. This may occur for particular industries or occupations for which the index has been developed for, or applied to, specifically. Care must always be taken, therefore, when using an index to ensure that it is not being applied out of context.

Indices have been developed by many researchers, over many years, for different circumstances and different applications. In general three types of approaches have evolved, namely 'rational', 'empirical' and 'direct'.

Types of thermal indices

Rational

Rational (or analytical) thermal indices incorporate the principles of heat exchange and heat balance in assessing human response to hot, neutral and cold environments. If a body is to remain at a constant temperature the heat inputs to the body need to be balanced by the heat losses. The body heat balance equation previously quoted (Equation 12.1) can be rearranged as:

$$M \pm K \pm C \pm R - E = S \qquad (12.13)$$

If the net heat storage (S) is zero the body can be

Form 1

Please answer the following questions concerned with *your thermal comfort*

1 Indicate on the scale below how you feel *now*

Hot	
Warm	
Slightly warm	
Neutral	
Slightly cool	
Cool	
Cold	

2 Please indicate how you would like to be *now*

☐ Warmer   ☐ No change   ☐ Cooler

3 Please indicate how you *generally* feel at work

Hot	
Warm	
Slightly warm	
Neutral	
Slightly cool	
Cool	
Cold	

4 Please indicate how you would *generally* like to be at work

☐ Warmer   ☐ No change   ☐ Cooler

5 Are you generally satisfied with your thermal environment at work

☐ Yes   ☐ No

6 Please give any additional information or comments which you think are relevant to the assessment of your thermal environment at work (e.g. draughts, dryness, clothing, suggested improvements etc.)

Thank you

Fig. 12.3 Example of a thermal comfort questionnaire. From British Occupational Hygiene Society (1990).

said to be in heat balance, i.e. in a neutral thermal environment, and hence the internal body temperature can be maintained constant. If S is positive the core temperature will rise depending on the value of S and the time of exposure to the conditions. Similarly if S is negative the core temperature will fall.

Analysis procedures require the values represented in the equation to be calculated from a knowledge of the physical environment, clothing and activity. Rational thermal indices use heat transfer equations along the lines previously quoted (and sometimes mathematical representations of the human thermoregulatory system) to 'predict' human response to thermal environments.

A comprehensive mathematical and physical appraisal of the heat balance equation represents the approach taken by Fanger (1970) in relation to thermal comfort. This is the basis of ISO 7730 *Moderate Thermal Environments* (International Organization for Standardization, 1984). This approach enables conditions to be predicted which should provide 'comfort' or neutrality for differing levels of activity and clothing.

Similarly, ISO 7933 *Hot Environments — Analytical Determination of Thermal Stress using Calculation of Required Sweat Rate* (International Organization for Standardization, 1989) assesses heat stress conditions by the ability of the body to lose sufficient heat to the environment by the evaporation of sweat via a thorough analysis of the heat balance equation.

Empirical indices

Empirical thermal indices are based upon data collected from human subjects who have been exposed to a range of environmental conditions. Examples are the effective temperature (ET) and corrected effective temperature (CET) scales. These scales were derived from subjective studies on US marines; environments providing the same sensation were allocated equal ET/CET values. These scales take into account the thermal conditions (but simplify radiation effects) and two levels of clothing ('lightly clad' and 'stripped to the waist'). Variation in activity was not allowed for in the original approach. Thus, they are not fully compre-

hensive in relation to the six thermal parameters — partly to simplify the approach and partly because the scale was originally devised for particular circumstances (i.e. marines on ship decks in warm/hot conditions).

For this type of index, the index must be 'fitted' to values which experience predicts will provide 'comfort' or a degree of stress, e.g. a certain value (or range of values) of CET is recommended for a given occupational activity.

Direct indices

Direct indices are measurements taken by a simple instrument which responds to similar environmental components to which humans respond. For example a wet, black globe with a thermometer placed at its centre will respond to air temperature, radiant temperature, air velocity and humidity. The temperature of the globe will therefore provide a simple thermal index, which with experience of use can provide a method of assessment of hot environments. Other instruments of this type include the temperature of a heated ellipse and the integrated value of wet bulb temperature, air temperature and black globe temperature (the WBGT scale). The application of direct indices is thus empirical in nature.

Selection of appropriate thermal indices

The first action in the selection of a thermal index is to determine whether a heat stress, comfort or cold stress index is required. Numerous thermal indices have been developed and most will provide a value which will be related to human response (if used in the appropriate environment). An important point is that experience with the use of an index should be gained in a particular occupation or industry. In practice it is advisable to gain experience initially with a simple direct index; this can then be used for day-to-day monitoring. If more detailed analysis is required, a rational index can be used (again experience should be gained in a particular industry) and if necessary both subjective and objective measurements taken. There may be circumstances when conditions are particularly extreme and lie outside the range of the index selected. In such cases a suitable alternative index must be selected, or the problem be examined from first principles and direct physiological measurements made (e.g. of core temperature and heart rate).

Heat stress indices and standards

The purpose of a heat stress index is to provide the means for assessing hot thermal environments to predict their likely effect on people. In theory a heat stress index will take account of all environmental factors to produce a single index number which, when considered in relation to a person, their clothing and metabolic rate, will enable the stress, strain or risk to them to be assessed. In practice many indices will not consider all factors, or will deal with fixed values of one or more of the parameters in order to simplify the approach.

Empirical indices do not readily permit detailed consideration of the individual components of the thermal environment but, being practically derived, they are more widely used as the basis for standards. Theoretically derived standards allow detailed consideration of the factors controlling the body's heat balance and are therefore useful when assessing changes or control measures, but because their basis is theoretical they are often more complex to apply.

There are a number of indices which have been used to assess heat exposure. They are principally intended to prevent the deep body temperature from exceeding 38°C; they do not necessarily protect against the milder or chronic effects of heat. Control is achieved either by limiting environmental conditions in which exposure or work is permitted, or by limiting the time of exposure.

No index or standard is applicable in all circumstances since they have varying quantitative effects to changes in the individual components of the thermal environment. Thus, the application of different indices or standards to a particular environment often produces differing results. Also, a standard which is intended to provide a safe environment for all people will be far more restrictive than one aimed at young, fit people. A number of the more commonly used indices are described.

Heat stress — empirical and direct indices

Wet bulb temperature

Wet bulb temperature alone may be used in certain circumstances. For example, a maximum wet bulb temperature of 27°C has been quoted as a standard for tunnelling work where radiant heat is rarely a problem but humidity is often high. Also, in the cotton industry, where humidity is often high, prohibition of work in weaving sheds may occur when the wet bulb temperature exceeds 27°C.

Oxford index

The Oxford index (WD) (derived by A.R. Lind, 1957) predicts tolerance times for fit men working for short periods in extreme conditions. It was derived from tolerance times of mines rescue personnel, wearing breathing apparatus, at different metabolic rates (up to $180\,\mathrm{W\,m^{-2}}$) and is calculated from:

$$WD = 0.15\,DB + 0.85\,WB \qquad (12.14)$$

where DB is the dry bulb temperature and WB is the wet bulb temperature. Tolerance times are given with the index. Caution needs to be exercised in the use of this index as some people will be at risk at the recommended values.

Effective temperature and corrected effective temperature

Effective temperature (ET), developed in the 1920s by subjective tests on US marines, takes account of wet bulb temperature, dry bulb and air velocity. The corrected effective temperature (CET) was 'corrected' (by H.M. Vernon and C.G. Warner in the 1930s) to take into account radiation conditions, by incorporating the globe (150 mm) thermometer temperature in place of the dry bulb temperature. Two levels of clothing are considered ('normal', i.e. lightly clad and 'basic', i.e. stripped to the waist) and subsequent developments also allowed for varying work rate. CET is not generally used nowadays to predict heat stress, although it is still applied, for instance, in coalmining industries, in preference to other thermal standards. The CET normal chart is shown in Fig. 12.4.

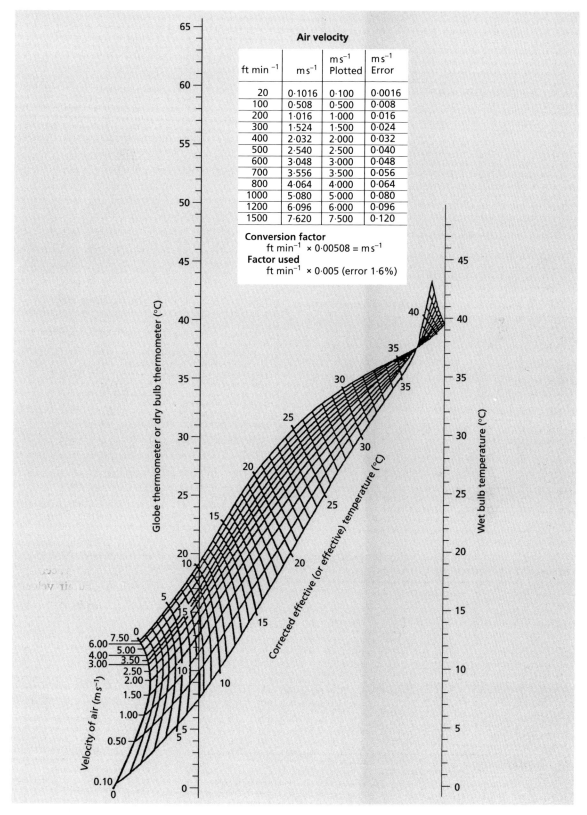

Fig. 12.4 Chart of corrected effective (or effective) temperature (i.e. CET or ET), normal scale (i.e. for persons lightly clad).

Wet bulb globe temperature

Wet bulb globe temperature (WBGT) is the most widely accepted heat stress index and forms the basis of many standards, most notably threshold limit values of the American Conference of Governmental Industrial Hygienisis (ACGIH) in the USA (American Conference of Governmental Industrial Hygienists, 1994), ISO 7243 (International Organization for Standardization, 1982 and 1989) and BS EN 27243 (British Standards Institution, 1994b).

WBGT is calculated from:

$$WBGT = 0.7\,WB + 0.3\,GT \quad \text{indoors} \qquad (12.15)$$

or

$$WBGT = 0.7\,WB + 0.2\,GT + 0.1\,DB \quad \text{outdoors} \qquad (12.16)$$

where WB is the wet bulb temperature (natural), GT is the globe thermometer temperature (150 mm diameter globe) and DB is the dry bulb temperature. The outdoors formula reduces the influence of the globe contribution from direct sun.

The WBGT index was originally derived to reduce heat casualties in the USA during military training. It takes account empirically of radiant and air temperatures, humidity and low air velocities (principally via the natural wet bulb and partly via the globe reading). The index alone does not provide guidance to exposure; it must be used with empirical recommendations based on the body core temperature not exceeding 38°C.

Table 12.3 and Fig. 12.5 reproduce the standards for exposure as specified by ISO 7243 (International Organization for Standardization, 1982 and 1989) using WBGT. These figures are generally conservative and indicate a level which is likely to be safe for most people who are physically fit and in good health. It is to be noted that different values are quoted for persons acclimatized and not acclimatized to heat. This standard is based on clothing worn being light summer clothing (clo value 0.6) and does not allow for variations in clothing, in particular the wearing of personal protective equipment (e.g. full respirator suit). It is assumed that rest periods are at the same thermal conditions as the activity and there is adequate water and salt intake. If conditions of exposure fluctuate, an appropriate time-weighted average exposure value should be derived.

The ACGIH quote the WBGT index for heat stress in their annual threshold limit values (TLV) listings (e.g. American Conference and Governmental Industrial Hygienists, 1993). Included in their guidance is a table for work–rest regimes (Table 12.4) and correction factors which can be applied for different clothing regimes (Table 12.5).

WBGT is also used as the basis for another exposure limit: the physiological heat exposure

Table 12.3 Reference values of wet bulb globe temperature (WBGT) heat stress index from ISO 7243. If the reference values are exceeded then measures must be taken to either reduce the WBGT value or implement a work–rest regime (see Fig. 12.5 and Table 12.4). After International Organization for Standardization (1989)

Metabolic rate class	Metabolic rate M Related to a unit skin surface area (W m^{-2})	Total (for a mean skin surface area of 1.8 m^2) (W)	Reference value of WBGT Person acclimatized to heat (°C)	Person not acclimatized to heat (°C)
0 (resting)	$M < 65$	$M < 117$	33	32
1	$65 < M < 130$	$117 < M < 234$	30	29
2	$130 < M < 200$	$234 < M < 360$	28	26
3	$200 < M < 260$	$360 < M < 468$	25[*] (26[†])	22[*] (23[†])
4	$M > 260$	$M > 468$	23[*] (25[†])	18[*] (20[†])

[*] No sensible air movement.
[†] Sensible air movement.
Extracts from ISO 7243 (1989) are reproduced with the permission of BSI. Complete copies can be obtained by post from BSI Sales, 389 Chiswick High Road, London, W4 4AL; tel: 0181 996 7000.

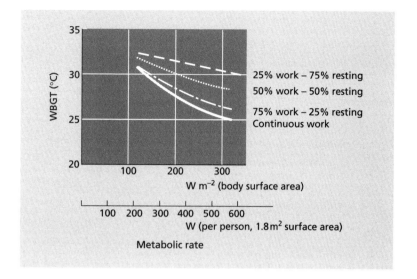

Fig. 12.5 Curves showing reference values of wet bulb globe temperature (WBGT) established for various work–rest cycles (on an hourly basis) for an acclimatized person. From ISO 7243 (International Organization for Standardization, 1989).

limit (PHEL) devised by A.R. Dasler in 1977. This permits exposure for short periods of time to temperatures higher than those permitted by ISO 7243.

Table 12.4 Examples of work–rest regimes (hourly) for acclimatized workers for values of wet bulb globe temperature (WBGT). Adapted from ACGIH TLV listing (American Conference of Governmental Industrial Hygienists, 1994)

Work–rest regimen (each hour)	Workload		
	Light	Moderate	Heavy
Continuous work	30.0	26.7	25.0
75% work–25% rest	30.6	28.0	25.9
50% work–50% rest	31.4	29.4	27.9
25% work–75% rest	32.2	31.1	30.0

See original documentation for application.

Table 12.5 Correction factors for clothing (in degrees Celsius) for wet bulb globe temperature (WBGT) index. Adapted from ACGIH TLV listings (American Conference of Governmental Industrial Hygienists, 1994)

Clothing type	Clo value	WBGT correction
Summer work clothes	0.6	0
Cotton coveralls	1.0	−2
Winter work clothes	1.4	−4
Water barrier, permeable	1.2	−6

See original documentation for application.

PHEL aims to provide safe working conditions for 95% of fit young men under 45 years of age and is limited to metabolic rates of $85–150\,W\,m^{-2}$ and WBGT values of 31–50°C. It therefore needs to be applied with great caution, with medical agreement and under good supervision.

Heat stress — rational/analytical indices

Required sweat rate — ISO 7933

Various indices have been developed to predict thermal strain on the body by applying the heat balance equation: namely balancing the heat inputs from the environment and metabolic rate against heat loss by the evaporation of sweat. The most developed of these is given in ISO 7933 (International Organization for Standardization, 1989), which can be used for predicting heat strain from a very wide range of factors by determining the required sweat rate. The procedure requires knowledge of all the environmental parameters, work rate and clothing. It also takes into account the evaporative efficiency of sweat rate and uses the concept of skin wettedness, previously referred to. Recommendations for exposure are based on limiting the rise of core temperature and on assessing the strain induced by the sweating process. Whilst being the most extensive and detailed of the methods for predicting heat strain and the effects of the different components of the thermal environment, ISO 7933 is complex and difficult to use. It is generally not suitable for occasional or casual use; a computer program is given in the standard to facilitate calculations.

Heat stress index

An earlier analytical index is the heat stress index (HSI) developed by H.S. Belding and T.F. Hatch (in the 1950s). This is orientated towards assessment via knowledge of environmental conditions and heat balance, and is often referred to as an 'engineering' approach as individual components of the environment can then be modified to provide control. The method for calculating the HSI is based on the heat transfer equations which have been previously discussed, and is as follows:

$$HSI = \frac{E_{req}}{E_{max}} \times 100 \qquad (12.17)$$

where E_{req} is the required evaporative (i.e. sweat) loss in $W\,m^{-2}$ and E_{max} is the maximum evaporative (i.e. sweat) loss in $W\,m^{-2}$. E_{req} is calculated by:

$$E_{req} = M - R - C \qquad (12.18)$$

where M is the metabolic rate $(W\,m^{-2})$. R is the radiation loss $(W\,m^{-2})$ and $= 4.4(35 - t_r)$ (clothed) or $7.3(35 - t_r)$ (unclothed), where t_r is the mean radiant temperature (°C). C is the convection loss $(W\,m^{-2})$ and $= 4.6v^{0.6}(35 - t_a)$ (clothed) or $7.6\,v^{0.6}(35 - t_a)$ (unclothed), where v is the air velocity $(m\,s^{-1})$ and t_a is the dry bulb (i.e. air) temperature (°C). E_{max} is calculated by:

$$E_{max} = 7.0\ v^{0.6}(56 - p_a)\ \text{clothed} \qquad (12.19)$$

or

$$E_{max} = 11.7\ v^{0.6}(56 - p_a)\ \text{unclothed}\quad (12.20)$$

where p_a is the water vapour pressure (mb). E_{max} has an upper limit of $390\,W\,m^{-2}$.

HSI is the ratio of the required heat loss to the maximum loss available by evaporation (taken as $390\,W\,m^{-2}$, equivalent to 1 l sweat loss per hour). It is expressed as a number between 0 and 100, representing stress and hence indicating strain. Conditions giving an HSI of below 40 are not considered to pose a risk to health; above 40 the risk increases; and 100 is the maximum tolerated by fit, acclimatized young men, where heat gain matches the maximum heat loss by evaporation.

Fig. 12.6 (*Facing page*) Nomogram for determining the predicted 4 h sweat rate (P4SR). The procedure is as follows:
1 Add the following correction to the wet bulb if the globe temperature differs from the dry:

$$\text{Correction} = 0.4(t_g - t)$$

2 Add a correction to the wet bulb temperature if the work rate exceeds $63\,W\,m^{-2}$, according to the table below.

Activity	Approximate metabolic rate (M) $(W\,m^{-2})$	Correction (°C)
Sedentary	76	0.6
Light	116	2.2
Moderate	192	3.3
Heavy	262	4.2

3 Add 1.0°C to the wet bulb temperature if the subject is wearing light clothing. If they are wearing shorts, add nothing.
4 Using the chart, draw a straight line between the globe or dry bulb temperature (where applicable) which appears on the left-hand side of the chart and the intersection between the modified wet bulb temperature and the air velocity appearing on the block on the right-hand side. The basic 4 h sweat rate (B4SR) can be read from the intersection of this line with the air velocity lines on the B4SR block appearing in the centre.
5 The P4SR can be calculated from the equations:

P4SR = B4SR + 0.012 $(M - 63)$ for a person wearing shorts,
P4SR = B4SR + 0.25 for a person at rest wearing overalls over shorts, and
P4SR = B4SR + 0.25 + 0.017 $(M - 63)$ for a person working, wearing overalls over shorts.

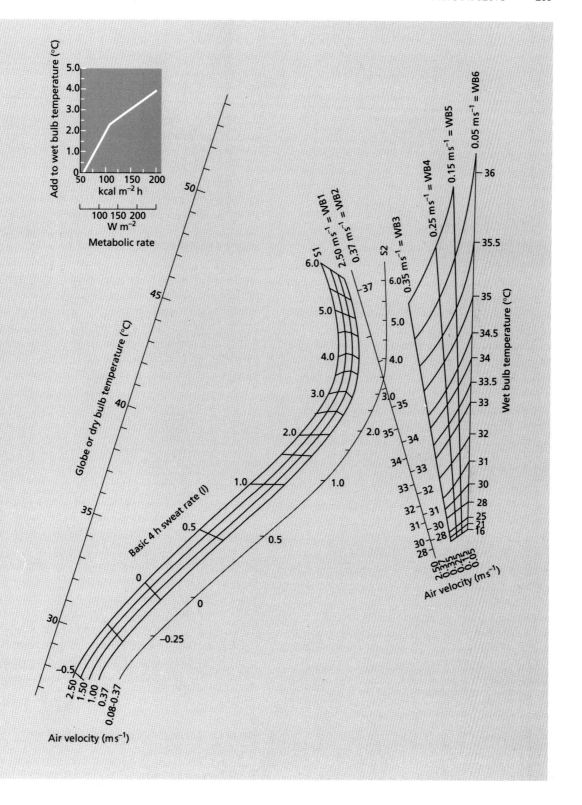

Over 100 there is a net heat gain to the body and the core temperature will rise unless the exposure time is limited. The maximum allowable exposure time (AET) in minutes is calculated from:

$$\mathrm{AET} = \frac{2440}{E_{\mathrm{req}} - E_{\mathrm{max}}} \qquad (12.21)$$

This equation is derived from the principles of heat storage (for a typical adult), with a maximum allowable body temperature rise due to heat storage of 1.8°C within an hourly period, combined with a rest period to allow for stored heat to be lost.

Predicted 4 h sweat rate

In contrast to the HSI, the predicted 4 h sweat rate (P4SR) index is 'physiologically' based, enabling a nominal sweat rate (i.e. strain) to be predicted from criteria relating to the environment and individual. Limiting values for various circumstances are recommended by different organizations. Typically, the recommended upper limit of P4SR for fit acclimatized young men is 4.5 l, whereas for clothed industrial workers the limiting figure is 2.7 l. The procedure for determining the index is shown in Fig. 12.6.

The use and application of heat stress indices

An index does not predict working conditions which are completely safe, as even at moderately elevated temperatures there will be some risk of the milder medical effects, and also, individuals vary considerably in their susceptibility. For most applications, ISO 7243 (International Organization for Standardization, 1982 and 1989) (i.e. WBGT) provides a relatively safe baseline, below which the risk of serious medical effect is very small to most people, whether working continuously or for short periods. However, even the conservative standards of this index will not provide sufficient protection in all cases. In particular, ISO 7243 cannot be assumed to apply to work or activities carried out in impervious protective clothing, and it may not fully reflect the risk if radiant temperature or air temperature and air velocity are high.

In circumstances where ISO 7243 does not apply, or where exposure to more extreme environments

may occur, other indices can be used. Since the risk increases with temperature, they should be applied with great caution and in conjunction with other precautions, particularly medical screening, supervision and, if advised by a doctor, medical monitoring (e.g. ISO 9886 (International Organization for Standardization, 1992)). The most appropriate index or indices which take adequate account of all relevant environmental conditions, clothing, metabolism, etc. should be used. If possible, it is advisable to compare the results of several indices. The required sweat rate approach (ISO 7933 (International Organization for Standardization, 1989)) will provide the most comprehensive assessment of conditions, although other indices may have practical benefits in particular situations. However, some exposure conditions lie outside the range of any of the indices, in which case the problem needs to be viewed from first principles and is likely to call for direct physiological monitoring. A summary of parameters involved, and recommendations given, for the more widely used heat stress indices is shown in Table 12.6.

Indices for comfort

Empirical

The corrected effective temperature (CET) scale, previously described under heat stress indices, has also been used as a single figure index for comfort. There are recommended levels for comfort in differing occupations, e.g. CET should lie in the range 16–18°C for comfort in typical office environments. However, the values quoted depend on who quotes them, for instance those quoted in the UK are typically 2–4°C lower than those quoted in the USA.

CET has been superseded generally now as it is considered to overemphasize the importance of humidity in relation to comfort, as well as not being sufficiently comprehensive.

Analytical: Fanger analysis and ISO 7730

A comprehensive mathematical, physical and physiological appraisal of the heat balance equation was made by Fanger (1970), and forms the basis of

Table 12.6 Summary of factors and recommendations involved with five heat stress indices

Parameter	Index				
	WBGT (ISO 7243)	Required sweat rate (ISO 7933)	HSI	P4SR	CET
Air temperature	0.1 DB	Yes	Yes	G/DB	G/DB
Radiant temperature	0.2/0.3G	MRT	MRT	G	G
Humidity	NWB	VP	VP	WB	WB
Air movement	no	$m\,s^{-1}$	$m\,s^{-1}$	$m\,s^{-1}$	$m\,s^{-1}$
Clothing	1 level	clo value	2 levels	clo value	2 levels
Activity	3 levels	$W\,m^{-2}$	$W\,m^{-2}$	$W\,m^{-2}$	1 level (corrections)
Recommendations	Work–rest regimes	Exposure time	Exposure time	Sweat rate limits	Empirical

CET, corrected effective temperature; DB, dry bulb; G, globe; HSI, heat stress index; MRT, mean radiant temperature; NWB, natural wet bulb; P4SR, predicted 4 h sweat rate; WB, wet bulb; WBGT, wet bulb globe temperature; VP, vapour pressure.

ISO 7730 *Moderate Thermal Environments* (International Organization for Standardization, 1984). This approach enables conditions which should provide 'comfort' or neutrality to be predicted for differing levels of activity and clothing. This is usually presented graphically, where air temperature, MRT and air velocity are combined as variables, with relative humidity (RH) assumed to be constant at 50%. (Fanger established that RH variations from 30–70% — the range usually found in buildings — have very little effect on thermally comfortable conditions.) Comfort conditions can be expressed graphically for different levels of activity and clothing, as shown in Fig. 12.7.

Fanger also expressed comfort in terms of the 'predicted mean vote' (PMV), via the standard subjective voting scale:

−3 cold
−2 cool
−1 slightly cool
 0 neutral
+1 slightly warm
+2 warm
+3 hot

For given thermal conditions, Fanger's work predicts what the average vote on the scale will be (for a group of persons), i.e. the PMV for the group, and also the percentage of persons satisfied or dissatisfied with the environment, i.e. the predicted percentage dissatisfied (PPD). For example, if the PMV is +1.0 or −1.0, then the PPD will be 26%, i.e. this percentage of the group is predicted to be dissatisfied with the environment; a PMV of +2.0 or −2.0 gives a PPD of 75%. This relationship between PMV and PPD can be expressed graphically, as in Fig. 12.8. It should be noted that if the PMV is 0.0 (i.e. the ideal thermal environment), then 5% are still dissatisfied. ISO 7730 suggests for comfort that the limits for PMV in practice should be +0.5 to −0.5, giving a PPD of 10%. The Annex of the standard quotes examples of particular conditions which are predicted to satisfy this limit.

Heat balance alone is not a sufficient condition for thermal comfort. Localized discomfort on parts of the body can still occur even though the body as a whole may be in thermal balance. Individual components of the environment (e.g. air movement) must remain within limits and asymmetry of conditions must be controlled. This applies particularly to vertical temperature gradients and vertical and horizontal radiation effects. The discomfort sensation of air movement is also dependent on the turbulence of the air. Recommendations for limits in relation to localized conditions, e.g. to air movement, temperature gradients, etc. are given in the Annex to ISO 7730.

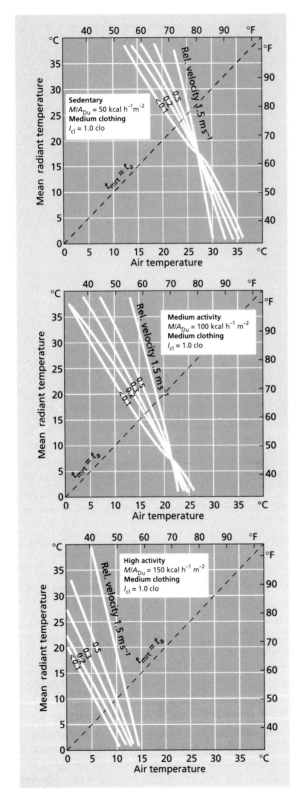

Direct index: dry resultant temperature

This is an index recommended by the UK Chartered Institution of Building Services Engineers (CIBSE, 1987), and represents a straightforward approach which nevertheless encompasses all aspects. The dry resultant temperature (DRT) is the value taken up by a 100 mm globe thermometer in 'still air', i.e. it integrates air temperature and MRT (with RH assumed to be 40–60%), with small corrections to be made for increasing air movement. There is also a 'wet' resultant temperature, where the surface of the globe is kept moist. This index is similar to the conventional 'wet bulb' and in isolation can be used as a heat stress index. DRT is usually referred to simply as 'resultant temperature'.

For the 100 mm globe, the globe temperature, i.e. resultant temperature (RT), is defined by:

$$RT = 0.5\,AT + 0.5\,MRT \qquad (12.22)$$

where AT is the air temperature and MRT is the mean radiant temperature, i.e. a simple average of the two. Corrections for air movement need to be made; typical values are: for $0.2\,\mathrm{m\,s^{-1}}$, add 1.0°C to RT; for $0.4\,\mathrm{m\,s^{-1}}$, add 1.5°C to RT; and for $0.6\,\mathrm{m\,s^{-1}}$, add 2.0°C to RT. RH is assumed to be 40–60% (i.e. as normally found in buildings).

Recommended resultant temperatures for various types of spaces or building are given by the CIBSE, where typical clothing and activity in these spaces are assumed, e.g. 21°C for living rooms and 20°C for offices. A tolerance of ±1.5°C is usually considered allowable. Quoting a resultant temperature (instead of, for example, a 'simple' temperature or the air temperature) ensures that all the parameters are considered, although the individual components may not be expressed.

ASHRAE (the American Society of Heating, Refrigeration and Air Conditioning Engineers) have their own standards — similar to Fanger's approach, namely '*ASHRAE 55-1981 Thermal Environment Conditions for Human Occupancy*' (ASHRAE, 1981).

Fig. 12.7 Examples of Fanger comfort graphs — for medium clothing and sedentary, medium and high levels of activity. Reproduced by permission of McGraw-Hill Book Co. from Fanger (1970).

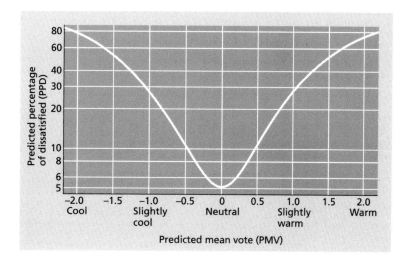

Fig. 12.8 The relationship between the predicted mean vote (PMV) in the range cool to warm, i.e. −2.0 to +2.0, and the predicted percentage dissatisfied (PPD) for a large group of subjects.

Indices for cold stress

Standards relating to work performance, thermal balance and exposure duration in cold environments are not as well developed and validated as those for heat exposure. It is generally more difficult to assess the stress of cold climates, possibly because of the potentially greater part played by behavioural thermoregulation in maintaining body temperature conditions. The objectives of standards for cold exposure are to avoid core temperature falling below 35°C and to prevent cold injury to the extremities such as hands and feet. More widely used examples are given.

Still shade temperature

The still shade temperature (SST) takes actual outdoor conditions and expresses them as an 'equivalent' temperature where there is no solar heat exchange and no wind effect. A correction is applied for the solar heat absorbed by the body (allowing for clothing type, posture, etc.), which in full sunshine can amount to two or three times the resting metabolic rate. Further corrections are required to convert conditions to 'still', i.e. with an air velocity of zero, taking metabolic rate into account. Thus any set of conditions can be converted to a single index figure. It is still necessary to have empirical recommendations to relate exposure to the index in a similar way to, e.g., WBGT for heat stress.

Wind chill index

The wind chill index (WCI) is an index of heat loss from the body and was developed by P.A. Siple and C.F. Passel in 1945 in order to identify the potential risk resulting from the combined cooling effect of wind and cold conditions. It is an empirical approach, based on an artificial model for the human, namely on the cooling characteristics of a warm (33°C), water-filled tin cylinder hoisted on a pole in a station in Antarctica under different conditions of windspeed and temperature. The index is found to correlate well with human reactions to cold and wind and is successful in identifying conditions of potential danger when skin surfaces are exposed. It is of particular value in estimating the local cooling of hands, feet and head that may produce deterioration of physical performance and cold injury.

The relationship between windspeed and cooling power is non-linear. It is based on the forced convection type formulae quoted previously. In broad terms, the most significant increase in cooling is produced by air movement increasing from calm to $2\,\text{m s}^{-1}$, while for changes at higher velocities, e.g. from 10 to $15\,\text{m s}^{-1}$, there is no great increase, as can be seen from Fig. 12.9.

The WCI does not take into account the amount of clothing worn, which is necessary to express theoretically the effect of wind on heat loss of subjects. The proven usefulness of the WCI in practice is probably because tolerance of cold

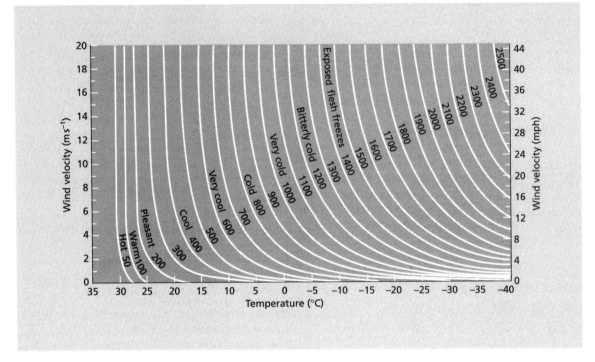

Fig. 12.9 The wind chill index (WCI). Values marked against the curves are the rate of cooling in kcal m^{-2} h^{-1} (multiply by 1.16 to convert to W m^{-2}) at different combinations of wind velocity (m s^{-1}) and temperature (°C).

conditions, given adequate nutrition, is ultimately determined by the reaction of parts of the unprotected body. Complete protection of exposed areas by the use of suitable face mask and gloves would, in effect, make the WCI inapplicable. This contrasts with the approach of Required Insulation (I_{REQ}) (see below).

The WCI is defined by the following empirical formula:

$$\text{WCI} = (33 - t_a)(10v^{0.5} - v + 10.45) \quad (12.23)$$

where WCI is the cooling power of the environment in kcal m^{-2} h^{-1}, t_a is the ambient temperature (°C) and v is the air velocity in m s^{-1}. Values are usually expressed graphically (see Fig. 12.9) or as an equivalent 'chilling temperature' (Table 12.7).

Required clothing insulation

The important role of clothing insulation, omitted in the WCI, is used in the required clothing insulation (I_{REQ}) approach to express cold stress in

Table 12.7 The 'chilling temperature' (t_{ch}) defined as the ambient temperature which, under calm conditions (< 1.8 m s^{-1} windspeed), produces the same cooling power as the actual environmental conditions. Values of corresponding wind chill index (WCI) are also given

WCI (W m^{-2})	t_{ch} (°C)	Effect (typical)
1160	−12	Very cold
1392	−21	Exposed flesh freezes after 60 min
1624	−30	Exposed flesh freezes after 20 min
1856	−40	Exposed flesh freezes after 15 min
2088	−49	Exposed flesh freezes after 10 min
2320	−58	Exposed flesh freezes after 8 min
2552	−67	Exposed flesh freezes after 4 min
2784	−76	Exposed flesh freezes after 1 min

terms of general body cooling and the insulation required to maintain thermal balance. Since there is an upper limit to the amount of clothing insulation possible, a duration period for limiting exposure on the basis of acceptable levels of body cooling may also be calculated for the available clothing.

I_{REQ} is a rational approach to assessing cold stress, based on the heat balance equation (Equations 12.1 and 12.13). It is defined as the minimal thermal insulation required to maintain body thermal equilibrium under steady state conditions when sweating is absent and peripheral vasoconstriction is present. The minimal value of I_{REQ} describes the net insulation required to maintain the body in a state of thermal equilibrium at normal levels of body temperature. The higher the value of I_{REQ} at any given activity level, the greater the cooling power of the environment. Alternatively, increasing energy expenditure in the working environment will reduce I_{REQ}. The procedure does not fully cover local cooling of the head, hands and feet; these may require separate consideration, e.g. via the WCI. I_{REQ} is the basis of an ISO standard under development. The thermal characteristics of clothing, reliable information on which is clearly required to put I_{REQ} into practice, are given in ISO 9920 (International Organization for Standardization, 1995).

SURVEYING THE THERMAL ENVIRONMENT

Objective measurements and instrumentation

Assessment of the thermal environment requires the accurate knowledge of the physical quantities involved. The fundamental parameters describing the environment, with the usual units involved, are:
- air temperature (°C);
- mean radiant temperature (°C);
- relative humidity (%) or absolute humidity of the air (pressure, Pa) (100 Pa = 1 mb);
- air velocity ($m\,s^{-1}$).

These can be measured individually, or in combined form to give an 'integrated' parameter or index figure direct. Information is usually also required relating to the activity and clothing of personnel involved. These values are normally estimated rather than measured and usually relate to fixed 'categories' within the index being applied (e.g. low, medium or high rates of activity). However, techniques are available for assessing these in detail, for example see ISO 8996, 9886 and 9920

(International Organization for Standardization, 1990, 1992 and 1995).

The thermal environment also varies with time due to the action of controls, cyclic changes in processes or the influence of varying external conditions. Furthermore, there are likely to be variations throughout the space, particularly near to windows and air inlet and extract grilles or localized sources of heat or cold. Measurements therefore should normally be made at various positions throughout a room and at three heights: ankle height (0.1 m), abdomen level (0.6 m in sitting areas and 1.1 m in standing areas) and head height (1.1 m in sitting areas and 1.7 m in standing areas). It is usual to weight these values 1 : 2 : 1 to reflect the body burden. Knowledge of the variation of parameters with position is also of importance in assessing the asymmetry of conditions, especially in relation to comfort. Measurements should be carried out over the cycling period of the process (see Chapter 17), operation or of the heating/cooling controls and, where external solar conditions affect the internal environment, at different times during the day.

In cases of heat and cold stress, individual circumstances need to be taken into account when selecting positions for measurement. In general, the position should reflect the thermal load on the individual concerned. The concept of 'personal' monitoring, where equipment is attached to the individual, is not currently generally applicable in the thermal environment for practical reasons, but may need to be undertaken in special circumstances, e.g. to assess the radiant heat load experienced by fire-fighters, or to obtain real time information on the medical condition of the individual, e.g. heart rate and core temperature.

Air temperature

Air temperature (also referred to as the dry bulb temperature) can be measured with a suitable thermometer: mercury/alcohol in glass, electrical resistance, thermistor, thermocouple or differential expansion type. The relative properties of the different types are given in Table 12.8. In summary, simple glass thermometers are relatively low cost, accurate (in the case of the mercury type typically

Table 12.8 Relative properties of temperature sensing probes and instruments. From British Occupational Hygiene Society (1990)

Property	Thermocouple*	Thermistor	Platinum resistance thermometer	Semiconductor junction[†]	Mercury in glass
Long-term stability	Variable	Ages	Stable	Stable	Stable
Signal for 1°C change	$10-60\,\mu V$	1% of resistance (linearized)	$40\,\mu V$ (at 1 mA current)	$2.3\,mV$	–
Speed of response	Fast	Fast	Moderate	Moderate	Slow
Relative cost[‡]	1	4	5	2	3
Mechanical stability	Robust	Moderate	Moderate	Robust	Poor
Reproducibility	Moderate	Good	Very good	Poor	Very good
Linearity	Moderate	Linearized versions required	Good	Good	Good
Accuracy (typical)	± 2°C	± 1°C	± 0.1°C	± 1°C	± 0.1°C (NPL calibrated)

* Cold junction or compensated circuit required.
[†] High self-heating effect.
[‡] Relative cost: 1, cheap; 5, expensive.

to ±0.2°C) and reliable, but are fragile and inflexible in use. The three electrical types provide more versatility (e.g. with purpose-designed air or surface probes) but accuracy is often less than the mercury in glass type (although resolution to 0.1°C is often presented on the display) and regular calibration is required. The differential expansion principle is most commonly found in continuous recording devices.

Although the instruments themselves are relatively straightforward in operation, many precautions need to be taken when using a thermometer and when measuring air temperature in particular. Examples are given below.
- The probe should be shielded from radiation sources (hot or cold), e.g. with aluminium foil, but air movement must be allowed through the foil.
- The air should be sampled by creating air movement, enhancing convective transfer relative to radiation exchange.
- An appropriate response time is required.
- If measuring varying air temperatures, for instance from air-conditioning systems, a fast response probe is required.

- Purpose-designed air probes (electrical) have a rapid response sensor in an open-ended metallic cylinder for radiation shielding and physical protection; such probes are essential for testing for fluctuations in air temperature.
- Probes should be kept dry (and clean).
- The reading being taken should be appropriate for the circumstances involved, e.g. a room air temperature may vary by a few degrees from a window to near a radiator, and from floor to ceiling.
- There are likely to be vertical temperature gradients, particularly in tall spaces and at mezzanine levels, hence appropriate sampling should be undertaken.
- Readings should not be influenced by the measurer's own body.
- Electrical thermometers have standard potential problem areas, including batteries, drift, calibration and the issue of display resolution versus instrument accuracy.

Radiant temperature

Radiant temperature can be measured indirectly

with a globe thermometer or directly with pyro-meters, thermopiles or non-contact thermometers. It can also be assessed via surface temperature measurements and calculation. The mean radiant temperature (MRT) is the temperature of a uniform imaginary enclosure in which the radiant heat transfer to an object in the enclosure is equal to the radiant heat transfer in the actual space. It results from the summation and averaging of all the surface temperatures around a point. It can be determined by measuring all these surface temperatures (e.g. walls, windows, lights, etc.) and then calculating appropriately. However, this is usually impractical and in practice it is usually measured by instruments which allow the radiation from the walls of the enclosure to be integrated into a mean value.

Two-sphere radiometer

MRT can be measured directly using a two-sphere radiometer. In this method, two spheres with different emission coefficients (one black and one polished copper) are used. The two spheres are heated to the same temperature so that they will be exposed to the same convective heat loss. As the emissivity of the black sphere is higher than that of the polished one, there is a difference in the heat supplied to the two spheres to maintain the same temperature. This gives a measure of the incoming radiation. The mean radiant temperature can be calculated from:

$$(t_r + 273)^4 = (t_s + 273)^4 + \frac{(P_p - P_b)}{\sigma(E_b - E_p)} \quad (12.24)$$

where t_r is the mean radiant temperature (°C), t_s is the sensor temperature (°C), P_p is the heat supplied to the polished sphere (W m^{-2}), P_b is the heat supplied to the black sphere (W m^{-2}), E_p is the emissivity of the polished sphere, E_b is the emissivity of the black sphere and σ is the Stefan–Boltzmann constant (5.67 × 10^{-8} W m^{-2} K^{-4}).

Globe thermometer

The globe thermometer temperature can be used to determine the MRT indirectly, or used as a measure of radiant conditions in its own right to be used directly in an index (e.g. as in the WBGT index).

The globe thermometer is a matt black, hollow copper sphere (original size 150 mm diameter) with a simple thermometer projecting into the centre of the sphere. The sphere is suspended freely and allowed to come into thermal equilibrium with the surroundings (this takes approximately 20 min) to give the globe or 'black bulb' temperature. This can be converted into the MRT value with knowledge of the air temperature and air velocity, either by using appropriate nomograms (Fig. 12.10), or by calculation. The globe heats or cools due to radiation exchange, but its final temperature is also a function of heat transfer by convection. The temperature of the globe (t_g) at thermal equilibrium allows the MRT (t_r) to be determined:

for natural convection (150 mm globe)

$$t_r = [(t_g + 273)^4 + 0.4 \times 10^8 (t_g - t_a)^{0.25} \times (t_g - t_a)]^{0.25} - 273 \quad (12.25)$$

for forced convection

$$t_r = [(t_g + 273)^4 + 2.5 \times 10^8 \times v^{0.6} \times (t_g - t_a)]^{0.25} - 273 \quad (12.26)$$

where t_r is the mean radiant temperature (°C), t_g is the black globe temperature (°C), t_a is the air temperature (°C) and v is the air velocity (m s^{-1}). In order to decide whether the equations for natural or forced convection should be used it is first necessary to evaluate the coefficient of heat transfer:

for natural convection

$$h_{cn} = 1.4 \left(\frac{t_g - t_a}{D}\right)^{0.25} \quad (\text{W m}^{-2}°\text{C}^{-1}) \quad (12.27)$$

for forced convection

$$h_{cf} = 6.3 \frac{v^{0.6}}{D^{0.4}} \quad (\text{W m}^{-2}°\text{C}^{-1}) \quad (12.28)$$

where h_{cn} is the coefficient of heat transfer for natural convection, h_{cf} is the coefficient of heat transfer for forced convection and D is the diameter of the globe (m). If $h_{cn} > h_{cf}$ use the natural convection formula and if $h_{cf} < h_{cn}$ use the forced convection formula.

The heat transfer mechanisms occurring with the globe thermometer are illustrated by the following example. Assume the globe is placed in an environment where the MRT is greater than the air

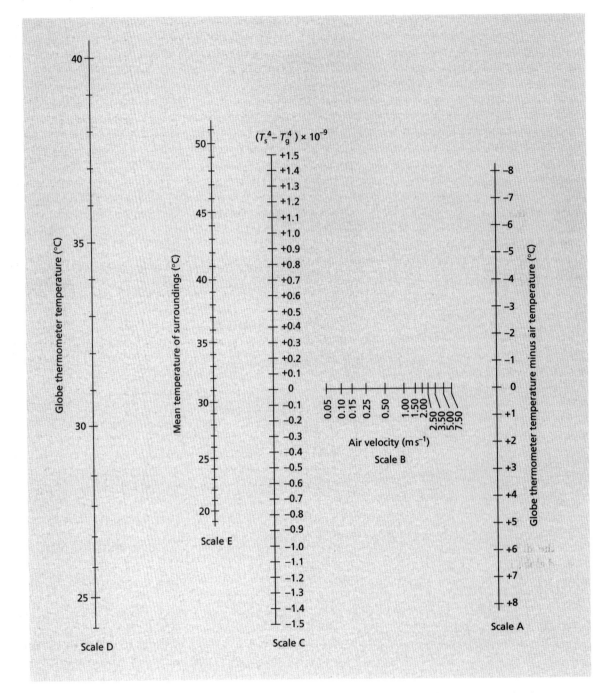

Fig. 12.10 Example of a nomogram for determining the mean radiant temperature (MRT) from the globe thermometer reading. Air temperature and air velocity are also required.

temperature (AT), e.g. walls at 40°C and AT 20°C, and the globe itself starts at 20°C in still air conditions. Initially there will be a net radiation gain from the wall surfaces to the globe and it will begin to rise in temperature. However, as soon as the globe rises above the AT, natural convection losses will take place. After some time (e.g. 20 min) an equilibrium will occur between net radiation gain and convection losses, with the globe being typically at 30°C for the conditions quoted. If air movement increases, convection losses will also increase with a resulting lower globe value, e.g. 28°C in the example quoted for air movement of 2 m s^{-1}. Alternatively, if the AT is 20°C and globe 30°C in high air movement conditions then the MRT will be several degrees higher than 40°C.

The thermometer is at the centre of the globe and heat transfer to the thermometer bulb must take place (this affecting the time taken to come to equilibrium) via the following processes: conduction through the walls of the globe (being made of copper, this occurs readily); natural convection exchange from the inner walls to the air inside the globe and to the thermometer; radiation exchange between the inner walls themselves and with the thermometer. There may also be some conduction from the globe to its support/stand which should be minimized.

These heat exchange processes can be quantified using heat transfer equations for radiation and convection to predict theoretically the temperature that the globe will read, as given in Equations 12.25–12.28. The mechanisms are also dependent on the diameter of the globe. If a non-standard sized globe is used, then the appropriate equations are:

for natural convection

$$t_r = \left[(t_g + 273)^4 + \frac{0.25 \times 10^8}{\varepsilon} \right. $$
$$\left. \left(\frac{t_g - t_a}{D} \right)^{0.25} (t_g - t_a) \right]^{0.25} - 273 \qquad (12.29)$$

for forced convection

$$t_r = \left[(t_g + 273)^4 + \frac{1.1 \times 10^8 \, v^{0.6}}{\varepsilon \, D^{0.4}} (t_g - t_a) \right]^{0.25} - 273$$
$$(12.30)$$

where ε is the emissivity. In general, for different sized globe thermometers at nominal zero air movement ($<0.1 \, \text{m s}^{-1}$) the following relationship applies:

$$T(\text{globe}) = g \times \text{MRT} + (1 - g) \times \text{AT} \qquad (12.31)$$

where g is a factor in the range 0–1. In the simplest case, for a 100 mm globe, $g = 0.5$, i.e.

$$T(\text{globe}) = 0.5 \times \text{MRT} + 0.5 \times \text{AT} \qquad (12.32)$$

as applicable for the dry resultant temperature quoted previously. g is smaller for smaller globes (e.g. ~0.3 for the 40 mm globe), i.e. more weight is given to the AT, and larger for the 150 mm globe (e.g. ~0.6).

In using the globe thermometer it should be suspended in an appropriate position, and not influenced by the assessor's own body. As readings for 150 mm globes take typically 20 min, only a limited number can usually be taken. The 40 mm globe responds more rapidly but may give different readings to the 150 mm globe as it is more affected by air movement, i.e. convection losses.

The globe thermometer is not appropriate for obtaining the radiant temperature of a localized radiation source. It measures the overall radiation conditions of all its surroundings, i.e. the MRT. Pyrometers and thermopiles are suitable for measuring the radiation temperature (i.e. surface temperature) of particular surfaces, e.g. reaction vessels, furnaces, cold roofs, etc. They are otherwise known as 'radiation thermometers', 'non-contact surface thermometers' or 'infrared thermometers'. When pointed directly at a surface they give an instantaneous read-out of the temperature of the surface (provided that the surface emissivity is known). The size of target area increases with distance. Alternatively, the surface temperature can be measured directly with an appropriate contact probe, but this technique is often impractical, hazardous or time consuming.

Humidity conditions

Humidity conditions can be assessed via the relative humidity (RH), usually measured as a percentage figure directly (%), or via the wet bulb and dry bulb temperatures. It can also be expressed as

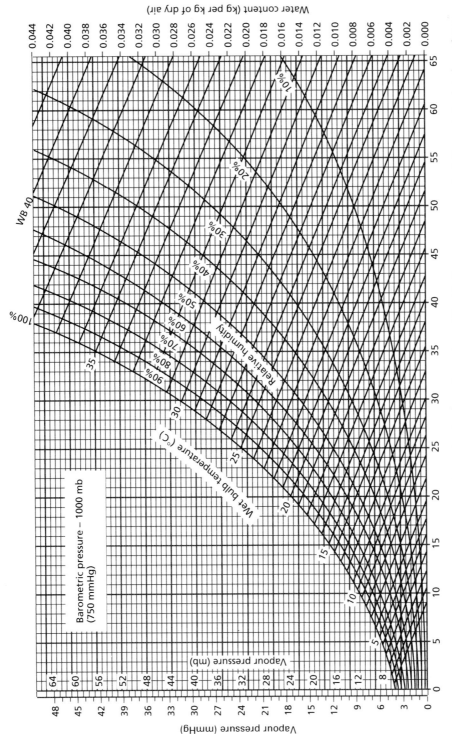

Fig. 12.11 The psychrometric chart showing the relationship between dry and wet (sling) bulb temperatures and relative and absolute humidities. Note, for vapour pressure 1 mb = 100 Pa.

absolute humidity either in kg of water per kg of air, or as a vapour pressure (in Pa or kPa). The interrelation of these parameters is given by the psychrometric chart (Fig. 12.11). Common types of hygrometers are: wet and dry bulb, dew point, moving fabric, electronic and chemical.

Wet and dry bulb methods

Water evaporating freely from a thermometer will cause a cooling effect termed the 'wet bulb depression' with the resulting temperature known as the 'wet bulb' (cf. the 'dry bulb'). The extent of this cooling is a function of how freely the water can evaporate, i.e. on the relative humidity of the surrounding air and the local air movement. Slide rules, tables or the psychrometric chart provide the RH value for given wet and dry bulbs. There are two types of measured wet bulb, described by the terms: 'natural', i.e. unaspirated, screen, Masons or sheltered; and 'forced', i.e. aspirated, sling, whirling or draught. The value given by the natural wet bulb is influenced by local air movement and is thus less predictable than the forced version. However, it is easier to measure, and in reflecting localized conditions it may be more applicable, e.g. as used directly in the WBGT index.

There are three common instruments based on the wet and dry bulb principle. The Masons hygrometer has two static thermometers. One has a wick dipped into a reservoir to give the natural wet bulb; air movement can be induced around the wet bulb to create forced conditions. The whirling hygrometer has air movement induced by whirling. The wet bulb should be read first as this temperature rises after motion stops (except at 100% RH). The Assman hygrometer is a laboratory-based instrument for calibration purposes. Airflow is induced by a motor and fan at a known speed ($\sim 4\,m\,s^{-1}$) and there are radiation shields to the thermometers. The wet and dry bulb principle can also be employed with electrical thermometer sensors.

General precautions to be applied in using wet and dry bulb hygrometers are as follows:
- distilled water should be used;
- the wick should be clean, and replaced when necessary;
- the wick should have a firm fit, not too tight or slack, and cover the whole of the sensor;
- the air velocity over the wick should be at least $4\,m\,s^{-1}$ for the forced bulb;
- typically a whirling time of 2 min is required to obtain the initial forced wet bulb reading;
- the dry bulb must be kept dry;
- the thermometers should be shielded from radiation sources;
- the wet bulb should be read first, before it starts to rise in temperature;
- at least three readings should be taken.

Dew point apparatus

A silvered surface (mirror) is cooled by the evaporation of ether, or a similar chemical, in a reservoir in direct contact with the mirror. The dew point (i.e. the temperature when condensation occurs) is determined by cooling and then warming of the mirror. Using the psychrometric chart, the dew point value gives the RH or absolute humidity for known air temperatures. The mirror can be cooled electrically (by the Peltier effect) and condensation detected automatically by light-scattering techniques.

Moving fabric hygrometers

Some materials change in length in a manner which is directly proportional to relative humidity — examples being hair, skin and timber. This movement can be translated to a lever arm for recording humidity, e.g. in the thermohygrograph. This instrument records temperature and relative humidity on a continuous basis (temperature is sensed by a bimetallic strip). When measuring RH directly it is essential also to measure air temperature to interpret variations in RH (i.e. whether they are solely temperature related). Such instruments must be regularly calibrated, e.g. against a whirling hygrometer, and handling the sensing element should be avoided as grease and dirt alters the response to RH.

Electrical resistance or capacitance

Some materials change their electrical resistance

Table 12.9(a) Typical occupational situations where heat stress could occur*

	Temperatures			Air velocity	Metabolic rate	PPE[†]
	Radiant	Air	Wet bulb			
Manufacturing						
Tops of furnaces	h	h	m	m	m	+
Handling molten metal, rolling and forging	H	m	m	m	h	+
Knockout and fettling	h	h	m	m	h	
Metal refining	h	m	m	m	h	
Welding, brazing, etc.	h	m	m	m	m	+
Glass making	H	h	m	low	h	+
Boiler and furnace maintenance	h	h	m	low	h	+
Metal finishing, pickling, galvanizing, degreasing	m	m	h	m	m	
Mining and tunnelling						
Face work, deep mines	m	h	m	low–m	h	(+)
Face work, highly mechanized mines and tunnels	m	h	h	low–m	h	
All work in very deep mines	h	h	m	m	m	
Mine rescue work — fire-fighting	m	h	h	low	h	+
Miscellaneous						
Laundries	m	m	h	low	m	
Kitchens	h	h	h	low	m	
Fire-fighting	h	h	h	low–m	h	(+)
Asbestos removal	m	h	(h)	low	h	+
Boiler-rooms, compressor houses — electricity generation	h	h	m	m	m	
Shipping and armed services						
Ships, boiler-rooms, ships' guns	h	h	h	low	m	
Tanks	h	h	m	low	m	+
Fighting aircraft	m	h	m	low	low	
Outdoor work in hot places						
Agriculture, quarrying, outdoor marketing	H	h	m	m	h	

* H, high with red heat or above; h, high; m, medium.
† Situations where required personal protective equipment may contribute significantly to heat strain are indicated by +.

or capacitance as a function of relative humidity, e.g. alumina (aluminium oxide) and complex ammonium salts. This principle can be applied to give a measure of RH directly. Sensors must be regularly calibrated as their response is readily distorted by pollutants. They are used mainly in industrial (e.g. food processing), laboratory and air-conditioning humidity control applications. There are many portable instruments available using this principle, but care is required in their use; sensors can be reliable in the middle RH range, e.g. 40–80%, but outside this range their accuracy decreases. Calibration can be undertaken with 'pots' of known RH value. Another electrical device is based on phase change properties of lithium chloride.

Table 12.9(b) Typical occupational situations where cold stress could occur*

	Temperatures			Air velocity	Metabolic rate	Water[†]
	Radiant	Air	Wet bulb			
Outdoor						
Quarrying, tipping, agriculture, stockyards, railways, local authority maintenance	low	low	low	h	–	m
Sea fishing, oil rigs, shipping, armed services	low	low	low	h	–	h
Indoor						
Deep freeze stores	low	low	low	low–m	–	low
Mining in intake airways	low	low	low	h	–	low
Diving[‡]	low	low	low	low	low	h

* h, high; m, medium.

[†] Refers to situations where heat loss due to water conduction or evaporation from wet clothing occurs.

[‡] Also has high respiratory heat loss.

Air velocity

Anemometers based on a range of principles are available, i.e. katathermometer (cooling), electrical resistance and thermistor types (cooling), moving vane types (mechanical action) and tracer techniques (e.g. smoke). Air movement associated with thermal environments is often very low, i.e. $< 0.2\,\mathrm{m\,s^{-1}}$, and this limits the selection of a suitable anemometer. Traditionally the katathermometer satisfies this criterion.

Katathermometer (cooling or 'down' thermometer)

The katathermometer bulb is heated in hot water and its cooling time between two fixed temperatures measured. This is converted to an air velocity using an appropriate chart knowing the surrounding air temperature and the calibration factor for the katathermometer (Fig. 12.12). If radiation sources are present, then a silvered bulb should be used. Katathermometers of different cooling ranges are available, giving different scales for measured velocity. The instrument provides multidirectional airflow measurement, averages out fluctuations and can measure to very low airspeeds and is thus suited to the measurement of general room air movement.

Cooling resistance/thermistor anemometer

A wire coil or thermistor bead is heated to approximately 100°C above ambient, and the electrical current required to maintain it at this temperature is monitored. This is a function of the air velocity and air temperature. These instruments are widely used for measuring high air movement (e.g. $> 0.5\,\mathrm{m\,s^{-1}}$), but can also be configured for lower values but at relatively high cost. Information on air turbulence, which is relevant for comfort studies, can also be provided.

Moving vane type instruments (e.g. the rotating vane anemometer) are best suited to directional air movement of $> 0.3\,\mathrm{m\,s^{-1}}$. Tracer methods (the most common being smoke) are essential for identifying and demonstrating airflow patterns in spaces, the effects of ventilation or air-conditioning systems and to identify draughts.

Integrating meters

Meters are available which will measure all, or a selection, of these parameters and combine them

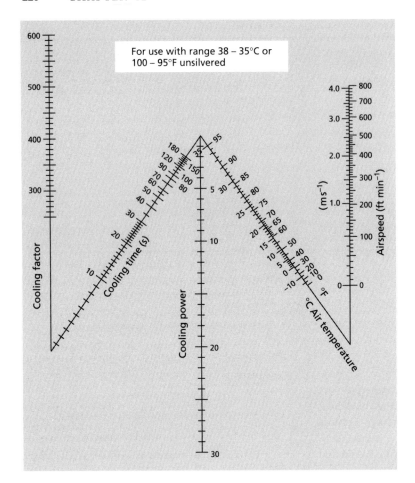

Fig. 12.12 Example of a chart for determining the air velocity from the katathermometer cooling time. Chart selection involves kata cooling range and type of bulb (silvered or non-silvered).

as appropriate into a single figure scale. For example a wet bulb globe thermometer (WBGT) meter measures air temperature (dry bulb), globe temperature (40–150 mm, depending on the model) and unaspirated wet bulb temperature, i.e. natural wet bulb (NWB). (This may be aspirated if required for other measurements.) These are then combined to give a single figure value. They can be used for continuous remote monitoring and may be linked to alarm systems.

A further device is the thermal comfort meter which is based on Fanger's work and enables the predicted mean vote (PMV) or percentage of people dissatisfied (PPD) with a particular environment to be measured. Other devices, e.g. indoor climate analysers, are specifically designed to assess individual parameters, e.g. factors affecting discomfort, such as measurement of radiation asymmetry and air movement perceived as a draught.

Further details on measurement techniques are given in BS EN 27726 (British Standards Institution, 1994a) and ISO 7726 *Thermal Environments — Instruments and Methods for Measuring Physical Quantities* (International Organization for Standardization, 1985).

PRINCIPLES OF CONTROL

Typical occupational activities which can lead to heat or cold stress problems are shown in Table 12.9. The relative contribution of the four environmental factors plus activity (metabolic rate) and clothing (where protective clothing, respirators, etc. can add to the thermal burden) are also given.

Principles of control are discussed in the following sections for heat and cold stress. Control in relation to thermal comfort is generally an issue of the fine-tuning of conditions, and is discussed separately.

Control for hot conditions

The effects of heat stress can be controlled in a number of ways. The planning of work can minimize the length and extent of exposure. Modifying the environmental conditions can reduce the body burden. Appropriate supervision and training is essential for the health, safety and welfare of individuals. Finally, special protective clothing can be of value, whilst protective clothing for other hazards, e.g. toxic contaminants, can lead to exacerbation of heat stress problems.

Planning

Exposure to conditions which could lead to heat strain are best avoided or minimized by careful planning whenever possible. This applies in particular to work activities such as maintenance and repair of hot equipment, replacement of insulating materials on steam pipes, etc. and other work of short duration which can often be planned ahead.

If exposure is unavoidable then the risk should be controlled to an acceptable level, preferably by environmental control. Figure 12.13 illustrates the points to be considered when planning for hot work. Where, despite all reasonable environmental control measures, conditions are still likely to lead to heat strain, then additional precautions will be required to reduce personal risk, e.g. medical pre-selection and acclimatization, supervision and training, restriction of work periods and thermal protective clothing.

Environmental control

Modifying the thermal parameters which are contributing to the heat stress conditions can be considered as follows.

Control of the source

Where heat is released by a particular process or source, the temperature of the source itself should be reduced. This may be done by direct temperature reduction, surface insulation, radiant heat emission control or a combination of these factors.

Ventilation, air-conditioning and air movement

Ventilation can be used for thermal environment control either by removing or diluting hot/humid air and replacing it with cooler/drier air, or by increasing air movement over the body. Cooling effects from air movement result from heat loss/gain from convection and loss from evaporation. However, as the air temperature rises, losses are reduced and may become gains. As a rule of thumb, for hot conditions, if the wet bulb temperature is below 36°C, increasing air velocity over the body is beneficial, but above 36°C, it is detrimental.

Evaporative cooling

Air temperature can be reduced *in situ* (via evaporative cooling) by the use of fine water sprays or wetted elements. Whilst this can reduce the air temperature, it also increases relative humidity and these two factors must be balanced when evaluating the potential benefits. Health risks associated with potential microbiological activity with such processes should also be assessed.

Radiation shields and barriers

Radiant heat from high-temperature sources can be reduced by radiation barriers positioned between the source and the subject. Ideally, such barriers should be of a material with good insulating properties and have surfaces of low emissivity (i.e. high reflectivity) so that they do not themselves become hot, reradiate and present a contact hazard. Reflected radiation from the heat source should be directed so as to avoid contributing to the heat load. Metal grids, chains or transparent reflective materials such as partially silvered glass or clear plastics can be used where it is necessary to view the heat source itself. Cold surfaces, e.g. water-cooled panels, can also be used as radiation sinks.

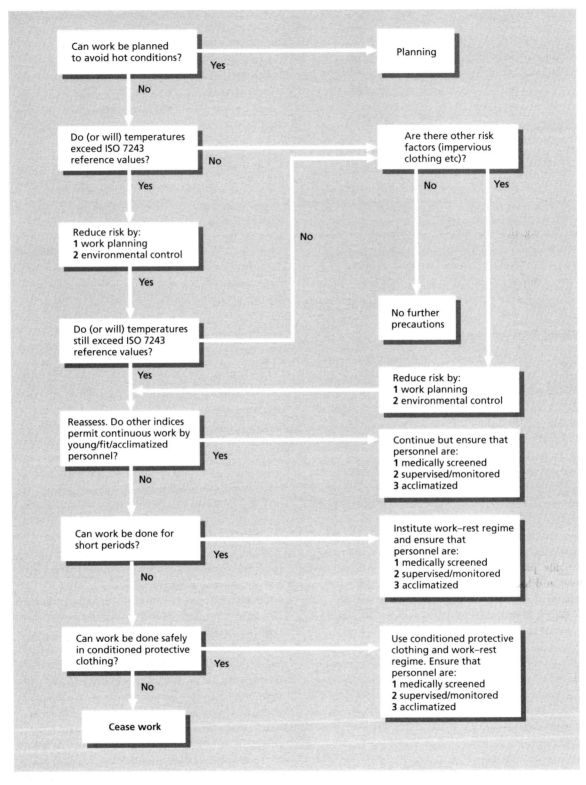

Fig. 12.13 Flow chart for use in planning for hot work. From British Occupational Hygiene Society (1990).

Managerial aspects

Supervision and training are essential whenever work is to be carried out in hot environments, to ensure that potential heat casualties are detected quickly and immediately removed to a place for recovery. Personnel should not be allowed to work alone and unsupervised in such conditions.

Restricted work periods (work–rest regimes) invariably require to be implemented, e.g. as recommended by an appropriate heat stress index. Such recommendations may be conservative in nature, e.g. the rest area in ISO 7243 (International Organization for Standardization, 1982 and 1989) is assumed to be at the same WBGT value as the work itself; for cooler rest areas recovery would be expected to be more rapid. Hence, more pragmatic approaches based on physiological monitoring may be appropriate.

Protective clothing and equipment

Clothing, especially protective clothing (including respirators), often has an adverse effect on the body's heat balance in hot environments by insulating the body and also reducing evaporative heat loss. Impervious clothing particularly impedes heat loss and the wearing of such clothing may present some risk if physically demanding work or exercise is carried out at air (dry bulb) temperatures as low as 21°C, especially if the wearer is unfit, not acclimatized or otherwise susceptible.

In some circumstances, clothing is required to provide protection against general heat, radiant heat and localized burns (e.g. from molten metal splashes). Heat-resistant protective clothing will only give protection for limited periods and may have a detrimental effect over long periods. If continued exposure is necessary in circumstances where it would not otherwise be permitted, the use of cooled or conditioned protective clothing may allow longer periods of exposure. Examples are ice-cooled jackets, air-cooled suits and liquid (water)-cooled suits. It should be noted that wearing the jacket or suit can in itself lead to an increase in the metabolic rate and thus thermal strain. Because cooled or conditioned clothing is used in circumstances where exposure would not otherwise be permitted, its use should be restricted to those who are medically fit and there should be a high standard of supervision since, in the event of its failure, the user will be exposed to an unacceptable environment and will need to be removed immediately.

Control for cold conditions

The principles of control for thermal protection necessary to ensure comfort and well-being in the cold are determined by two sets of factors: personal and environmental. Personal factors include bodily activity (metabolic rate), clothing insulation worn and available, and duration of the exposure. Environmental factors are ambient air temperature and wind velocity in particular, but also radiant conditions and the presence of precipitation.

Clothing

If shelter is not available, clothing is the most important means of protection against cold stress for people living or working in cold environments. The thermal insulation provided by clothing is a result of the fibrous structure of the clothing itself and air trapped between layers of clothing. Clothing also has to protect against wind which can penetrate and negate the insulating property of the trapped air. It is therefore necessary for an effective cold weather assembly to be windproof by having an outside layer made of tightly woven or impermeable material.

Clothing which is waterproof is also essential in cold, wet environments because of the rapid cooling produced by the combined effects of evaporation and wind-chill. However, a serious disadvantage of waterproofing is that the clothing is also impermeable to water vapour escaping from the skin surface. If it cannot escape, this water vapour will condense beneath the impermeable layer in cold weather and reduce the insulation effects of the trapped air, as well as being a source of discomfort. This effect is increased if the individual is physically active and sweating. In environments with temperatures below 0°C, trapped water in clothing may freeze. Impermeable clothing is mainly useful for people who are not very active. Loosely fitted, with openings around the neck and inbuilt air vents, the garments rely on a bellows effect to vent and reduce water vapour build-up. For active personnel, clothing with special external fabric which is both windproof and waterproof, but allows water vapour transfer, should be used.

The other important consideration with respect to clothing is protection of the extremities and head. Thick, insulating gloves are of little use when fine hand movements are required, and, furthermore, insulation around small-diameter cylinders, like the fingers, is difficult to achieve. Mitts, with all the fingers enclosed together and only the thumb separate, provide more effective insulation. Under survival situations these weaknesses in insulation can be overcome by withdrawing the hands and arms into the body of the jacket (ensuring that loose sleeves are constrained and made airtight). Local cold injury to the hands and face is especially likely to occur since these areas are the most frequently exposed and particular care must therefore be applied, such as providing local heating to the areas.

Work activity

Clothing insulation must be balanced against work performed. However, if work is intermittent (the usual case) then problems can arise, e.g. a worker dressed for thermal protection during periods of inactivity will be overdressed for hard work, and hence providing clothing for operators engaged in intermittent work schedules can present some difficulty.

Work–rest regimes

Warm shelters should be available for rest and recovery for work performed continuously in a cold environment with an equivalent chill temperature below −7°C. During rest periods it is recommended that dry clothing be provided as necessary and body fluids replaced (preferably by warm, sweet drinks and soups) to combat dehydration. Alcohol and caffeine-containing beverages are not advisable as these have adverse diuretic and circulatory effects.

In environments of −12°C or below, e.g. in many cold stores, it is necessary for workers to be under constant observation or supervision. Work rates should not be so high as to cause heavy sweating, but if this is unavoidable, more frequent rest pauses in the warm for changing into dry clothes should be taken. Sitting or standing still for long periods in the cold should be avoided. Air movement from air blast coolers should be minimized by properly designed air distribution systems and should not exceed $1\,m\,s^{-1}$ at the work site. Out of doors in snow or ice-covered terrain, eye protection should be provided from blowing ice crystals, whilst safety goggles and exposed skin treatment are needed to protect against ultraviolet radiation and glare.

Control and comfort

In recent years, much attention has been concentrated on the 'quality' of internal working environments, particularly offices. Thermal comfort represents one area contributing to such 'quality', or lack of, and standards for thermal comfort are well established (e.g. ISO 7730, International Organization for Standardization, 1984). However, buildings themselves and thermal control systems can influence conditions detrimentally, whilst the lack of perceived control by occupants can also be an important contributing factor. Issues which are likely to influence the thermal conditions occurring within a space or building include: the building location, orientation (particularly with respect to sunpaths), fabric, the active internal temperature-modifying systems (heating, air-conditioning, etc.) with associated controls and the influence of people, lighting and equipment.

Ideally, the building fabric itself will moderate the external climate to produce internal conditions which are more comfortable. However, the fabric may exacerbate conditions, for instance internal overheating arising from solar gain through large areas of glazing (i.e. the greenhouse effect). Control by the fabric (known as 'passive' control) is influenced by many factors; these include the areas and orientation of glazing, the type of glazing (insulation value and radiation transmission properties), the thermal insulation values of the building fabric (walls, floors and roof) and the speed of response of the fabric to heat gains or losses. The speed of response is governed by the thermal mass of the fabric and structure (which is closely linked to the actual mass) but is also affected by the position of thermal insulation in the fabric. Thermal mass providing slow response helps to even out temperature fluctuations caused, for instance, by solar gain through windows in hot weather conditions, but also influences the rate at which the building reaches acceptable occupancy temperatures via the internal heating system during the heating season. Whether a building is best suited to be thermally heavyweight (slow response) or lightweight (fast response) is thus an interrelation of many factors.

Passive thermal control will only provide suitable internal thermal conditions for occupancy during relatively moderate external conditions. At other times 'active' control will be required to heat or cool the building, whilst ventilation may also need to be achieved actively (i.e. mechanically) if the building is, for instance, deep-plan or work areas require special climate control.

In relation to simple heating, control of conditions may be achieved by modifying the air temperature, the radiant temperature or a combination of both, e.g. by warm air blowers or radiant/convector heaters. In such cases the temperature parameter which is not being modified directly, alters indirectly with a time delay. For example, with a warm air system, the radiant temperature gradually changes as surface temperatures slowly follow the changing air temperature.

Relative humidity may also be separately controlled during heating, usually to avoid the air becoming too dry (less than 40% RH), primarily for general comfort (e.g. relating to dry skin and eyes, etc.) rather than specifically for thermal comfort. Air movement requires to be moderated or controlled in order to avoid the sensation of draughts. These are more noticeable if they are associated with air of low temperature, e.g. air dropping from a cold, glazed surface. An upper limit of air movement over the body of $0.15\,\mathrm{m\,s^{-1}}$ is usually recommended for comfort when a building is in the heating mode.

In hot external conditions, maintaining suitable conditions inside may be simply a function of providing enhanced air movement (via windows and/or fans) for increasing convection (and evap-

oration) losses to the body and also taking advantage of the thermal mass of the building to provide some degree of natural cooling (on a 24 h cycle basis). However, artificial (i.e. mechanical) cooling may be required, particularly if the building is deep-plan, there are high internal gains or processes require close temperature control. In such cases cooling is most commonly achieved by supplying air at reduced temperature (typically 14°C) to spaces (via 'air-conditioning'), allowing also the control of RH, if required, by dehumidification. In such applications, air movement over people needs to be controlled, typically to a maximum of $0.25\,\mathrm{m\,s^{-1}}$. Less commonly, cooling can be provided by radiant means, e.g. via chilled ceilings, where circulating chilled water cools exposed surfaces to provide a radiation 'sink'. Care must be exercised in such applications to avoid condensation occurring on the cold surfaces. It should be noted that the application of air-conditioning to buildings can have considerable financial implications in relation to capital and running costs, as well as being regarded somewhat unfavourably in relation to environmental issues, such as energy consumption and atmospheric gaseous emissions.

The internal activities in a bulding can have an important bearing on conditions arising, and the need and type of active thermal control. People, artificial lighting and equipment (e.g. computers and terminals) produce significant heat gains to spaces which can contribute usefully in the heating season but may lead to overheating effects at other times of the year. Thus, they require assessment, alongside the passive and active systems themselves.

Finally, the means of control over the thermal environment (including ventilation) that can be exercised by occupants can have a marked effect on perceived comfort. If no means of control is provided, i.e. occupants have an environment imposed upon them (e.g. in an open-plan air-conditioned office), this can exacerbate occupant dissatisfaction.

Thus, thermal comfort in buildings is a complex issue where any factor, or combination of factors, may require attention to improve a thermally unsatisfactory environment. A summary of typical actions to assess conditions can be found in BOHS

Technical Guide No. 8 (British Occupational Hygiene Society, 1990). It is likely that a range of personnel will be required for investigations of comfort, in particular those responsible for the design, operation and maintenance of the mechanical services plant (building services engineers) and for the building and fabric itself.

REFERENCES

American Conference of Governmental Industrial Hygienists (1994). *Threshold Limit Values for 1994–95.* ACGIH, Cincinnati.

ASHRAE (1981). *American Society of Heating, Refrigeration and Air-conditioning Engineers, Standard SS — 1981.* ASHRAE, Atlanta.

British Occupational Hygiene Society (1990). *The Thermal Environment.* BOHS Technical Guide No. 8. Science Reviews, Leeds.

British Standards Institution (1994a). *Thermal Environments — Instruments and Methods for Measuring Physical Quantities.* British Standards Institution BS EN 27726.

British Standards Institution (1994b). *Hot Environments — Estimation of the Heat Stress on a Working Man, based on the WBGT-Index.* British Standards Institution BS 27243.

CIBSE (1987). *Chartered Institution of Building Services Engineers, Guide A.* Balham, London.

Fanger, P.O. (1970). *Thermal Comfort.* Danish Technical Press, Copenhagen and (1972) McGraw-Hill, New York.

International Organization for Standardization (1982) (revised 1989). *Hot Environments — Estimation of the Heat Stress on a Working Man, Based on the WBGT-Index.* International Standard ISO 7243.

International Organization for Standardization (1984). *Moderate Thermal Environments — Determination of the PMV and PPD Indices and Specification of the Conditions for Thermal Comfort.* International Standard ISO 7730.

International Organization for Standardization (1985). *Thermal Environments — Instruments and Methods for Measuring Physical Quantities.* International Standard ISO 7726.

International Organization for Standardization (1989). *Hot Environments — Analytical Determination and Interpretation of Thermal Stress Using Calculation of Required Sweat Rate.* International Standard ISO 7933.

International Organization for Standardization (1990). *Ergonomics — Determination of Metabolic Heat Production.* International Standard ISO 8996.

International Organization for Standardization (1992). *Evaluation of Thermal Strain by Physiological Measurement.* International Standard ISO 9886.

International Organization for Standardization (1995). *Ergonomics of the Thermal Environment — Estimation of the Thermal Insulation and Evaporative Resistance of a Clothing Ensemble.* International Standard ISO 9920.

FURTHER READING

Chrenko, F.A. (ed.) (1974). *Bedford's Basic Principles of Ventilation and Heating.* H.K. Lewis, London.

Clark, R.P. and Edholm, O.G. (1985). *Man and his Thermal Environment.* Edward Arnold, London.

Edholm, O.G. (1978). *Man — Hot and Cold.* Edward Arnold, London.

National Institute for Occupational Safety and Health (1986). *Criteria for a Recommended Standard — Occupational Exposure to Hot Environments, Revised Criteria 1986.* NIOSH, Cincinnati.

Parsons, K.C. (1993). *Human Thermal Environments.* Taylor and Francis, London.

CHAPTER 13
Non-ionizing Radiation

B.J. Maddock

INTRODUCTION

Electric and magnetic fields, radio waves, light, X-rays and gamma rays are all manifestations of the same phenomenon — electromagnetism. Its unifying theoretical foundations, provided by James Clerk Maxwell, formed the great triumph of nineteenth century physics. The frequency of the oscillations of a field best characterizes its nature. These frequencies cover an enormously wide range from essentially zero, for static fields such as that of the Earth, to 10^{22} hertz (Hz or cycles s^{-1}) and beyond for the most energetic gamma rays. The complete spectrum is shown in Fig. 13.1.

Electromagnetic fields do not require any medium for their existence or transmission (as sound waves do), but various materials can influence their propagation by processes such as absorption, reflection, refraction and diffraction. The universal speed of electromagnetic waves in 'free space' is $3 \times 10^8\,\mathrm{m\,s^{-1}}$. This speed ($c$) is related to the frequency (v in hertz) and the wavelength (λ in metres) of the wave by:

$$c = v\lambda \qquad (13.1)$$

The wavelength is the distance between any two successive crests in the sequence of waves. If the wave is travelling in some material, the speed is in general reduced (by an amount which may depend on the frequency) and the wavelength is shorter accordingly. The change for propagation in air can usually be neglected.

For frequencies above about 10^5 Hz, radiating fields, in which energy is transported away from the source, predominate — hence the term 'radi-

ation' in the title of this chapter. At yet higher frequencies, typically when the visible part of the spectrum is reached, the quantum nature of the radiation begins to become apparent. As the late Professor Feynman remarked, 'energy comes in lumps'; it is not possible to have indefinitely smaller amounts. The smallest unit or quantum ('photon' for electromagnetic radiation) depends upon the frequency according to the famous formula:

$$E = hv \qquad (13.2)$$

where E is the energy (J), h is Planck's constant (6.63×10^{-34} J s) and v is the frequency (Hz). These energies are extremely small in everyday terms, so the 'lumps' do not become obvious until one reaches the gamma ray part of the spectrum where the radiation behaves much more as particles than as waves.

Because these photon energies are small, it is often convenient to use a smaller energy unit which is more appropriate to the interaction of the radiation with matter. This is the electronvolt (eV), which is the energy acquired by a single electron being accelerated through a potential difference of 1 V. $1\,\mathrm{eV} = 1.6 \times 10^{-19}$ J, so the photon energy for a frequency of 3×10^{15} Hz (a wavelength of 100 nm) is 12.4 eV — the energy required to remove an electron from a hydrogen atom. This lies near the middle of the ultraviolet (UV) region and it is generally taken as the divide between non-ionizing and ionizing radiation. Increasingly above this point, the photons have sufficient energy to eject electrons from atoms, leaving the latter charged or 'ionized'. Such ionization can lead to effects in

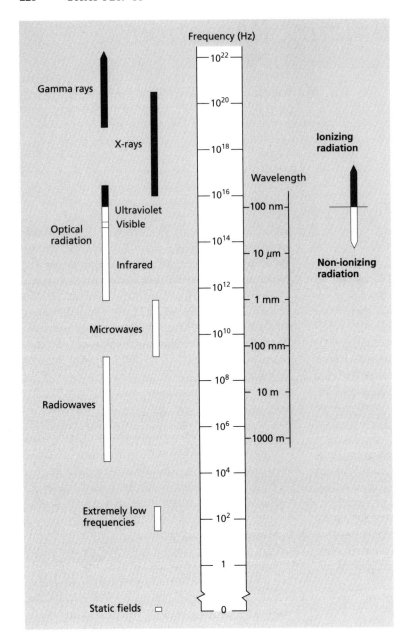

Fig. 13.1. The electromagnetic spectrum covers an enormously wide range of frequencies – from zero for static fields to 10^{22} Hz and beyond for the most energetic gamma rays. Note the divide between non-ionizing and ionizing radiation, generally taken as 3×10^{15} Hz (a wavelength of 100 nm near the middle of the UV region).

biological materials (see Chapter 14) which are quite different from those which follow absorption of lower-frequency radiation.

Radio engineers have for a long time divided their part of the spectrum into decade ranges. This has subsequently been extended both ways to run from below power frequencies right up to the beginning of the infrared (IR) region (Table 13.1).

Electromagnetism and the technology based upon it have brought immense benefits to modern society and have contributed in many ways to improvements in health and working conditions. This chapter provides detailed background material on the major segments of the non-ionizing part of the electromagnetic spectrum – low frequencies, radiofrequencies (RF) and optical wavelengths (IR,

Table 13.1 Ranges and selected uses of low and radio frequencies

Frequency range	Uses
30–300 Hz ELF Extremely low frequency	Electric power systems, railways, industrial processes, metal melting, motors, appliances
300–3000 Hz VF Voice frequency	Electric furnaces, induction heating, hardening, soldering, melting, refining
3–30 kHz VLF Very low frequency	Very long-range communications, radio navigation, induction heating, hardening, melting
30–300 kHz LF Low frequency	Radionavigation, radiolocation, electro-erosion, induction heating and melting, power inverters
0.3–3 MHz MF Medium frequency	AM broadcasting, marine radiotelephone, radionavigation, RF welding, industrial RF equipment
3–30 MHz HF High frequency	Short-wave, citizens and amateur radio, medical diathermy, MRI, dielectric heating, wood drying and gluing
30–300 MHz VHF Very high frequency	FM broadcasting, police, fire, air traffic control, MRI, plastic welding, food processing, plasma heating
0.3–3 GHz UHF Ultra high frequency	TV broadcasting, microwave communications, mobile radio, radar, medical diathermy, cooking
3–30 GHz SHF Super high frequency	Radar, satellite communications, microwave relays, anti-intruder alarms
30–300 GHz EHF Extremely high frequency	Radar, radionavigation, satellite communications, microwave relays

MRI, magnetic resonance imaging; RF, radiofrequency.

visible and UV) — noting, in the context of occupational hygiene, possible adverse effects. There is also a section on lasers.

LOW FREQUENCIES

The frequencies considered here extend from zero (static fields) to about 100 kHz. This upper bound is arbitrary, but is chosen because below it there is essentially no radiation ('non-ionizing *radiation*' is an inappropriate label here), while above it one enters the range of radio broadcasting. In the low-frequency part of the electromagnetic spectrum the electric and magnetic components need to be considered separately.

Sources of static magnetic fields include the Earth, permanent magnets, magnetic resonance imaging (MRI) equipment, electrolytic processes using direct currents, some railway traction systems and the electromagnets used in guiding beams of nuclear particles. Static electric fields arise wherever there is an accumulation of electric charge, for example in thunder clouds, on synthetic fibres, on VDU and TV screens and near high-voltage DC (direct current) power systems.

Fields which oscillate at power frequencies — sometimes called ELF (extremely low frequency) (see Table 13.1) — are found wherever electricity is supplied and used. For example, they are produced by appliances, office equipment, electrical machinery, supply wiring, power lines and some electric railways. The magnetic field arises from the alternating currents (AC), while the electric field arises from the alternating voltage used. The frequency is usually 50 Hz, though 60 Hz is used in North America, parts of Japan and some other areas. Some European railways use $16\frac{2}{3}$ Hz, while aircraft power systems usually operate at 400 Hz. Higher-frequency fields (tens of kilohertz) are produced by industrial equipment, such as in some metal heating and melting plants, by some security and anti-theft systems and by the line-scanning circuits of cathode-ray tube VDUs (these VDUs also produce ELF fields from their frame-scanning and power circuits).

Fields are not easy to imagine since they are rather abstract concepts used to describe how a source of some electric or magnetic effect influences another object. However, they are often thought of as lines of force which may sometimes be visualized as in Fig. 13.2.

Field waveforms are not always sinusoidal because of components at harmonics of the fundamental frequency in the current or voltage sources. The field may then be analysed in terms of its harmonics or treated as a complex waveform if rapidly changing parts are of interest.

Electric fields are expressed in volts per metre $(V\,m^{-1})$ and magnetic fields in amperes per metre $(A\,m^{-1})$. However, for magnetic fields the flux density — in teslas (T) — is frequently used because this quantity best characterizes the interaction of magnetic fields with conducting objects. It is also more simply related to the older unit: the gauss (G). The tesla is a large unit, hence the milli, micro and nano sub-multiples (mT, μT and nT) are often used. The relation between these magnetic units is: $1\,mT \equiv 10\,G$, and $\cong 796\,A\,m^{-1}$ (except in magnetizable material). For alternating fields, the root-mean-square (rms) value is almost always used which, for sinusoidal waves, is the peak amplitude (measured from the zero line) divided by $\sqrt{2}$.

The field strengths encountered cover a very wide range. At 50 Hz for example, they range from about $1-100\,V\,m^{-1}$ and $0.01-1\,\mu T$ in an office away from equipment, up to at least $10\,kV\,m^{-1}$

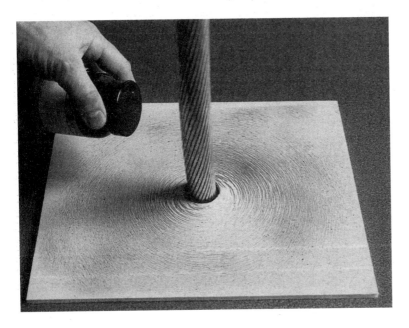

Fig. 13.2 Iron filings reveal the circular pattern of magnetic field surrounding a conductor carrying a current. (Photograph by courtesy of National Grid.)

and 1 mT near heavy electrical plant. In fact the field depends critically on the distance from the source – it falls off rapidly as one moves away – and this is illustrated, in terms of a magnetic field, in Fig. 13.3. Electric fields also decay rapidly with distance, but the behaviour is more complex because of the presence of nearby objects and the ground.

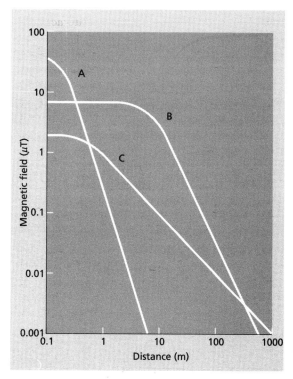

Fig. 13.3 The magnetic field falls quite rapidly as one moves away from the source. Graph A is for a compact source such as an electric motor, B is for an extended source with equal 'go' and 'return' currents such as a power line, and C is for a single long current-carrying conductor. For each, the field is that along a path passing close to the source at a distance roughly equal to the centre of the curved portion of the respective graph. Well away from the source, the variation is as $1/d^3$ for A, $1/d^2$ for B and $1/d$ for C, where d is the distance from the source. At the larger distances, therefore, there is likely to be a 'background' field composed of the various contributions from single currents – net currents in electrical cables for example.

Physical interactions

Static electric fields exert weak attractive forces by inducing charges on the surface of objects. If an object in the field is not well-connected electrically to the Earth, it will take on a voltage with respect to the Earth. Static magnetic fields can exert strong attractive forces on magnetizable material.

Similarly, an alternating electric field (E) induces charges and voltages on an object. The induced, alternating positive and negative charges at the surface give rise to a small alternating current (I) in the object, proportional to the frequency (f) and the size of the object:

$$I = 2\pi\varepsilon_0 EfA \qquad (13.3)$$

where A is the effective area of the object (about 5 m^2 for a person standing in a vertical field) and ε_0 is the permittivity of free space (8.85×10^{-12} F m^{-1}). A field of 1 kV m^{-1} at 50 Hz creates a total current through the feet of a person of average size of about 15 μA. The resulting 'internal' electric field (given by the local current density multiplied by the conductivity of the body) is usually negligible, being at least a millionfold lower than that outside. Heating is also negligible.

The voltage induced on a person by an electric field is likely to be different from that induced on some nearby object – for example, a steel structure or a vehicle – so that a small spark may occur at the instant of touching the object. Such spark discharges are akin to those experienced when touching a metal filing cabinet after walking across a synthetic carpet in dry conditions. If contact with the object is maintained, a current continues to flow. In practice, such currents are unlikely to exceed a milliampere at power frequencies, unless the field is particularly strong and the object large. Earthing of the object, or other measures to equalize the potentials, generally removes any difficulties which could arise from such situations.

An alternating magnetic field (flux density B) induces an electric field which, if present in a conducting object, drives a circulating current around the object with a magnitude proportional to the frequency and the radial position (r). If large, as they can be in a metal, these currents give rise to heating. The local current density (J) in $A\,m^{-2}$ in a circular object perpendicular to the field is:

$$J = \pi Bfr\sigma \qquad (13.4)$$

where σ is the electrical conductivity of the object. For a person $(\sigma \sim 0.2\,S\,m^{-1})$ the heating is negligible and the pattern of current flow depends on the relative direction of the field (Fig. 13.4).

The magnetic field can sometimes have a direct influence causing, for example, vibration of nearby steel or, through forces on the electron beam, 'wobbling' of VDU displays. Repositioning or re-orienting the VDU can often alleviate this problem.

Physiological effects

Strong electric fields may sometimes be perceived through a tingling of exposed skin or, at power frequencies, by vibration of fine hairs on the back of the hand or neck. Occasionally, small discharges between the edges of clothing or spectacle frames and the skin may be experienced. If persistent and strong, these effects can be annoying but they do not have any lasting physiological consequences. Individual sensitivity varies greatly, but it is rare to reach the threshold for annoyance.

Induced or contact currents may be felt if they are strong enough to stimulate nerve or muscle cells. The threshold for this is lowest in the range $10-1000\,Hz$ at about $1\,A\,m^{-2}$, a level not reached by induction in any reasonable field. Because of the small conducting cross-section of a finger or arm, contact currents may be felt. As the frequency rises to $100\,kHz$, the threshold current density rises approximately in proportion and the sensation eventually changes to one of warmth.

An interesting effect occurs for currents in the narrow frequency range of about $10-100\,Hz$ flowing through the retina of the eye. Faint, flickering visual sensations occur which are known as 'magnetophosphenes' when they are caused by magnetic fields and as 'electrophosphenes' if they arise from injected current. The corresponding threshold current densities have been estimated to be in the range $10-100\,mA\,m^{-2}$, which is only reached in unusually strong magnetic fields.

Effects on health

For some years, the question has been asked whether or not there may be more subtle effects, including harmful effects on health, at the much

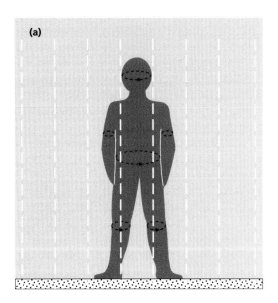
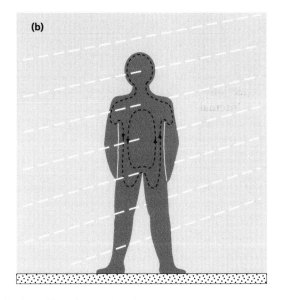

Fig. 13.4 Small imperceptible circulating currents (signified by the dotted lines) are induced in a person when they are in an alternating magnetic field (dashed lines:([a] vertical field, (b) horizontal field). The current flows in loops perpendicular to the direction of the field.

lower levels of induced current and fields to which persons are ordinarily exposed in daily life. A wide range of *in vitro* biological investigations, animal studies and epidemiological studies have been carried out, but, despite 20 years of research, no clear picture has emerged and no adverse effects have been established. The epidemiological findings suggest an association between childhood cancer and the proximity of homes to overhead power lines, but with no supporting biological evidence. The findings also point to an increased incidence of certain cancers in 'electrical' workers, though whether this has any connection with electric or magnetic fields remains open. There is great uncertainty in the assessment, especially retrospectively, of exposure to these fields.

For persons fitted with active, implantable devices such as pacemakers, some caution may be needed in a few situations. Although these devices are designed to cope with electrical interference, strong fields may occasionally affect their operation. In a particular case, advice should be sought from the manufacturer of the device and from those responsible for implanting it.

Exposure standards

A few countries have developed guidance or standards for occupational exposure to low-frequency electric or magnetic fields and there is one international set of guidelines for power frequencies from the former International Non-ionizing Radiation Committee (INIRC) of the International Radiation Protection Association (IRPA). The successor body, the International Commission on Non-ionizing Radiation Protection (ICNIRP), reaffirmed these in 1993 and issued advice concerning static fields in 1994. In addition, the Commission of the European Union (CEU), CENELEC (the European Committee for Electrotechnical Standardization, 1995) and the Institute of Electrical and Electronics Engineers (IEEE) on behalf of the American National Standards Institute (ANSI) are developing standards. Those standards which provide an explicit rationale focus on established interactions and particularly on induced currents; they set field levels a factor of 10 to a 100 below the levels corresponding to nerve and muscle stimulation. A higher magnetic field is sometimes indicated for limbs, partly because of

their smaller size and hence lower induced currents for a given field.

Control

Electric fields are fairly easily reduced or screened, either near the source or near the person, by arrangements of metallic wires, mesh or sheeting. In extreme cases, such as when working directly on live high-voltage power lines, conducting suits are used. Magnetic fields in the low-frequency range are more difficult to control, sometimes requiring impracticably thick sheets of steel or aluminium, at least at power frequencies, to obtain a significant reduction. A better approach is to arrange for all 'go' and 'return' currents to be as close together as possible (to increase field cancellation) and as distant from the working location as feasible. For electrical machines and transformers, good design can ensure that the leakage field is small. Occasionally, active screening systems are used in which an additional cancelling field is generated.

Measurements

The measurement of static electric fields requires quite sophisticated equipment and, as with alternating fields, considerable care since the field is so easily perturbed by the presence of nearby objects, including the person using the instrument. Most low-frequency electric-field meters consist essentially of two plates and a device to measure the capacitively-induced current between them.

A variety of flux-gate magnetometers and Hall effect devices are available for measuring static magnetic fields and some of these have a response up to several hundred hertz and beyond. The simplest and most common meters for low-frequency alternating magnetic fields are based on measuring the voltage induced in a coil, which must be oriented so that its axis is parallel to the field. To avoid this necessity, devices are available which contain three orthogonal coils with electronic circuits to sum the three signals correctly. Such devices may also be conveniently employed to measure the 'elliptically-polarized' fields produced by electrical systems using three-phase currents.

It is important to check that any meter which is

used for a magnetic field is not adversely affected by the presence of an electric field (and vice versa), or by any radiofrequency fields which may also be present. Fields often vary markedly from point to point, so it is necessary to decide which is the most appropriate location for a measurement or over what volume it is appropriate to average the field. Fields also vary with time, as the source voltage or current changes. Therefore, some average over time must be chosen.

RADIOFREQUENCIES

Strictly, 'radiofrequency' (RF) denotes any frequency at which electromagnetic radiation is useful for telecommunication. Here it is used for the region 100 kHz to 300 GHz, which includes microwaves. This region encompasses frequencies with a wide range of uses. These uses may roughly be divided into those which rely on the radiated nature of the waves – radio and television broadcasting for example — and those where the electromagnetic fields are either used close to the source or are confined in some way, typically being used for heating. See Table 13.1 for some applications of radiofrequencies. The strengths of the fields used in these applications vary over many orders of magnitude, from minuscule to potentially hazardous.

At the lower frequencies in this range, the electric and magnetic fields must still be considered separately but, as the frequency rises, they become increasingly coupled together until true radiation predominates. Which regime applies in a given situation depends on the wavelength, the distance from the source and the size of the source. The region close to a radiating source is known as the 'near field'. The pattern of fields is complex, often varying strongly from point to point, and consists of both non-propagating components ('reactive', or 'inductive' if the magnetic field dominates) and radiating components. At some distance from the source (the 'far field'), only these latter persist (Fig. 13.5). The field intensities then vary inversely with distance, hence the power density varies inversely as the square of the distance. Incident power densities are usually given in watts per square metre (W m^{-2}), while absorption, particularly in biologi-

cal tissue, is characterized by the specific energy absorption rate (SAR) in watts per kilogram (W kg^{-1}). For absorption in thin layers (as occurs at the higher frequencies), an absorbed power density is used (W m^{-2}).

Physical interactions

Just as for the low frequencies discussed above, radiofrequency fields can induce voltages on objects which, if touched, may cause 'RF burns' from the discharge current. Currents are also induced in conducting objects, including persons, with consequent heating if the fields are sufficiently strong. As the frequency rises, the magnitudes of these currents, and hence the power absorbed, increase such that the absorption is increasingly concentrated in the surface layer. A 'skin or penetration depth' (d) may be defined for non-magnetic material as:

$$d = \sqrt{(1/\pi f \sigma)} \qquad (13.5)$$

at which the power absorption has fallen to 14% ($1/e^2$) of its value at the surface. For biological tissue this depth is 60–600 mm at 100 MHz and 3–30 mm at 10 GHz. The shallower depths are for high-water-content tissue (e.g. muscle, skin) and the deeper are for low-water-content tissue (e.g. fat, bone). Two other factors become important as the frequency increases: (1) when the wavelength of the field becomes comparable to that of the object, various resonances can occur; and (2) reflections from neighbouring objects can give rise to complex field patterns because of interference.

It is convenient to divide the frequency range into four regions to correspond with the major features of the power-absorption processes involved (Fig. 13.6). In the first, the 'sub-resonance range', the absorption increases with increasing frequency, proportionally to begin with and then more rapidly, because of the increasing induced currents. Thus, the possibility of significant heating arises in strong fields, particularly in narrow regions such as the ankles where the current density is high. Next is the 'resonance range', where the body dimensions are of the order of a quarter to a half of a wavelength, and in which strong absorption takes place, with a marked peak when the electric field com-

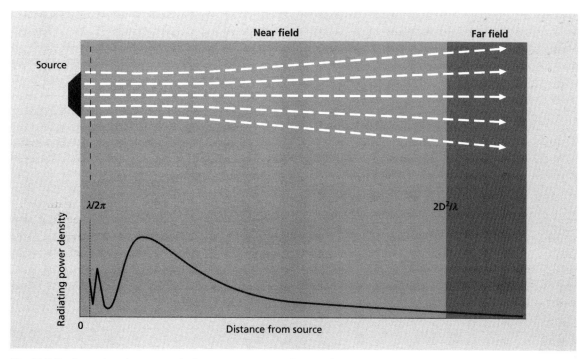

Fig. 13.5 In the region close to a radiofrequency source — the near field — the radiating power density varies markedly both along the beam (as shown here for a square aperture) and across it. In the far field — beyond a distance of about $2D^2/\lambda$ from the source (λ is the wavelength and D is the largest dimension of the source aperture, usually several times λ) — the pattern is smooth becoming almost a plane wave, with the inverse square law reduction in power density established by that distance. Very close to the source, within a distance of the order of λ, there are also nonradiating reactive fields which fall off more rapidly with distance than do the radiating fields, but which dominate the latter within about $\lambda/2\pi$ of the source. In the context of human exposure, these reactive fields are usually of consequence only for wavelengths greater than about 1 m. In this figure the power density and distance scales are linear.

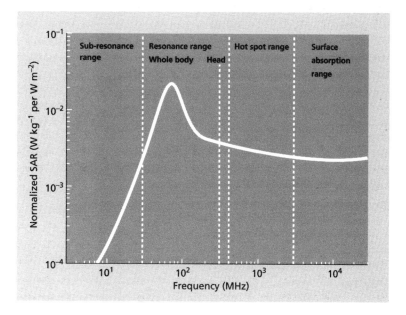

Fig. 13.6 The absorption of radiofrequency energy in a person needs to be considered in terms of several frequency ranges corresponding to the different absorption processes involved. A typical variation of the specific energy absorption rate (SAR) with frequency is shown here. The peak in the resonance range occurs when the electric field is parallel to the long dimension of the body.

ponent of the radiation is aligned with the major axis of the body. Partial body resonances, such as in the head, also occur. Then follows the 'hot-spot range', where local heating is more affected by the variation in the electrical properties of the body from point to point, and by shape and refraction effects. Finally, one reaches the 'surface absorption range', in which the fields penetrate only a few millimetres with the consequence that the heating is largely superficial.

Physiological effects

The principal physiological effect of any power absorption is an increase in body temperature. For modest inputs, the thermoregulatory system of the body can adjust and raise the heat lost by increasing the blood flow to surface areas, and by increasing the evaporation of moisture. However, above a level of about $4\,W\,kg^{-1}$ this becomes progressively more difficult and hyperthermia may result. If the absorption is confined to a restricted region, a limb for example, substantially higher values can be tolerated. There are, however, some regions (the eye in particular, where removal of heat by the blood system is poor) for which lower levels need to be ensured. This is primarily a problem at the higher frequencies where the absorption is superficial.

One rather different phenomenon is that of 'microwave hearing'. If a person is in the beam of a pulsed transmission, such as from a radar set, and the instantaneous power during the pulses is high enough (even though the average power may be quite small) and the pulses short enough, a buzzing or clicking sound may be 'heard', which is related to the pulse repetition rate of the equipment. This effect is thought to be caused by minute thermo-elastic-expansion pulses generated in the head by the pulses of energy absorbed. It is not known to be deleterious but is considered best avoided.

Effects on health

Significant overheating of tissue clearly poses a health hazard. However, as for exposure to low-frequency fields, there have been suggestions of potentially harmful effects at levels of field or power density well below those at which heating occurs and these are consequently referred to as 'athermal' effects. They have proved equivocal and the present consensus is that no adverse effects have been established beyond those which arise from excessive heating.

The operation of some cardiac pacemakers and other active, implantable devices may be affected by radiofrequencies below 'thermal' levels but this is primarily an electromagnetic compatibility problem and progressively is being addressed by the manufacturers.

Exposure standards

More countries have guidelines or standards for exposure to radiofrequency fields than for low-frequency fields, reflecting the existence of a real hazard from excessive heating at these frequencies. There used to be a wide divergence of views as to what levels were tolerable, but in recent years there has been considerable convergence. It is becoming generally accepted that a whole-body specific energy absorption rate of $0.4\,W\,kg^{-1}$, about one-tenth of the level at which significant changes in body temperature occur, is reasonable. There is still some disagreement over whether an even larger factor is necessary for some classes of persons. Higher values can be permitted when the absorption is confined to restricted regions of the body. Averaging over times reflecting the corresponding thermal time constants is also usually specified.

Many studies and calculations have been made concerning the translation of a specific energy absorption rate into measurable quantities, such as power density and field strength, and this too is now fairly well defined. Guidelines or standards have been published, or are being developed, by the IRPA, National Radiological Protection Board (NRPB), IEEE/ANSI, CEU, CENELEC and others.

Control

Much can be done to avoid excessive exposure to radiofrequency fields by careful design and siting of the source: for example, the use of directional aerials with controlled side lobes for broadcast and communication systems, the reduction of stray fields from industrial heating equipment and the correct earthing of equipment and metallic objects.

Screening may sometimes be needed and in principle this is not difficult for radiofrequencies. Metallic meshes are effective, provided the mesh size is considerably smaller than the wavelength — witness the perforated screens on the doors of microwave ovens. Absorptive material may sometimes be required to avoid undesirable reflections. In certain cases it is necessary to exclude personnel from high-field regions. To achieve effective control, measurements need to be made regularly in areas where exposure levels could approach or exceed guidelines and personnel need to be trained in correct work practices.

Measurements

Equipment for measuring radiofrequency radiation is broadly of two types. In the first, the field (usually the electric field) is sensed and the result displayed in terms of power density assuming plane-wave conditions. In the other, power is absorbed and the resulting temperature rise determined by a thermistor or thermocouple and displayed as a power density. Often, three orthogonal sensors (e.g. three small dipoles) are incorporated to give an isotropic response, thus eliminating the need to orient the device according to the direction and polarization of the incident wave. For near-field measurements, instruments which determine specifically the electric and/or magnetic field are required. Most instruments respond over a fairly broad band of frequencies, which is convenient, but care is needed if it is necessary to distinguish between more than one soure. Some devices are easily overloaded, and even damaged, so frequent checks on correct operation as well as calibration are advisable. For pulsed and modulated sources, consideration should be given to appropriate averaging times.

OPTICAL RADIATION

In the optical part of the electromagnetic spectrum, the radiation is usually characterized by its wavelength. This is partly because the wavelength is easier to determine than the frequency, but also because some important optical processes, such as

diffraction, depend critically on the relationship between the wavelength and the size of the features of an illuminated object. The optical range is customarily taken to run from a wavelength of 1 mm (the top of the radiofrequency range) through the IR, visible and UV regions to a wavelength of about 10 nm, overlapping the bottom of the soft X-ray region. However, the region from 100 nm to 10 nm is generally taken to belong to the ionizing part of the spectrum.

Both the IR and UV regions may be sub-divided in various ways, but the most appropriate here is that defined by the International Commission on Illumination (CIE) and based broadly on the biological effects of the radiation. The various ranges are given in Table 13.2. The Earth's atmosphere absorbs all incident solar UV radiation shorter than 280 nm and, in addition, absorption in the ozone layer limits the amount of UVB which reaches the Earth's surface. Below about 180 nm, propagation of UV radiation in air is not possible because of strong absorption.

All bodies emit optical radiation over quite a wide spread of wavelengths depending on their temperature. For a so-called 'black body' (a fair approximation for many hot bodies), the peak emission occurs at a wavelength (λ in μm) given by Wien's law:

$$\lambda = \frac{2898}{T} \qquad (13.6)$$

where T is the absolute temperature. Thus, a relatively high temperature is needed to achieve signifi-

Table 13.2 The principal wavelength regions of optical radiation as defined by the International Commission on Illumination

Region	Wavelength
UVC	100 to 280 nm
UVB	280 to 315 nm
UVA	315 to 380−400 nm
Light*	380−400 to 760−780 nm
IRA	760−780 to 1400 nm
IRB	1.4 to 3.0 μm
IRC	3.0 μm to 1 mm

*The limits for the human eye vary between individuals over the ranges indicated.

cant optical output. For a conventional tungsten-filament lamp, for example, $T \sim 2800$ K, so the peak is in the near IR, though some tungsten-halogen lamps can emit biologically-significant amounts of UV radiation. Even for the sun $(T \sim 6000$ K), by far the most important source of optical radiation for mankind from a hygiene point of view, about half the radiation reaching the Earth's atmosphere is still in the IR.

There are also sources whose output tends to be concentrated in narrow spectral regions. These use an electrical discharge in a gas or vapour. A fluorescent lamp is a typical example, in which mercury vapour produces a strong emission in the UV at 253.7 nm (4.9 eV). Most of this is absorbed by the phosphor coating which then fluoresces at several wavelengths in the visible range. Multicomponent phosphors are needed to give a good approximation to white light. Sodium lamps radiate directly in the visible yellow region at 589 nm and by increasing the pressure of the vapour the energy levels are broadened, thereby broadening the range of wavelengths produced and improving the colour.

Some indication of the range of intense sources which may be encountered is given in Table 13.3. Lasers are considered in a later section. It should be noted that when short-wavelength (less than about 250 nm) UV radiation is transmitted through air, ozone is produced.

Physical interactions

The way optical radiation is absorbed depends on the wavelength; in the far IR (wavelengths greater than a few tens of micrometres), the electric field of the radiation interacts with induced or residual electric dipole moments of molecules to increase rotational oscillations, while at the shorter IR wavelengths, the action is to increase internal motions such as flexing and stretching vibrations. In all these cases, the energy absorbed is progressively shared with adjacent molecules and amongst all the modes of oscillation and motion. This is manifest as a rise in temperature of the absorbing material. Thermal effects are thus to be found throughout the IR and into the red end of the visible region. Apart from transmission to the back of the eye, the absorption of optical radiation by

Table 13.3 Typical sources of optical radiation

Lamps	Incandescent (including tungsten halogen)
	Low-pressure gas discharge
	Fluorescent
	Low-pressure sodium
	'Blacklight'
	Mercury vapour
	High-pressure sodium
	Metal halide
	Xenon
Industrial processes	Arc and gas welding
	Hot and molten metal
	Glass working
	Electrical discharges
Natural	Solar

the human body is almost entirely superficial. Therefore, local cooling by thermal diffusion and by nearby blood flow are important in determining whether the temperature reached is high enough to cause damage. At shorter wavelengths, beginning towards the blue end of the visible region, but particularly in the UV regions, the energy absorbed may raise electrons to higher energy states within the molecules. This can lead to photochemical reactions in which the energy alters chemical bonding.

Quantities frequently used in characterizing optical radiation include irradiance (the power per unit area incident on a target surface), radiant exposure (the energy absorbed per unit area of the target) and, for extended sources, radiance (the power emitted per unit area per unit solid angle by a source). The corresponding quantities expressed per unit wavelength are used in more detailed spectral analyses. These can be multiplied by a spectral weighting function, variously known as a 'response', 'action' or 'hazard function', which characterizes the relative variation of the biological response with wavelength, to obtain a measure of the actual biological response to be expected from the radiation in question.

Biological effects

There are many vital and life-sustaining benefits of optical radiation which should not be forgotten, but here the focus is on the potentially adverse effects which may arise from excessive exposure to certain sources. Many sources radiate over a broad band of wavelengths and any hazards they pose need to be considered for each region of the spectrum separately and also collectively to allow for any synergistic effects.

For prolonged exposure to far IR radiation, particularly in the B and C regions, there is a possibility of thermal stress when the temperature-regulating system of the body can no longer maintain adequate control. However, most attention with regard to optical radiation needs to be given to possible direct effects on the eye and the skin. The main effects that may occur are summarized in Fig. 13.7 in terms of the relevant spectral regions.

The eye

In the far IR (IRC), corneal burn is the only effect that may arise since the cornea is essentially opaque in this region, thus shielding the rest of the eye.

The natural tear film provides an important cooling mechanism at the corneal surface, so those persons who suffer from 'dry-eye' are at a disadvantage in the presence of strong IRC sources. In the IRA and part of the IRB ($< 2 \mu m$) regions, the corneal absorption is lower so that significant absorption occurs in the lens and adjacent material. Prolonged exposure in this region may lead, years later, to enhanced lenticular opacities — commonly referred to as 'cataracts' and first recognized as a hazard for glass-blowers many years ago. Improved working conditions have apparently eliminated the incidence of this affliction in this occupation and there is little evidence that more modern sources, such as welding arcs, are a cause of cataracts.

In the IRA and visible regions the radiation reaches the retina, and is usually focused on it, giving a much increased irradiance. Therefore, an intense source can lead to retinal damage through local burning. At the blue end of the spectrum, there is also the possibility of photochemical injury

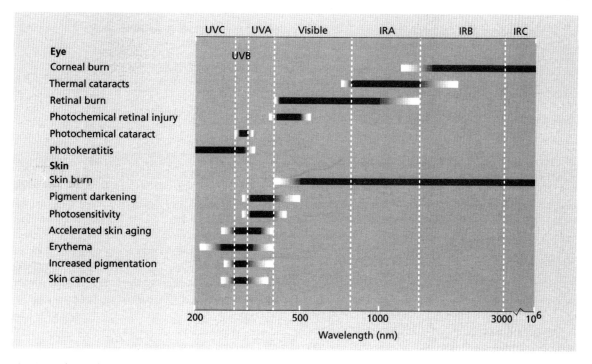

Fig. 13.7 The predominant biological effects of optical radiation are listed here according to the wavelengths at which they may occur. The first three effects for the eye are thermal in origin and the shift of them to progressively shorter wavelengths arises from the diminishing absorption with reducing wavelength of first the cornea and then the lens.

to the retina. However, the normal reflex reactions to a bright source (blinking, eye movement and turning of the head) provide good protection, except for intense laser sources. Of course, vision itself depends on photochemical reactions in the rod and cone photoreceptors of the retina.

Data from animal studies show that UVB wavelengths in the range 295–315 nm can induce both temporary and permanent lenticular opacities, the latter only at a radiant energy density or radiant exposure of about 5000 J m^{-2} and above. Human data are sparse. More significantly, photokeratitis (inflammation and damage to the surface of the cornea) and conjunctivitis may occur throughout the UV region, but especially in the UVB and UVC ranges, with a threshold of about 30 J m^{-2}. 'Snow-blindness' (from the strong, scattered blue and UV radiation) and 'welder's flash' are typical instances. For exposures just above the threshold, the effects appear some hours after the exposure with the symptoms perhaps persisting for only a few days. Fortunately the outermost epithelial cells of the cornea are constantly renewed on a time scale of a day or two, but deeper damage takes longer to be repaired. Effects of this type are characterized by a dose, essentially the exposure level multiplied by the exposure time. However, there is usually some lower threshold for the effect and, at low levels of exposure, repair can keep pace. For direct sunlight (but not necessarily for industrial sources of UV) the cornea is reasonably protected by the recessed position of the eye and the glancing incidence of the radiation. Little UV radiation reaches the retina because of absorption in the anterior part of the eye. For those persons (aphakes) who have had a lens removed (and for children), there can be a retinal hazard from UVA radiation.

The skin

Thermal skin burn is possible throughout the IR and much of the visible regions at high irradiances. UVA photosensitive reactions may occur in some individuals when certain chemicals (e.g. in cosmetics or therapeutic agents) either have been applied to the skin or have been ingested and subsequently transported sufficiently close to the skin surface to be able to absorb the incident radiation. Some pigment darkening may result from exposure at the shorter-wavelength end of the visible region and in the UVA region. Increased pigmentation ('tanning') — the production of extra melanin and the migration of melanin from deeper to shallower layers in the skin — occurs primarily as a result of UVB exposure. Much of the ageing of skin — the drying, coarsening and wrinkling — is now attributed to the effect of chronic exposure to sunlight, principally the UV fraction. Sunburn is however, the most obvious result of excessive exposure to UV radiation, the UVB component being mainly responsible. A complex set of photochemical and biochemical reactions produce the initial reddening (erythema), usually accompanied by some tanning.

The most serious long-term consequence attributed to UV exposure is an increase in skin cancers. It is now generally accepted that solar UV radiation is a causal agent in the production of human non-melanoma skin cancers. For the less common, but more serious, malignant melanomas, epidemiological evidence indicates that high levels of exposure to solar UV, particularly at an early age, may be a contributory factor.

Standards

For IR and visible radiation there are as yet no internationally agreed standards for exposure from non-laser sources. The American Conference of Governmental Industrial Hygienists (ACGIH) does, however, include recommended guidelines in its annual booklet of threshold limit values and these now extend to the IRB as well as the IRA and visible regions (American Conference of Governmental Industrial Hygienists, 1994). Avoidance of thermal injury to the eye and photochemical injury to the retina form the basis of these guidelines.

For UV radiation, the former INIRC (now the ICNIRP) has published comprehensive guidelines, similar to those of the ACGIH. The principal restrictions given by the INIRC are: (1) the effective radiant exposure on unprotected skin for all UV wavelengths and on unprotected eyes for UVB and UVC should not exceed 30 J m^{-2} within an 8 h period; and (2) the total incident radiant exposure for UVA on unprotected eyes should not exceed

$10^4 \mathrm{J\,m^{-2}}$ within an 8 h period. When examined in detail, these various guidelines are necessarily complex because they have to take account of the different biological effects within this part of the spectrum and the often marked dependence of each effect on the wavelength of the radiation (Fig. 13.8).

Control

The general rule 'engineering controls first, administrative controls and special working procedures next, and personal protective equipment last' applies to exposure to optical radiation for which the major concern is the protection of the skin and eyes.

Emission may be controlled by using enclosures, screens and, for UV especially, appropriate absorbing glass or plastic. Some modern light sources, such as tungsten-halogen lamps, need additional filters if they are used near the body. If reflective screens are used, care must be taken to ensure that the problem is not just moved to another place. In general, at distances comparable with the size of the source, the irradiance is inversely proportional to the distance from the source, while with increasing distance there is a gradual change to an inverse

square law. Exposure can often be reduced substantially, simply by being further away from the source. For retinal injury, however, this is not necessarily so because of the focusing action of the eye. Outdoors, appropriate sunglasses, hats, clothing and shading should be used if prolonged exposure to sunlight is likely. Not all fabrics provide adequate shielding for UV, especially when wet.

For some tasks, personal protective equipment is essential, such as reflective clothing for extreme radiant heating, and goggles for use where there are intense unshielded light sources. Occasionally, the energy absorbed by the glass in the goggles may raise their temperature sufficiently to radiate longer-wavelength heat directly to the cornea. An outer reflective coating can be advantageous in these circumstances. Helmets with simple filter windows have long been used when arc welding or plasma spraying. Now, improved designs with auto-darkening filters are available which allow the welder still to see the work immediately prior to striking the arc. Their use also removes the necessity for constantly raising and lowering the helmet. Detailed standards for these are still being developed and it is necessary to ensure that the darkening speed is fast enough for the work being done. Switching times as short as $100\,\mu s$ are possible.

Measurements

Because the biological effects of optical radiation depend greatly on the wavelength, the complete assessment of a source or a location may require the use of quite sophisticated spectroradiometers to obtain the irradiance as a function of the wavelength. In many situations simpler equipment can be used, either in conjunction with filters to separate the spectral regions, or directly if its response is tailored to match the appropriate 'action spectrum' or biological spectral response factors. The angular response of the instrument can also be an important feature. Instruments which effectively integrate the received radiation over a period of time are useful in providing a measure of dose for those conditions where this is a suitable quantity, for instance when assessing the likelihood of erythema from a UV source. The simplest of these is like a film badge and incorporates a polysulphone film to

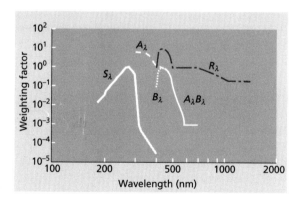

Fig. 13.8 To take account of the sharply varying biological effectiveness of optical radiation with wavelength, especially for broadband sources, various spectral weighting factors are used. S_λ is the relative spectral effectiveness of UV radiation for both the eye and the skin; R_λ is the retinal thermal hazard function; B_λ is the blue-light hazard function (for retinal photochemical injury) and A_λ is the aphakic hazard function (i.e. B_λ adjusted for persons who have had a lens removed).

indicate UV dose through a change in coloration, though its spectral response does not accurately match the erythemal action spectrum. Being worn, though, means that better account is taken of the person's movements with respect to the source which, through self-shielding for example, may influence the effective dose.

For the longer IR wavelengths, measuring devices are normally 'thermal', in that they rely on the absorption of the incident energy increasing the temperature of the sensing element. This in turn may be detected electrically to produce a signal proportional to the incident radiation power. Such instruments are inherently broadband and tend to be slower in response and not particularly sensitive. 'Photonic' detectors — semiconductor photodiodes or photomultipliers for example — respond to the photons of the incident radiation and can be very sensitive and fast but with narrower bandwidths.

LASERS

Optical radiation usually consists of a large number of photons emitted spontaneously, and hence randomly in time, by the atoms or molecules in the source. The essence of laser action is the stimulation of the atoms or molecules so that the individual photons are emitted in phase with each other. The radiation oscillations are then to a great

extent coherent in time and in space (i.e. both along and across the beam). The result is that the radiation has a very specific wavelength. Lasers are now available in most parts of the optical spectrum (Table 13.4). LASER is an acronym for Light Amplification by Stimulated Emission of Radiation. In fact, most lasers act as oscillators — amplifiers with internal positive feedback — but 'losers' is hardly an appealing label.

A laser has three basic components: the 'lasing' medium, a 'pump' and an optical cavity. The medium contains particular atoms or molecules which have a set of internal energy levels such that many of the atoms or molecules can be pumped up to a higher, metastable level and then stimulated to emit energy by returning to a lower level. The medium may be a gas (e.g. a mixture of helium and neon), a liquid (e.g. ethanol containing rhodamine 6G dye) or a solid (e.g. gallium arsenide or yttrium aluminium garnet containing neodymium). The pump is the initial source of the energy and may be optical (e.g. a flash tube), electrical (e.g. a current through the medium) or chemical (a chemical reaction leaving the lasing molecules in the higher energy state). The optical cavity, which resonates at the wavelength to be produced, is usually formed by placing a mirror at each end of the medium. The radiation then travels back and forth many times, being amplified as it does so. One of the mirrors is

Table 13.4 A summary of commonly used lasers and examples of their applications

Laser	Emission (nm)	Applications
Excimer	193–351	Laser surgery, material processing
Helium-cadmium	325, 442	Alignment, surveying
Dye lasers	350–1000	Instruments, dermatology
Argon ion	350, 458–514.5	Holography, retinal surgery, displays
Krypton ion	568, 647	Instruments, displays
Helium-neon	632.8	Alignment, surveying, holography
Ruby	694.3	Ranging, dermatology
Gallium arsenide	850–950	Optical fibre communications, ranging
Neodymium glass/YAG	1060	Material processing, radar/ranging, surgery
Carbon dioxide	10 600	Material processing, radar/ranging, surgery

only partially reflecting, thus allowing part of the energy to emerge in a well-collimated beam. This last feature means that lasers have a high brightness or radiance. Some lasers operate as continuous wave (CW) sources, others are pulsed — some producing extremely short pulses of very high peak power.

Uses

In about 30 years, lasers have progressed from invention to widespread application in industry, business, commerce, construction, transport, medicine, research and the home, as well as by the military. Each of these exploits one or more of the key features of lasers: narrow, almost parallel beams; narrow wavelength spread; coherence and high powers and power densities. Some of the references at the end of this chapter contain more details.

Hazards

Some lasers are potentially very hazardous because of their high radiance (brightness) and the high energies which they can deliver to the body, particularly the eye, and also because of their long range. The coherence and narrow band properties, except in so far as they contribute to the narrow beams, do not pose any new hazard. Outside the visible region, though, the absence of any associated broadband and partly visible radiation means that the laser may be more easily overlooked. Inadvertent reflections must also be avoided, otherwise the beam may be redirected into what would have been a safe zone.

All the biological interactions of optical radiation described previously apply to laser radiation, with the obvious proviso that damage from absorption may be more severe because of extreme localization and high-energy densities. Absorption of intense, short pulses can generate thermoacoustic pressure transients which may lead to ablation of tissue. At extremely high intensities (usually only met in sub-nanosecond pulses) the electric field of the optical radiation can interact directly with cells and molecules and cause their disruption, even in transparent material.

Classification

The hazards of lasers were recognized early and, over the years, a classification system has been developed which greatly contributes to their safe use and to reducing the effort that might otherwise be needed on the part of those responsible for safety where the laser is operated. Most users will not need to make exposure measurements and can concentrate on establishing safe working practices appropriate to the classification of the laser being used. The hazard classification scheme (IEC 825−1 (International Electrotechnical Commission, 1993) and EN 60825−1 (European Committee for Electrotechnical Standardization, 1994)) is akin to an emission standard and takes account of the capabilities of the laser itself and also the protective features provided — the extent to which the radiation is confined within the installation for instance. Manufacturers must determine the class to which a particular laser belongs, label it accordingly and provide the necessary user information. The classes may be summarized as shown below.

Class 1 lasers are those that are inherently safe because of their low power or are safe by virtue of the protective features incorporated into the design of the product.

Class 2 lasers are low-power devices that emit visible radiation; they are not intrinsically safe but eye protection is normally afforded by aversion responses including the blink reflex. They are not capable of causing injury to the skin.

Class 3A lasers emit higher levels of radiation. They differ from class 2 products in that they emit a higher power but in a beam of larger cross-section, so that when the output is viewed directly, the power of the beam entering the eye does not exceed that of a class 2 product. If the beam is viewed with an optical aid (e.g. a binocular telescope) then the hazard is increased. Hence, more stringent precautions are required.

Class 3B lasers are capable of causing eye injury either because their output is invisible and therefore aversion responses are not activated or because the beam power is such that damage is done in a time shorter than the blink reflex ($\sim 0.25\,\text{s}$). Higher-power lasers in this class may also cause skin burns but, for lasers other than those which emit UV radiation, it would be usual to expect that sufficient discomfort would arise from skin exposure to cause withdrawal of the exposed skin.

Class 4 is the most hazardous laser classification. Laser products in this class are high-power devices capable of causing an immediate injury to the eyes and skin. Exposure to diffuse reflections even may be hazardous.

Figure 13.9 shows these classes for continuous-wave lasers. Variations in the detail of this scheme may be found in some national recommendations.

Standards

Standards defining limits of exposure to laser radiation are complex, and consequently some-times difficult to interpret. This is because of the wide range of biological interactions possible, their dependence on wavelength, energy, power, pulse duration, beam geometry and so on. Standards or guidelines have been drawn up by various international (viz IEC (International Electrotechnical Commission)/CENELEC, IRPA/INIRC) and national bodies.

Controls

In addition to ensuring that a laser is properly classified and that any associated requirements are met, it is advisable to consider several other matters as follows, depending on the classification.

For class 2: the positioning and mounting of the laser from the point of view of the likelihood of the beam reaching a person's eye; the absorption of the beam at the end of its useful path; the provision of suitable warning signs.

For class 3A: the prevention of direct viewing of the beam with optical instruments; the training and approval of operators; and as for class 2 above.

For classes 3B and 4: control of access to the area in which the laser is operated (special consideration needs to be given to outdoor use); the removal of specularly reflecting surfaces from near the beam path; the appointment of a Laser Safety Officer; and as for classes 2 and 3A above.

In some cases, personal protective equipment (special clothing and eyewear) may be required. If eyewear has to be used, it is important to ensure that it is acceptable and always used, that it does not impair normal visibility seriously and that it is adequate for the power and wavelength of the radiation in question.

There are some secondary potential hazards associated with lasers (particularly high-power devices) which should be borne in mind, such as fumes and flying debris from the target, electric shock from power supplies, possible explosions in

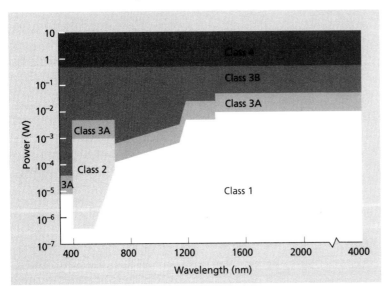

Fig. 13.9 There is a well-established classification system for lasers based on the hazards which their use may entail. The details are complex but a simplified presentation for continuous-wave lasers is shown here in terms of the accessible power emission limits and the wavelength. From International Electrotechnical Commission (1993) and European Committee for Electrotechnical Standardization (1994).

capacitor banks, and the toxic chemicals used in some lasers.

Measurements

The measurement of laser radiation is not easy because of the wide range of conditions met and there are many possible sources of error. It is recommended that some of the references listed below are consulted. The general types of instrument needed have been outlined above but, in addition, special techniques are required to resolve the time course of the nanosecond and sub-nanosecond pulses which some lasers produce.

REFERENCES

American Conference of Governmental Industrial Hygienists (1994). *Threshold Limit Values and Biological Exposure Indices.* ACGIH, Cincinnati.

European Committee for Electrotechnical Standardization (1994). *Safety of Laser Products, Equipment Classification, Requirements and User's Guide.* EN 60825-1: 1994. CENELEC, Brussels.

International Electrotechnical Commission (1993). *Safety of Laser Products, Equipment Classification, Requirements and User's Guide.* IEC 825-1: 1993. IEC, Geneva.

FURTHER READING

Advisory Group on Non-ionising Radiation (1994). Health effects related to the use of visual display units. *Documents of the NRPB*, **5**,(2), 1-75.

Duchêne, A.S., Lakey, J.R.A. and Repacholi, M.H. (ed.) (1991). *IRPA Guidelines on Protection against Non-ionizing Radiation.* Pergamon Press/McGraw Hill, New York.

European Committee for Electrotechnical Standardization (1995). *Human Exposure to Electromagnetic Fields, Low Frequency (0 Hz-10 kHz).* ENV 50166-1: 1995. CENELEC, Brussels.

European Committee for Electrotechnical Standardization (1995). *Human Exposure to Electromagnetic Fields, High Frequency (10 kHz-300 GHz).* ENV 50166-2: 1995. CENELEC, Brussels.

Green, M.W. (ed.) (1992). *Non-ionizing Radiation.* IRPA, Vancouver.

International Non-ionizing Radiation Committee in collaboration with The International Labour Office (1993). *The Use of Lasers in the Workplace.* Occupational Safety and Health Series No. 68. International Labour Office, Geneva.

McKinlay, A.F., Harlen, F. and Whillock, M.J. (1988). *Hazards of Optical Radiation. A Guide to Sources, Uses and Safety.* Adam Hilger, Bristol and Philadelphia.

National Radiological Protection Board (1993). Restrictions on human exposure to static and time varying electromagnetic fields and radiation. *Documents of the NRPB* **4**(5), 1-69.

Repacholi, M.H. (ed.) (1988). *Non-ionizing Radiations: Physical Characteristics, Biological Effects and Health Hazard Assessment.* IRPA, Melbourne.

Sliney, D. and Wolbarsht, M. (1980). *Safety with Lasers and Other Optical Sources. A Comprehensive Handbook.* Plenum, New York and London.

Suess, M.J. and Benwell-Morison, D.A. (ed.) (1989). *Non-ionizing Radiation Protection.* WHO Regional Publications, European Series, No. 25. Copenhagen.

World Health Organization (1979). *Environmental Health Criteria 14: Ultraviolet Radiation.* WHO, Geneva.

World Health Organization (1982). *Environmental Health Criteria 23: Lasers and Optical Radiation.* WHO, Geneva.

World Health Organization (1984). *Environmental Health Criteria 35: Extremely Low Frequency (ELF) Fields.* WHO, Geneva.

World Health Organization (1987). *Environmental Health Criteria 69: Magnetic Fields.* WHO, Geneva.

World Health Organization (1993). *Environmental Health Criteria 137: Electromagnetic Fields (300 Hz to 300 GHz).* WHO, Geneva.

CHAPTER 14

Ionizing Radiation: Physics, Measurement, Biological Effects and Control

R.F. Clayton

INTRODUCTION

'Ionising', or the alternative spelling 'ionizing', radiation can be defined as radiant energy which, either directly or indirectly, produces ionization of the matter through which it passes. It is encountered both as part of the electromagnetic spectrum and as particulate matter. The term 'radiation' correctly applies to all forms of radiant energy: radio waves, heat, light, sound, etc. However, as this chapter is concerned only with ionizing radiation, for simplicity it will be referred to as 'radiation'. Since the advent of nuclear weapons, nuclear energy and irradiation of foodstuffs by gamma rays, 'radiation' has become an emotive word with the general public, being associated with all the undesirable effects of ionizing radiations. There is also widespread confusion between what is meant by the terms 'radioactive' and 'radiation'. 'Radioactive' is the name given to the property of a substance which undergoes spontaneous disintegration and emits 'radiation' during the process of disintegration. Ionizing radiations include:

- X-rays generated by electrical devices;
- X-rays and gamma rays emitted by radioactive material;
- alpha and beta particles emitted by radioactive material;
- neutrons generated during nuclear fission and fusion processes;
- high-energy particles produced in accelerators.

Although much ionizing radiation is artificially produced, by far the greater proportion of the exposure of the general public is to naturally occurring radiations from radioactive materials in the Earth's crust, radioactive gases in the atmosphere and cosmic radiation from outer space.

To understand the production of radiation from radioactive material requires an elementary knowledge of atomic structure and the phenomenon of radioactivity. This concept will be explained in the next section.

SOURCES OF IONIZING RADIATION

X-rays

X-rays were discovered in 1895 by Dr Röntgen who showed that they penetrated matter opaque to visible light and that they ionized air, enabling it to conduct electricity. They are part of the electromagnetic spectrum, having a shorter wavelength than visible light and ultraviolet radiation. Most X-rays are produced in apparatus specifically designed for that purpose, such as medical and industrial X-ray sets. They may also be produced in any electrical apparatus in which there is a heated cathode emitting electrons and a potential difference of a few thousand volts accelerating the electrons so that they bombard an anode. Most of the energy of the electrons absorbed in the anode appears as heat and a small proportion as X-rays. The energy of these X-rays lies between 60% and 70% of the accelerating voltage used in the apparatus. Thus, in an apparatus with an accelerating voltage of 50 kV (kilovolts), the X-ray energy will lie in the range 30–35 keV (kiloelectronvolts). Examples of such devices are: cathode-ray tubes (TV tubes), radio valves, valve rectifiers, electron beam welders, electron microscopes, mass spectrometers, gyrotrons and all types of accelerators. With few exceptions, any apparatus which has an accelerating potential in excess of 5 kV may be considered as having the potential to give rise to an ionizing radiation hazard.

Some X-rays may be emitted during the disintegration of radioactive material or when beta particles emitted by radioactive material are stopped in some absorbing material. These latter are a special case and will be defined later in the chapter.

Atomic structure

As stated in the introduction, a simple explanation of the structure of the atom and nuclear disintegration is necessary to understand the phenomenon of radioactivity and the production of ionizing radiations from this source. An atom may be considered to consist of a nucleus, which carries a positive electric charge of the order of 5×10^{18} coulombs per cubic centimetre $(C\,cm^{-3})$, surrounded by negatively charged orbiting electrons, rather like a miniature solar system, with a sun (the nucleus) and orbiting planets (the electrons). The electrons are held in discrete orbital shells, each having its own energy level. The orbital shells are identified by letters, the innermost shell being called the 'K' shell, the next the 'L' shell, and so on. The nucleus is made up of densely packed, positively charged protons and neutrons which do not carry any electrical charge. It is very small, having a radius of about 10^{-12} cm, compared to the radii of atoms which are about 10^{-8} cm. As the nucleus contains virtually all the mass of the atom, it must have a very high density of about $10^{14}\,g\,cm^{-3}$. In an atom in its normal state, the number of orbiting electrons equals the number of nuclear protons so that the atom as a whole appears uncharged.

The neutron has the additional property of being capable of dividing into a positively charged proton and a negatively charged electron. This electron should not be confused with the orbital electrons, although they are physically similar. Other properties of the nuclear particles are summarized in Table 14.1.

The number of protons in the nucleus of a particular atom determines its atomic number (Z) and

Table 14.1 Properties of the nuclear particles

Particle	Relative mass	Electrical charge
Proton	Approximately 1	Positive (+1)
Neutron	Approximately 1	Uncharged (0)
Electron	Approximately $\dfrac{1}{1840}$	Negative (−)

thus determines the element and its chemical nature. Examples are:

$Z = 1 =$ hydrogen (H),
$Z = 3 =$ helium (He),
$Z = 24 =$ chromium (Cr).

The number of neutrons (N) in a nucleus is about the same as the number of protons (Z) in the case of the lighter elements (carbon-12, $Z = 6$, $N = 6$; cobalt-59, $Z = 27$, $N = 32$), but somewhat greater in the case of the heavier elements such as uranium. There may be up to about 50 extra neutrons in the heaviest nuclei (uranium-238, $Z = 92$, $N = 146$; $N - Z = 54$). The number of neutrons can vary slightly between the atoms of the same element; the sum of the number of neutrons and protons in a nucleus determines the atomic weight of the element A; (thus $Z + N = A$). The precise number of neutrons in a particular atom of an element also determines the isotope of the element or which nuclide is the nucleus. These isotopes or nuclides are not always radioactive; for example oxygen isotopes with the atomic weights of 16, 17 and 18 are not radioactive, but oxygen-19 is. The Z number of an element is indicated by a subscript in front of the chemical symbol (thus $_1$H) and the atomic weight of the element by a superscript also in front of the chemical symbol (thus ^{1}H). The two combined showing both the Z and A numbers are written thus: $_1^1$H. In reports and correspondence, instead of using the scientific representation as shown in the previous sentence, it is usual and acceptable to use the form cobalt-60, or carbon-14. A pseudo-scientific method is to use the chemical symbol and the isotope number, for example Co-60 or C-14.

Radioactivity

Radioactivity was discovered in the late nineteenth century by the Curies and other workers. Radioactivity may be defined as the property possessed by some atomic nuclei of disintegrating spontaneously, with the loss of energy through the emission of a charged particle such as an alpha or beta particle and electromagnetic radiation such as gamma and/or X-rays. For legislative purposes such as the Radioactive Substances Act 1993 and the Ionising Radiations Regulations 1985, radioactivity may be defined more narrowly. Radioactivity occurs when there is an imbalance of energy in the nucleus. This is usually due to a disparate proton to neutron ratio for the particular nuclide and the mass/energy relationship among the parent nucleus, the daughter nucleus and the emitted particle which gives rise to divergent atomic packing fractions and nuclear binding energies. Virtually all nuclides with an atomic number greater than 83 are radioactive.

Radioactive decay is a random process. Therefore a radioactive nucleus is likely to decay at any time, however long it has existed. The probability of disintegration is not affected by external factors such as temperature, pressure, its state of chemical combination, etc. The probability per unit time of a nucleus decaying is called the 'decay constant' and is represented by the symbol λ. It varies enormously from one radionuclide to another. The decay constant has the dimensions of 1/time and is usually expressed in s^{-1}. To establish the basic formula for radioactive decay it is assumed that at a given time there are N radioactive nuclei present and that the average number decaying per second is λN. Hence:

$$\frac{dN}{dt} = -\lambda N \qquad (14.1)$$

from which the basic formula for radioactive decay is derived:

$$N = N_0\, e^{-\lambda t} \qquad (14.2)$$

where N_0 is the number of atoms present when $t = 0$.

The mean life of the nuclei of a certain nuclide can be represented by the formula $\tau = 1/\lambda$. However, it is more usual to express the rate of radioactive decay in terms of the half-life (T). This is the time elapsing before half of the original radioactive nuclei have decayed. It can be derived from the formula $N = N_0\, e^{-\lambda t}$ by putting:

$$\frac{N}{N_0} = \frac{1}{2} = e^{-\lambda T}$$

therefore $\ln 2 = \lambda T$, and

$$T = \frac{\ln 2}{\lambda} = \frac{0.693}{\lambda} = 0.693\tau \qquad (14.3)$$

thus the mean life of the nuclei is 1/0.693 or 1.443 times as long as the half-life of the radionuclide.

TYPES OF IONIZING RADIATION DUE TO RADIOACTIVITY

The three basic types of ionizing radiations emitted by radioactive material are: the alpha particle (α); the beta particle (β); and the gamma ray (γ). Each radioactive nuclide emits one or more of these radiations and each has an energy characteristic of the decaying nuclide. An alpha particle is composed of two protons and two neutrons, and therefore is the nucleus of a helium atom. A beta particle is essentially an electron, usually carrying a negative charge, but occasionally it may carry a positive charge and is then called a 'positron'. A positron is defined as the antiparticle of the electron and is the only antiparticle currently considered to have any significance in radiation protection or nuclear power.

Some radioactive materials may emit neutrons and some will emit X-rays. The latter are more likely to be emitted from the orbital electron shells rather than from the atomic nucleus. This occurs when an electron from the inner shell of 'K' electrons is captured by the nucleus. The excess energy arising from the loss of the electron into the nucleus appears as X-ray emissions. This form of radioactive decay is known conventionally as 'K capture'.

Neutrons are emitted from some of the heavier atoms, such as plutonium, due to spontaneous fission of the atom. Specially prepared material, such as americium/beryllium alloys in which the alpha particle emitted by the americium displaces a neutron from the beryllium atom, are available as discrete neutron sources.

Of all five types of radiation, only alpha and beta particles are directly ionizing since they carry an electrical charge. The other types of radiation do not carry an electrical charge and produce ionization by their interaction with the target material.

The energy of all types of radiation is measured in electronvolts (eV) but this being such a small quantity, the energy is more usually expressed in kiloelectronvolts (keV) or megaelectronvolts (MeV).

Alpha radiation

Alpha radiation is emitted mainly by radioisotopes of the heavy elements such as thorium, radium, uranium and plutonium. Alpha radiation, from whatever source, consists of heavy, doubly charged particles and results in the original element being transformed into an element which is two atomic numbers (Z) lower and four atomic mass numbers (A) lower. For example, plutonium-239 ($Z = 94$, $A = 239$) emits an alpha particle and is transformed into uranium-235 ($Z = 92$, $A = 235$).

The alpha particle from each radioisotope has its own characteristic energy or energies. In most cases, all such emission is at one discrete energy, but in some cases two or even three energy levels are detected. For example, the alpha particles from uranium-235 have energies of 4.18 MeV and 4.56 MeV, whereas the alpha particles from uranium-238 have only one energy level at 4.2 MeV. Most alpha-emitting elements also emit either an X-ray or gamma ray as an energy-adjusting mechanism when the newly formed atom settles from an excited state to a ground state.

Beta radiation

Beta radiation is emitted mainly by radioisotopes of the intermediate and lighter atomic weight elements, although some isotopes of the heavier elements also emit beta particles. Examples of the latter are plutonium-241, uranium-237 and some of the radioactive daughters in the decay chain of the naturally occurring radioactive elements radium and thorium. A beta particle is essentially an electron, but originates from the transformation of a neutron in the nucleus into a proton and an electron and has a mass of 1/1840 of a proton. They are not to be confused with the orbital electrons. The beta particle is usually represented by the symbol β, but sometimes by either β^+ or β^-. The latter two symbols are to differentiate the more common, negatively charged particle from the less

common, positively charged particle (positron). The β^- is produced when there is a neutron excess in the originating nucleus and the β^+ when there is a neutron deficiency. Beta radiation, from whatever isotope, consists of light, singly charged particles. In the case of negative beta radiation, the original element is transformed into an element with a numerically one higher Z number but with the same A number. For example, cobalt-60 ($Z = 27$, $A = 60$) emits a β^- and is transformed into nickel-60 ($Z = 28$, $A = 60$). In the case of an element which emits a positively charged beta particle, the original element is transformed into one with a lower Z number but with the same A number. For example, when zinc-63 ($Z = 30$, $A = 63$) emits a positron (β^+) it is transformed into copper-63 ($Z = 29$, $A = 63$). Beta radiation from each beta emitter has its own spectrum of energies, not a discrete energy level as in the case of alpha particles. Each spectrum, however, has a characteristic maximum, for example yttrium-90 (the daughter of strontium-90) has a maximum at 2.27 MeV, whereas phosphorus-32 has a maximum at 1.71 MeV. Most beta emitters also emit an energy-compensating gamma or X-ray.

Gamma radiation

Gamma radiation, which is part of the electromagnetic spectrum, is emitted as an accompaniment to most alpha and beta emissions; there are no 'gamma only' emitters. Gamma radiation, not being particulate and not carrying an electrical charge, does not ionize other matter directly. It only does so by its interaction with the molecular or atomic structure of the irradiated material. Its emission from a radioactive substance does not bring about any transformation in the emitting element. It occurs when the excess energy present in an atom following its transformation is released, when it settles from the excited state following the transformation into its ground state. For example, when cobalt-60 decays to nickel-60, the two gamma rays having energies of 1.33 MeV and 1.17 MeV normally used to identify the presence of cobalt-60 are in fact emitted by the daughter nickel-60 atom settling to its ground state.

X-radiation

X-radiation is similar to gamma radiation but is less penetrating and has a longer wavelength. It is produced in radioactive material as a result of the release of excess energy when a daughter atom settles to its ground state. It may also be released when there is a disruption in the orbital shells, such as when a 'K' shell electron is captured by the nucleus or when an electron falls from a higher-energy shell to a lower-energy shell.

Bremsstrahlung radiation

When beta particles are attenuated in matter, some of the energy appears as X-radiation which in this case is termed 'bremsstrahlung' ('braking radiation', from the German 'bremsen', to brake or slow down and 'strahlung', radiation). Generally, bombardment of a material by X-rays or gamma rays does not result in the irradiated material becoming radioactive. When the energy of the radiation is in excess of about 6 MeV, then some activation may occur depending on the nature of the material being irradiated.

Neutron radiation

Neutron radiation is emitted from some fissile material when it undergoes spontaneous fission resulting in the formation of fission products which are usually radioactive and a release of energy which may appear as heat, X-rays, gamma rays and beta rays. Examples of elements undergoing significant spontaneous fission are californium-252,
plutonium-240 and curium-244. Other transuranic elements undergo spontaneous fission to a lesser degree. Neutrons are also emitted from radioactive sources specifically manufactured for this purpose, such as americium-241 alloyed with beryllium. Neutrons are also produced in nuclear reactors, some accelerators and nuclear fusion experiments.

Although not directly ionizing, they do bring about ionization by their interaction with matter. More importantly they make the irradiated material radioactive, thereby producing an extra source of ionization due to the radioactive decay of the isotopes produced.

PROPERTIES OF IONIZING RADIATION

Alpha and beta particles, because they are particulate and carry an electric charge, interact both mechanically and electrically with the atoms of the materials irradiated by them. Because they progressively lose their energy they have a finite range. Table 14.2 summarizes the properties of the various types of radiation discussed in this section.

Alpha radiation

An alpha particle has approximately 7360 times the mass of a beta particle (electron), twice the electric charge and travels more slowly. Therefore it loses its energy much more quickly and thus deposits all its energy over a very short path. It has a range of only a few centimetres in air at STP (standard temperature and pressure) and only a few micrometres in tissue. The short range and low

Table 14.2 Properties of types of ionizing radiation

Type of radiation	Nature and symbol	Relative mass	Electrical charge	Approximate energy range	Approximate maximum range in air (at STP)
Alpha	α particulate	4	+2	2 to 8 MeV	Few centimetres
Beta	β particulate	$\frac{1}{1840}$	−1 or +1	keV to 5 MeV	Few metres
Gamma	γ electromagnetic	0	0	keV to 7 MeV	Very long range
X-rays	X electromagnetic	0	0	keV up to 20 MeV	Very long range
Neutrons	n particulate	0	0	eV to 20 MeV	Long range

penetrating power of an alpha particle mean that it is difficult to detect, can be shielded completely by very thin material such as paper and does not penetrate the dead, outer layers of the human skin. These properties mean that alpha particles originating from a source outside the human body do not present any radiological hazard. Because they deposit all their energy over a very short range in tissue they are extremely hazardous when released from radioactive material deposited inside the body.

Beta radiation

Beta radiation is more penetrating than alpha radiation and has a longer range in air (the range depending on the energy of the particle). The energy of beta particles varies enormously, from about 18 keV in the case of beta radiation from tritium (hydrogen-3) to about 3.6 MeV in the case of potassium-42. The energies of beta emissions from some fission products are even higher. Despite the high maximum energy of some beta particles, they can be efficiently shielded by relatively light materials such as 'Perspex', aluminium and glass. Because their path in tissue is much longer than that of an alpha particle and therefore they do not deposit so much energy per unit length in the absorbing material, they do not represent such a great hazard as an alpha particle when released from radioactive material deposited inside the body. The hazard however is not insignificant.

A danger which must be guarded against when designing shielding for beta radiation is the production of bremsstrahlung X-rays in the material used for shielding. In the case of large beta sources with high energy maxima, such as tera-becqueral (TBq), peta-becquerel (PBq) and strontium-90/yttrium-90 sources, substantial thicknesses of heavy shielding may be required to attenuate the bremsstrahlung X-rays.

Gamma radiation and X-radiation

Both gamma and X-radiation are electromagnetic radiation and have short wavelengths. Being uncharged they are not deflected by magnetic fields and as a result have long ranges in air. They are very penetrating and will pass through the body, irradiating all internal organs in their path. Heavy shielding is required to attenuate them, often up to several centimetres of lead or a few metres of concrete.

Neutron radiation

Because they are uncharged, neutrons cannot be deflected by magnetic fields, but their energy is dissipated when they undergo collisions with the atoms of the irradiated material which then becomes radioactive. Because of the manner in which they interact with matter, they may deposit their energy in the target material over a relatively short distance and can produce significant doses of ionizing radiation. This is due first to their immediate atomic interactions in which they may produce electrons and heavy particles and then to radiation from the radioactive material produced in the target. Because they interact with targets and make them radioactive, storage and transport containers for neutron sources will become radioactive.

RADIOLOGICAL PROTECTION TERMINOLOGY

In addition to knowing the terms for describing the properties of radiation and radioactivity, persons working with ionizing radiation should become familiar with the various terms used in the field of radiological protection.

External radiation   The term used to identify radiation arising from sources outside the body, whereas the term *internal radiation* is applied to sources of radiation deposited inside the body. X-ray sets can produce only external radiation hazards, even though the effects of the exposure effects to the radiation are on the internal organs of the body. Radioactive material produces external radiation when it is outside the body, but internal radiation if any is deposited inside the body as a result of an accident (for example, where radioactive material is breathed in and deposited in the lungs).

Sealed sources or *closed sources*   Sources which remain intact under all circumstances, whether in routine use or during emergency situations.

They may be radioactive material sealed in some form of encapsulation or may be non-friable solid radioactive material. Before being defined as a sealed or closed source, they have to satisfy certain strict criteria such as not breaking under pressure or when dropped or when subjected to high temperatures. They must not show any sign of leaching or leakage when immersed in water for extended periods.

Unsealed sources or *open sources*   Sources which are in a form capable of giving rise to radioactive contamination on or in any other material with which they come into contact. They include any source which does not satisfy the rigid criteria required of sealed or closed sources. They include powders, dusts, solutions, liquids, gases, vapours, friable solids or solids from which the surface such as an oxide layer can be removed easily.

Radioactive contamination   This is normally thought of as unwanted radioactive substances on surfaces or in the air in the workplace. Contamination is also present if the wrong material is present in an operating zone, such as a glove box or fume cupboard. X-rays, gamma rays or a sealed source in contact with a surface will not give rise to contamination. Neutron sources and very high-energy X-rays will make materials exposed to them radioactive, which is a different matter altogether from becoming contaminated.

MEASUREMENT

The relevant authority for advising on the use of units in radioactivity and radiation measurement and in the field of radiological protection is the International Commission on Radiation Units and Measurements (ICRU). In 1975 the ICRU advised that the International System of units formulated in 1960 (SI units) should be used throughout the field of radiological protection, radioactivity and radiation measurements. Since 1975 it has been a statutory requirement in the UK for all radiation dose-rate meters to have their readings displayed in SI units. This requirement does not apply to contamination monitors or instruments such as installed alarm monitors, whose sole purpose is to detect the presence of ionizing radiations.

Although the use of the traditional units has been largely superseded, they are still occasionally encountered. Old radioactive sources may be labelled in the traditional units and the specifications of old X-ray sets may be written in the old units. Some knowledge of them may still be required for persons who may be engaged in the decommissioning or decontamination of old installations, disposing of old radioactive sources or dealing with old X-ray sets.

Units of radioactivity

Materials demonstrating radioactivity disintegrate at a certain rate per unit of time, usually per second (s^{-1}), which is the reciprocal of the SI unit of time. The special unit of radioactivity is the becquerel (Bq). The radioactivity of a material which is decaying at a rate of 1 disintegration per second $(1 s^{-1})$ is one becquerel (1 Bq). Because this is such a small quantity it is more usual to encounter amounts such as the kilobecquerel (kBq), the megabecquerel (MBq) or even higher values.

The traditional unit, the curie (Ci), was originally defined as the number of disintegrations per second (dps) associated with 1 g of radium-226 in equilibrium with its daughters. It was later defined as being that amount of radioactivity giving rise to 3.7×10^{10} dps. Fractions and multiples of the curie were used, e.g. the millicurie (mCi = 3.7×10^{7} dps) and the megacurie (MCi = 3.7×10^{16} dps). The becquerel is approximately equivalent to 2.703×10^{-11} of a curie; thus 1 MBq = 1 μCi and 1 mCi = 37 MBq.

Units of radiation dose

The derived SI unit for the measurement of radiation dose absorbed in any irradiated material has the dimensions of joules per kilogram and is called a gray (Gy). One gray dose is equivalent to the deposition of one joule per kilogram in the irradiated material:

$$1 \, Gy = 1 \, J \, kg^{-1} \qquad (14.4)$$

The special derived SI unit for describing the dose equivalent is the sievert (Sv) and is the absorbed dose in Gy multiplied by a quality factor (Q) to take account of the different degrees of harm likely to result from unit dose to tissue due to different types of radiation. The quality factor is dimensionless and therefore the dose equivalent still has the dimensions of joules per kilogram:

$$1\,Sv = 1\,Gy \times Q \qquad (14.5)$$

Multiples or fractions of the primary units are commonly used such as a millisievert (mSv) (1 mSv = 1/1000 of a sievert) or a microsievert (1 µSv = 1/1 000 000 of a sievert).

The traditional unit of the röntgen is now very rarely encountered except in the use of X-rays and in the specification of old X-ray tubes. Strictly it is a measure of X-ray exposure rather than absorbed dose. It is not applicable to any other type of radiation, except perhaps gamma radiation up to about 3.0 MeV. It was defined in terms of ionization produced in air at STP and was given the symbol R:

$$1\,R = 2.58 \times 10^{-4}\ \text{coulombs kg}^{-1}$$
$$= 87.7\ \text{ergs g}^{-1} \qquad (14.6)$$

Exposure to one röntgen resulted in an absorbed dose of 95 ergs g^{-1} of irradiated material.

The unit used for the measurement of absorbed dose was the rad, which are the initials of 'röntgen absorbed dose'. It is a measure of the absorbed dose, or deposited energy, in any material from any type of radiation and has the numerical equivalent of 100 ergs g^{-1}:

$$1\,\text{rad} = 100\,\text{ergs g}^{-1} \qquad (14.7)$$

To measure the effectiveness or harm of a radiation dose to human tissue, the unit used was the rem, the initials of 'rad equivalent man'. This is the absorbed does in rads multiplied by a quality factor. The quality factor here has the same function as that described earlier.

$$1\,\text{rem} = 1\,\text{rad} \times Q \qquad (14.8)$$

By applying the conversion factors for ergs to joules and grams to kilograms, it will be seen that 1 Gy = 100 rad.

Units of radiation dose rate

The above units are measures of accumulated dose and are the result of being exposed in a radiation field for a finite time. To be able to calculate a potential dose it is necessary to measure dose rate. This is measured in dose per unit time, usually per hour, for example microsievert per hour (µSv h^{-1}). Dose rates in the main beam of X-ray sets, for example, may be given in dose per minute or second (Sv min^{-1} or mSv s^{-1}).

INSTRUMENTATION

No one type of instrument can be used to detect or measure all types of radiation. It is necessary to make a distinction between those which detect radiation and require some interpretation of the readings and those which will read directly in dose rate or accumulated dose. Passive radiation detectors are the film badge and the thermoluminescent dosimeters which when processed will indicate accumulated dose.

Radiation detection or measuring instruments are all based on one of four types of detector which, with associated electronic circuitry, may be used to indicate count rate, dose rate or accumulated dose.
1 The ionization chamber.
2 The proportional counter.
3 The Geiger–Müller tube.
4 The scintillation counter.
The instruments may be either portable or installed in fixed positions. All the instruments depend on their response to ionization produced due to the interaction between ionizing radiation and matter. Alpha and beta radiation are detected by their direct ionizing properties so that the media in which they move becomes ionized and thus electrically conducting. X-rays and gamma rays produce electrons when they pass through matter and it is these electrons which are detected. Neutrons, when reacting with matter, produce a variety of charged particles, and again it is these which are detected. The detectors are connected to electronic circuitry to amplify their signal to enable it to be displayed as either an audible or visual response.

An ionization chamber consists of a volume of air enclosed in a vessel with two electrodes with a potential difference between them. The incident radiation ionizes the air and the ions formed are attracted to the electrodes. The current flowing is measured and can be converted to give a direct reading of the absorbed dose.

A *proportional counter* functions in a way similar to an ionization chamber but operates at a higher potential difference and is more sensitive. Because it operates at the higher voltage the ions produced are accelerated and cause further ionization: a phenomenon known as 'gas multiplication'.

A *Geiger–Müller tube*, more commonly known as a *Geiger counter*, operates at an even higher potential difference and as a result ions produced are accelerated to higher velocities and therefore it produces many more secondary ions than either the ionization chamber or the proportional counter. The current produced is no longer proportional to the dose because the enormous number of ions produced results in a relatively large pulse arriving at the electrode in comparison to that produced by the initial incident radiation.

Scintillation detectors rely on the ability of certain substances to re-emit, as light, energy they absorb from incident ionizing radiations. The emitted light is amplified by a photomultiplier before being fed into the electronic circuitry of the instrument and displayed as either a visual or audible signal. Scintillators may be either solid or liquid, the latter being used to detect very low-energy beta particles such as those emitted by tritium (hydrogen-3). Alpha radiation is difficult to detect because of its short range in air and in solid or liquid matter. Alpha detectors usually utilize a scintillation detector coupled with a photomultiplier. The window of the detector must be light tight to prevent spurious readings being obtained, but thin enough to allow the passage of alpha particles. The window is extremely fragile and therefore great care is required when using an alpha detector because even a minute hole in it destroying its light tightness will render the instrument inoperative. The scintillator also is very thin, usually being a coating of a substance, such as zinc sulphide, on a screen transparent to light. Because of the thinness of the scintillating material, it is not significantly affected by other radiations.

Scintillation detectors are used also to detect beta radiation, X-radiation and gamma radiation, but because these are more penetrating, the windows can be made of thicker material and consequently they are less fragile than those used in alpha particle detectors. They must still maintain light tightness.

A sophisticated type of instrument incorporating a scintillation detector and suitable electronic circuitry is used to distinguish between the energies of incident radiations.

Instruments using any one of the types of detectors described are available in various forms for a variety of uses. Those used essentially for external radiation assessment may be described as radiation meters, dose rate meters, rate meters, etc. Pocket sized instruments such as the quartz fibre electroscope based on a miniature ionization chamber or electronic instruments utilizing small Geiger–Müller tubes are available. The latter are now available in a variety of forms, ranging from those only giving warning of the presence of radiation to sophisticated types capable of giving dose rates, integrated doses and having pre-set alarm indication when selected dose rates or integrated doses are detected.

Some instruments are designed specifically for monitoring surfaces for radioactive contamination. It should be noted that there is no completely satisfactory instrument for monitoring directly for tritium contamination. The information from contamination monitors is usually displayed in counts per second. It is necessary to convert these readings into quantities of radioactive contamination per unit area. As the response of the instrument is dependent on the energy of the emissions from the contaminant, it is necessary to have some form of conversion table or graph. Most instrument suppliers provide this information in the manuals supplied with the instrument.

It is a statutory requirement that portable instruments are checked by a qualified person to ensure that they remain within specified calibration limits at least once in every 14 months and whenever they may have been repaired or been subject to treatment which may have resulted in damage to the instrument.

Film badges and thermoluminescent dosimeters are used primarily for monitoring cumulative radiation doses to personnel but they may also be installed to monitor accumulated doses in occupied and unoccupied areas. The recorded cumulative personal doses are to be held as the legally required dose records for radiation workers. The film badge when processed provides a visual record of the person's dose and by reason of various filters in the film badge holder can differentiate between beta radiation, gamma radiation, X-radiation and doses due to neutrons of thermal energies. It should be remembered that either of these dosimeters only records the dose to the dosimeter and therefore only to the part of the body on which it is worn. If it is suspected that extremities of the body may be exposed to short-range beta radiation then special extra dosimeters should be worn.

BIOLOGICAL EFFECTS OF RADIATION

The biological effects of ionizing radiations can be considered at varying biological levels: to the body as a whole, to individual cells of the body and even down to biological material such as the chromosomes and genes.

The effect on the body as a whole can be either acute, as in the case of very high doses being received in a short time, or long term. Short-term effects due to very high doses delivered in a short space of time (from seconds to hours) may give rise to: changes in the blood count, the number of some cells such as the leucocytes being reduced (at 0.25 Sv); sickness (at 1.0 Sv); failure of blood-forming organs (at 4.0 Sv); damage to the intestinal tract linings; and damage to the central nervous system (at 6.0–12.0 Sv). Any whole-body dose in excess of 6 Sv is almost certain to prove fatal. Visible effects to the skin are hair loss (4.0–5.0 Sv) and erythema of the skin to serious skin burns (from 6.0 to > 10.0 Sv). The long-term effects may result in the production of cancers, in either the blood (leukaemia), bone or soft tissue.

The effect on individual cells may be to cause the cell to die, it may slow down its speed of reproduction or it may cause damage to the genes or chromosomes in the cell. If the DNA (deoxyribonucleic acid) in the sex cells in either the male sperm or the female ova is damaged, then damage may be passed on to offspring.

Damage sustained by an irradiated individual is termed the 'somatic' effect and that passed on to descendants is called the 'hereditary' effect. 'Deterministic', or 'non-stochastic' effects as they were originally called, are those which will not occur until a certain threshold of dose is exceeded. 'Stochastic' effects are those for which there is a probability of them occurring, with no dose threshold apparent and an increasing probability of occurrence with increase in dose.

CONTROL

Legislative control

Within a decade or so of the discovery of radioactivity and radiation it became apparent that they presented a potential hazard to persons working with them and that some sort of control on exposure was required. National bodies eventually united to form an International X-ray and Radium Protection Committee in 1928, which eventually developed into the International Commission on Radiological Protection (ICRP). The ICRP has a number of technical committees advising on various aspects of radiological protection, their findings being published in the *Annals of the ICRP*. Their latest general recommendations, based on revised risk assessments calculated from the long-term effects on Hiroshima and Nagasaki atomic bomb survivors and other data accumulated since their previous publications in 1975, appear in ICRP Publication 60 (International Commission on Radiological Protection, 1991a). The recommendations of this publication are intended to prevent the occurrence of deterministic effects and limit the probability of stochastic effects, both to individuals and their immediate and second generation offspring, to an acceptable level. Table 14.3 summarizes the dose limits recommended by *ICRP 60* which should achieve the aims stated above.

The ICRP recommends no special occupational dose limits for women who are not pregnant, the limits being the same as for men. Once pregnancy has been declared, the ICRP recommend that the dose to the woman's abdomen should be restricted to 2 mSv for the remainder of the pregnancy.

The same overriding principal established in earlier publications, of keeping doses 'as low as reasonably achievable' (the ALARA principle),

Table 14.3 Summary of ICRP 60 dose limits.* From International Commission on Radiological Protection (1991)

Radiation workers	50 mSv in any 1 year period but not more than 100 mSv in any 5 year period (implied average dose of 20 mSv per year)
General public	1 mSv per year, but in special circumstances a higher effective dose could be allowed in a single year, but the average dose must not exceed 1 mSv per year during the person's lifetime

* There is no change to the dose limits for individual organs or for the eye lens.

economic and social factors being taken into account, still remains. As a method for achieving their recommendations, the ICRP commended the following practices:
• no practice should be adopted unless its introduction produces a positive net benefit;
• all exposures should be kept as low a reasonably achievable;
• none of their recommended dose limits should be exceeded.
National governments such as the UK Parliament, and organizations such as the European Commission, take note of these recommendations and incorporate them in their legislation.

Legislation to control exposures not only requires control of doses to those persons exposed in the course of their employment but also to members of the general public. In the UK the principal pieces of legislation are the Ionising Radiations Regulations 1985 (IRR85) Statutory Instrument 1985 No. 1333 made under the Health and Safety at Work etc. Act 1974 and the Radioactive Substances Act 1993 (RSA93). The former is administered by the Health and Safety Executive (HSE) and the latter by Her Majesty's Inspectorate of Pollution (HMIP). The IRR85 is concerned primarily with the safety of workers. The RSA93 controls the use of radioactive material and the disposal of all forms of radioactive waste, thus exercising some control on the exposure of the general public due to radioactivity discharged into the environment.

Within the UK there is the National Radiological

Protection Board (NRPB), a government organization which advises parliament and government departments on radiological protection. They also run training courses, dosimetry services and advisory services for industry.

Until 1960 there were no statutory regulations governing the use of radioactivity or radiation and those made in the 1960s only applied to factories. Other places such as hospitals, research and teaching establishments, dental and veterinary practices followed their own Codes of Practice. The Ionising Radiation Regulations 1985 and their accompanying Approved Codes of Practice (ACOP) formed the first comprehensive set of regulations which covered all users of ionizing radiation and radioactivity. The new ICRP recommendations cannot be embodied into the present IRR85 without parliamentary approval. To take note of the ICRP recommendations, the HSE issued a Part 4 ACOP which advises on stricter constraints on radiation exposures, requiring investigations and subsequent reports to HSE if doses exceed 75 mSv in any 5 year period. Table 14.4 summarizes the Ionising Radiations Regulations 1985 legally permitted dose limits. It should be noted that both the ICRP recommendations and the statutory limits embodied in regulations exclude radiation doses incurred as a result of medical or dental practices and as a result of exposure to natural background radiation. Exceptions to the latter appear in the NRPB publi-

Table 14.4 Summary of UK permitted annual dose limits (mSv). From Ionising Radiations Regulations 1985

	Whole body	Individual organs	Lens of eye
Radiation workers	50	500	150
Trainees under the age of 18	15	150	50
Non-radiation workers and members of the general public*	5	50	15

* The dose limit to the abdomen of a woman of reproductive capacity is 13 mSv in any consecutive 13 week period. The dose limit to the abdomen of a woman who is pregnant is limited to 10 mSv during the period of the pregnancy.

cation *Documents of the NRPB*, Vol. 4, No. 2 (1993), which recommends that some form of control may be necessary for persons who may be exposed to:

- materials containing elevated levels of natural radionuclides;
- cosmic rays to aircrew and other frequent fliers in jet aircraft;
- radon and its daughters.

There is again the overriding requirement that doses are to be kept to 'as low as reasonably practicable'; different terminology but the same principle as the ICRP ALARA.

The Radioactive Substances Act 1993 requires that before a person uses radioactive material, that person must register with HMIP and obtain authorization to use the material, to store the material and to accumulate and dispose of radioactive waste arising from their operations. A number of Statutory Instruments allow some exemptions from the requirements of the Act.

Administrative measures for controlling exposure to ionizing radiation

Before any work with ionizing radiation or radioactivity is started, a hazard assessment to determine the potential risk to the workforce is required. When significant amounts of radioactivity are to be used, there may be a requirement also to assess the potential hazard to the environment and the general public living in the neighbourhood of routine operations and discharges of radioactive waste, as well as the effects of an accident. The latter may require the development of an emergency plan in co-operation with the local emergency services such as the police and fire services. Liaison with government departments such as HMIP, the Ministry of Agriculture, Fisheries and Food, local Health departments, etc. may be required. Due regard for the ICRP recommendations, NRPB recommendations and legal requirements is absolutely necessary.

Following the assessment, which will indicate the degree of hazard, the degree of control can be determined. The establishment of areas must be considered. These are usually defined by boundary demarcation and notices, but may be defined by

clear description in documents and require differing levels of control, for which adequate records are necessary. Deciding which members of the workforce are to be designated as classified radiation workers and arranging for their medical surveillance and personal dosimetry must be done at an early stage. Radiation protection supervisors (RPS) and radiation protection advisors (RPA) must be appointed and their training arranged. Training of the personnel who will be working with radiation and/or radioactive material must also be arranged. Radiation and contamination monitoring programmes are to be designed and the necessity for air sampling considered. In some circumstances it may be necessary to provide personal air samplers. Monitoring programmes of waste streams whether solid, liquid or gaseous must also be considered. Local rules for each laboratory or plant, describing the precautions to be taken, must be prepared and made available to every member of the workforce. A copy of the rules is to be displayed at the workstation. If the main document is long or complicated, a summary of the rules may be displayed at the workstation, but every operator must still have access to the main document.

Practical measures for controlling exposure to ionizing radiation

Practical control of exposure to ionizing radiations, as with other potential hazards, requires both foresight and planning. Methods to protect persons from any potential harm are to be designed and developed to deal with the hazard. Control of radiation and radioactive material can be conveniently dealt with by considering the hazard from external radiation (radiation from sources outside the body) and internal radiation (radiation from sources inside the body) separately although in practice concurrent precautions may be required.

Control of external exposure

External radiation can arise from sealed or unsealed radioactive sources, X-ray equipment, accelerators or any electrical device capable of accelerating electrons to greater than 5.0 MeV. There are three classical methods which can be applied to reduce exposure to external ionizing radiation: time, distance and shielding.

Time

Since cumulative dose is a function of exposure time and dose rate (just as cumulative distance travelled is a function of time and speed), reducing the time spent in a field of radiation will reduce the total dose received. In other words, do not spend any more time in a radiation field than is required to perform the task in hand. Do not conduct discussions in a radiation field unless absolutely necessary; adjourn to an area of low background.

Distance

The greater the distance between oneself and a source of radiation, the lower the dose rate which will be encountered and consequently the total dose received will be reduced. It is not always advantageous to put the maximum distance possible between oneself and an exposed source. For example, manipulation of a source using 2 m long tongs is much more difficult than when using 1 m long tongs and therefore the amount of time necessary to complete the task may well offset the advantage gained from the increased distance. In physics, there is a law called the 'inverse square law' which states that if the distance between a point source of radiation and the object being irradiated is doubled, the dose rate at the target is reduced to a quarter of the original dose rate.

Example: if the dose rate at point 'A', 1 m from a source of radiation, is $10 \, \text{mSv h}^{-1}$, then the dose rate at point 'B', 2 m from the source, will be reduced to $2.5 \, \text{mSv h}^{-1}$, and at point 'C', 3 m from the source, it will be reduced to $1.1 \, \text{mSv h}^{-1}$

$$D_B = \frac{10}{2^2} = \frac{10}{2 \times 2} = 2.5 \, \text{mSv h}^{-1}$$

and

$$D_C = \frac{10}{3^2} = \frac{10}{3 \times 3} = 1.1 \, \text{mSv h}^{-1}$$

thus

$$D_B = \frac{D_A}{d^2} \qquad (14.9)$$

where D_B is the dose rate at point 'B', D_A is the dose rate at point 'A' (which must be a unit distance from the source, e.g. 1 m or 1 cm, etc.) and d is the distance from the source to the point of interest such as point 'B' or 'C'. The converse is true, so that on halving the distance between a source and the irradiated body, the dose rate is increased fourfold. It is for these reasons that it is always advised that radioactive material should not be manipulated by hand, the use of some form of handling device should always be used. As an example, if a beta source is manipulated with a gloved hand giving an estimated distance of 1.0 mm between the source and the hand, the dose rate at 100 mm will only be about one ten-thousandth of that encountered at 1.0 mm

Shielding

The best method of ensuring that doses are kept to a minimum is to introduce shielding material between the radiation source and the person likely to be irradiated. The thickness of the shield required will depend on the energy of the radiation, the amount of radiation present and the required dose rate at the point of interest. Currently the aim to is keep dose rates in the occupied zones to below $2.5 \, \mu\text{Sv h}^{-1}$ and below $1.0 \, \mu\text{Sv h}^{-1}$ if reasonably practicable. The more energetic the radiation and the higher the dose rate present, then the thicker the shielding material required to provide the necessary degree of protection. The thickness of the shield required will also depend on the shield material. Thus for radiation of a specific energy and similar dose rate, only half the thickness of lead will be required to provide the same degree of protection as that provided by steel of a certain thickness. Concrete ($2.35 \, \text{g cm}^{-3}$) is commonly used for shielding large sources. Shielding for neutron sources is usually complex, comprising a neutron moderator to reduce the energy of the incident neutrons, followed by a neutron capture material to stop the lower energy neutrons and finally a gamma shield to attenuate gamma radiation associated with the neutron source as well as gamma radiation produced in the neutron shields. When designing shielding for beta sources, consideration must be given to shielding against bremsstrahlung X-rays produced in the beta shield material or within the beta source itself due to self-absorption of beta particles in the source material

Radiation monitoring

An adequate monitoring programme should be designed. This could include monitoring with hand-held portable instruments or installed monitors which may be fitted with remote reading and alarm systems in addition to giving local indication of dose rate and/or integrated accumulated dose.

Control of internal radiation

Internal radiation arises from radioactive material deposited inside the body and there are four routes by which radioactive material can enter the body:
1 Inhalation: inhaling contaminated air.
2 Ingestion: by taking radioactive material in through the mouth.
3 Injection: by radioactive material entering the body via wounds or medical conditions such as eczema causing skin lesions.
4 Absorption: through the intact skin or by radioactive material penetrating through the intact skin. This is a particular problem when working with tritium (hydrogen-3). Approximately 30% of any intake of tritium oxide (tritiated water) is by absorption through the skin, where exposure is due to airborne tritium. Where the skin is wetted by tritium-contaminated water, the intake by absorption is almost 100%.

Radioactive material will only enter the body if it escapes from the facility in which it is manipulated and contaminates surfaces, becomes airborne or contaminates food and drink. To prevent this occurring it is necessary to provide some form of containment. Examples of containment vary from fume cupboards, which rely on an adequate airflow into them to prevent dispersal into the workplace, up to sealed glove boxes working under negative pressure.

There should always be a system of 'defence in depth'. The apparatus in which the work is done should be in some form of primary containment, such as a fume cupboard or glove box. This primary containment should be in an area which has an appropriate classification, either a 'controlled' or 'supervised' area as defined in the IRR85, and there

should be a buffer area surrounding it incorporating personal monitoring and washing facilities.

It is necessary to ensure that an adequate monitoring programme is introduced. This may include air sampling as well as surface contamination monitoring. The issue of personal air samplers may be required. The results of the monitoring programme are to be compared with 'derived limits' for both air and surface contamination. Derived limits for inhalation and ingestion are found in ICRP Publications 30 and 61 (International Commission on Radiological Protection, 1981 and 1991b). The limits at which an area must be designated as a 'controlled area' as defined in the IRR85 due to the risk of internal radiation appears in Schedule 2 of that document.

A wide variety of monitoring techniques are available for assessing the amount of radioactive contamination on surfaces, ranging from direct monitoring to taking smear or wipe samples, collecting samples on adhesive tape and measuring the amount of material deposited on deposition trays. Many of the techniques available are described in the International Atomic Energy Agency (IAEA) Technical Reports Series No. 120, *Monitoring of Radioactive Contamination on Surfaces* (1970).

When unsealed radioactive sources are being manipulated, local rules should prohibit eating, drinking, applying cosmetics or the use of tobacco in any form in the designated area. The use of mouth-operated apparatus must also be banned. In areas in which there is a serious risk of contamination, personal belongings should be left in the changing room. Nothing should leave a contamination controlled area unless it has been monitored and certified clear of significant contamination. Personal monitoring, washing and hygiene must be strictly enforced.

Transport of radioactive material

National and international regulations governing the transport of radioactive material exist, most of them being based on the International Atomic Energy Agency (IAEA) Safety Series No. 6, *Regulations for the Safe Transport of Radioactive Materials* (1985) and associated advisory material. In addition to these, individual carriers impose their own restrictions on the types and amounts of radio-active material which they will transport. Reference to these should be made before transporting radioactive material. Carriers and their regulations involved are: the Post Office, British Railways, Inland Waterways Authority, International Air Transport Association (IATA), Merchant Shipping (Dangerous Goods) Regulations (the Blue Book), etc. The Radioactive Material (Road Transport) Act 1991 and Statutory Instrument No. 1729 Radioactive Substances (carriage by road) (Great Britain) (Amendment) Regulations 1985, introduced the 1985 IAEA Safety Series No. 6 into UK law. So far no regulations made under the Act have been published. There is also the European Agreement concerning the International Carriage of Dangerous Goods by Road (ADR) which includes the carriage of radioactive materials.

BACKGROUND SOURCES OF RADIATION

Radioactivity was discovered towards the end of the nineteenth century, but humans have been exposed to radiation from natural sources since their first appearance on the planet. It is interesting to consider the magnitude of doses due to natural background radiation and lifestyles (Table 14.5). The largest dose of radiation, about 87% of the total, received by a person living in the UK is due to 'natural background' radiation. Other radiation comes from food, lifestyle, radioactive material in the body, etc.

Table 14.5 Magnitude of doses of radiation due to natural background radiation and lifestyles

Natural background (87%)	Cosmic radiation from outer space
	Gamma radiation from radioactive materials in the ground and buildings
	Radioactive gas in the air (radon gas)
	Radioactive materials in the body (potassium-40 in the skeleton)
Food and drink	Natural radioactive materials in food and drink (radium in Brazil nuts)
Medical exposure (11%)	Diagnostic X-ray examinations and therapeutic irradiations
Lifestyle (0.5%)	TV, air travel, luminous watches and instruments

REFERENCES

Health and Safety Executive (1985). *The Ionising Radiations Regulations 1985 Statutory Instrument No. 1333* and associated *Approved Codes of Practice*. HMSO, London.

International Atomic Energy Agency (1970). *Monitoring of Radioactive Contamination on Surfaces*. IAEA Technical Report Series 120, Vienna.

International Atomic Energy Agency (1985). *Regulations for the Safe Transport of Radioactive Materials*. IAEA Safety Series No. 6.

International Commission on Radiological Protection (1981). *Annals of the International Commission on Radiological Protection*, Vol. 6. ICRP Publication 30, *Limits for Intakes of Radionuclides by Workers*.

International Commission on Radiological Protection (1991). *Annals of the International Commission on Radiological Protection*, Vol. 21, Nos 1–3. ICRP Publication 60, *Recommendations of the ICRP on Radiological Protection*.

International Commission on Radiological Protection (1991). *Annals of the International Commission on Radiological Protection*, Vol. 21, No. 4. ICRP Publication 61, *Limits for Intakes of Radionuclides by Workers*. (Taking account of Dose Limits in ICRP Publication 60.)

National Radiological Protection Board (1993). *Documents of the NRPB*, Vol. 4, No. 2.

Radioactive Material (Road Transport) Act, 1991. Chapter 27.

The Radioactive Substances Act, 1993. Chapter 12. HMSO, London.

FURTHER READING

HMSO. *The Ionising Radiations (Outside Workers) Regulations 1993. Protection of Outside Workers against Ionising Radiations*. HMSO, London.

Hughes, D. (1993). *The Control of Sources of Ionising Radiation*. HHSC Handbook No. 12.

International Atomic Energy Agency (1990). *Advisory Material for the IAEA Regulations for the Safe Transport of Radioactive Materials*, (3rd edn.) IAEA Safety Series No. 37.

CHAPTER 15

Ergonomics

K.C. Parsons

DEFINITIONS AND ORIGINS

Ergonomics places knowledge of human attributes, characteristics, capabilities and limitations at the centre of any consideration of the design and assessment of work. It is an interdisciplinary subject involving human psychology, anatomy and physiology, mathematics, physics and related disciplines. In application it integrates knowledge in these areas to deal with practical problems in the design and evaluation of systems involving people.

The word 'ergonomics' was invented by an interdisciplinary group of British scientists in Oxford in 1949. The need for such a subject had been perceived in the period up to and during the Second World War where multidisciplinary teams had successfully worked together to solve important practical problems. Experience had been gained in both military and industrial settings.

There followed a great interest in, and rapid expansion of, the subject both nationally and internationally. The establishment of the Ergonomics Research Society in the UK was a landmark and had as one of its aims the dissemination of the results of scientific research for use in industrial applications. It later changed its name to the Ergonomics Society, reflecting that not only did ergonomists carry out research but also that much work was conducted on applied projects for and within industry.

There are now national ergonomics societies throughout the world and most contribute to the International Ergonomics Association (IEA) which was set up in 1959. Although there are a number of scientific publications associated with the subject,

the two recognized and established journals are *Ergonomics* and *Applied Ergonomics*. In the USA the term 'human factors' was adopted to describe ergonomics activity. The worldwide acceptance and expansion of ergonomics, however, resulted in the Human Factors Society changing its name to The Human Factors and Ergonomics Society.

There are a number of definitions of ergonomics and the Ergonomics Society brochure *Ergonomics in Action* provides the following definition.

> 'Ergonomics is about fit. Ergonomics is concerned with the fit between people, the activities they wish to carry out, the tools, machines and systems they use to aid them and the environments in which they are performed. A chair must be the correct height for the occupant, a computer program must be understandable, the instruments in an aircraft must be readable by the pilot and the lighting in a factory must be adequate. If this fit is achieved, we would expect the performance of the user to be better than if it were not'.

Stranks (1992) provides four definitions, but these are (inevitably) inadequate. However, to provide a closer understanding, it is helpful to consider how they are inadequate. These are listed below with comments.

1 'Ergonomics is the scientific study of the interrelationships between people and their work'. This is rather vague and although probably does cover most of ergonomics, it also covers other subjects. The focus on work must be taken in a general way, to encompass the range of contexts covered by ergonomics.

2 'Ergonomics is fitting the task to the individual'.

This is only a small part of ergonomics and although it correctly concentrates on the individual, it misses the general philosophy. For example, it is perfectly acceptable also to fit the individual to the task, using training methods.

3 'Ergonomics is the scientific study of work'. This refers more to work study, or time and motion study, than to ergonomics.

4 'Ergonomics is the study of the man–machine interface'. This is also true, but is only a part of ergonomics activity. It focuses very much on equipment design but does not include organizational issues, environment and other aspects.

ERGONOMICS AND OCCUPATIONAL HYGIENE

Occupational hygiene is concerned with how peoples' health may be affected by their work. This chapter provides a description of useful ergonomics data and methods and also provides examples in some specific areas of application that will be of interest in occupational hygiene. For further information and reading on the subject, a list of publications is provided at the end of the chapter.

Ergonomics data

Ergonomics data concerns information about human characteristics, capacities, capabilities and so on. In any occupational hygiene application it can be used to provide the 'human data' for use in workplace design. Ergonomics databases are now available on computer. ERGOBASE from the USA for example, provides anthropometric data for 44 global civilian and military populations and data on specialist populations, such as wheelchair users, pregnant women and the elderly. Body forces and strength (static, isometric, dynamic) and aerobic capacities are also provided. There are also a number of other anthropometric databases and availability of such data on computers has led to easy access and use of computer-aided design of workplaces.

Anthropometry is only one characteristic of humans and there are many others. For convenience, these are considered below in terms of body size, sensing capacity, information processing

or mental capacity and output capacity. Very little data can be presented in a short chapter such as this and there is much more. An important point, however, is that an ergonomics database will never be complete. Ergonomics methods, therefore, not only include the use of data but also how to collect and use it in specific applications and contexts. The practise of ergonomics also includes user evaluation methods for the design and assessment of products, systems and workplaces. Ergonomics methods are discussed later in this chapter.

Data representation

Whatever the data of interest, whether it be body height, maximum grip force or visual performance in a driving simulator, there will be differences, both between people and groups of people (inter-individual differences) and with any person over time (intra-individual differences). Therefore, ergonomics data is often presented to quantify these differences. It is often assumed that individual differences, over a wide range of parameters, are normally distributed (Fig. 15.1). It can be seen that the average (50th percentile) value over the responses or characteristics of individuals bisects the frequency distribution curve. This value could

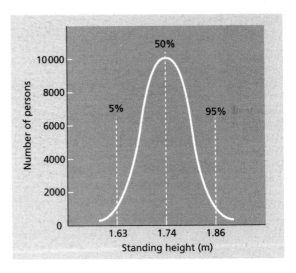

Fig. 15.1 Frequency distribution of ergonomics data. Standing height of British males is shown, but similar presentations could be made from sitting height, hand size, performance, etc. From Grandjean (1988).

be used to design for the average person (e.g. in terms of sitting height). To design a vehicle seat such that 95% of people would not make contact with the vehicle roof, then the height of the roof should be greater than the 95 percentile sitting height. To select drivers so that 95% of the population can reach the pedals, the seat adjustment should allow contact by 95% of drivers and hence the drivers should have a greater leg length than the 5 percentile driver. Thus ergonomics data can be used in design and evaluation.

Useful ergonomics data are presented throughout this chapter in Tables 15.1 to 15.11 and Fig. 15.2 to 15.11. For further information and data the reader should consult the references provided at the end of the chapter.

Body size

Body size can be presented in lengths, areas and volumes as well as mass, proportions, body composition and so on. Body sizes that are relevant

Table 15.1 Anthropometric data for British men and women aged 19–65 years. All values in millimetres. From Grandjean (1988), after Pheasant (1986)

	Men			Women		
	5th %ile	50th %ile	95th %ile	5th %ile	50th %ile	95th %ile
Standing height	1625	1740	1855	1505	1610	1710
Eye height	1515	1630	1745	1405	1505	1610
Shoulder height	1315	1425	1535	1215	1310	1405
Elbow height	1005	1090	1180	930	1005	1085
Hip height	840	920	1000	740	810	885
Knuckle height	690	755	825	660	720	780
Fingertip height	590	655	720	560	625	685
Sitting height	850	910	965	795	850	910
Sitting eye height	735	790	845	685	740	795
Sitting shoulder height	540	595	645	505	555	610
Sitting elbow height	195	245	295	185	235	280
Thigh thickness	135	160	185	125	155	180
Buttock–knee length	540	595	645	520	570	620
Buttock–popliteal length	440	495	550	435	480	530
Knee height	490	545	595	455	500	540
Popliteal height	395	440	490	355	400	445
Shoulder breadth (bideltoid)	420	465	510	355	395	435
Shoulder breadth (biacromial)	365	400	430	325	355	385
Hip breadth	310	360	405	310	370	435
Chest (bust) depth	215	250	285	210	250	295
Abdominal depth	220	270	325	205	255	305
Shoulder–elbow length	330	365	395	300	330	360
Elbow–fingertip length	440	475	510	400	430	460
Upper limb length	720	780	840	655	705	760
Shoulder–grip length	610	665	715	555	600	650
Head length	180	195	205	165	180	190
Head breadth	145	155	165	135	145	150
Hand length	175	190	205	160	175	190
Hand breadth	80	85	95	70	75	85
Foot length	240	265	285	215	235	255
Foot breadth	85	95	110	80	90	100
Span	1655	1790	1925	1490	1605	1725
Elbow span	865	945	1020	780	850	920
Vertical grip reach (standing)	1925	2060	2190	1790	1905	2020
Vertical grip reach (sitting)	1145	1245	1340	1060	1150	1235
Forward grip reach	720	780	835	650	705	755

Table 15.2 Pheasant's five fundamental fallacies. From Pheasant (1986)

---

1 The design is satisfactory for me, it will therefore be satisfactory for everyone else

2 The design is satisfactory for the average person, it will therefore be satisfactory for everyone else

3 The variability of human beings is so great that it cannot possibly be catered for in any design, but since people are wonderfully adaptable it doesn't matter anyway

4 Ergonomics is expensive and since products are actually purchased on appearance and styling, ergonomic considerations may conveniently be ignored

5 Ergonomics is an excellent idea. I always design things with ergonomics in mind but I do it intuitively and rely on my common sense so I don't need tables of data

---

in the design and assessment of workplaces are presented in Table 15.1. The data are taken from Pheasant (1986) and apply to British males and females. The reader should refer to Pheasant (1986) for data on other populations and dimensions. It is interesting to note that 'secular trends' occur. For example, average standing height may increase over a number of years as nutrition and quality of

life improves. Pheasant (1986) also lists what he terms the 'five fundamental fallacies' (Table 15.2). These apply to ergonomics and user-centred design in general and are commonly articulated by a range of professionals in a number of forms. Pheasant discusses these in detail and it is left to the reader of this chapter to consider them and identify them as fallacies in the area of occupational hygiene. An important point is that there is no average person. Someone of average height will not be average in all other respects. For example, if we design a door to allow only average (or less) height *and* width persons through, then some of those with average height (width) will be too wide (tall) to pass through the door. Further useful data relating to body size, are presented in Tables 15.3 to 15.5 and in Figs 15.2 to 15.5.

Sensory capacity

The senses of the body detect and relay information concerning the external world to the brain. They respond to light, temperature, pressure, taste, smell and sound and involve some specialized organs (eye, ear, etc.) The physical levels of environmental stimuli are detected and interpreted by the

Table 15.3 Mean and 90% confidence interval (CI) of hand and wrist dimensions for young German men and women. Values in millimetres. From Grandjean (1988), after Jurgens (1973)

	Men		Women	
	Mean	90% CI	Mean	90% CI
Circumference of hand	211	193–230	187	175–201
Breadth of hand	106	98–113	–	–
Circumference of wrist	171	155–188	161	143–179
Maximum grip (circumference of thumb and forefinger)	134	120–153	–	–

Table 15.4 Maximum height of reach for men and women. Values in millimetres. From Grandjean (1988)

	Men			Women		
	5th %ile	50th %ile	95th %ile	5th %ile	50th %ile	95th %ile
To fingertip	2040	2180	2310	1890	2000	2120
Grasping height	1920	2060	2190	1790	1900	2020

Table 15.5 Preferred visual display unit (VDU) workstation settings and eye levels during work. Visual angles and screen inclination are related to the horizontal plane. Values in millimetres or degrees. $N > 50$ subjects. From Grandjean (1988)

	Mean	Range
Seat height	480	430–570
Keyboard height above floor	790	710–870
Screen height above floor	1030	920–1160
Visual down angle: eye to screen centre	−0.9°	+2° to−2°
Visual distance, eye to screen	760	610–930
Screen upward inclination	94°	88°–103°
Eye level above floor	1150	1070–1270

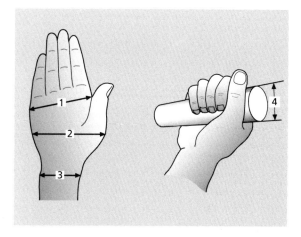

Fig. 15.3 Indication of measurements listed in Table 15.3. 1, circumference of hand; 2, breadth of hand; 3, circumference of wrist; 4, maximum grip. From Grandjean (1988), after Jurgens (1973).

body. Knowledge of the dynamic characteristics (capacities and limitations) of these sensing systems is important in ergonomics assessment. Examples are provided in Tables 15.6 and 15.7 and Figs 15.6 to 15.9. It is important to remember that there is a 'human transfer function'. Physical levels of the environment are not directly related to levels of sensation and perception. This is the origin of the dB(A) unit, for example, where the 'A-weighting' is an attempt to simulate human perception of noise. Perception is also greatly influenced by experiences and disposition of individuals. Whether a level of noise is annoying or not, for example, will depend upon not only noise level but the source of the noise, the receiver's attitude to the source and what they are doing at the time.

Mental capacity

Mental capacity is of great importance in ergonomics assessment, especially where tasks and jobs have significant mental components involving decision-making, reasoning, memory and so on. There will be problems if a job were designed involving the memory of 20 individual items when people generally can memorize only seven. Cognitive performance depends upon many factors and is

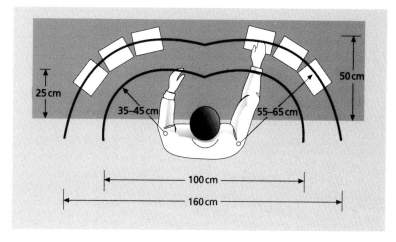

Fig. 15.2 Horizontal arc of grasp and working area at tabletop height. The grasping distance takes account of the distance from the shoulder to the hand; the working distance only from the elbow to the hand. The values include the 5th percentile, and so apply to men and women of less than average size. From Grandjean (1988).

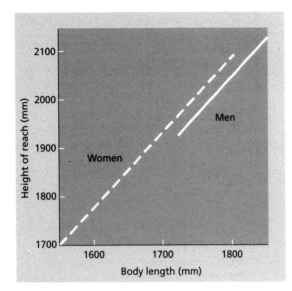

Fig. 15.4 Height to which a free-standing person can reach and place a hand flat on a shelf. From Grandjean (1988).

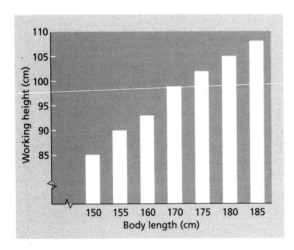

Fig. 15.5 Working heights for light work while standing, in relation to body length. From Grandjean (1988).

Table 15.6 Average near point at different ages. From Grandjean (1988)

Age (years)	Near point (mm)
16	80
32	120
44	250
50	500
60	1000

Table 15.7 Recommended heights of lettering and proportions of letters or figures*. From Grandjean (1988)

Distance from the eye (mm)	Height of small letters or figures (mm)
Up to 500	2.5
501–900	5.0
901–1800	9.0
1801–3600	18.0
3601–6000	30.0

* Width of letters or figures should be 2/3 × height for both lower and upper case. Lower case height should be 2/3 × upper case.

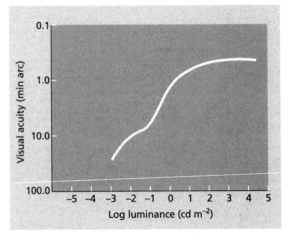

Fig. 15.6 The variation in visual acuity with luminance. From Grandjean (1988).

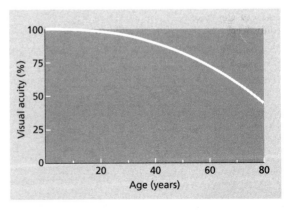

Fig. 15.7 Decrease of visual acuity with age. From Grandjean (1988).

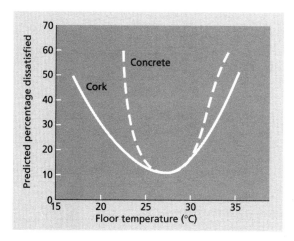

Fig. 15.8 The predicted percentage dissatisfied (PPD) for people standing with bare feet on cork or concrete floors. After Olesen (1977).

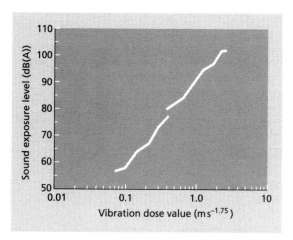

Fig. 15.9 Contours showing the median subjective equivalence between sound and vibration. After Griffin (1990).

related to personal factors such as mood, motivation and state of arousal. Mental performance always involves activity of a number of mental components. Considering mental capacity in terms of characteristics of component parts, such as memory, reasoning, etc., is therefore inadequate when considering the whole. The capacities and properties of each component are interrelated with the activity and capacities of others and the performance of the whole will also be affected by the general state of the person, in terms of mood for example. Mental models are often used to describe the mental performance and requirements of individuals when performing mental tasks. Such models are always simplifications and are useful only in specific contexts.

Human data are presented below, however such data will always be insufficient in application. Uptake of information, memory and vigilance are considered, but there are other factors such as logical reasoning, level of knowledge, expertise and training and scenario testing that will be relevant. Ergonomists often identify the 'mental model' of the user population (and that required for a job). This refers to the internal representation of 'the world' that a person brings to tasks. It is important that this mental model is appropriate for the task being performed. As a simple example, consider an operator's mental model of a system involving a submarine hatch, where it is concluded from the model that lifting a lever closes the hatch, when in fact it opens the hatch.

Uptake of information

The ability of humans to take in information is of great importance in ergonomics design. Only a small proportion of all information available can be transmitted to the brain and it is often considered that attention to information is based upon a single channel capacity. Information from two spoken sources at once, or visual and auditory information presented simultaneously, will not produce optimum performance as one input will not be attended to, or a sharing of the single channel will take place. The single channel also has a limited rate of information uptake. This will depend upon factors such as fatigue. The design of an aircraft cockpit is a classic example where this must be taken very seriously. Another important area is in the design of process control rooms for chemical plants or nuclear power stations. The reduction or filtering of information from sensory detection to lasting impression in the brain is shown in Table 15.8.

Memory

Memory represents the ability to 'store' information for later recall and is often considered

Table 15.8 Estimated information transfer by a person: from reception from the outside world to storage for lasting impression. From Grandjean (1988)

Process	Information stream (bits s^{-1})
Detection by the sense organ	1 000 000 000
At nerve junctions	3 000 000
Conscious awareness	16
Lasting impression	0.7

in terms of short-term memory and long-term memory. Short-term memory is concerned with the storage of information from a few seconds to a few hours. If the information is to be stored for longer it must be transferred to long-term memory. The capacity to remember something depends upon a number of factors and has been extensively studied. Association of information greatly increases effectiveness. While we may be able to remember on average only about seven individual items, if information is grouped correctly we can remember the seven groupings and hence much greater individual amounts of information. The design of control panels and of computer software often uses this characteristic of memory to advantage.

Vigilance

Vigilance is the ability to stay alert and hence attend to and respond to stimuli. The reaction to stimuli can be measured in terms of reaction time. 'Simple reaction time' is the time to respond to a single, simple stimulus and is about 0.25 s. 'Choice reaction time' varies with the number of choices available and times are shown in Table 15.9.

The reaction times will depend upon the nature of the stimulus and the response, and the level of expectation and alertness of the individual.

Table 15.9 Relationship between number of possible answers and choice reaction time (1/100th of a second). From Grandjean (1988).

Number of possible answers	1	2	3	4	5	6	7	8	9	10
Reaction time	20	35	40	45	50	55	60	60	65	65

Vigilance performance can be greatly decreased if a person is bored and does not know quite when to expect a stimulus and especially if he or she is not quite sure what to look for. Ship watch-keeping is a classic example of this, but monitoring the state of warning signals in control rooms or driving at night along deserted roads provide other examples. Figure 15.10 shows the relationship between frequency of signals and percentage of signals noticed. The inverted U shape of the curve, showing 'underload', 'optimum' and 'overload', is a classic finding. The following conclusions can be drawn.

1 Sustained alertness decreases with time, especially after 30 min.

2 Observational performance is relatively improved if signals are more frequent and stronger, the observer is given feedback on performance and signals are clear.

3 Performance is relatively worse if intervals between signals vary, the observer is under physical stress or just woken from sleep and there are unfavourable environmental conditions.

Output capacity

The reaction time discussed above is concerned with sensory detection and perception, information processing and output in terms of response. The 'output capacity' of the body includes the speed, accuracy and force if muscular output is considered. Speech and signalling are other forms of output.

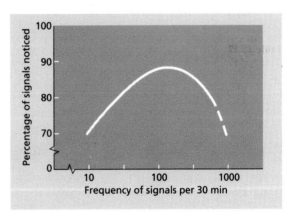

Fig. 15.10 Relation between frequency of signals requiring reaction and the observed performance. From Grandjean (1988).

The ability to operate controls will depend upon output capacity. Recommended distance between adjoining controls is shown in Table 15.10 and the maximum muscular force for men and women is shown in Table 15.11. The effect of age on maximum muscular power is presented in Fig. 15.11. Recommendations for maximum acceptable loads are based upon output capacity data and are provided in Tables 15.12 and 15.13.

Ergonomics methods

No data concerning humans will ever be complete and therefore ergonomists require methods for collecting relevant data and for the correct use of data that are available. For a comprehensive text on ergonomics methods, see Wilson and Corlett (1990). For convenience, in this chapter, methods are divided into four types as described overleaf.

Table 15.10 Distance apart of adjoining controls (mm). From Grandjean (1988)

Control	Method of operation	Minimum	Optimum
Push button	One finger	20	50
Toggle switch	One finger	25	50
Main switch	One hand	50	100
	Both hands	75	125
Hand wheel	Both hands	75	125
Rotating knob	One hand	25	50
·Pedal	Two pedals with same foot	50	100

Table 15.11 Mean and standard deviation (SD) maximum muscular force for men and women. From Grandjean (1988), after Hettinger (1960)

Function	Men Mean maximum force (N)	SD	Women Mean maximum force (N)	SD
Hand clasp	460	120	280	70
Kicking (knee bent at 90 degrees)	400	60	320	50
Stretching the back	1100	160	740	160

Table 15.12 Maximum acceptable loads (N) for young men while lifting for not more than once per minute. From Grandjean (1988), after Davis and Stubbs (1977)

Condition	Grasping distance as a fraction of arm length $\frac{1}{4}$	$\frac{1}{2}$	$\frac{3}{4}$	$\frac{4}{4}$
Standing up				
Two-handed lift, frontal	350	250	150	100
One-handed lift, frontal	300	220	140	100
One-handed lift, sideways	270	200	130	100
Seated				
Two-handed lift, frontal	270	170	120	110
One-handed lift, frontal	350	220	140	100
One-handed lift, sideways	330	210	140	90

Table 15.13 Maximum acceptable loads (upright standing posture) under various lifting conditions (N). From Grandjean (1988), after Davis and Stubbs (1977)

	Men				Women			
	Under 50		Over 50		Under 50		Over 50	
	Occ.*	Freq.†	Occ.	Freq.	Occ.	Freq.	Occ.	Freq.
Two-handed lift; compact load, close to the body, within preferred range of heights	300	210	240	140	180	130	140	100
One-handed lift; compact load close to body	200	140	120	80	120	80	70	50

* Occ. = occasional lifts, <1 lift per min.
† Freq. = frequent lifts, >1 lift per min.

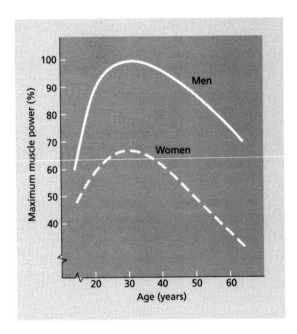

Fig. 15.11 Muscle power in relation to age and sex. From Grandjean (1988), after Hettinger (1960).

1 *Objective methods*: where a direct measurement is made of a human response (e.g. heart rate, sweat loss, skin temperature, electroencephalography (EEG), electromyography (EMG), analysis of blood, nitrogen in urine, speed and accuracy of performance, seat pressure, eye movements, maximum grip strength, etc.).

(a) Possible advantages: direct and quantifiable measure of response that may clearly relate to applications (e.g. human performance, comfort, health and safety).

(b) Possible disadvantages: inconvenient, expensive and may interfere with what is being measured.

2 *Subjective methods*: where people report their impressions, usually verbally or on scales and questionnaires (e.g. sensation, comfort, preference, difficulty, stress, perception, etc.).

(a) Possible advantages: often quick, convenient, easy to quantify and relates directly to psychological phenomena such as comfort and preference.

(b) Possible disadvantages: people may not give a useful answer, in terms of health and safety for example. Can have significant bias and provides little information about why subjects report in the way they did.

3 *Behavioural methods*: where the behaviour of people is observed (by a trained person, video, two-way mirror, etc.) and inferences drawn (e.g. frequency of passengers sitting in seats in a bus, route people take in a hospital or shopping centre, fidgeting in a classroom, etc.).

(a) Possible advantages: non-interference with what is being measured, direct and realistic evaluation of a design.

(b) Possible disadvantages: difficult to establish and interpret measure. Time-consuming in data collection and difficult to quantify results for formal analysis.

4 *Modelling methods*: where a physical or mathematical (computer) model of a human system is used to make predictions about a human response (e.g. empirical models involving databases or regression equations based upon the responses for human subjects rational models based upon an 'engineering' approach to biomechanics, heat transfer, etc.). An anthropometric model is shown in use in Fig. 15.12.

(a) Possible advantages: quick, consistent response to be used in the early stage of design and in preliminary assessment. Can be used in computer-aided ergonomics (design).

(b) Possible disadvantages: models will always be relatively inaccurate and an oversimplification of human systems. Possible misuse if predictions misinterpreted or taken too literally.

Design of ergonomics investigations

To collect data in an efficient and effective way, ergonomics investigations should be designed according to established principles. It is important to spend some time on this to ensure a successful investigation. People are often used to assess products (systems, job designs, environments, etc.) and they should be selected so that they are representative of the user population of interest, and of sufficient number to give meaningful results. Statistical sampling techniques are therefore used. Other methods of design to avoid bias when collecting data include methods to reduce order effects and to minimize interference with what is being measured. There are many texts on investigation design and Drury (1990) specifically considers the design of ergonomics studies and experiments.

User performance and evaluation

An expanding field in occupational hygiene is to use ergonomics methods in the user evaluation of products such as safety software or protective clothing. A representative sample of users (people who will use the product, system, etc.) would carry

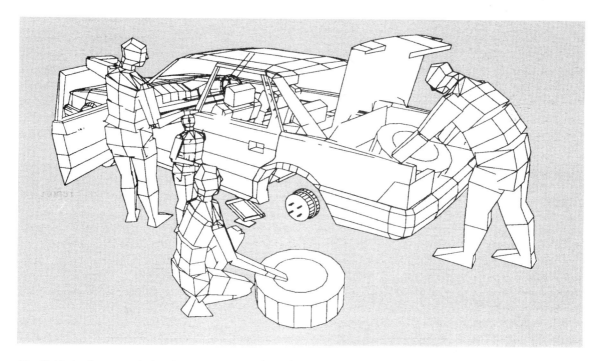

Fig. 15.12 Anthropometric data (SAMMIE or System for Aiding Man–Machine Interaction Evaluation) used in the design and evaluation of a car. A hierarchical data structure enables functional as well as geometrical relationships to be modelled, thus all moving parts of the model can be made to function. For example, the car's doors, bonnet and boot can be made to open and close. Inside the car it is possible to adjust the seat and steering wheel within the design specification.

out representative tasks and performance would be compared with criteria of acceptance. User performance tests for software, for example, would use people who will use the software in investigations to determine how well they can use it. This can be performed on a prototype design to give feedback and hence improve a future prototype for testing (iterative approach to design) or on a finished product where the level of performance of users is compared with what is considered as required and acceptable.

User performance tests should be 'correctly' designed and will typically involve a number of types of ergonomics method. To evaluate computer software for example, the number of keystrokes used, the speed and accuracy of performance and eye movements could be objective methods complemented by subjective measures of preference and ease of use. For protective clothing, a user performance test could involve a representative task, and environment and measurements of heart rate and sweat loss (objective) and ratings of stickiness and discomfort (subjective). A behavioural measure could be to observe who uses what clothing and in what way, given a free choice and a task to perform. Ergonomics in user testing has become so important and widespread that there are now a number of specialized 'usability' laboratories across the world. For further information on user tests and trials the reader is referred to McClelland (1990).

Task analysis

Task analysis is a fundamental ergonomics tool and, as it suggests, identifies tasks involved in jobs and the tasks required to complete a job successfully. The analysis of tasks can reveal human requirements necessary to complete the job and this can be compared with human capabilities and limitations. If these are exceeded then the job will not be completed; a system may then fail leading to the loss of productivity or an accident. Techniques of task analysis are therefore now widely used in the design and assessment of complex systems, such as in nuclear power stations. Its origins could be said to stem from the early work of Taylor on work study. However task analysis takes

this concept much further. It considers not only physical demands but also such things as information uptake, sensory requirements, mental and behavioural requirements and output requirements.

Task analysis techniques produce information that can contribute to the design of a new system or the evaluation of an existing one. The information is collected based upon an analysis of the human task requirements and behaviour. For a new system, systems diagrams and simulated tasks involving users may be employed. For existing tasks, systems diagrams may have to be created and jobs identified and described from observation of workers (e.g. pen and paper, computer and video methods of collection). For a more detailed description the reader is referred to Stammers, Carey and Astley (1990).

Systems ergonomics and the organization

In the 1960s and early 1970s it was generally recognized that jobs, machines, management, production workers, supporting staff and products were all connected and that all operate within 'systems' and should be considered as such. Systems therefore had objectives and goals, and if jobs were to be designed effectively then systems characteristics and objectives should be considered. The systems philosophy has many applications and engineers considered systems engineering and production systems, managers considered management systems and so on. This penetrated many applied disciplines and hence 'systems ergonomics' was developed. For a detailed description see Singleton (1974). This holistic systems philosophy was applied by ergonomists to provide a broader context in which to view man−machine−environment systems. Later developments included the effects of the organization, ergonomics not only considering the capacities and characteristics of individuals but also of groups and organizations and hence involving knowledge of social psychology and management. The modern ergonomist, therefore, would use the systems approach and involve the organization. Systems and information flow diagrams and organograms would be used, stakeholders identified and cost-effectiveness and marketing would also be considered.

There has been a convergence of subjects in this area. For example, occupational hygienists are encouraged to use a systems approach looking at safety systems and systems for the management of occupational health. Modern management studies include the design and management of jobs and organizations. All three disciplines have been greatly involved in organizational change brought about by the introduction of information technology. For further information on the ergonomics approach to information technology and organizational change, and so-called sociotechnical systems, see Eason (1988).

Examples of ergonomics investigation

It should be clear that ergonomics has a wide range of applications and it is important to recognize that it brings a user-centred philosophy to bear upon problems. Ergonomists sometimes give the impression that it is the solution to many problems and this is clearly not true. Ergonomics can, however, combine with other disciplines to contribute to solutions. In recent years a number of important developments (e.g. European directives) have promoted an interest in ergonomics. Some are closely related to occupational hygiene and a few of these are considered below with an attempt to identify the ergonomics contribution to the area.

Computer workstations

The development of information technology and in particular the wide availability and use of personal

Table 15.14 Seating and posture for typical office tasks

Seat back adjustability
Good lumbar support
Seat height adjustability
No excess pressure on underside of thighs and backs
  of knees
Foot support if needed
Space for postural change, no obstacles under desk
Forearms approximately horizontal
Minimal extension, flexion or deviation of wrists
Screen height and angle should allow comfortable
  head position
Space in front of keyboard to support hands/wrists
  during pauses in keying

computers, especially in offices, has had a great effect on the type of jobs and activities people perform. Areas of interest include the design of the computer hardware and workstation layout (leading to EEC directives and regulations), visual requirements and requirements for the design of computer software.

Ergonomics data concerning anthropometry (see Table 15.1), visual performance, postural control and related fatigue, key spacing on keyboards (see Table 15.10) and more, contributed to the formation of regulations for workstation design. Table 15.14 provides areas listed by the Health and Safety Display Screen Equipment Regulations, 1992 (Health and Safety Executive, 1992a).

Software design has also been considered in detail and has led to the expansion of what is termed 'cognitive ergonomics'. The design of software in structure will depend to a large extent upon the cognitive requirements and capabilities of users. Task analysis is used widely in this area. The requirements for the computer software interface design led to the publication of lists of ergonomics (human factors) guidelines. The limitations in available ergonomics data led to the development of methods of 'usability' testing, prototyping and also the construction of 'usability' laboratories. Systems approaches identify user requirements and software specification. Initially consumer and market pressure (only usable products were bought) led software development. Later, the importance of 'usable software' in complex and critical (e.g. safety) systems stimulated the production of regulations for software design.

Manual handling

Mital, Nicholson and Ayoub (1993) estimate that the direct costs for manual handling injuries in the USA is approximately 15 billion dollars annually and that indirect costs would be much more. Ergonomists can provide ergonomics data regarding lifting/lowering, carrying and pushing/pulling (see Table 15.12). An ergonomics systems approach may lead to the avoidance of the requirement to perform manual handling. Subjective, objective and modelling methods have been used to provide data. Regulations exist in the USA and Europe. In the

UK, the Health and Safety Executive Manual Handling Operations Regulations, 1992 apply (Health and Safety Executive, 1992b). Ergonomics data have been used to set limits, however each situation is unique and involves many variables (posture, twisting, what is lifted, person lifting, etc.). User tests and trials are possible, but there are important issues of safety and ethics. They must be carefully controlled to ensure that no injury occurs to subjects. Task analysis and improved equipment and job design may remove the necessity for manual materials handling. Some ergonomists propose that 'no lifting' should always be a design aim and that this starting position should only be moved from if necessary and by as little as possible.

Protective clothing and equipment

Protective clothing and protective equipment should protect the body against hazards. Comfort and performance are important but secondary concepts (although if a person is not comfortable the clothing may not be worn). An ergonomics systems approach may determine what would be an optimum solution, where the person can be separated from the hazard, thus obviating the use for personal protection. A task analysis can identify wearer requirements. Ergonomics data can provide information concerning restriction to vision, hearing, touch and manual dexterity. Data concerning physiological responses of wearers can contribute to predictions of heat stress and thermal discomfort. User trials are becoming widely accepted. Representative wearers perform tasks in representative environments (without the hazard!) and objective and subjective responses are measured and compared with criteria for acceptance. This will contribute to protective clothing and equipment design, evaluation and certification.

Other areas

An ergonomics approach can contribute to many other areas and includes environmental design and assessment, equipment design, evaluation of consumer products and work-related upper limb disorders, designing for maintenance, design of control rooms or vehicles, and many more.

REFERENCES

Davis, P.R. and Stubbs, D.A. (1977). Safe levels of manual forces for young males. *Applied Ergonomics*, **8**, 141–50.

Drury, C. (1990). Designing ergonomics studies and experiments. In *Evaluation of Human Work*, (ed. J.R. Wilson and E.N. Corlett), pp. 101–30. Taylor & Francis, London.

Eason, K.D. (1988). *Information Technology and Organisational Change*. Taylor & Francis, London.

Grandjean, E. (1988). *Fitting the Task to the Man*, (4th edn). Taylor & Francis, London.

Griffin, M.J. (1990). *Handbook of Human Vibration*. Academic Press, London.

Health and Safety Executive (1992a). *Display Screen Equipment Work*. Health and Safety (Display Screen Equipment) Regulations, 1992. HMSO, London.

Health and Safety Executive (1992b). *Manual Handling*. Manual Handling Operations Regulations, 1992. HMSO, London.

Hettinger, T. (1960). Muscle strength for men and women. *Zentralblatt Arbeit und Wissenschaft*, **14**, 7–84. (Cited in Grandjean (1993).)

Jurgens, H.W. (1973). Korpermasse. In *Ergonomie*, Band 1, (ed. H. Schmidtke). Carl Hanser Verlag, Munich. (Cited in Grandjean (1993).)

McClelland, I. (1990). Product assessment and user trials. In *Evaluation of Human Work*, (ed. J.R. Wilson and E.N. Corlett) pp. 218–47. Taylor & Francis, London.

Mital, A., Nicholson, A.S. and Ayoub, M.M. (1993). *Manual Materials Handling*. Taylor & Francis, London.

Olesen, B.W. (1977). *Thermal Comfort Requirements for Floors Occupied by People with Bare Feet*. ASHRAE Transactions, No. 83, Part 2.

Pheasant, S.T. (1986). *Bodyspace: Anthropometrics, Ergonomics and Design*. Taylor & Francis, London.

Singleton, W.T. (1974). *Man–Machine Systems*. Penguin, London.

Stammers, R.B., Carey, M.S. and Astley, J.A. (1990). Task analysis. In *Evaluation of Human Work*, (ed. J.R. Wilson and E.N. Corlett). Taylor & Francis, London.

Stranks, J. (1992). *A Manager's Guide to Health and Safety at Work*, (2nd edn). Kogan–Page, London.

Wilson, J.R. and Corlett, E.N. (ed.) (1990). *Evaluation of Human Work*. Taylor & Francis, London.

FURTHER READING

Bailey, R.W. (1982). *Human Performance Engineering*. Prentice-Hall, London.

Boyce, P.R. (1981). *Human Factors in Lighting*. Applied Science Publishers, London.

Chaffin, D.B. and Andersson, G. (1984). *Occupational Biomechanics*. John Wiley & Sons, New York.

Galer, I.A.R. (1987). *Applied Ergonomics Handbook*, (2nd edn). Butterworth, London.

Grandjean, E. (1987). *Ergonomics in Computerized Offices*. Taylor & Francis, London.

Health and Safety Executive (1992). *Work Equipment*. Provision and Use of Work Equipment Regulations, 1992. HMSO, London.

Health and Safety Executive (1992). *Personal Protective Equipment at Work*. Personal Protective Equipment at Work Regulations, 1992. HMSO, London.

Helander, M. (ed.) (1988). *Handbook of Human–Computer Interaction*. North-Holland, Amsterdam.

Kvalseth, T.O. (ed.) (1983). *Ergonomics of Workstation Design*. Butterworth, London.

Parsons, K.C. (1993). *Human Thermal Environments*. Taylor & Francis, London.

Putz-Anderson, V. (ed.) (1992). *Cumulative Trauma Disorders*. Taylor & Francis, London.

Van Cott, H.P. and Kinkade, Ph.D. (1972). *Human Engineering Guide to Equipment Design*. McGraw-Hill, Washington.

Wickens, C.D. (1984). *Engineering Psychology and Human Performance*. Merrill, Columbus.

CHAPTER 16
Biological Monitoring

T-C. Aw

INTRODUCTION

Biological monitoring is a tool that is available in occupational health practice to assess the extent of exposure, uptake and metabolism of chemicals in the workplace. It relies on the analysis of biological samples to provide an index of exposure and therefore gives an indication of possible risks to health. Biological monitoring complements environmental monitoring as a method for risk assessment and prevention of occupational ill health due to workplace chemical exposures.

DEFINITIONS AND TERMINOLOGY

Different definitions used for the term 'biological monitoring' include a variety of procedures for the health surveillance of workers in occupational heath practice. Some authors use the term to refer to any procedure used to monitor exposed workers, e.g. periodic X-rays, symptom enquiry or blood and urine tests. Others include tests indicating special effects, such as detecting the presence of DNA adducts in biological samples. Zielhuis (1985) drew attention to the confusion in terminology, and suggested that there should be some uniformity in the use of the term and its concepts. There is a need to distinguish biological monitoring from biological effects monitoring and health effects monitoring. The following definitions were advocated.

Biological monitoring. This is 'the measurement and assessment of workplace agents or their metabolites either in tissues, secreta, excreta, expired air or any combinations of these to evaluate exposure and health risk compared to an appropriate measure'. This definition restricts the term to the detection of chemical substances, or their breakdown products, in biological samples. It requires that there is an adequate and valid method for measurement, and that there is a means to decide on the extent of exposure and risk to health from the results obtained. While this definition confines it to workplace agents, the methods and application may also be used for non-occupational environmental exposure to chemicals. Biological monitoring does not include detection of alterations in enzyme levels or other biochemical changes in such samples. This is covered by the term 'biological effect monitoring'.

Biological effect monitoring. This term was proposed by Zielhuis and Henderson (1986) to refer to 'the measurement and assessment of early biological effects, of which the relationship to health impairment has not yet been established, in exposed workers to evaluate exposure and/or health risk compared to an appropriate reference'. The effect may not by itself be adverse to health but it would be an indication of a workplace agent causing some detectable biochemical alteration. An example of this is the detection of free erythrocyte protoporphyrin (FEP) in blood, or δ-aminolaevulinic acid in urine (ALA-D), of workers exposed to inorganic lead. FEP and ALA-D do not cause any direct pathological damage to the individual but increased levels of these chemicals reflect excessive exposure to, and absorption of, inorganic lead.

In occupational exposure to cadmium, the excretion of β-2 microglobulin (a small molecular weight protein) in the urine may be a transient or persistent effect. Its presence suggests renal tubular dysfunction. However, there are limited epidemiological data to show whether increased urinary levels of this small molecular weight protein lead to clinically significant renal damage. Detecting β-2 microglobulin in the urine for cadmium-exposed workers would therefore fall into the category of biological effect monitoring.

Acetylcholine is produced in the transmission of nerve impulses between nerves and muscles and is inactivated by an enzyme — acetylcholinesterase. Reduction in acetylcholinesterase activity is a biological effect that occurs with exposure to organophosphorus pesticides such as Diazinon, Malathion and Parathion, and to nerve agents such as Sarin and Soman. In exposure to these compounds the inhibition of cholinesterase is irreversible, whereas exposure to pesticides belonging to the carbamates group produces reversible inhibition. In the use of cholinesterase levels for biological effect monitoring, consideration has to be given to whether these levels are determined in red blood cells or in serum or plasma.

Health effects monitoring (health surveillance). This is 'the periodic physiological or clinical examination of exposed workers with the objective of protecting and preventing occupationally related diseases'. Examples of physiological tests are spirometry and audiometry. Clinical examination includes regular examination of the skin for chromate-exposed workers, and periodic review of symptoms to detect early clinical effects for workers exposed to glutaraldehyde or other respiratory sensitizers.

The UK Control of Substances Hazardous to Health regulations (COSHH) included biological monitoring under health surveillance, instead of keeping the two terms distinct. The American Conference of Governmental Industrial Hygienists (ACGIH) include biological monitoring and biological effect monitoring together for their list of biological exposure indices (BEIs).

INDICATIONS FOR BIOLOGICAL MONITORING

The main advantage of biological monitoring over environmental monitoring is that it assesses exposure from all routes — respiratory, dermal and oral, and not just airborne exposure alone. Key indications for considering biological monitoring are given below.

1 The occurrence of several routes of exposure and absorption of a chemical, e.g. organic solvents such as xylene, can be absorbed by inhalation and through the skin. Where the circumstances of workplace use of a chemical suggests that the route of absorption is likely to be through the skin and ingestion rather than by inhalation, ambient air monitoring as an indicator of exposure is less useful than biological monitoring.

2 The existence of valid laboratory methods for detecting the presence of the chemical or its metabolites.

3 The availability of reference values for interpreting the results obtained.

Biological monitoring can be used to confirm the efficacy of control measures, including the use of personal protective equipment. Where control measures have been instituted, the reduction or elimination of systemic absorption of a chemical can be confirmed by the absence of the substance or its metabolites in biological samples.

Biological monitoring is also useful when there are several sources of exposure to a chemical. These sources could be occupational and non-occupational. For example, a painter working with paint stripper in a poorly ventilated garage could have an increase in blood carboxyhaemoglobin due to several factors. The poor ventilation, and therefore poor supply of oxygen, could lead to the inadequate combustion of carbon compounds producing carbon monoxide in the garage. Methylene chloride in the paint stripper is metabolized to produce carboxyhaemoglobin. If the painter is a cigarette smoker, this will contribute to increased blood carboxyhaemoglobin. In this situation environmental monitoring for carbon monoxide will not give a complete indication of the risk to health. Biological monitoring for carboxyhaemoglobin levels in blood will be a better indicator.

TYPES OF BIOLOGICAL SAMPLES

The range of biological samples that theoretically can be obtained and analysed includes blood, urine, breath, fat, hair and nail, milk, faeces, sweat, saliva and semen. For biological monitoring in occupational health practice, it is primarily blood and urine samples that have been most widely used. Breath sample analysis is being developed increasingly for a number of organic solvents. Hair, nail and fat sample analysis are of limited use. There is scant published experience on the analysis of other samples for occupational exposures. Table 16.1 shows some examples of the types of biological samples that can be collected, and chemicals encountered in occupational settings and metabolites that can be identified in those samples.

Urine

Urine samples can be used to determine exposure by detecting the amount of the parent compound present, e.g. metals such as lead, mercury or cadmium. It can also identify the amount of

Table 16.1 Types of biological samples and analytes

Biological sample	Examples of parent compounds	Examples of metabolites
Urine	Heavy metals, e.g. organic lead, mercury, cadmium, chromium, cobalt Metalloids, e.g. arsenic Ketones, e.g. methyl ethyl ketone, methyl isobutyl ketone Other compounds, e.g. fluorides, pentachorophenol	Aromatic compounds, e.g. phenol (for benzene and phenol), hippuric acid (for toluene), methylhippuric acids (for xylenes), mandelic acid (for styrene and ethyl benzene) Chlorinated solvents, e.g. trichloroacetic acid (for trichloroethylene, perchloroethylene, 1,1,1-trichloroethane) Dialkylphosphates (for organophosphorus pesticides) 2,5-Hexanedione (for n-hexane)
Blood	Heavy metals, e.g. inorganic lead, mercury, cadmium, cobalt Aromatic compounds, e.g. toluene Chlorinated solvents, e.g. trichloroethylene, perchloroethylene, 1,1,1-trichloroethane	Carboxyhaemoglobin (for methylene chloride and carbon monoxide) Trichloroethanol (for trichloroethylene)
Breath	Aromatic compounds, e.g. benzene, toluene, ethyl benzene Chlorinated solvents, e.g. trichloroethylene, perchloroethylene, 1,1,1-trichloroethane, carbon tetrachloride, methylene choride	
Hair and nail	Arsenic, mercury	
Fat	Polychlorinated biphenyls	

metabolites of specific chemicals, e.g. organic solvents such as benzene (which produces phenol in the urine), toluene (hippuric acid), xylene (methyl hippuric acid) and styrene (mandelic acid). Alkyl phosphates are another example of metabolites which are detected in urine samples from workers exposed to organophosphate pesticides.

The main advantage of using urine samples is the ease of collection compared to blood or other biological samples. Exposed workers are also less likely to decline to co-operate when asked to produce urine samples rather than blood. However, urine samples are open to external contamination, and clear instructions must be given to the workers to wash their hands and ideally to shower and change out of their work clothes into clean clothes before providing a sample.

Several factors have to be considered before deciding on using urine samples for biological monitoring over other biological samples. Relevant factors are the specific chemical of interest, whether it is organic or inorganic and its valency state, as well as the period and duration of exposure. The following examples indicate when urine samples are used instead of blood for biological monitoring.

1 For metallic mercury, urine is the biological sample of choice for assessing longer-term (over a 3–4 week period) exposure. For recent, acute exposure (over 1 or 2 days) blood mercury gives a better indication of exposure.

2 In the case of exposure to inorganic lead, blood lead is preferred over urinary lead. However, for exposure to organic lead compounds the situation is reversed, with urinary lead as a better index than blood lead.

3 With exposure to chromium compounds, metabolism results in chromium being excreted in the urine in the trivalent form, regardless of whether exposure and absorption includes hexavalent as well as trivalent forms. Hence, total chromium in the urine will not indicate the relative exposures to different species of chromium compounds of different valency states.

Blood

Blood samples can also be collected to identify parent compounds or their metabolites. For ex-

posure to heavy metals such as lead, mercury and cadmium, blood levels are often determined for biological monitoring. For organic solvents such as perchloroethylene and trichloroethylene, the solvents themselves can be identified in blood. For other solvents, their metabolites can be detected in blood (e.g. free trichloroethanol for exposure to trichloroethylene) and in urine (e.g. trichloroethanol and trichloroacetic acid for exposure to trichloroethylene). Examples of metabolites from other organic solvents are shown in Table 16.1.

The disadvantages of using blood samples for biological monitoring include poorer co-operation from the workforce because of the discomfort of the procedure, especially if venepuncture is required on a regular basis. Some individuals may faint during venepuncture or even at the thought of the procedure. Facilities have to be in place to deal with this possibility. For those with veins that are not prominent, a degree of skill and experience is required to collect successfully a suitable quantity of blood. Otherwise a haematoma may result which can discourage the individual and his or her colleagues from future participation in biological monitoring.

Care must be taken to prevent external contamination of the blood sample, especially when the parent compound is to be determined. The site of venepuncture has to be adequately cleaned. For determining chromium levels in blood, the use of chromium-free needles has been suggested. Also, all precautions should be taken by the occupational health practitioner to prevent direct skin contact with the collected blood samples, therefore diminishing the risk of acquiring blood-borne infections. Practitioners who are regularly involved in collecting blood samples for biological monitoring should be fully immunized against hepatitis B, and use universal precautions in handling blood samples. All equipment used for venepuncture must be properly disposed of.

Breath

The model for breath sample analysis is the detection of alcohol in the breath by use of a breathalyser. The same principles can be used for detecting and quantifying other volatile organic compounds that are excreted in the breath. The process involves either breathing out into a direct reading instrument or into a glass pipette, aluminium tube, sampling bag or other collection device before dispatching the collected sample to a laboratory for analysis. The advantages of breath analysis are that the collection of samples is non-invasive, and repeated samples can be taken within a short period of time. The disadvantages include current lack of agreement on how samples have to be collected, standardization on the type of collecting device used, and laboratory methods for analysis. Analytical instruments for breath samples that can be used at the work site or for field studies are currently not widely available.

The ACGIH has indicated that exhaled breath samples are suitable for detection and determination of the following substances: benzene, toluene, carbon monoxide, ethyl benzene, n-hexane, methyl chloroform (1,1,1-trichloroethane), perchloroethylene and trichloroethylene (American Conference of Governmental Industrial Hygienists, 1993). The German Commission for the investigation of health hazards of chemical compounds in the work area (Deutsche Forschungsgemeinschaft) mentions alveolar air analysis for carbon tetrachloride, methyl chloroform (1,1,1-trichloroethane) and perchloroethylene. The ACGIH distinguishes between mixed-exhaled air and end-exhaled air and refers to the difference between these two types of breath samples in amounts of solvent detected during exposure and after exposure. Those with impaired lung function may not provide a suitable breath sample for such analysis. Cigarette smoking and endogenous compounds from dietary sources can also affect the breath levels of some compounds. Acetaldehyde concentrations in breath are higher in smokers than in non-smokers. Ammonia in breath can be derived from protein metabolism.

Hair and nail

Analysis of hair and nail samples has been used to assess exposure to arsenic and mercury. The rationale for this is that as hair and nail growth occurs, absorbed arsenic or mercury is incorporated into a segment of the hair or nail. In theory, providing that the rate of hair and nail growth is known,

this allows an estimation of when the exposure to these chemicals occurred. However, while hair grows at the rate of about 1 cm per month, there are periods of active as well as slow growth. This make any extrapolation of amounts of chemicals detected to the timing of exposure difficult.

Hair and nail analysis is seldom used in occupational health practice for biological monitoring as there are several practical difficulties, including cost and consistency of the analysis. External contamination of the hair and nail may give an erroneous indication of the amount absorbed systemically. Contamination may occur from occupational and non-occupational activity, and the use of hair dyes and shampoos can also affect the subsequent analysis. Procedures to wash and clean the samples before analysis may not adequately remove contaminants adsorbed onto the surface of the samples. The difference between amounts in head versus pubic hair, or in fingernail versus toenail samples, may indicate the extent of surface contamination. There are limitations in the interpretation of the results obtained, particularly for individuals rather than groups. Such analysis has also been tainted by apparent mail-order attempts at diagnosing and treating mineral deficiency and/or chemical overexposure, from hair and nail samples sent through the post.

Fat

Samples of body fat have been used for determining the extent of exposure to polychlorinated biphenyls (PCBs). PCBs are present in industrial transformers and have been documented as causing chloracne and liver damage. Besides the toxicity of PCBs and their contaminants, they are not easily biodegradable and therefore persist in the environment and in adipose tissue. Fat samples are obtained by needle biopsy or by surgical excision. The quantity of fat required for the assay of PCB content is several hundred grams. The amount of PCB determined is in parts per billion or parts per trillion quantities. Any contamination or error will cause a considerable difference in the estimate from the true value. It is not practical to collect fat samples periodically nor is it likely to attract many volunteers. This method, therefore, has considerable limitations for use in practical biological monitoring.

PRACTICAL CONSIDERATIONS

Timing of sample collection

For some substances, especially those with long half-lives, the timing of collection of the biological sample is not critical. This applies to blood lead and urinary cadmium. The half-life of a substance refers to the time required for clearance of 50% of the substance from the medium. For some chemicals, samples have to be taken at critical times during the working week. Examples of samples to be collected at the end of the work shift include urinary mandelic acid for styrene exposure, and urinary methylhippuric acid for xylene exposure. Samples to be collected towards the end of the working week include urine for arsenic levels, and urine for trichloroacetic acid from trichloroethylene exposure. For styrene in blood, ACGIH has produced sets of reference values which apply to: (1) samples obtained before the next work shift; and (2) those collected at the end of a work shift. The critical times for collection are in part related to the reference values established for interpreting the results (see Table 16.2).

Selection of the correct container for the biological samples

Precautions have to be taken to use a suitable container for the biological sample. The container must be able to hold a sufficient amount of the biological sample. The amount needed for analysis will be indicated by the laboratory. For urinalysis, 20–25 ml of urine is usually adequate for a spot sample; 24 h urine samples are collected in clinical practice but rarely for occupational health purposes because of the logistics of obtaining such samples for individuals at work. As little as 5 ml of blood may be sufficient for blood samples for most compounds. For breath samples, the volume collected depends upon the device provided by the laboratory. Most laboratories provide or recommend appropriate containers to use for biological samples.

Chemicals such as mercury can be adsorbed onto the surface of some polypropylene or polyethylene containers and this could result in the detection of a lowered urinary mercury level. For such chemicals, the use of a glass container would be better than a plastic bottle.

Chemical plasticizers used for plastic containers or bottle caps can interfere with the analysis for PCBs. Hence, in the collection of blood or adipose tissue samples for determining PCB levels, plastic receptacles should not be used. Because the quantities of PCBs determined are small, eliminating any interference with the analysis is critical to avoid considerable errors in the results.

The choice of a proper container also applies to blood samples. If serum samples are required, no anticoagulant is needed. If whole blood is required, then heparin or ethylenediamine tetra acetic acid (EDTA) should be present as an anticoagulant. However, since EDTA chelates metals, it would not be appropriate for whole blood determination for metals, e.g. chromium in red blood cells. Preservatives are also used for urine samples, especially if there is likely to be some delay between collection and delivery to the laboratory and subsequent analysis.

The amount of solvent in a blood sample is usually analysed in the laboratory by head-space analysis. This technique requires the volatile components in the sample to equilibrate with the atmosphere in the closed container. An aliquot of the air, containing the solvent vapour above the blood level in the container, is then injected into a gas chromatograph. Incomplete filling of the container with blood can lead to loss of solvent from the sample, resulting in a lower blood solvent result. It is therefore necessary, for this analysis, to fill the container up with as much blood as possible without spillage.

Contact with the laboratory

The choice of a suitable laboratory for analysis of biological samples is essential for obtaining valid results. Laboratories should have sufficient experience in analysing samples from occupational health, belong to a quality control scheme and have a quality assurance programme. In the USA, there is an Occupational Health and Safety Admin-istration (OSHA) list of laboratories for blood lead determinations. In the UK the Occupational Medicine and Hygiene Laboratory of the Health and Safety Executive (HSE), independent toxicology laboratories and those within the health service provide analysis of biological samples for a range of chemicals. Advice from the laboratory should be obtained on the quantity of the sample required, what special precautions are needed and how it is to be stored and delivered to the laboratory. Certain samples have to be kept at a low temperature and dispatched to the laboratory as soon as possible after collection. All samples should be adequately and securely labelled and packed. A large 'pooled' sample of urine due to breakage from poor packing, or a number of labels separated from their samples, is to be avoided.

INTERPRETATION OF RESULTS

Results from biological monitoring of similarly exposed workers are subject to intra- and inter-subject variation. Factors which have to be taken into account in the interpretation of results include:

1 those related to the individual (age, sex, body mass index, genetic differences in the metabolism of compounds, pregnancy state, exercise and physical activity, smoking, medication, con-sumption of alcohol and other dietary factors, and the presence of any existing lung, liver or kidney disease or other illness);
2 factors related to the exposure (timing and intensity of exposure in relation to timing of col-lection of the biological sample, mixed exposures which may affect the metabolism of the compounds absorbed, and routes of exposure);
3 factors related to the chemical of interest (half-life, where and how it is metabolized and excreted).

Reference values

In the UK, occupational exposure limits for air-borne substances are published annually in an HSE document — EH40. However, reference values for biological monitoring are not produced by the HSE in a similar format. Hence, other references,

including various documents produced by the HSE, will have to be consulted for interpreting the results of biological monitoring. The HSE Occupational Medicine and Hygiene Laboratory has an internal handbook with some information on interpreting such results. The HSE Guidance Notes (Medical Series) is another reference source. Scientific staff of the laboratory and employment medical advisers are available to assist with interpretation of biological monitoring data. Other analytical laboratories may provide some guidance on the interpretation of the results. The philosophy behind the determination of reference values has to be appreciated in order to use the values appropriately.

In the USA, BEIs are published annually by the ACGIH. BEIs are described as in general represent-ing 'the levels of determinants which are most likely to be observed in specimens collected from a healthy worker who has been exposed to chemi-cals to the same extent as a worker with inhalation exposure to the TLV', where 'TLV' is the threshold limit value. They are not meant as indicating a sharp distinction between hazardous and non-hazardous exposures. Exceeding these values do not necessarily indicate harmful effects or overt occupational disease, nor do levels below these values necessarily indicate a lack of adverse effect.

The list of BEIs appears together with the list of TLVs. Thirty-nine different substances or groups of substances are included in the 1993–1994 ACGIH booklet on TLVs and BEIs (American Conference of Governmental Industrial Hygienists, 1993). For each substance there is an indication of when the sample should be collected, whether the parent compound or the metabolite should be determined and what the BEI is. Where applicable, notations are also provided to indicate increased susceptibility for some individuals, the presence of background levels of some determinants in non-occupationally exposed groups, non-specificity of some findings and the semi-quantitative nature of some sub-stances measured. Also indicated are substances for which there is the intention to establish or change the indices. Further details of the BEIs are provided in the relevant ACGIH references.

The German Commission for the investigation of health hazards of chemical compounds in the work area (Deutsche Forschungsgemeinschaft) promulgate maximum permissible concentrations for airborne chemicals in the workplace (MAK values) (Forschungsgemeinschaft, 1993). It also proposes technical exposure limits (TRK values) particularly for carcinogens and mutagens, and biological tolerance values (BAT values) for biological monitoring. BAT values are defined as the maximum permissible quantity of a chemical compound, its metabolites or any deviation from the norm of biological parameters induced by these substances in exposed humans. In this context, the German Commission has included biological monitoring together with biological effect monitoring. The BAT list includes values for more than 30 different chemicals.

Table 16.2 provides a comparison of some values published by different organizations. It demonstrates the variation in values, units of expression and timing of sample collection.

Specificity of metabolites

In the interpretation of the results from biological monitoring it is essential to be aware of whether the compound detected in the biological sample is specific to the exposure of concern, or whether it may result from several sources of exposure. Some compounds produce mainly a single, specific metabolite, e.g. xylene is metabolized to methylhippuric acid in the urine, and this is not derived from other sources. Other compounds produce two or more metabolites, e.g. styrene is metabolized to mandelic acid and phenylglyoxylic acid. Phenylglyoxylic acid is also a metabolite of ethyl benzene. Benzene is metabolized to phenol in the urine, but this can also occur from phenol exposure. Hippuric acid in the urine can come from exposure to toluene, and also from ingestion of benzoic acid. Foods and drinks that contain benzoic acid as a preservative can therefore form a dietary source of urinary hippuric acid. Trichloroethylene exposure results

Table 16.2 Reference values for biological monitoring: some examples for blood, urine and exhaled air samples

Chemical	HSE	ACGIH	DFG
Blood lead	70 µg per 100 ml	50 µg per 100 ml	70 µg per 100 ml for men and 30 µg per 100 ml for women < 45 years of age
Blood carboxyhaemoglobin for carbon monoxide exposure	—*	3.5% at end of shift	5% at end of exposure or end of shift
Urine inorganic mercury	120 nmol mmol^{-1} creatinine	35 µg g^{-1} creatinine for preshift sample	200 µg l^{-1}
Urine methylene dianiline	50 nmol mmol^{-1} creatinine	—	—
Urine mandelic acid for styrene exposure	—	800 mg g^{-1} creatinine for end of shift sample	2 g l^{-1} at end of exposure or end of shift
Perchloroethylene in end-exhaled air	—	5 ppm for sample prior to last shift of work week	9.5 ml m^{-3} at the beginning of the next shift
Carbon monoxide in end-exhaled air	—	20 ppm for end of shift sample	—

* Dashes indicate that no specific reference value has been specified.
HSE, Health and Safety Executive; ACGIH, American Conference of Governmental Industrial Hygienists, Inc.; DFG, Deutsche Forschungsgemeinschaft.
For values for other substances see American Conference of Governmental Industrial Hygienists (1993) and Forschungsgemeinschaft (1993).

in the metabolites trichloroethanol and trichloro-acetic acid. About 1–2% of absorbed perchloro-ethylene is also excreted in the urine as trichloro-acetic acid. Xylene is metabolized to the specific metabolite methylhippuric acid which is not pro-duced from dietary sources. There are three dif-ferent isomers of xylene (ortho-, meta- and para-) and it is possible to detect three related isomers of methylhippuric acid in urine from exposure to a mixture of isomers of xylene.

Units of expression for results

The data from Table 16.2 shows that different units are used for expressing the results from bio-logical monitoring. This tends to add confusion when interpreting results. Blood results are nor-mally expressed in $mg\,l^{-1}$. Urinary levels of com-pounds are often expressed in mg or μg per unit volume of urine, which has the disadvantage of being affected by urinary concentration or dilution. Expressing urine results in terms of the specific gravity of the urine sample has been suggested and used. However, most of the proposed reference values for substances in urine are not published in this way; 24 h urine samples will even out the fluctuations in urine concentration throughout the day and indicate the total amount of a compound excreted in the 24 h period. Whilst this is possible with hospital in-patients, it is impractical for biological monitoring of worker populations. Creatinine correction has therefore been used to overcome these limitations. Creatinine is a protein excreted in the urine. It is an indication of muscle mass and is affected by fever and compromised renal function. The daily excretion is, however, fairly independent of urine concentration or di-lution and is relatively constant at $15-20\,mg\,kg^{-1}$ for females and $20-25\,mg\,kg^{-1}$ for males. There is an attempt now for reference values for many chemicals or their metabolites in urine to be expressed in terms of $mg\,g^{-1}$ creatinine, or $mmol\,mmol^{-1}$ (SI units) of creatinine. As a rough guide for converting $mmol\,mmol^{-1}$ creatinine to $mg\,l^{-1}$ the following formula has been suggested:

$$mg\,l^{-1} = (mmol\,mmol^{-1}\,creatinine) \times (mol.\,wt\,of\,chemical) \times 10$$

This is based on the assumption that 1 l of urine contains about 10 mmol of creatinine.

Interference by concomitant exposure to other chemicals

Consumption of alcoholic beverages can interfere with the biological monitoring for certain com-pounds such as the organic solvents. In addition to causing additive, synergistic or antagonistic clinical effects, ethanol may delay the rate of metabolism of compounds by competing for the liver enzymes involved. Ethanol is metabolized by liver dehydrogenases, catalase and mixed-function oxidases. The competition for acetaldehyde de-hydrogenase between ethanol and trichloroethylene delays the metabolism of trichloroethylene to trichloroacetic acid and causes the clinical phenomenon 'degreaser's flush' which is seen in trichloroethylene-exposed workers who have recently consumed alcohol. A similar facial flush occurs in exposure to N,N-dimethylformamide, cyanamide and carbon disulphide. Competition for enzymes can increase the blood level of the solvents xylene, toluene and trichloroethylene if there is occupational exposure and concomitant alcohol consumption during the work shift. This will also cause a decrease in the amount of urinary metabolites of these solvents.

Where several metabolites are produced from exposure to one chemical, ethanol may have a differential effect on the rate of production of these metabolites. Alcohol ingestion with concomitant styrene exposure leads to a greater reduction in mandelic acid than in phenylglyoxylic acid (both are metabolites of styrene) in blood and urine. Poorly metabolized compounds, such as perchloro-ethylene and 1,1,1-trichloroethane, are not affected by alcohol ingestion.

However, regular alcohol consumption can cause induction of microsomal enzymes in the liver. Because of their non-specificity, these enzymes can speed up the metabolism of certain organic solvents (e.g. styrene). Alteration in the rate of metabolism will mean that the timing of collection of biological samples in relation to the period of exposure can be crucial in interpreting the results of biological monitoring. As a recognition of the variation in the nature and extent of the effect of alcohol on metabolism of some chemicals, it has been suggested that alcohol consumption should be avoided on days when biological monitoring is to be performed.

Cigarette smoking can affect enzymatic activity in lung parenchymal cells and in alveolar macrophages and may alter the rate of metabolism of inhaled compounds. This may explain the difference in acetaldehyde levels in the breath in exposed smokers compared to non-smokers.

Aspirin consumption can affect the metabolism of xylene. It reduces methylhippuric acid concentration in the urine by competing for glycine. This amino acid is essential for conjugation in the metabolism of both aspirin and xylene. Other medications such as barbiturates are known to induce liver enzymes, and can alter the rate of hepatic breakdown of absorbed chemicals.

OTHER PRACTICAL, LEGAL AND ETHICAL ISSUES

Training of staff to collect biological samples

Occupational health practitioners who have to carry out biological monitoring should have adequate training in how to collect the biological samples, especially blood samples. Experience in phlebotomy is essential, including the need to take all necessary precautions during collecting, handling and transport of samples, and disposal of equipment used. Those who collect biological samples should also be capable of explaining the reasons for the procedure, indicate what tests will be done on the samples and reassure the workers on what tests will not be performed, e.g. HIV testing on blood samples. They should also have the means to interpret the results and be aware of extraneous factors that can affect these results. Within the UK, biological monitoring is usually performed by an occupational physician or occupational health nurse. Occupational hygienists and other occupational health practitioners with relevant training can acquire the necessary competence to participate in biological monitoring.

However it is essential to recognize when outside assistance may be required.

Notification of biological monitoring results

The individual worker is entitled to his or her own results with an explanation of what they indicate. This is the responsibility of the occupational health professional carrying out the monitoring. The results should also be communicated to the person's family physician (general practitioner) for inclusion into the health records, since the individual may raise this with his or her doctor on subsequent visits to the surgery. Management and unions can be provided with grouped data, taking the necessary precautions to retain confidentiality by removing specific identifiers. Feedback should also be provided to other occupational health and safety practitioners, and where required to the appropriate regulatory agencies. Occupational hygienists would find the results valuable to complement findings from environmental monitoring, and to confirm satisfactory control measures for reduction of exposure.

Storage of biological monitoring results

The UK COSHH regulations require that where biological monitoring as part of surveillance is performed, the results are kept for at least 40 years from the date of last entry. If such records are properly collected, recorded and stored, they can be of value in future epidemiological studies. Where companies cease operations, current advice is for the collected results of biological and environmental monitoring to be offered to the Health and Safety Executive.

CONCLUSIONS

Biological monitoring will be used to a greater extent for assessing occupational exposure to chemicals as new methods are developed for detecting and quantifying substances or metabolites in biological samples. Advances in laboratory technology will allow smaller quantities of chemicals to be detected in biological samples with greater sensitivity and specificity. Reference values will have to be agreed to allow clear and uniform interpretation of results. Recognition of the limitations of the process and the many factors that can affect the results is essential. More occupational health practitioners may endeavour to carry out biological monitoring to complement environmental monitoring, but the precautions needed, and the skills required have to be considered. In the future, the techniques of biological monitoring may be extended from occupational exposures to non-occupational environmental exposures. This would aid in risk assessment in occupational and environmental settings and would be a useful tool for the prevention of occupational and environmental ill health from chemical exposures.

REFERENCES

American Conference of Governmental Industrial Hygienists (1993). *1993–1994 Threshold Limit Values for Chemical Substances and Physical Agents and Biological Exposure Indices.* ACGIH, Cincinnati.

Forschungsgemeinschaft (1993). *MAK and BAT-Values 1993.* Commission for the Investigation of Health Hazards of Chemical Compounds in the Work Area. Report No. 29. VCH Verlagsgesellschaft, Weinheim.

Zielhuis, R.L. (1985). Biological monitoring: confusion in terminology. (Editorial.) *American Journal of Industrial Medicine,* **8**, 515–16.

Zielhuis, R.L. and Henderson, P.T. (1986). Definitions of monitoring activities and their relevance for the practice of occupational health. *International Archives of occupational and Environmental Health,* **57**, 249–57.

FURTHER READING

Aitio, A., Järvisalo, J., Riihimäki, V. and Hernberg, S. (1988). Biological monitoring. In *Occupational Medicine: Principles and Practical Applications,* (2nd edn.), (ed. C. Zenz), pp. 175–97. Yearbook Medical Publishers, Chicago.

Fiserova–Bergerova, V. (1993). Interference of alcoholic beverage consumption with biological monitoring of occupational exposure to industrial chemicals. *Applied Occupational and Environmental Hygiene,* **8**(9), 757–60.

Health and Safety Executive (1992). *Biological Monitoring for Chemical Exposures in the Workplace.* HSE Guidance Note Environmental Hygiene Series EH56. HMSO, London.

Kneip, T.J. and Crable, J.V. (ed.) (1988). *Methods for Biological Monitoring: a Manual for Assessing Human Exposure to Hazardous Substances.* APHA, Washington DC.

Lauwerys, R.R. (1983). *Industrial Chemical Exposure: Guidelines for Biological Monitoring.* Biomedical Publications, Davis.

Lowry, L.K. (1986). Biological exposure index as a complement to the TLV. *Journal of Occupational Medicine,* **28**(8), 578–82.

Monster, A.C. (1986). Biological monitoring of chlorinated hydrocarbon solvents. *Journal of Occupational Medicine,* **28**(8), 583–8.

Notten, W.R.F., Herber, R.F.M., Hunter, W.J., Monster, A.C. and Zielhuis, R.L. (ed.) (1988). *Health Surveillance of Individual Workers Exposed to Chemical Agents.* Springer-Verlag, Berlin.

Wilson, H.K. (1986). Breath analysis: physiological basis and sampling techniques. *Scandinavian Journal of Work, Environment and Health,* **12**, 174–92.

CHAPTER 17
Sampling Strategies

K. Gardiner

INTRODUCTION

The actual measurement of workplace contaminants must always be seen as only part of a holistic approach to the prevention or reduction of ill health at work (Health and Safety Executive, 1991). The major purpose of a sampling strategy is that by careful consideration of the issues involved (which are discussed below), the validity of the data generated will be maximized and thereby the inferences drawn will be strengthened. This should also ensure the most cost-effective approach.

This chapter attempts to highlight and integrate the many issues which need to be considered before embarking on a sampling programme (whether one or thousands of samples are to be taken), but is not meant to be a definitive exposition of the mathematical derivation of sampling methodologies. These issues are applicable to the measurement of any workplace contaminant, however, this chapter will draw mainly on the requirements for the measurement of airborne contaminants. Safety issues, such as the assessment of flammability or the ability of an environment to sustain life, are not covered.

The fundamental questions referred to above are given below and should be, and are, addressed in turn. As all of these issues are integrated, it is not prudent to address any one in isolation.

Questions to address

1 Why sample?
   Level of approach?
2 What to measure?
3 How to sample?
4 Whose exposure should be measured?
5 Where to collect the sample?
6 When to measure?
7 How long to sample for?
8 How many measurements/readings?
9 How often to sample?
10 What to do with the data?
11 What to record?

WHY SAMPLE?

This is the most fundamental question of all and needs a satisfactory answer before proceeding. There are many reasons for taking measurements (some of which are given below) and the strategy by which the data has to be collected for each is different.

In a perfect world there would be no exposure to any toxic substances. However, it is not perfect and there are exposures to toxic substances. In a nearly perfect world, everyone doing the same job would receive the same exposure. Again this is not true, as in real life exposure is variable and the magnitude of its variability is dependent upon such factors as: the nature, density and intensity of activity/process/people, the contaminant(s) of interest and environmental components such as temperature, windspeed, wind direction, humidity, etc. (Fig. 17.1).

As alluded to at the beginning of this chapter, our primary concern is the prevention or minimization of occupationally induced ill health and therefore the elimination and control of workplace contaminants is our ultimate aim. To this end, one

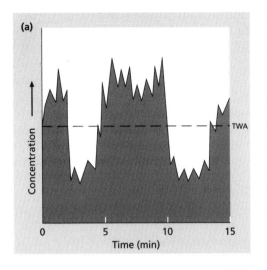

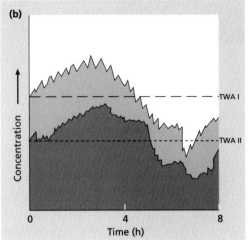

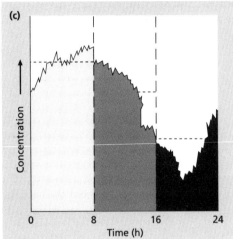

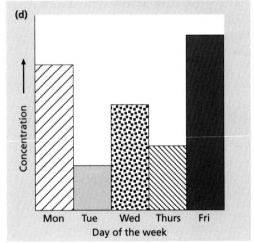

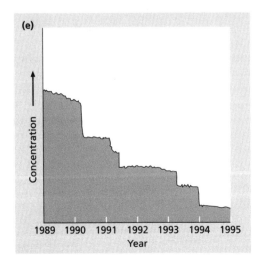

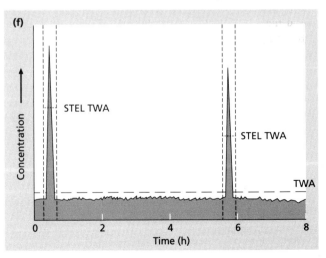

must ask the question 'Why sample at all?'. If something is clearly wrong and readily rectifiable without the taking of measurements then it would be prudent to do so, thereby avoiding additional expense and delay. However, below are some examples where the taking of measurements may be justified.

- Assessment of compliance.
- Assessment of health risk.
- Epidemiological study.
- Selection of control requirements.
- Assessment of control performance.
- Litigation.

Assessment of compliance

The most common reason for sampling is to determine whether an individual's or a group of individuals' exposure exceeds an occupational exposure limit (OEL). This usually requires the a priori selection of part of the workforce which is undertaking a task using certain contaminants, and is usually designed to be a 'worst case scenario'. If the exposure of these individuals is significantly less than the standard, then by default, everyone else's will be as well.

However, exposure can vary greatly, both within and between individuals, days, shifts, etc. (see Fig. 17.1) and therefore this approach can be limited and generate misleading results. It is necessary to look carefully at the wording and meaning of the legislation in each country. In the UK there are two standards: occupational exposure standards (OESs) and maximum exposure limits (MELs). A MEL is the maximum concentration of an airborne substance to which employees may be exposed and it is the employer's duty to reduce and keep exposure as far below the MEL as is reasonably practicable. Exposure measurements should be taken to show that the MEL is not normally exceeded, i.e. 'that an

occasional result above the MEL is without real significance and is not indicative of a failure to maintain adequate control' (rather than the actual measurement being statistically significantly above the standard). In comparison, for those substances assigned an OES, 'if exposure by inhalation exceeds the OES, then control will still be deemed to be adequate provided that the employer has identified why the OES has been exceeded and is taking appropriate steps to comply with the OES as soon as reasonably practicable' (COSHH, 1994). It is therefore clear that, unlike in the USA, there is no requirement for compliance testing in the UK. However, despite this, there is an expectation by enforcers and employers that exposure can be characterized by the measurement of a few individuals on a single day doing a limited number of different tasks. As a result, potentially incorrect and costly decisions may be made.

There are a number of substances where there is a clear legislative requirement to take measurements, such as vinyl chloride monomer, chromic acid, lead and asbestos. With these substances there is less flexibility in terms of sample location, frequency, etc., but the same philosophy in terms of comparison with an OEL is present.

Assessment of health risk

A great deal of the legislation currently emanating from the European Community requires the 'assessment of risk' – in this case to health (COSHH, 1994). This can be both quantitative and qualitative, thereby moving away from the prescriptive and limited comparison of exposure levels with exposure standards. Therefore, a sampling strategy designed to assist in the assessment of health risk must relate to the biological phenomena which dictate the risks of disease.

These include the rate of uptake (inhalation,

Fig. 17.1 (*Facing page*) Examples of the variability of exposure: (a) hypothetical personal exposure as measured by continuous monitoring and the integrated 15 min time-weighted average (TWA) exposure; (b) hypothetical continuous trace and integrated TWA personal exposure for two individuals undertaking the same work over an 8 h period; (c) hypothetical continuous trace and integrated TWA personal exposure for three individuals undertaking the same work on different shifts over a 24 h period; (d) hypothetical 8 h TWA personal exposures for an individual undertaking the same work over a period of a week; (e) hypothetical trace of weekly TWA personal exposures for an individual undertaking the same work over a number of years; and (f) hypothetical trace of personal exposure and 8 h and 15 min TWAs of a contained process with occasional fugitive omissions.

skin absorption and ingestion), the rate of elimination and therefore the burden (dose), and the rate of repair (Rappaport, 1991). Clearly, different approaches are needed for acute or chronic toxicants than for substances which may have very serious short-term effects or for those that are irritant and/or narcotic.

Epidemiological study

The main objective of an epidemiological study (see Chapter 20) is to determine if exposure to a contaminant affects the health status of a group of individuals. The requirements of the sampling strategies are therefore often more akin to those of health risk assessment than to those of compliance, as one is more interested in the precise estimation of mean group exposure from low- to high-exposed groups than in the measurement of specific individuals undertaking specific tasks. Again, the study design (which should reflect the nature of the contaminant), whether it be prospective, cross-sectional or retrospective (see Chapter 18), will dictate the sampling strategy. If sampling prospectively, epidemiological requirements are likely to be different from those of compliance testing as, for example, one is likely to be concerned with contaminants believed to be harmless at the time, and/or to be well below the current OEL.

Selection of control requirements

If it has been decided that a contaminant and/or process is not under adequate control, it may be necessary to take measurements to determine how much exposure needs to be reduced by. Unfortunately, actual measurements are often needed to justify capital expenditure. Examples include the choice of face velocities, hood design, volume flow rates, etc. for ventilation systems (see Chapter 22), respirator selection (see Chapter 23) and octave band analysis for the choice of noise control (see Chapter 9).

Assessment of control performance

Once a contaminant and/or process is deemed to be under control it may be necessary to ensure the continued performance of the system. This can be either by the measurement of the contaminant or by direct assessment of the process itself. However, simple techniques such as the Tyndall beam or dust lamp may be sufficiently effective but significantly cheaper and faster.

Litigation

It is unfortunate that exposure to contaminants may cause detrimental health effects, but in these litigious times some redress is being found. However, the measurement of the contaminant(s) of interest and the strategy for its collection may have an impact for both the plaintiff and the defendant.

LEVEL OF APPROACH

Having determined the reason for sampling, it is necessary to determine the need or importance of the answer, thereby prioritizing which contaminants and/or processes are associated with the highest degree of risk (Corn, 1985). Some risk determinants include: the number of potentially exposed individuals; the toxicity of the substance(s); the quantities used over some arbitrary reference period; the likely duration and concentration of exposure (plus exposure via routes other than inhalation), i.e. dose; existence and confidence in control measures; likelihood and magnitude of change to the process and its control; and the presence of substances which may be potentiators or act synergistically or antagonistically with contaminants.

Occupational hygiene surveys can be broken down into four levels relative to the level of priority assigned: an initial assessment, a preliminary survey, a detailed survey and routine monitoring. The level of survey is obviously related to the importance associated with the answer (as described above) and the magnitude of the survey relative to the factors involved (numbers of people, variability, etc.). Figure 17.2 is a self-explanatory flow diagram to aid in the visualization and understanding of this process. Greater detail of the information needed or obtained by these various levels is available elsewhere (British Occupational

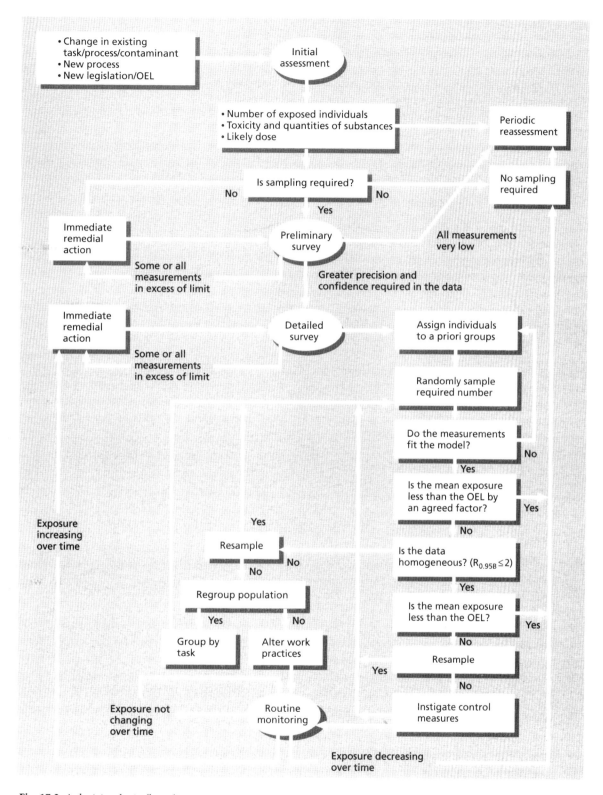

Fig. 17.2 A decision logic flow diagram.

Hygiene Society, 1993; Health and Safety Executive, 1989).

Providing specific answers (who, which, etc.) for the general areas given above (compliance, health risk, etc.) is outside the remit of this chapter and the reader needs to determine whether the issue and/or the data provided is relevant for their purpose.

WHAT TO MEASURE?

Rarely in industrial situations is only one substance used and therefore a decision must be made as to which, of potentially many, contaminants should be measured? Reference to the original aim of sampling will assist (i.e. compliance or health risk). There are three main options which involve the assessment of: (1) all, or many, of the contaminants; (2) the 'mixture' as a whole; or (3) reference/surrogate substance(s).

1 The increasing availability of techniques able to identify and quantify large numbers of contaminants has improved the possibility of measuring multicontaminant mixtures. However, this process will certainly be expensive. For compliance purposes there may be a number of substances in the mixture with OELs and with the same site of action, thereby necessitating this approach along with the use of the additive equation:

$$\frac{Conc_1}{OEL_1} + \frac{Conc_2}{OEL_2} + \frac{Conc_n}{OEL_n} \leq 1 \qquad (17.1)$$

This approach may also be necessary where the components in the mixture and their relative ratios are constantly changing.

2 Instead of breaking down a mixture into its component parts (as in (1) above), the contaminant of interest is by definition a mixture (e.g. rubber, foundry or welding fume). The OEL is therefore set and assessed on this basis. Again, this approach may satisfy the needs of compliance testing but not those of health risk assessment. For example with welding, issues such as the proportion of hexavalent chrome may be important for both compliance and health risk assessment. Other examples are the measurement of non-specific dusts (either respirable or total inhalable) whose values are compared to the respirable and total dust standard of 5 and $10 \, mg \, m^{-3}$ respectively.

3 Where a mixture has been well characterized in terms of its constituents and relative ratios throughout a process, it is possible to measure one or a limited number of these as a surrogate for the whole. The choice of which one(s) may be dictated by the difficulty or ease of measurement and analysis, and/or the state of toxicological knowledge and existence of OELs.

If approach (3) is to be undertaken, issues such as the type of standard (OES or MEL) and the basis on which they have been set, the toxicity of the various components (e.g. whether carcinogenic), the proportion of each component in the bulk material and the volatility and thereby likely airborne concentrations of each component should be addressed (British Occupational Hygiene Society, 1982). It is believed that by using this method (3), if the concentration of the most volatile and/or toxic substance is under control, then by default so should all other contaminants.

A useful means of combining both the OEL (ppm) and the volatility of a substance (which is temperature dependent) is the 'vapour hazard index or ratio' (see Chapter 6):

$$VHR = \frac{Saturation \; concentration \; (SC)}{OEL} \qquad (17.2)$$

HOW TO SAMPLE?

This chapter will not reiterate the techniques of sampling covered in other chapters. However, it is necessary to discuss some of the requirements in selecting the appropriate method from those available.

Depending on the question being addressed, and the level of approach required, it is not always necessary to use the technique that has the greatest accuracy, precision, sensitivity and specificity. Not foresaking practical issues, such as the intrinsic safety, user acceptability (i.e. weight and size) and performance (i.e. flow rate range and battery longevity) of the equipment, the sampling and analytical methods chosen should meet the requirements of the sampling strategy and not vice versa (Rappaport, 1991).

With reference to compliance testing, it is possible to determine crudely the specificity and sensitivity requirements of a sampling technique. Figure 17.3 shows the relationship between method requirements and concentration relative to the OEL, with the widest and darkest parts of the figure being those most relevant to their definitions. All measuring techniques are subject to error, certainly random error and perhaps systematic error. Knowledge of this for all parts of the sampling train and subsequent analyses is necessary to ensure that it is minimized and that comparability is maximized. This may include the: contaminant stability; sampling device (i.e. dust head); sampling media and its stability (i.e. absorber/adsorber or filter); tubing; pump (i.e. flow rate fluctuations); and analytical technique. The potential and magnitude of the error varies within a sampling train, and between the sampling trains required for different contaminants. For example, the flow rate can easily be set incorrectly relative to the requirements of the instrument (i.e. cyclones) or in absolute terms (i.e. the rotameter reads $2.01\,m^{-1}$ but in reality it is $1.81\,m^{-1}$).

WHOSE EXPOSURE SHOULD BE MEASURED?

In a workplace with a few staff all doing similar jobs, the need to separate people into groups as the basis for individual selection is small, however, in large workforces undertaking a multitude of different tasks the need is greater. (This issue is inextricably linked with the number of samples, which is discussed below.) If specific groups are being focused upon, then consideration of the following may be of use: those already unwell (i.e. asthmatics using sensitizers); those working for extended periods (i.e. greater than 8 h); those working at an elevated rate (i.e. they will potentially be breathing more in) and those undertaking maintenance and related unscheduled tasks. As discussed previously, the option of which of the worker groups to sample is dictated by the reason for sampling; but first, it is necessary to determine the means by which the groups are defined.

If the strict definition of homogeneity is that all the exposure distributions of all workers have the same means and standard deviations (which is almost unheard of) then one is left with the contentious issue of how homogeneity can be defined and tested in a manner that is useable and achievable. There are two main methods by which the population to be sampled can be grouped and assessed for homogeneity and they are prospective and retrospective employee groupings.

Prospective employee grouping

Prospective employee grouping relies on the ability of the occupational hygienist to assign individuals to a group or 'zone' before sampling, on the basis of the following criteria: similarity of tasks; exposure to the same range of airborne contaminants; similarity of the environment (i.e. process equipment, exposure and controls); and the ability to identify an individual with a specific zone (Corn and Esmen, 1979). Although this technique was developed for epidemiological purposes, it lends itself to the

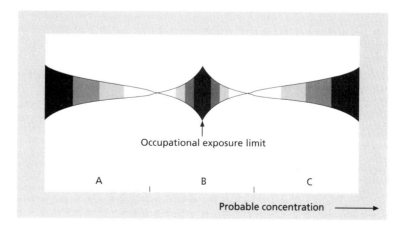

Fig. 17.3 The requirements of the measuring technique relative to the exposure concentration: A, technique requires good sensitivity and reasonable specificity; B, technique requires good specificity and reasonable sensitivity; C, technique does not necessarily require either good sensitivity or specificity.

Occupational exposure limit

A   B   C

Probable concentration ⟶

needs of compliance testing. The major benefit is that when the measurement of personal exposure confirms the homogeneity of the group, this allows decisions on compliance, control, etc. to be made with greater confidence. The zones in a workplace can be redefined but this should also be a prospective exercise.

Care needs to be taken in the selection of certain individuals, such as those involved in maintenance or non-routine tasks. These individuals are also likely to be at the higher end of the exposure profile and may need to be grouped separately. There has not been a rigid definition of homogeneity but it clearly relates to the variability of the data. Therefore, measures such as the standard deviation or geometric standard deviation (where log-normality is known or has been determined) are used for sizeable data sets and non-parametric measures, such as the inter-quartile range, are used for small data sets. The Health and Safety Executive (1989) state a crude but useful rule, that is: if an individual's exposure is less than half, or greater than twice, the group mean then they should be reassigned to another group.

Retrospective employee grouping

It has been proposed that instead of prospectively allocating individuals into groups before sampling, the whole exposed population should be sampled randomly with groups created retrospectively (Rappaport, 1991). It was felt that this technique was the most appropriate means of assessing chronic exposure and effect (i.e. health assessment and/or epidemiology) as it is not always possible to identify individuals by inspection. Unlike for compliance testing, where the highest exposure is usually of interest, for health assessment and epidemiology the precise estimation of the mean exposure and the within and between worker variability are of importance (Kromhout, Symanski and Rappaport, 1993; Rappaport, Kromhout and Symanski, 1993).

After random sampling of the workforce, the data must be grouped. (In the main, occupational hygiene data is log-normally distributed, but if possible its distributional form should be tested.) However, it is necessary first to identify the

components of exposure variability. The exposure to an airborne contaminant of all workers on all days ('total distribution') has a geometric mean μ_c and geometric standard deviation $\sigma_{g,T}$. Each individual has their own personal distribution of day to day exposures ('within worker distribution') which can be characterized by individual geometric means $\mu_{c,W}$ and geometric standard deviation $\sigma_{g,W}$. To assess these, one would need to undertake repeat measurements over a period of time on the same individuals. In addition, there are differences in mean exposure between the individuals ('between worker distribution') and this has the same geometric mean value (μ_c) as the distribution of all exposures. However, the geometric standard deviation of the 'total distribution' ($\sigma_{g,T}$) is larger than the between worker geometric standard deviation ($\sigma_{g,B}$) as it represents the combination of both the within and between worker components of exposure variability (Fig. 17.4).

As previously mentioned, 'useable' homogeneity has no strict definition but Rappaport (1991) has arbitrarily defined a 'monomorphic group' with reference to the between worker distribution. A 'monomorphic group' is one in which 95% of the individual mean exposures lie within a factor of 2. This implies that the ratio of the 97.5th percentile to the 2.5th percentile ($R_{0.95B}$) is not greater than 2 and would have a between worker geometric standard deviation ($\sigma_{g,B}$) of ≤ 1.2.

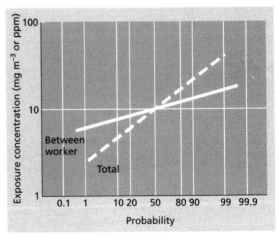

Fig. 17.4 Hypothetical probability plot showing the difference between total and between worker distributions.

In practice this arbitrary factor of 2 may be too restrictive as inferred by the Health and Safety Executive (HSE) in the UK. They recommend that individuals' mean exposure should be within a range of 0.5–2 times the group mean (Health and Safety Executive, 1989). It is clear that the HSE values (0.5–2) relate to the minimum and maximum means and not the 2.5th and 97.5th percentile. However, if this factor of 4 (2/0.5) was for the 2.5th and 97.5th percentile then this would correspond to a monomorphic group with $R_{0.95B} \leq 4$ and a between worker geometric standard deviation $(\sigma_{g,B})$ of < 1.4.

If used for epidemiological purposes, inhomogeneity can result in overlapping exposure distributions and hence misclassification, which ultimately leads to the tendency to underestimate the relationship between exposure and health outcome. However, the insistence and use of absolute criteria for (in-)homogeneity may not always be necessary, as it is feasible for the exposure distributions of two or more inhomogeneous groups $(R_{0.95B} > 2)$ not to overlap. Under these circumstances, the estimate of the relative risk at a certain exposure level will be unbiased although lacking precision (Heederik, Kromhout and Burema, 1991).

It is also suggested that comparison of within and between worker geometric standard deviations can be used to indicate the source of the exposure variability. A comparatively large within worker geometric standard deviation indicates that the exposure is governed primarily by the process or environmental conditions shared by all (thereby the observational or prospective approach should provide a valid assessment of exposure) and comparatively large between worker geometric standard deviations indicate that individual tasks or practices are important determinants of exposure. It is these differences in individual practices which are difficult to observe and thereby limit the validity of the prospective approach.

WHERE TO COLLECT THE SAMPLE?

The occupational hygienist has two main choices with regard to the location of the sampling device: either to place the equipment on the individual (personal) or to fix it to a tripod and for it to be static over the duration of sampling (static). If an assessment of compliance or health risk is being undertaken, the preferred location is personal as this is most likely to reflect the individual's exposure. In fact, for all but a few substances (e.g. cotton dust, the annual MEL for vinyl chloride monomer and subtilisins (proteolytic enzymes)) the OELs are specific to personal exposure.

It is conventional to call the microenvironment to which an individual will be exposed the 'breathing zone' and this is defined as approximately 20–30 cm from the nose and mouth (Fig. 17.5(a)). However, recent work has brought into question this concept and reliance on the results from it. One study (Vaughan, Chalmers and Botham, 1990) showed that when a dust sampler was placed equidistant from the nose and mouth on each lapel there was a twofold difference between the results in 5% of the cases. It is also known that substances with a high degree of thermal buoyancy, such as welding fume and colophony (from rosin core pyrolysis or flow solder baths), generate a reasonably well-defined plume which rises sharply. A significant proportion of this may miss the lapel-located sampler, but, as a result of the nature of the work and therefore the required body position, will generate significant exposure. The welding head sampler is therefore mounted on a cranial cap or on the inside of airstream welding helmets (Fig. 17.5(b)). Perhaps colophony fume would be sampled better by the use of 13 mm open-faced heads located on safety spectacles, thereby again more accurately reflecting true exposure. Clearly, consideration of the work activity must be given before placement of the equipment, and discussion with the worker with regard to wearability may be fruitful.

As there is a poor relationship between static samples and real personal exposure their use is less prevalent, however, they do have specific uses. The main one is in the assessment of the requirements and performance of control measures. The fixed location of the sampler strengthens the validity of comparing concentrations pre- and post-control intervention without the variability inherent with personal samples. Some measuring devices are large and barely portable, let alone suitable for personal sampling. This is especially true for continuous monitoring devices or where very large volumes of

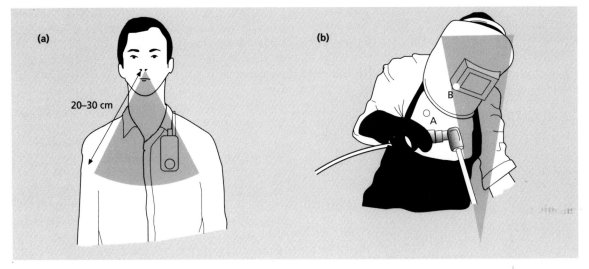

Fig. 17.5 Location of sampler: (a) breathing zone highlighted with sampler located in its 'normal' lapel position; and (b) well-defined plume missing the 'normal' lapel position (A), and sampler located underneath welding helmet next to nose/mouth (B). From Health and Safety Executive (1989 and 1990). Crown copyright is reproduced with the permission of the Controller of HMSO.

air are needed to be sampled due to the low ambient concentrations. Occasionally static samples can be used as a surrogate for personal exposure, especially where the nature of the work may make the wearing of additional sampling equipment more hazardous, or where a clear relationship between static measurements and personal exposure has been defined (e.g. on return roadways in coalmines).

WHEN TO MEASURE?

This question can relate to when to sample within a day or shift, or on which day of the week or shift to sample. Processes can be split into three main types — continuous, cyclic or random — whether they are considered within a day or over a number of days. In fact, most major processes will have elements of all three (i.e. in a carbon black plant the production part is continuous, the packaging of the material is cyclic and the maintenance work is random). A degree of familiarity of the process is necessary for this to be known and should greatly improve the validity of the measurements.

Depending on the reason for taking the measurements, the sampling should reflect the nature of the process. For example, if the process is continuous it will not matter greatly if the sampling is continuous, cyclic or random. In comparison, if the

process is cyclic, the time and/or day on which samples are taken is critical. This is because the period over which the measurement is taken could exactly match the duration of the peaks or troughs, however, if the duration of the process cycles is much shorter than the duration of the sampling cycles then this is of less importance. Obviously for health risk assessment and epidemiological purposes, the random choice of when to sample is more appropriate, provided the frequency of sampling is great enough. This is to ensure that tasks rarely undertaken are likely to be included.

HOW LONG TO SAMPLE FOR?

In the main, for the purposes of compliance testing, the duration over which the sample should be taken is dictated by the reference period of the OEL. In the UK, there are both long-term 8 h time-weighted average (TWA) exposure limits and short-term 15 min TWA exposure limits (STEL) (the reference period of 15 min for the STEL recently having been changed from 10 min). However, for well-controlled, continuous processes with very little variability, periods shorter than the 8 h reference period may be sufficient as a surrogate of the whole work period. Also, it is not uncommon for two or more quite different tasks to be undertaken within one day and therefore two separate samples are taken and the TWA then calculated relative to an 8 h reference period. Compliance testing against a STEL is difficult, due to the lack of sensitivity and precision of most techniques when the ambient concentration is low and the flow rate of the instrument is either limited (i.e. low flow pumps for adsorbent tubes) or set (cyclones). If the magnitude of the outcome of failure to control exposure to the STEL is great then it may be preferable to use continuous monitoring devices.

Chronic toxicants

The issues of how long to sample for with regard to health risk assessment and epidemiology is more complex. Rappaport (1991) has used the toxicokinetic properties of substances to produce a model that indicates that exposure variability must be transmitted through to body burden and ultimately damage if it is to affect the risk of disease. For those substances with a chronic effect, the transmission of day-to-day variation in exposure diminishes rapidly if its biological half-life $(T_{1/2})$ is $10\,h < T_{1/2} < 100\,h$, so that less than half of the variability is expected to reach the tissues when $T_{1/2} > 40\,h$. This value of $T_{1/2}$ can be used as a strategic benchmark to identify contaminants for which day-to-day variation in exposure is unlikely to be important (Rappaport, 1988 and 1991). This means that tissue damage, the very entity we are trying to assess and ultimately prevent, would be related to the mean exposure and time. However, this presumes linear kinetics, but issues such as synergistic or antagonistic effects (from concurrent exposure to other contaminants), allergic reactions to sensitizers or from an upward-curving burden damage relationship (from periods of intense exposure saturating the normal clearance processes) may mean that the translation of exposure to damage is non-linear.

The major benefits of this are that instead of taking five 8 h samples over the period of a week, fewer samples taken over a longer duration (e.g. a week) may be possible (depending on the ambient concentration and sampler overload). Clearly, however, information relating to compliance, task-specific short-term fluctuations and control will be lost.

Acute toxicants

For substances with an acute effect, their rate constants for biological elimination and repair are in the range of seconds to hours and therefore the transfer between exposure and tissue damage occur within the time frame of a single shift. In addition, the transmission of exposure variability to the site of damage (the tissues) is likely to be efficient. Non-linearity together with acute responses means that short-term exposure variability cannot be ignored as it is likely to be the primary determinant of acute response.

As mentioned above, the required sensitivity and precision of the measuring techniques are often not capable of accurately characterizing exposure whether it be for compliance or assessment of health risk and therefore continuous monitoring may be more appropriate. However, it may be advantageous to differentiate between those acute responses that lead to potentially irreversible effects (phosgene–pulmonary oedema) and temporary effects such as irritation or narcosis (sulphur dioxide, xylene) as well as the likely variability of the process or job. In epidemiological studies, it may be necessary to look carefully at the profile of the exposure; for example, it has been postulated that it is in some way the 'peakiness' of the exposure to sensitizers that causes sensitization rather than the dose (Gardiner, 1995).

It is often thought that instead of struggling to measure short-term exposure it may be better to concentrate on elimination or control of the problem — which is the philosophy with which we started.

HOW MANY MEASUREMENTS/ READINGS?

Hopefully, it is becoming apparent that the variability of exposure data is such that taking one or two samples on one day is insufficient to reach any conclusions about the workplace. Therefore, in the main, the greater the number of samples taken the better. However, everyday constraints, such as time and money, mean that in large workforces (i.e. more than 10 people doing the same job) the exposure of only a proportion can be assessed. The number of samples taken is also dependent upon the pre-existing knowledge of within and between person exposure variability as most methods rely on group homogeneity, as has already been defined. For example, instead of having a workforce of 100 with the generic title of lathe operator, you may have 10 homogenous sub-groups of varying sizes. The following are some examples of the means by which the number of samples can be calculated and, not withstanding the reason for sampling, increased in sophistication and hence reliability.

If no information is available on the cohort of interest then general guidance is required. The HSE (Health and Safety Executive, 1989) suggest at least one in 10 individuals are sampled (this is perhaps suitable for a very large population) and Corn (1985) suggests that at least three samples should be taken from the population of interest and if the difference between them is greater than 25% then additional samples should be taken. It is often stated that an occupational hygienist can 'cope' with between 5 and 10 'sampling trains' at the same time. It would therefore be prudent to define the homogenous group to be sampled in such a way that the 5–10 samples constitutes as large a proportion as possible (i.e. if possible sample everyone, but the greater the proportion the better).

The National Institute for Occupational Safety and Health (NIOSH) promulgated a method by which one could decide that one wanted at least one measurement from the sampled population to be in the top T% with C% confidence (Leidel, Busch and Lynch, 1977). This was designed specifically as a compliance tool but has been used in epidemiological studies as a means of calculating a 'reasonable proportion' of a workforce in 18 separate locations with five comparable job categories without any a priori knowledge of exposure (Gardiner et al., 1992). Tables exist wherein one specifies the upper fraction of exposure (e.g. top 10%) and the confidence with which one wants to find an exposure measurement in that fraction (e.g. 95% confidence). The total number of individuals in the defined homogenous group is determined (group size) and then the required number of samples to be taken in that day is read off (Table 17.1). These values are not dependent upon knowledge of distributional form. These values can be calculated by the following:

for large populations (infinite size $(N = \infty)$)

$$n = \frac{\ln \alpha}{\ln (1 - \tau)} \tag{17.3}$$

Table 17.1 Sample size selection (NIOSH)

Top 20% with 90% confidence (Use $n = N$ if $N \le 5$)		Top 20% with 95% confidence (Use $n = N$ if $N \le 6$)		Top 10% with 90% confidence (Use $n = N$ if $N \le 7$)		Top 10% with 95% confidence (Use $n = N$ if $N \le 11$)	
Size of group (N)	No. of samples required (n)	Size of group (N)	No. of samples required (n)	Size of group (N)	No. of samples required (n)	Size of group (N)	No. of samples required (n)
6	5	7–8	6	8	7	12	11
7–9	6	9–11	7	9	8	13–14	12
10–14	7	12–14	8	10	9	15–16	13
15–26	8	15–18	9	11–12	10	17–18	14
27–50	9	19–26	10	13–14	11	19–21	15
51–∞	11	27–43	11	15–17	12	22–24	16
		44–50	12	18–20	13	25–27	17
		51–∞	14	21–24	14	28–31	18
				25–29	15	32–35	19
				30–37	16	36–41	20
				38–49	17	42–50	21
				50	18	∞	29
				∞	22		

for groups of size N $(N < \infty)$

$$\alpha = \frac{(N - N_0)!}{(N - N_0 - n)!} \times \frac{(N - n)!}{N!} \qquad (17.4)$$

where N is the group size, n is the sample size, $1 - \alpha$ is the confidence $(C\%/100)$, τ is the proportion of the group $(\tau = \text{top } T\%/100)$ and N_0 is $N.\tau$.

It is clear that with small groups, the proportion needed to be sampled is greater than for large population sizes and that as the selection criteria becomes tighter, the proportion of the bigger group sizes to be sampled gets greater. Care needs to be taken as there is a probability $(100 - C\%)$ of missing workers in the top $T\%$ and to ensure that there are no repeat measurements.

Knowledge of the geometric mean and geometric standard deviation from previous surveys can be used to calculate the required number of samples. If no data are available, then mean exposures and their standard deviations can be either estimated or extracted from published data for comparable industries. It is preferable to overestimate rather than underestimate the geometric standard deviation as this will maximize the sample size (i.e. > 2). Therefore, the number of samples required (n) can be calculated from these data using the formula:

$$n = \left(\frac{t\,\text{CV}}{E}\right)^2 \qquad (17.5)$$

where CV is the coefficient of variation (SD/mean), E is the acceptable or chosen level of error and t is the t-distribution value for the chosen confidence level and $n_0 - 1$ degrees of freedom.

For example, normally distributed carbon black data with an arithmetic mean of $6.0\,\text{mg m}^{-3}$, standard deviation of $2.0\,\text{mg m}^{-3}$, chosen error limit of 5%, 95% confidence level and $t = 1.960$ (degrees of freedom ∞):

$$n = \left(\frac{1.960 \times 2.0/6.0}{0.05}\right)^2$$

$$n = 171 \text{ samples}$$

Therefore, to estimate the mean concentration of the population within 5% of the 'true' mean with 95% confidence, 171 samples from the same group would be needed! Clearly, the greater the hom-

ogeneity and acceptable/allowable error and the less the confidence required, the smaller the number of samples needed.

It is suggested that if the data are known or suspected to be log-normally distributed the same formula can be used. This is because the central limit theorem states that the distribution of means is approximately normal, even for log-normally distributed data sets.

An alternative formula can be used if the population of interest is small, i.e. when $10\,n < N$ (where N is the population size):

$$n\,\frac{(N - 1)}{(N - n)} = \left(\frac{t\,\text{CV}}{E}\right)^2 \qquad (17.6)$$

If compliance testing is being undertaken then it is possible to choose the number of samples relative to the required degree of compliance to the OEL. Rappaport and Selvin (1987) have promulgated an equation to test the arithmetic mean exposure against the OEL with a certain statistical significance and power and thereby provide the required sample size needed (Table 17.2). Again, it is clear that the greater the variability and the closer the mean value is to the standard, the greater the number of samples required.

For sample durations of less than the complete shift, it has been postulated that approximately 25% of the exposure duration should be sampled (with the proviso that there are no significant systematic variations in exposure). However, if the fixed duration of the sampling device is 1 min, then

Table 17.2 Sample size requirements for testing the mean exposure from a log-normal distribution of 8 h TWAs (95% significance and 90% power)

Mean/OEL	Geometric standard deviation for sample size (n)				
	1.5	2.0	2.5	3.0	3.5
0.1	2	6	13	21	30
0.25	3	10	19	30	43
0.5	7	21	41	67	96
0.75	25	82	164	266	384
1.25	25	82	164	266	384
1.50	7	21	41	67	96
2.00	2	6	11	17	24
3.00	1	2	3	5	6

Table 17.3 Minimum number of samples required per shift relative to the predetermined sample duration

Sample duration	Minimum number of samples per shift
10 s	30
1 min	20
5 min	12
15 min	4
30 min	3
1 h	2

in an 8 h shift 120 samples would be required. In reality this is not feasible and sufficient statistical stability is reached with 20 samples per shift. Table 17.3 shows the minimum number of samples as a function of sample duration.

In epidemiology, the numbers of samples required to be taken often relies on detailed information about the partitioning of the exposure variability before a study commences formally. For example, in studies where everyones exposure is measured, then the number of repeat measurements per worker can be calculated (along with prediction of the bias in the regression coefficient) by use of the within to between worker variance ratio (Boleij *et al.*, 1995):

$$\beta^\star = \frac{\beta}{\left(1 + \dfrac{\lambda}{n}\right)} \tag{17.7}$$

where $\beta^\star$ is the observed regression coefficient, β is the true regression coefficient, λ is the variance ratio (within to between worker variance) and n is the number of measurements per individual.

HOW OFTEN TO SAMPLE?

'How often to sample' within a day has been covered under 'when to sample'? However, there still remains the issue of over how many days, etc. should samples be taken. Equation 17.5 can also be used to determine the number of days on which measurements need to be taken to estimate an individual's true mean exposure within a certain error limit and confidence. For example, the following respirable dust data (mg m^{-3}) were collected over eight days: 1.27, 1.33, 1.36, 1.49, 1.67, 1.75,

1.80, 2.48. Therefore:

Geometric mean (GM)   = 1.61 mg m^{-3},
Geometric standard
deviation (GSD)   = 1.24 mg m^{-3},
Arithmetic mean (AM)   = 1.64 mg m^{-3},
Arithmetic standard
deviation (ASD)   = 0.39 mg m^{-3},
Minimum variance
unbiased (MVU) AM   = 1.64 mg m^{-3},
Minimum variance
unbiased (MVU) SD   = 0.36 mg m^{-3},
Coefficient of variation
(from MVU estimators)   = 0.22.

With a 10% error limit and 90% confidence, Equation 17.5 provides the number of days on which samples need to be taken as:

$$n = \left(\frac{1.645 \times 0.22}{0.1}\right)^2$$

$$n = 14 \text{ days}$$

Note: always round the figure up for the number of samples or days.

If it is felt that it is not acceptable to determine the precision of the estimation of the arithmetic mean and instead an estimate of the geometric mean is required with the same precision, then the coefficient of variation (CV) can be replaced by the ratio of the natural log of the geometric standard deviation (GSD) to the natural log of the geometric mean (GM) (see Equation 17.8):

$$n = \frac{\left(t\,\dfrac{\ln \text{GSD}}{\ln \text{GM}}\right)^2}{E} \tag{17.8}$$

$$n = \frac{\left(1.645\,\dfrac{\ln 1.24}{\ln 1.61}\right)^2}{0.1}$$

$$n = 56 \text{ days}$$

If the same data are used as in the previous example (GSD of 1.24 mg m^{-3}) it would suggest that 56 samples are required in order to have 90% confidence and that the natural log of the sample geometric mean will be within 10% of the true geometric mean. In this case, a 10% range for the natural log GM is from 1.54 to 1.69 mg m^{-3} which is perhaps an excessive degree of precision, thereby explaining the radical increase in the number of samples from 14 to 56. As previously discussed, geometric standard deviations are rarely as low as 1.24 and therefore the number required to be sampled would normally be even higher (Dewell, 1989).

Routine monitoring

For some substances and processes, a long-term routine monitoring programme based over the period of a year or longer may be appropriate. The frequency of sampling can be determined by deciding what annual sample size, n, is sufficient to obtain acceptable estimates of the parameters of the finite population $(n = pA)$, where p is the number of individuals chosen for each trial and A is the number of trials per annum. For most purposes, the mean and variance of the distribution should be estimated.

There are a number of schemes by which the frequency of monitoring can be related to the ratio of mean exposure to the OEL. It has been suggested by Roach (1977) that the closer the measured exposures are to the OEL, the greater the frequency of sampling and that those values either significantly above or below the OEL need to be sampled less frequently. The frequency of sampling, per 10 employees, is given in Table 17.4.

The Comité Européen de Normalisation (CEN) have suggested a scheme which also uses action levels (N1 to N4) as determinants of sampling activity (Comité Européen de Normalisation, 1992); this is given in Table 17.5. The action levels are:

N1 = 0.4 OEL:
N2 = 0.7 OEL;
N3 = 1.0 OEL;
N4 = 1.5 OEL;

and the scheme is as outlined below.

- Once the need for periodic measurements has been decided the first one is carried out within 16 weeks. The maximum time until the next sample depends on the previous result.
- If the exposure is < 0.25 OEL then the sample interval is 64 weeks.
- If the exposure is > 0.25 OEL but < 0.5 OEL then the sample interval is 32 weeks.
- If the exposure is between 0.5 OEL and the OEL then the sample interval is 16 weeks.

Care needs to be taken to ensure that the same job is not being sampled each and every time and that seasonal effects are avoided.

Table 17.4 Minimum frequency of regular monitoring

Shifts to be sampled (per 10 employees)	Exposure/OEL
1 per month	1–2
1 per quarter	0.5–1 or 2–4
1 per annum	0.1–0.5 or 4–20
None	< 0.1 or > 20

OEL; occupational exposure limit.

Table 17.5 Measurement frequencies relative to action levels N1–N4

Exposure relative to action level	Sampling activity
C ≤ N1 twice consecutively	Omit the following three measurements
C ≤ N2	Continue basic schedule
* N2 < C ≤ N4	A new measurement is taken during the next time unit
* N2 < C ≤ N4 for two consecutive units	An additional measurement is done in the four subsequent programmed intervals. If this is one time unit, immediate action should be taken to reduce exposure
N3 < C ≤ N4 twice consecutively	Take immediate action to reduce exposure
C > N4	Immediate action to be taken to reduce exposure

* If C > N3 appropriate measures to improve control should be identified and implemented

WHAT TO DO WITH THE DATA?

It is hoped that, because the reason for sampling was identified before embarking on the measurement programme, it is known what we are going to do with the data now it has been collected. Unfortunately, this is not always the case and one is reminded of the adage: 'don't ask a question if you don't know what to do with the answer'.

The belief exists, in the profession, that almost all data are log-normally distributed, however, this assumption is rarely tested. It is possible to test the skewness and kurtosis of a distribution, but this is complex and not always informative. More readily interpretable, and certainly less complex, is the cumulative probability plot. This is a plot of the individual data points as a cumulative frequency curve where the percentage scale has been adjusted so that log-normal distributed exposure data will produce a straight line. The drawn line will summarize the characteristics of the population from which the samples were taken and enables generalizations and predictions to be made (Fig. 17.6).

To draw a log-probability plot, the data should be ranked in ascending order, the number of results counted, the appropriate plotting points taken from Table 17.6 and the results plotted against the corresponding point on log-probability paper (Chartwell 5575). If it is possible to draw a straight line 'by eye' then do so, but it is preferable to calculate the correct line. One method by which this can be done is by taking logarithms of the data, calculating the geometric mean (GM) and standard deviation (GSD) and then plotting $GM \times GSD^{1.65}$ against the 95th percentile and $GM/GSD^{1.65}$ against the 5th percentile. Draw a straight line between the two points and, as a check, see if the line passes through the geometric mean at the 50th percentile. Care needs to be taken as this is not a 'goodness of fit' test.

A number of useful measures such as the GM and GSD can be estimated from the plot (provided that this has not already been undertaken to calculate the line itself). The GM can be calculated by reading up from the 50th percentile until intersecting the line, and the concentration is then read off

Table 17.6 Log-probability plotting points

Rank order	5	6	7	8	9	10	11	12	13	14	15	16	17	18	19	20	Rank order
1	12.9	10.9	9.4	8.3	7.4	6.7	6.1	5.6	5.2	4.8	4.5	4.2	4.0	3.8	3.6	3.4	1
2	31.5	26.6	23.0	20.2	18.1	16.3	14.9	13.7	12.7	11.8	11.0	10.3	9.8	9.2	8.7	8.3	2
3	50.0	42.2	36.5	32.1	28.7	25.9	23.7	21.8	20.1	18.7	17.5	16.4	15.5	14.7	13.9	13.2	3
4	68.5	57.8	50.0	44.0	39.4	35.6	32.4	29.8	27.6	25.7	24.0	22.5	21.3	20.1	19.1	18.1	4
5	87.1	73.5	63.5	56.0	50.0	45.2	41.2	37.8	35.1	32.6	30.5	28.7	27.0	25.5	24.2	23.0	5
6		89.1	77.1	67.9	60.7	54.8	50.0	46.0	42.5	39.6	37.0	34.8	32.8	31.0	29.4	27.9	6
7			90.6	79.8	71.3	64.4	58.8	54.0	50.0	46.5	43.5	40.9	38.5	36.4	34.5	32.8	7
8				91.7	81.9	74.1	67.6	62.1	57.5	53.4	50.0	47.0	44.3	41.8	39.7	37.7	8
9					92.6	83.7	76.3	70.2	64.9	60.4	56.5	53.1	50.0	47.3	44.8	42.6	9
10						93.3	85.1	78.3	72.4	67.4	63.0	59.2	55.8	52.7	50.0	47.6	10
11							93.9	86.3	79.9	74.3	69.5	65.3	61.5	58.2	55.2	52.5	11
12								94.4	87.3	81.3	76.0	71.4	67.3	63.6	60.3	57.4	12
13									94.8	88.2	82.5	77.5	73.0	69.1	65.0	62.3	13
14										95.2	89.0	83.6	78.8	74.5	70.6	67.2	14
15											95.5	89.7	84.5	79.9	75.8	72.1	15
16												95.8	90.3	85.4	81.0	77.0	16
17													96.0	90.8	86.1	81.9	17
18														96.2	91.3	86.8	18
19															96.4	91.7	19
20																96.6	20

For sample size > 20: Plotting point $= \dfrac{\text{Rank order} - 0.3}{\text{Sample size} + 0.4} \times 100$

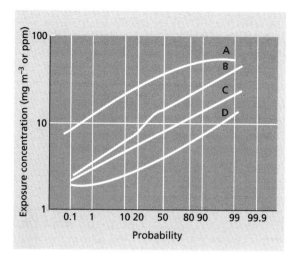

Fig. 17.6 Four hypothetical probability plots:
A, probability plot of a right-truncated distribution;
B, probability plot of a mixture of two distributions;
C, probability plot of a log-normal distribution;
D, probability plot of a left-truncated distribution.

the y-axis. The GSD is calculated by dividing the values gained from the 84th percentile by that gained from the 50th percentile. The gradient or slope of the line is therefore indicative of the variability of the results; the steeper the gradient the greater the variability (see Who to Sample? and Fig. 17.4).

Other valuable information which is readily obtainable from these plots includes a simple guide to the proportion of the population above or below a certain level of exposure. For example, the proportion of exposure measurements likely to be above 10 (arbitrary units) in Fig. 17.6, line C is about 30%. In addition, if the line is right-truncated (i.e. flattened to horizontal at the top) it is suggestive of the measuring device reaching the point of saturation (Fig. 17.6, line A), whereas if it is left-truncated (i.e. flattened to horizontal at the base) it is suggestive that the exposure is low and therefore the measuring device has reached its limit of detection due to insufficient sensitivity (Fig. 17.6, line D). If there appear to be potentially two distinct line segments then this is suggestive that in fact two separate populations have been measured (Fig. 17.6, line B). Lastly, two or more lines can be drawn on the same plot, perhaps to compare different systems of work or control techniques.

If compliance is being assessed, it is possible to take a pragmatic approach and simply divide the measured concentration by the OEL and make decisions based on this dimensionless index of exposure (Comité Européen de Normalisation, 1992). For example, if the value is 0.1 and the STEL conditions are fulfilled then compliance is assumed. However, when there is a high degree of variability in high-risk situations, incorrect conclusions may be drawn.

Another technique to determine compliance is to use the mean and variance of the exposure distribution to calculate the probability of a measurement exceeding the OEL. If the probability is $\leq 0.1\%$ then compliance is assumed, if the probability is $> 0.1\%$ but $\leq 5\%$ then the situation is probably compliant but more measurements are needed and, finally, if the probability is $> 5\%$ then the situation is not in compliance (Comité Européen de Normalisation, 1992).

These one-sided tolerance tests can be described for a log-normal distribution by the test statistic T_{u}:

$$T_{\mathrm{u}} = X_{\mathrm{L}} + K.S_{\mathrm{L}} \qquad (17.9)$$

where X_{L} is the geometric mean, S_{L} is the geometric standard deviation and K is a factor (the tolerance interval coefficient) determined by the level of confidence, the number of measurements and the percentage of measurement required to be within the tolerance interval. Unfortunately, a great number of samples are required as the proportion of measurements above the OEL increases. Table 17.7 gives an indication of the magnitude of the sampling effort required as the fraction of measurements above the OEL rises.

It has long been postulated that the mean ex-

Table 17.7 Number of measurements required to determine compliance with 95% confidence that less than 5% of all exposures are above the occupational exposure limit (OEL)

Percentage of exposure greater than OEL	Number of measurements required for a decision
0.1	8
1	22
2	50
3	Approximately 133
4	Approximately 600

posure is the best index of risk for chronic toxicants and Rappaport and Selvin (1987) have put forward an equation for the assessment of compliance, wherein if the mean exposure or some fraction of it is above the OEL then the situation is deemed to be non-compliant (based on log-normal distribution). The test statistic's distribution approximates that of a t distribution (with $n - 1$ degrees of freedom) and for compliance $T < t$ (t is taken from 't' values for the confidence level selected):

$$T = \frac{\bar{X}_c - OEL}{S_{\bar{X}_c}} \qquad (17.10)$$

where $\bar{X}_c$ is the maximum likelihood estimate of the mean concentration and $S_{\bar{X}_c}$ is the standard error of $\bar{X}_c$:

$$\bar{X}_c = \exp(\bar{x} + 0.5s^2)$$

where $\bar{x}$ is the mean of the log-transformed measurements and s^2 is the variance of the log-transformed measurements:

$$S_{\bar{X}_c} = \left[\mu_c^2 \frac{(S_L^2 + 0.5S_L^4)}{(n - 2)}\right]^{0.5}$$

where μ_c is the OEL.
Again, as the variance increases and the mean approaches the OEL, the required number of samples needed to determine compliance increases (see Table 17.2).

WHAT TO RECORD?

It is always necessary to record observations both at the time of sampling and in any subsequent reports. It is also advisable to record more information than one would have thought necessary at first, as on enquiry, the memory has often rapidly faded and if someone else is attempting to read and interpret the report, additional qualifying information is always of benefit.

Figure 17.7 is an example of a sample record sheet which is useful for both on-site recordings and for formalizing the information provided in a report. A plea from an occupational hygienist involved in epidemiological research is to state clearly the reasons for the measurement being taken, the person being chosen, when measurements were taken, etc., as retrospective reviews

and exposure assessments (see Chapter 18) of existing data are very difficult without this additional information.

OTHER ISSUES

Autocorrelation

It is necessary to be aware that sequential air samples may not be independent, i.e. the result of one measurement may affect the result of a subsequent one. This, the autocorrelation function $p(h)$, is often referred to as the third characteristic of a distribution (after the mean and variance) and defines the relationship between air concentrations separated by h intervals of time (h is the lag). A purely random series of results would have $p(h) = 0$ for all lags and a perfectly correlated series would have $p(h) = 1$ for all lags (Rappaport and Spear, 1988). If a high degree of autocorrelation does occur then invalid conclusions could be drawn about real exposure.

Periods of work greater than 8 h

The ever-changing requirements of employers in terms of the duration of work or their shifts may mean that potential difficulties arise when comparing exposures with OELs devised for five 8 h days per week. Clearly, the longer the day over which the contaminant is absorbed, the shorter the period of recovery before the next insult. For substances with very short half-lives this may not be a problem, but for those whose half-lives approach or exceed 16 h (the period of recovery for an 8 h working day) the body burden may rise over the week or shift period. A number of sophisticated models utilizing pharmacokinetics have been put forward but unfortunately they require a great deal of substance-specific information which is very rarely available. A more simplistic model by which OELs can be adjusted was postulated by Brief and Scala (1975) for longer working periods:

$$\text{OEL multiplication factor} = \frac{8}{H} \times \left(\frac{24 - H}{16}\right)$$
$$(17.11)$$

where H is the number of hours worked per day.

Monitoring Record Sheet

Author and Any Assistants	Tel. No.	Date of Sampling	Contaminant
Name of Occupier			CAS No.
Address of Premises/Location/Identity			Product/Trade Name
			Sampling/Analysis Details
			MDHS/NIOSH/ OSHA Ref.

Total No. of People on Site

Total No. of People in Area/Process of Interest

Ref. No.	Male/Female (M/F)	Personal Identifier	Sample Type Personal/ Static(P/S)	Sample Description (e.g. name/task /process /equipment)	Reason for Sampling (Compliance/ Random/Ratio etc.)	Exposure Modifier (e.g. other routes of absorption, confounding factors etc.)	Work Period (i.e. shift)	Start/ Stop Times	Duration (min)	1 Result	1 TWA ppm or mg m^{-3}	2 Result	2 TWA ppm or mg m^{-3}	3 Result	3 TWA ppm or mg m^{-3}
1															
2															
3															
4															
5															

Current Occupational Exposure Limits	8 hour
	15 min

Fig. 17.7 Sample record sheet.

Such a non-specific formula has limitations but at least it may afford the individual a degree of extra protection. However, the formula does not apply to continuous 24 h exposure, work periods of less than 7–8 h per day or 35 h per week, nor for concentration-dependent acute toxicants.

Work rate

As has been previously mentioned, the effect of chronic contaminants is dose dependent. It is therefore unfortunate that little or no account is taken of the individual's work rate. It is possible for the depth and rate of respiration to triple during arduous physical activity and therefore so will the amount of inhaled contaminant, although the absorbed dose will vary between contaminants. The measurement of personal exposure is simply an estimate of the airborne concentration within the individual's breathing zone and may not reflect the true absorbed dose and hence biological monitoring should also be undertaken (see Chapter 16). Care also needs to be taken with particulates as the change in the rate and depth of respiration will affect the amount and sites of deposition.

SUMMARY AND CONCLUSIONS

It is hoped that a reasonable exposition of the various issues involved in the construction or development of a comprehensive sampling strategy has been made. Probably of most importance is to decide exactly what question you are trying to answer by the taking of measurements and once this has been decided the other aspects fall into place. It is also hoped that both those who request the taking of measurements (employers) and those who have to take the measurements (occupational/industrial hygienists) will realize that sampling individuals who happen to be around on a particular day will provide little more information than that, and that extrapolation to any other person, day, shift, equipment, location, etc. is often ill-advised.

REFERENCES

Boleij, J.S.M., Buringh, E., Heederick, D. and Kromhout, H. (1995). *Occupational Hygiene of Chemicals and Biological Agents.* Elsevier, Amsterdam.

Brief, R.S. and Scala, R.A. (1975). Occupational exposure limits for novel work schedules. *American Industrial Hygiene Association Journal*, **36**, 467–9.

British Occupational Hygiene Society (1982). *Hydrocarbon Distillate Vapour Composition: Prediction by Microcomputer.* BOHS Technical Guide No. 2. British Occupational Hygiene Society, Derby.

British Occupational Hygiene Society (1993). *Sampling Strategies for Airborne Contaminants in the Workplace.* BOHS Technical Guide No. 11. British Occupational Hygiene Society, H & H Scientific Consultants Ltd., Leeds.

Comité Européen de Normalisation (1992). *Workplace Atmospheres — Guidance for the Assessment of Exposure to Chemical Agents for Comparison with Limit Values and Measurement Strategy.* prEN 689. CEN, Brussels.

Corn, N. (1985). Strategies of air sampling. *Scandinavian Journal of Work, Environment and Health*, **11**, 173–80.

Corn, M. and Esmen, N.A. (1979). Workplace exposure zones for classification of employee exposures to physical and chemical agents. *American Industrial Hygiene Association Journal*, **40**, 47–57.

COSHH (1994). *Control of Substances Hazardous to Health and Approved Code of Practice, Carcinogenic Substances.* The Control of Substances Hazardous to Health Regulations 1994, Approved Code of Practice. HMSO, London.

Dewell, P. (1989). *Some Applications of Statistics in Occupational Hygiene.* BOHS Technical Guide No. 1. British Occupational Hygiene Society, H & H Scientific Consultants Ltd., Leeds.

Gardiner, K. (1995). Editorial: exposure profiles and respiratory sensitizers. *Occupational Hygiene*, **1**, 243–5.

Gardiner, K., Trethowan, W.N., Harrington, J.M., Calvert, I.A. and Glass, D.C. (1992). Occupational exposure to carbon black in its manufacture. *Annals of Occupational Hygiene*, **36**, (5), 477–96.

Health and Safety Executive (1989). *Monitoring Strategies for Toxic Substances.* HSE Guidance Note EH42. Health and Safety Executive, HMSO, London.

Health and Safety Executive (1990). *The Control of Exposure to Fume from Welding, Brazing and Similar Processes.* HSE Guidance Note EH55. Health and Safety Executive, HMSO, London.

Health and Safety Executive (1991). *Successful Health and Safety Management.* Health and Safety Series Booklet HS(G)65. Health and Safety Executive, HMSO, London.

Heederik, D., Kromhout, H. and Burema, J. (1991). Letter to the Editor. *Annals of Occupational Hygiene*, **35**, (6), 671–3.

Kromhout, H., Symanski, E. and Rappaport, S.M. (1993). A comprehensive evaluation of within and between-worker components of occupational exposure to chemical agents. *Annals of Occupational Hygiene*, **37**, (3), 253–70.

Leidel, N., Busch, K. and Lynch, J. (1977). *Occupational Exposure Sampling Strategy Manual*. US DHEW, NIOSH Publ. No. 77–173. National Institute for Occupational Safety and Health, Cincinnati.

Rappaport, S.M. (1988). Biological considerations for designing sampling strategies. In *Advances in Air Sampling*, (ed. W. John), pp. 337–52. Lewis Publishers, Michigan.

Rappaport, S.M. (1991). Assessment of long-term exposures to toxic substances in air – Review. *Annals of Occupational Hygiene*, **35**, (1), 61–121.

Rappaport, S.M. and Selvin, S. (1987). A method for evaluating the mean exposure from a log normal distribution. *American Industrial Hygiene Association Journal*, **48**, 374–9.

Rappaport, S.M. and Spear, R.C. (1988). Physiological damping of exposure variability during brief periods. *Annals of Occupational Hygiene*, **32**, 21–33.

Rappaport, S.M., Kromhout, H. and Symanski, E. (1993). Variation of exposure between workers in homogenous exposure groups. *American Industrial Hygiene Association Journal*, **54**, (11), 654–62.

Roach, S.A. (1977). A most rational basis for air sampling programmes. *Annals of Occupational Hygiene*, **20**, 65–84.

Vaughan, N.P., Chalmers, C.P. and Botham, R.A. (1990). Field comparison of personal samplers for inhalable dust. *Annals of Occupational Hygiene*, **34**, (6), 553–73.

CHAPTER 18

Restrospective Exposure Assessment

T.J. Smith, P.A. Stewart and R.F. Herrick

INTRODUCTION

Chronic occupational diseases, such as cancers and some lung diseases, develop over long exposure periods. Direct measurements of each subject's workplace experiences over the whole time period of interest would give the most accurate assessment of exposure for an epidemiological study. However, this ideal has not been, and is not likely to be, achieved. Moreover, because of the long exposure or latency periods associated with these effects it is rare that there are data covering the period. Consequently, epidemiological studies of these diseases require the estimation of past exposures by a process called 'retrospective exposure assessment'.

Prior to the 1980s, most occupational hygienists and epidemiologists did not believe it was possible to make quantitative estimates of past exposures when there were no measurement data. Since then there has been a strong need to make such estimates for dose–response studies and a variety of approaches have been developed. These are technically difficult to use and may be costly in time and resources. As will be shown below, there are a number of elements that must be present for detailed quantitative retrospective estimation to be feasible. Approaches range from the simple separation of job titles into broad 'exposed' and 'unexposed' categories based on judgement, to elaborate statistical models and estimation strategies which predict a unique quantitative exposure for every job held by the subjects. The approaches also vary with the type of epidemiological study. Regardless of the strategy, the common goal of retrospective exposure assessment is to develop the most accurate and unbiased estimates of exposure within the limitations of the resources.

This chapter reviews the basic concepts involved in exposure measurement or assessment and then discusses the different approaches needed for retrospective assessment for each of the main types of epidemiological study. It concludes with a review of the reliability and validity of such procedures.

BASIC CONCEPTS

Dose indices for epidemiological studies

The goal in epidemiological studies is to approximate the dose to the target tissue as closely as possible because it is the cause of the adverse effect observed in the epidemiological outcome. A 'dose index' is a single number intended to summarize a part or all of a subject's exposure history that is relevant to the risk of an adverse outcome, such as the total dose of the suspected agent received by the subject. Conceptually the dose index is based on the pharmacological idea of an administered dose which has been widely used to characterize such exposure–response relationships. The epidemiological dose index that is closest to total administered dose is the 'cumulative exposure', which is the mean exposure in a job multiplied by the duration in the job summed over all jobs held. This has been a useful measure in many studies of chronic disease from asbestos, lead, cadmium and other agents. Other dose indices may also be important for the risk of a particular disease, such as the occurrence of peak exposures. The choice of an optimum dose index depends on the mechanism of the disease. Whatever dose index is used, it is important to recognize that exposure is not equivalent to dose. Some writers have used exposure and dose as interchangeable terms and created considerable confusion as a result.

Cumulative exposure as a dose index has the implicit assumption that long-term, low-intensity exposures are equivalent to short-term, high-intensity exposures. Since there are situations where short-term, high exposures, 'peaks', may produce more or less effects than moderate exposures, epidemiologists have explored a number of other dose measures to detect the effects of peaks. This is discussed in more detail below. See also Chapter 20.

Characteristics of job titles

Long-term exposures generally must be assigned to each subject based on his or her work history (a chronological listing of: date started; job title; and department or work site for each job held in a company). If an individual has worked for several companies then the work history from each should be obtained. The fundamental exposure assessment problem is one of converting job titles, department names and an industry type at a specific time period into exposure estimates (composition and intensity).

The 'job title' is the most common way to assign an exposure to a subject in an epidemiological study of long-term effects. Unfortunately, job titles are not standardized and have little intrinsic meaning for exposure, even at the extremes. For example, a job title such as 'clerk', which usually has little exposure, can be misleading because clerks can be located in production areas and be near emission sources. Conversely, the job title 'operator' in a chemical plant may have little exposure if the chemicals are all within the pipes and equipment so that the operator has little contact with them. The task activities and work locations are determined by the nature of the industrial process. However, the aggregation of those tasks and work locations under the definition of a job title is somewhat arbitrary and can vary across time, across plant site and across companies. As a result the evaluation of a job's tasks and work locations is a

critical part of retrospective exposure assessment.

A job title usually has a defined set of work activities (tasks) an individual has to perform at one or more locations. These activities are specified by the needs of the industrial or commercial process. Generally, these activities must be performed to meet the goal of the enterprise, such as making computer chips, recording insurance transactions or transporting petrol. However, the job title under which they are assigned is somewhat arbitrary and can vary among companies and can change across time when activities are reorganized. An example of the tasks and work locations associated with the job title 'petrol tanker driver' are given in Table 18.1. Some tasks have high exposure potential, such as loading, and some have none, such as paper work. The nature of the work site where the task is performed is also critical, such as delivering petrol to large underground tanks with remote venting versus delivering petrol to small tanks vented at eye-level directly into the operator's breathing zone.

Tasks may require less than a minute or several days to perform, and may be performed at a wide range of frequencies: many times per day; or less than once per month. Tasks also may vary widely in their exposure intensity. All of a job's tasks may contribute to the individual's long-term exposure, and all should be considered in a retrospective exposure assessment. Variability in both task frequency and exposure intensity over time are fundamental characteristics of jobs.

Epidemiological studies require estimates of exposure for all job titles in the subjects' work histories. Even where there have been exposure surveillance programmes, it is rare that all job titles and tasks with exposure potential have been characterized. Thus estimates must be made for both current jobs that have not been sampled and for past exposures prior to measurements.

Determinants of occupational exposure

An extrapolation rationale is needed that is compatible with the present and past data available to estimate exposures. The objective is to relate composition and intensity of exposure to deterministic factors that can be evaluated or estimated from

Table 18.1 Example of tasks and work locations associated with the job title of petrol tanker driver

Work location	Task activity	Duration	Frequency
Truck cab	Driving	5–60 min	2–12 per day
Loading facility	Loading truck tanks		
Top loading: no vapour control		15–30 min	2–12 per day
Bottom loading: vapour recovery		15–30 min	2–12 per day
Customer tanks	Delivery		
Underground tanks: remote venting		10–20 min	2–6 per day
Above ground tanks: vent at fill hole in breathing zone		5–15 min	2–10 per day
Office or cafe	Paper work and rest breaks	10–45 min	2–3 per day

NB: a typical situation will involve a mix of these tasks.

current and historical records. There are two simple paradigms that can guide this evaluation in a given situation:

1 the source–receptor model to describe the exposure process for a task, and

2 the task-specific time-weighted average exposure (task-TWA) as a description of a worker's overall average exposure from the combination of his or her task activities (task-TWA = the average task exposure multiplied by the duration of the task, summed over all tasks, divided by the total time in tasks).

Evaluation of a job title in an epidemiological study can use both of these models to identify the deterministic factors associated with the worker, the tasks and the work environment that determine exposures. A partial listing of the task factors is given in Table 18.2. If there are historical changes in these factors, there may be changes in the composition and/or intensity of exposures for a task. The task-TWA model allows us to combine data on a job title's tasks and determine their contributions to the overall TWA exposure for the job.

Table 18.2 Exposure process model: factors affecting exposure in a task

Source ------------------(Transport)------------> Worker			Setting
Process	Air	Location relative to source(s)	*Physical*
Materials	Surface	Duration	Room size
Output rate	Radiative	Energy demands	Sources and locations
Worker influence		Work habits and techniques	General controls
Source controls		Personal exposure controls	*Management*
			Pressure for production
			Concern for health and safety

Source–receptor model

This model of a task exposure is based on a concept borrowed from air pollution modelling: the source–receptor model, which describes the atmospheric transport of an air contaminant from an emission source to a receptor, e.g. an exposed population (see Chapter 21). In general, an industrial operation and its raw materials and products will define the sources, output strength and composition of airborne emissions (potential agents of effects). For example, a scrap brass refining operation requires scrap feed material, which may have some lead content, and the use of certain furnaces operated at defined temperatures over a specified production cycle, which in turn define the emission sources for lead fume. The intensity of exposure is determined by source output strength and configuration, air movements which transport and dilute the contaminants, effectiveness of local exhaust ventilation and the worker's proximity which is defined by his or her work task. Variability in the worker's exposure over time is a function of variability of source output, common composition and strength, variability of the transport processes (e.g. turbulent mixing), variability in the worker's position relative to the source and the effects of exposure controls at either the source or the worker (see Chapter 17). In many cases the worker's job activities control or contribute to the source, e.g. welding. Information about historical changes in materials, the process or the work site configuration can be used in the model to evaluate historical changes in exposure.

While the potential complexity of the factors determining an exposure are daunting, it is not necessary to characterize fully the deterministic relationship for all possible factors to use this approach. Identification of the major factors and their likely effects on exposure can be done qualitatively by examining the model for a given task. Then the effects of changes in factors can be described by multipliers. For example, the ratio of mean exposures for a task before and after changing a process from one type to another gives a multiplier to estimate the effects of this change without evaluating all of the component parts. It can also be argued that this ratio will apply to other situations which have not been measured. Thus the multipliers associated with past changes may be estimated from existing exposure measurements. Schneider et al. (1991) have developed this idea most extensively, but others have also used it. Thus, the model approach provides an explicit, powerful argument by analogy to estimate past operations that were never measured or characterized, if the emission sources and the exposure situation are comparable to an exposure that has been measured.

One limitation of the source–receptor model is that it works best for a single task performed near a defined source. In some cases a job comprises a single task, such as a packer who loads mineral wool products off the end of a production line, or a data clerk who works at a computer terminal all day. However, a job usually has more than one task and the model does not provide guidance about how the tasks may be combined to give an overall estimate of the mean. The task-specific TWA model provides this link to estimate the mean properly by weighting samples collected during various single-task activities or during a series of tasks.

Task-specific TWA model of job exposures

The worker's job title and work location are the connection points between the exposure assessment and the epidemiological evaluation. The task-TWA analysis provides two important insights: (1) it provides a method for extrapolating the effects of historic changes in the definition of a job and the task exposures associated with a job; and (2) it provides a vehicle for appropriately weighting short-term samples collected to characterize tasks with high-exposure potential. For example, a hygienist may collect 10 samples, five during 'normal' activities and five during activities with high-exposure potential. If the high exposures only represent 10% of the total activity time, the simple average of these 10 samples will outweigh the high-exposure activities.

The mathematical form of the task-TWA model is:

$$\text{Task-TWA} = \frac{\sum_{i=1}^{N} X_i \times t_i}{\sum_{i=1}^{N} t_i} \qquad (18.1)$$

The mean exposure for each task (X_i) is weighted by the total duration spent on the task (t_i). If the task is of short duration but repeated then the total duration is the average duration of each occurrence multiplied by the number of repetitions. In this case the concentration is not independent of the duration, for example high exposures may be associated with short duration. When this happens, each (j subscript) measured exposure must be multiplied by its duration $(X_{ij} \times t_{ij})$ to obtain the correctly weighted exposure-time product.

It is important to note the differences in this model from the common time-weighted average exposure, which is measured directly in an 8 h personal sample. The expression above is intended to cover all of the time period variations in tasks and exposures that will occur for a job title, not just 8 h. Some tasks are very infrequent, such as a periodic 6 month reactor cleaning, but these tasks may be very important contributors to health risk. Furthermore, as one considers increasing time spans in a chronic exposure study, changes in the definition of a job may occur where some tasks are excluded and new ones added. Effects of changes in process and production rate may increase or decrease task means.

The task weighting also provides a mechanism for utilizing occupational hygiene samples collected to describe peak exposures without distorting the overall distribution. Changes in job definitions have rarely been examined, but recent studies have identified important changes in lists of tasks and in the time required to accomplish tasks. The quantitative effects of historical changes in job exposures sometimes can be assessed given the duration and exposure intensity for the tasks. The task approach can also be used to group jobs that perform similar high-exposure tasks, and to identify and characterize jobs with 'peak' exposures.

A limitation of the task-TWA is the limited task data that may be available. Usually only tasks with high-exposure potential have been measured by hygienists. However low-exposure tasks can frequently be estimated with area samples which describe 'background' exposure levels.

Characteristics of exposure measurements

Exposures must have been measured at some point in time to anchor models for estimating past exposure. The estimation process is easiest and most accurate if there are multiple sets of measurements across time. While surveillance data can be extremely useful, they have several important limitations which must be addressed in building models or making exposure estimates.

1 Complex occupational exposures to chemicals are frequently difficult to characterize by sampling. Available data are often only rough indicators of exposure intensity for a specific agent. For example, total dust samples $(mg\,m^{-3})$ may indicate relative exposure intensity to a toxic component of the dust for a job's exposure. However, composition of the total dust often changes with work area, especially between high- and low-exposure areas. Assumptions about exposure composition should be clearly stated and carefully reviewed. (See Chapter 17).

2 Exposures are most often measured with techniques specified by regulations, but these techniques may not be directly relevant to current hypotheses about health risks. A classic example of this is using impinger counts of total dust (particles $> 1\,\mu m$) to characterize exposure for an effect caused by respirable crystalline silica dust (particles $< 3.5\,\mu m$). A conversion factor may exist in some situations, but the relationship is weak. In general, older methods may not be comparable with current approaches and technology. Studies may be needed to characterize the relationship between old and new methods.

3 Historical samples were often fixed location or area samples. While these may not directly estimate personal exposure, they may be very useful when combined with time–activity data on jobs and periods when both area and personal data were collected. For example, in a study of cadmium smelter workers, only area measurements were available from the 1940s to 1974, but there was an overlap of these samples with personal measurements for 1 year. The authors compared the area and personal measurements and used the ratio for each work area to adjust the area samples and make estimates of personal exposure. The authors of an aluminium smelter study also found differences between the two types of measurements, but resolved it by using the differences between the area and personal samples during the years of overlap to estimate earlier exposures.

4 Workers in some jobs may have used personal protective equipment, such as respirators. It is probably inappropriate to assume that this equipment dramatically reduces internal doses. Although laboratory studies have shown that well-fitted respirators may reduce inhalation exposure by tenfold or more, under normal day-to-day usage the protection factors are much less (see Chapter 23).

5 The sampling strategy for determining compliance with standards requires the hygienist to seek days that include situations or tasks with the highest exposure potential, when they can be identified (see Chapter 17). Consequently an unweighted mean of all full shift samples for a job may give a biased estimate of overall mean exposure. Data on the time workers spend in various situations and doing specific tasks can be obtained by interview and used to weight the full shift and task sampling data if the samples have adequate information on the sampling conditions.

Variability in worker exposures

Epidemiological studies of long-term exposures generally have assumed that all individuals performing the same job will have the same mean exposure. The mean for the job is assigned to everyone holding the job. This is based on the assumption that the primary source of variation in exposure samples was day-to-day variation in conditions experienced by all of the workers, and that averaging samples across time could control the variability. Recently that assumption has been challenged.

Rappaport, Kromhout and Symanski (1993) examined the variability in sampling data for a wide range of jobs. For a given job they contrasted the variability of between-worker means with the within-worker (day-to-day) variability, and found that in some jobs the between-worker variability can be a large component of the overall variability (see Chapter 17). Many factors can cause systematic differences in exposure between workers performing the same job, such as differences in the tasks performed, training, technical skill, work habits, posture or body size. An important aspect of these individual differences is the wide range of sensory sensitivity to irritants and other environmental stimuli. This heterogeneity can be important in limiting some individuals' exposures to adverse stimuli, such as eye, nose and throat irritation from airborne sulphur dioxide or formaldehyde. Figure 18.1 illustrates hypothetical sampling distributions for two jobs with the same overall sample means but different between-worker variability. As the variability between workers' means increases, epidemiological exposure groups become more heterogeneous and statistical comparison of job groups by their overall sample means will underestimate the variability between groups and overestimate differences between groups.

There is little the hygienist or epidemiologist can do to eliminate large between-worker variations in mean exposure. However, it can be an important source of misclassification and an explanation for a lack of apparent relationship between exposure

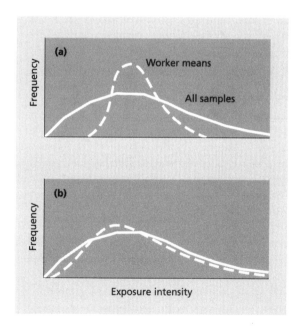

Fig. 18.1 Hypothetical sampling distributions for two jobs with the same overall sample means but different variability in individual mean exposures: (a) low between-worker variability; (b) high between-worker variability.

and health effects. Where there are known to be large differences between workers, it may be necessary to personalize exposure estimates, such as through collection of interview data about differences in performing key high-exposure tasks. This is similar to the collection of personal smoking data. These exposure differences may explain some of the variability observed in biological monitoring data on workers doing the same job, although biological indices also have other sources of variation.

APPROACHES TO RETROSPECTIVE EXPOSURE ASSESSMENT

The above section developed the basic concepts needed to support the extrapolation process to estimate both the composition and intensity of past exposures. This section takes those concepts and illustrates their application to the common epidemiological study designs, cohort and case–control, through the discussion of examples. Quantitative approaches are emphasized because they are more useful for hypothesis testing and for the development of exposure–response relationships.

Approaches for cohort studies

Cohort studies are designed to observe the disease experience of subjects chosen because they do, or do not, have an exposure of interest. With quantitative exposure estimates, cohort studies are useful for investigating exposure–risk relationships. The exposed subjects are chosen because they all have a common exposure situation at a point in time, such as they all worked for a given company during a 1 year period. Since the focus is a particular company, it is usually possible to obtain work history records from the company or a trade union, and data on company operations, materials used and changes over time. The company also may have collected exposure samples through its hygiene surveillance system which may be available.

If subjects have left the company but remain in the cohort then their subsequent exposure history has been lost. Commonly workers are asked about exposures prior to joining a company, but there is rarely follow-up to determine where they worked after leaving the company. It has been assumed that workers who left employment in a company went to other jobs and work locations at random, so there would be no differential contribution to their risk. However, it seems likely that exposure level while at the company might be correlated with exposure in the next job because workers will often choose jobs and industries where they have experience. Although it has not been done, employment data could be obtained through interviews of subjects or next of kin.

In cohort studies, the primary task is developing exposure estimates for all of the job titles in the work histories of the subjects. This problem can be separated into two components: (1) exposures in jobs not measured during periods with measurements; and (2) exposures in jobs in periods before there were measurements. Much more attention has been given to the second problem, where a variety of approaches has been used.

Unmeasured job titles – grouping similar jobs together

Based on extensive reviews of records in a number of large companies we have discovered that personnel lists of job titles are commonly more extensive than is needed by the operation. This occurs for a variety of personnel reasons unrelated to exposure. Consequently many titles in the personnel records are synonymous, with respect to exposure, and may be collapsed into a short list of 'generic' titles based on an assessment of job activities, tasks and work locations associated with exposures. This can substantially reduce the list of unmeasured jobs. Given the hygienist's bias toward measuring where there are likely to be significant exposures, most commonly the unmeasured jobs are those with background exposures or those with little likelihood of production area exposures, such as office workers. Jobs in peripheral areas can be assigned observed background levels distant from sources, or based on the absence of sources they may be assigned zero if they are in isolated areas.

Broad grouping of different jobs or industries can be done when the tasks and environments are judged to be sufficiently similar. This approach has been used to describe exposure zones or homogeneous exposure groups. For example, in a North Carolina study of dusty trade workers, all facilities within an industry were considered to be similar enough to combine all measurements across those facilities. Other investigators have also grouped jobs (Greife *et al.*, 1988) or facilities (Dodgson, Cherrie and Groat, 1987) to obtain a mean for a broader occupational group or for an industry category when monitoring data were unavailable for a number of the jobs or companies being evaluated. Investigators have provided varying levels of detail in their justifications of their grouping schemes. Grouping of jobs or industries, however, requires a careful evaluation of exposure factors to ensure that exposures are similar within the occupational group or industry. If exposures are not similar, combining jobs with heterogeneous exposures could result in subjects being assigned to the wrong exposure level (Rappaport, Kromhout and Symanski, 1993). As the grouping scheme becomes broader and has less detail on specific job activities and work settings, it becomes more likely that there are heterogeneous exposures within groups.

Assuming constant mean exposures

In some cases an operation has been essentially unchanged over a long period of time. When sufficient air monitoring data are available, means of job and area exposures obtained in a cross-sectional study or from recent surveillance sampling can be used as estimates of long-term exposure. This is an attractive approach that requires few assumptions if it can be documented that there were no changes in the operations and jobs. It does, however, require sufficient monitoring results to estimate all or most of the jobs. For example, one of us conducted a cross-sectional personal sampling study of major job types for a number of chemical exposures in a study of workers in a silicon carbide operation. Because few changes had occurred over the study period, the monitoring results were sufficient to be representative of historical exposures. All job titles in the work histories were assigned to one of the major job types.

In most workplaces, however, exposure levels have not been constant over time because of changes in the process, job tasks or engineering controls. Consequently the approach of using the current measured exposure and assuming that there has been no change is a poor estimator of long-term exposure.

Statistical approaches

Statistical models based on available monitoring data can be used to predict exposure levels in unmeasured jobs and past exposures based on factors if enough measurements exist across the jobs and over the years of the study to complete the missing data cells. This approach has the advantages of being straightforward and requiring few assumptions.

Analysis of variance has been used in studies of granite shed workers, styrene product workers and railroad workers. The models developed in these studies were based on the assumption that there were unspecified factors associated with the jobs and work sites that could be applied from general means to estimated means in situations that had not been measured. Regression techniques have been used in studies of asbestos workers (Dement *et al.*, 1983) and ethylene oxide workers (Greife *et al.*, 1988). Two problems may arise, however, in using statistical approaches. First, the workplace factors (variables) in the statistical model need to be a small number relative to the number of samples collected. Second, in a workplace with several hundreds to thousands of job titles, it is likely that most jobs will not have been monitored. Reduction of a large number of jobs to a small enough number for use in a statistical model may result in the formation of job categories with heterogeneous exposures, as noted earlier. The third problem is that all types of models are developed during periods with measurements and then applied to earlier time periods when the conditions used to create the model may not have existed. Unfortunately, this is a situation often encountered by investigators.

Calculation of means using tasks and time

Many historical data are area measurements and/

or of short duration. The use of these data as full-shift personal samples is problematic, as noted in the smelter study described above. To use short-term or area samples to develop estimates that are representative of full-shift exposures, some investigators have weighted short-term monitoring results by time. For example, in a study of asbestos workers, the authors used area measurements to calculate zone averages (Dement *et al.*, 1983; see Table 18.3 below). 8 h time-weighted average (TWA) exposures were then calculated by summing the products of each zone's average exposure and the time spent in that zone and adding task exposures where appropriate. This type of approach requires that the monitoring results are available for most tasks or areas in the study and that time spent in the zone or task can be estimated. Exposure effects of historic changes in job activities can be estimated using the task-TWA approach as described earlier.

Prediction from measurement data on other exposures

If there is an exposure that is parallel to the one of interest, measurements on that exposure may be used to predict the second exposure. This is only appropriate, however, when the relative level of exposure is expected to be the same for all the jobs being estimated. This approach was used in an aluminium smelter that had benzene-soluble materials (BSM) measurements over the study period and benzo(a)pyrene (BaP) measurements after 1976. The authors derived a ratio using BaP and BSM measurements from 1976 to 1983 for 19 occupational groups. Assuming the ratio remained the same over time, they applied this ratio to determine pre-1976 BaP levels.

Mixed methods based on data availability

In many situations a single approach, such as described above, is insufficient to estimate exposures in all of the jobs because the assumptions required are violated. It may be necessary to combine several approaches to make the estimates. For example, in an ongoing National Cancer Institute study of US acrylonitrile workers, although there were 16 000

hygienic measurements available to the investigators, they were from recent time periods and for only small numbers of the 3500 jobs in the study. For this reason, detailed and comprehensive procedures were developed to document how the exposure estimates were derived. For each exposed job, a detailed description was developed in a database that included: the process description the job was involved in; the location and tasks of the job; the occurrence of the major changes that took place in the workplace that were likely to have affected exposures; occurrence of overtime; the frequency of exposure; the frequency of peak and dermal exposures; the concentration of acrylonitrile in the liquid; personal protective use; reported health effects; the level of physical activity; and other exposures (Stewart *et al.*, 1992). A hierarchy of exposure assessment methods was then developed using several estimation methods because of the variability in the exposure data across jobs and through time. The methods included: calculation of means based on personal monitoring results where they were available; using a ratio method where the ratio of exposures of some jobs was applied to other jobs; calculation of exposure means for homogeneous exposure groups using the measurements of all the jobs within the group; and use of area measurements weighted by time. Formal criteria for using these methods were developed, as was a hierarchy of their use, based on their ability to predict the measurements. Each of the estimates was documented as to how it was derived and the assumptions made, which allowed reviewers to follow easily the decision-making process, using an interactive software package developed by Stewart and co-workers.

Estimates of exposure over time

Some investigators have attempted to develop an estimate for each year of exposure. Others have reduced the number of measurements necessary to specify an exposure by identifying time periods with no change, within which it is assumed that exposures remained constant. The source−receptor model strongly implies that exposures may be reasonably assumed to remain stationary over time periods when evidence indicates that no changes in exposure determinants occurred. The method for determining these stationary time periods has varied. For example, in the North Carolina dusty trades study, the silica monitoring results for each company were plotted by time and sample location. Any point in time when all measurements were above or below all successive measurements was considered as evidence of a change in the workplace environment. Mean concentrations were then calculated for before and after the change. If the plot of measurements showed no such pattern, the mean concentrations from all the years were averaged. Other investigators have developed time periods based on changes in the workplace which are identified from interviews of workers or from engineering and other production reports.

A few investigators used the sampling date or time period as an independent variable in a regression model. The time period variable was highly predictive of exposures so it remained in the model as an explanatory factor. The use of this model in an extrapolation of past exposures requires that the effect of time be bounded for exposures outside the measurement period. Information on such changes has also been used with professional judgment to derive exposure levels.

There is growing support for the deterministic model approach which is closely related to the source−receptor model. In the deterministic model, the major factors controlling exposure are specified, an estimate of the multiplier associated with each factor is obtained from a standard model based on first principles, and the history of changes in the factors for a workplace is determined. By combining the history with recent measurements of exposure, the multipliers can be used to estimate past exposures (Schneider *et al.*, 1991). For example, Dodgson, Cherrie and Groat (1987) estimated past synthetic mineral fibre exposures using estimates of factors associated with the workplace changes. The effects of two of the most important changes were also evaluated using an experimental design in an exposure simulation. Other less important factors were identified with estimated multipliers. The appropriate multiplier for each factor was then applied to each of the measurement means to derive the exposure estimates. Uncertainties arise from the effects of workplace idiosyncrasies, such

as placement of doors and windows, that may modify the effect of the standardized factors, such as emission rates. This approach has the advantage that it has a clear rationale for estimating past exposures that does not take a statistical model outside its database because the multipliers are derived from first principles or from experimental data.

Approaches for case−control studies

Case−control studies are useful because they can investigate rare diseases that are impractical to study in a reasonably sized cohort. The epidemiological analysis for case−control studies contrasts the histories of exposure for the cases and controls to identify differences that might represent causal factors. While this design is practical for the epidemiologist, it presents major difficulties to the exposure assessor because the subjects are chosen on the basis of their disease status, therefore, they generally have highly varied work histories representing a wide variety of workplaces and job titles. Case−control studies nested within cohort studies can take advantage of detailed exposure assessment done on the cohort.

Data collection

Since the subjects are not drawn from a single workplace, it is a major task to obtain exposure histories on the subjects and it is usually not feasible to obtain company records of work histories. The typical approach to collecting exposure information is to interview the study subject or next of kin for the jobs, employers and dates held by the subject. Qualitative analyses by a job title, or potential exposure inferred from a job title (from job exposure matrices) and semi-quantitative estimates of the probability of exposure (definite, probable, possible) or the level of exposure (low, medium or high) have been the traditional methods of exposure assessment. The limitations of these approaches are described below.

A major advance in assessing exposures in case−control studies has been described by Siemiatycki and Gerin (Gerin *et al.*, 1985). These investigators recognized that exposures are often idiosyncratic to the person holding the job, i.e., that everyone with the same job title does not necessarily have the same exposure. Siemiatycki and Gerin therefore used information on job activities, equipment and materials used and responses to occupation-specific questions for each individual study subject when assessing the exposures of each individual. These questions were keyed to local industries and their histories of operations. This method substantially increases the accuracy of assessments.

Estimation of exposures

Traditionally, exposure levels in case–control studies have been assessed by assigning an ordinal exposure score, e.g.: none; low; medium; or high, without a quantitative definition of the boundaries of each category. The literature that was reviewed by the industrial hygienist when developing the estimates has often been described, but investigators have rarely described in detail how estimates of exposure have been derived. A formal approach to evaluating exposures is now being developed by the National Cancer Institute. Because reports of occupational histories may be prone to error, particularly when reported by next of kin, evaluating the quality of the reported information may help to identify occupational histories that are likely to contain errors. If the reported information appears to be inconsistent or vague, the respondent could be recontacted or co-workers could be contacted. A third option would be to contact the employer of the subject, although the feasibility of this option has not been assessed.

Use of most chemicals varies even within a single industry, and therefore few chemicals are found at every worksite within the same industry. The probability that a job is exposed varies with the process and its environmental characteristics, the chemical being assessed and the tasks being performed in the job. Asking direct questions of the respondent may allow a definitive evaluation of the probability of exposure. If information still is not specific enough, the best estimate of the probability that exposure occurred may be based on the frequency of exposure in the population of workers holding the job in that industry. Such an estimate could be derived after reviewing existing databases.

In the USA, these include the Occupational Safety and Health Administration's Integrated Management Information System, the Environmental Protection Agency's TRI (toxic release inventory) system or the National Institute for Occupational Safety and Health's Job Exposure Matrix. These data sources offer an objective basis for quantitatively estimating exposure probability.

Estimating quantitative exposure levels in these types of studies is an enormous challenge for the industrial hygienist, but should be attempted. As described earlier, there are no standard methods to estimate exposures even in cohort studies and methods for the case–control design is even less developed. In addition, due to the complexity of the workplaces, it is unrealistic to evaluate all determinants affecting exposures. Five determinants from basic industrial hygiene principles considered to be central to exposure assessment have been identified and an approach to translate these determinants into quantitative exposure levels has been suggested by Stewart (1992).

Traditional exposure estimation approaches

Since case–control studies present major problems for exposure assessment, surrogate measures of exposure have been widely used, such as ever/never employed, duration of employment and semi-quantitative estimates. These were generally *ad hoc* evaluations based on assumptions about factors causing exposure. Limitations of these approaches have been described in detail elsewhere (Stewart and Herrick, 1991), but it is useful to review the limitations of these simpler approaches and some recent improvements to contrast them to the more expensive and time-consuming new quantitative methods developed for cohort studies.

Ever/never exposure classification

In many broad epidemiological studies, the study subjects were classified by whether they worked in a particular industry, or company, or job title. This type of classification may be highly accurate but, as noted above, employees within an industry or company or work area are likely to be exposed to a variety of chemicals at various levels, which often change over long time periods. If this exposure misclassification is random or non-differential, it may result in a decrease in the estimate of relative risk, and a causal association could be entirely missed. Even if an excess of some disease is identified, it is usually impossible to determine what workplace exposure may have been responsible for the excess without a more detailed assessment of exposures.

As an attempt to sharpen the ever/never analysis, some investigators have identified qualitative exposures to particular agents used in an industry, or company, or job title. Broadly applied, this approach may achieve limited accuracy when used by someone who is knowledgeable about an industry or plant. However, it is highly unusual for everyone in a plant or job title to have exposure to a particular agent, and certainly they do not all have the same level of exposure. When applied in depth to a single plant, better results may be obtained. In one study in the automobile industry, the investigators carefully reconstructed past operations, job activities and materials used in each work area by each job, for a study of machining fluid exposures. They were unable to make quantitative estimates of exposure because of practical limitations. They found relationships between cancer risks and some components of the machining

fluids, which will require further studies to develop exposure–response relationships.

Duration of employment or exposure

Traditionally, duration of employment in an industry or a job, or duration of exposure to a particular agent, has been widely used to investigate the existence of exposure–response relationships. Duration has two major advantages: (1) it is readily determined through a subject's work history obtained by interview or from the company records; and (2) duration usually has reasonable accuracy. Duration may be a satisfactory surrogate for cumulative exposure, but only under certain conditions. These are:

1 the exposure level is the same for all workers in an exposure category;

2 exposure levels have remained the same over time.

While these are reasonable, they are very difficult to verify and are commonly violated.

A study by Dement *et al.* (1983) illustrates a typical case in which these conditions were not met. Exposure monitoring data from a chrysotile asbestos plant were available back to 1930, and the ranges of estimated mean exposures for jobs within each department presented in Table 18.3 are de-

Table 18.3 Mean chrysotile asbestos levels (fibres cc^{-1}) and ranges in an asbestos plant by department and time period. From Dement *et al.* (1983)

Department	1930	1936–39	1945–46	1965–66	1971–75
Fibre preparation and waste processing	26–78*	—†	8–24	6–17	—
Carding	11–13	5–11	2–5	4–9	—
Ring spinning	7–8	—	—	7–9	5–6
Mule spinning	5–7	—	—	—	—
Foster winding	10–21	4–8	—	—	—
Twisting	25–36	5–8	—	—	—
Universal winding	4–8	—	—	—	—
Heavy weaving	5–31	1–8	—	—	—
Light weaving	3–7	—	—	—	—

* The report contained means of specific jobs within departments; the ranges of these means are shown.
† Dashes indicate no change from the earlier period.

rived from that report. Exposure levels varied widely, both within and across the different departments. Grouping subjects who were 'exposed' in the fibre preparation operation with subjects who were 'exposed' in light weaving with the same duration (of employment or exposure) would result in severe misclassification of actual exposures and long-term doses.

Table 18.3 also demonstrates that exposure levels may not remain static over time. If they change, they do not always drop and they do not remain at the same ranking relative to other jobs. In some departments, exposure levels remained essentially constant, e.g. mule spinning, universal winding and light weaving. Subjects who worked from 1930 to 1945 in the fibre preparation operation had much higher asbestos levels than subjects who worked their 15 years during 1960–1975 in that same department. Grouping subjects by duration alone, however, would put such subjects in the same analytical exposure category.

The arguments presented here are not to suggest that ever/never exposure or duration of employment should not be performed. These measures can be useful in hypothesis-generating studies, particularly when using readily available records. In addition, if the environmental conditions are met, duration can be a good measure of cumulative exposure in analytical studies. Moreover, detailed retrospective exposure assessment may not be possible or may require more financial or time resources than are available to the investigator. Investigators should recognize, however, that relying upon ever/never or duration of employment as the sole measures of exposure will probably result in misclassification, which will enhance the probability of missing associations.

Semi-quantitative expert estimates

The limitations of the simple methods presented earlier for evaluating exposure–response relationships have led some investigators to use a semi-quantitative approach. Experts knowledgeable about the past conditions, such as plant hygienists, create relative exposure categories, e.g. high, medium, and low, based on their expert judgement.

This type of analysis has been successful in finding associations, particularly in case–control studies. Unfortunately, few investigators have described in detail the procedures and rationale followed for the estimation of exposures.

There are several drawbacks to using semi-quantitative assessments without quantitative data. Exposure analyses require that ranked jobs be assigned weights to allow analysis by cumulative exposure (the sum of each exposure level multiplied by its duration). These weights are typically arbitrary, usually 1, 2 and 3, to designate low, medium and high exposure levels. Such an assignment assumes that a job in the medium category has twice the exposure level as a job in the low category and two-thirds the exposure level as a job in the high category. Other investigators have used geometrical scales to quantify exposures. However, it is not known if these weights better reflect reality.

In a study by Kromhout *et al.* (1987), air monitoring was conducted on various job tasks in five industries, and the sampling results were used to calculate an arithmetic mean for each task. These means were used to place each of the tasks into one of four exposure categories and to derive an overall mean for the exposure category. Independent of the monitoring, two occupational hygienists classified the tasks into four exposure categories ranging from no exposure (1) to high exposure (4). This study suggested that using weights based on judgement provides less accurate weights than directly estimating exposure levels. More investigation, however, is needed in this area.

Semi-quantitative relative ranking of exposure has another limitation: the ranks may not be comparable across sites and different companies. The relative ranks of job titles at a location may be appropriate at other locations, but the absolute levels may vary substantially so that the actual exposure of a 'high' job in one location may be equivalent to that in a 'low' job in another. For example, in one study there was a fixed relative ranking of dust exposures for different job titles within granite sheds and large differences in absolute exposures for similar job titles across the sheds.

Quantitative estimates from calibrated expert judgement

Recently, investigators have explored hybrid schemes where limited quantitative exposure data have been used to calibrate hygienists' professional judgement. The hybrid approach makes good use of limited measurement data in combination with expert judgement.

RELIABILITY AND VALIDITY ISSUES

The extrapolation of past exposures is not just a matter of having adequate measurement data to describe the composition and intensity of exposures. For a given study and exposure situation, there are a variety of data that can be used and which provide varying amounts of information. Evaluation of past exposures requires the investigator to take advantage of all of these data sources and blend them into an overall picture of historical exposures. As a result, within a given study the quality of information about exposures, its reliability and validity, can vary from job to job and over time periods.

Some researchers are uncomfortable with this approach and point out the probability of introducing errors when estimates are not based on actual measurements. This concern is valid, and undoubtedly some estimates result in misclassification of subjects. However, it is believed that the critical issue is not whether a quantitative approach results in misclassification, but whether the misclassification is greater than it would have been using some other approach, i.e. ever/never exposed, or duration of employment versus imprecise quantitative estimates. The authors believe that evaluating each job or job task for its possible exposure level and taking into account the relative differences between jobs is likely to ensure a better estimation of exposures and, therefore, less misclassification of subjects than other approaches.

Evaluation of the validity and reliability of the exposure estimates is important to the credibility of the study. Validity of estimates of past exposure is very difficult to determine because there may be no data with which to check them. A few studies have held some data aside to check the quality of estimates made with quantitative models (Griefe et al., 1988; Dodgson, Cherrie and Groat, 1987; Smith, Hammond and Wong, 1993). This has generally shown that the modelling approach produces reasonable estimates, generally within a factor of two of the measured exposures. However, it is not clear that the correlation of the estimates with current exposures is equivalent to that for past exposures. For case–control studies using several individuals to rate exposures, there have been some examinations of rater reliability. There have been a few studies to examine intra- and inter-rater reliability that have shown that reliable assessments can be obtained (Goldberg, Siemiatycki and Gerin, 1986; Hayes et al., 1986). However, this does not establish the validity of their evaluations.

Exposure misclassification is most likely to be non-differential in nature, that is, errors in exposure classification will occur throughout the study population, without regard to health or outcome status. In the simplest case, members of a study population who are truly exposed may be incorrectly classified as unexposed, and some exposed are classified as unexposed. In this case, the net result will be a bias in the study findings toward the null hypothesis of no association between exposure and response. In more quantitative exposure assessments, such as the assignment of individuals to rank ordered categories based upon cumulative lifetime exposure, non-differential misclassification between adjacent exposure categories can have an attenuating effect on an exposure response trend. Even when the exposure misclassification rate is only 20%, the true estimate of risk among the exposed can be substantially greater than the apparent relative risk (Checkoway, Savitz and Heyer, 1991). This holds whether the misclassification is between a simple exposed/unexposed dichotomy or between some more quantitative exposure classes. A misclassification rate of 20% would not be at all surprising in epidemiological studies, particularly when exposures must be estimated based upon a historical reconstruction for some members of a study population. In the few studies where estimates of historical exposures were compared with actual measurements of exposure from the past, agreement within 20% between estimates and measurements of past exposure would be considered to be very good. In many cases, much larger differences have been observed (Stewart and Herrick, 1991).

SUMMARY AND RECOMMENDATIONS

A fundamental exploration of the nature of exposure is needed in which sufficient data are collected to examine underlying relationships. For example, it is routinely assumed that time-weighted average measurements of exposure are log-normally distributed (most investigators qualify this assumption as a 'reasonable' first approximation). However, it has not been rigorously shown why this is so or, more importantly, when it is not so. Since much of our ability to extrapolate exposures, particularly high ones, depends on knowledge of the underlying distribution, this is a critical omission. Large data sets will be required to answer these distributional questions, and to determine how workplace factors affect exposures beyond broad categories. It is appalling how little investigation there has been of exposures to our most extensively studied health hazards (asbestos, lead and silica) compared to other areas of environmental science, such as the problem of atmospheric acid aerosol. This level of investigation is needed to characterize full complex industrial environmental processes.

Estimation of past exposures to potential health hazards is one of the most difficult problems for occupational hygiene research. Although it is very difficult, it is not impossible. Two conceptual models have been described that can guide the hygienist in this task: (1) the source–receptor model; and (2) the task-TWA model. In addition to estimating exposure when data do not exist, these two conceptual models may be useful for guiding evaluations of potential sources of error in estimates of past exposures. It is important to recognize that the steps in extrapolation of past exposures have variable magnitudes of uncertainty. Quantitative estimates of exposure intensity for the distant past generally have the highest uncertainty. However, large uncertainty in the intensity of exposure does not mean that qualitative exposures are equally uncertain. It is important to consider a variety of exposure measures because less quantitative measures derived from information on the nature of operations and job activities can be very useful in some cases.

ACKNOWLEDGEMENT

The authors wish to acknowledge the many contributions of others to the development of these ideas, especially our colleagues: Susan Woskie, Katharine Hammond, David Kriebel, Marilyn Hallock and Margaret Quinn.

REFERENCES

Checkoway, H., Savitz, D.A. and Heyer, N.J. (1991). Assessing the effects of nondifferential misclassification of exposures in occupational studies. *Applied Occupational and Environmental Hygiene*, **6**, 528–33.

Dement, J.M., Harris, R.L., Symons, M.J. and Shy, C.M. (1983). Exposures and mortality among chrysotile asbestos workers. Part I: exposure estimates. *American Journal of Industrial Medicine*, **4**, 399–419.

Dodgson, J., Cherrie, J. and Groat, S. (1987). Estimates of past exposure to respirable man-made mineral fibers in the European insulation wool industry. *Annals of Occupational Hygiene*, **31**, 567–82.

Gerin, M., Siemiatycki, J., Kemper, H. and Begin, D. (1985). Obtaining occupational exposure histories in epidemiologic case–control studies. *Journal of Occupational Medicine*, **27**, 420–6.

Goldberg, M.S., Siemiatycki, J. and Gerin, M. (1986). Inter-rater agreement in assessing occupational exposure in a case–control study. *British Journal of Industrial Medicine*, **43**, 667–76.

Greife, A.L., Hornung, R.W., Stayner, L.G. and Steenland, K.N. (1988). Development of a model for use in estimating exposure to ethylene oxide in a retrospective cohort mortality study. *Scandinavian Journal of Work, Environment and Health*, **14**, (Suppl. 1), 29–31.

Hayes, R.B., Raatgever, J.W., deBruyn, A. and Gerin, M. (1986). Cancer of the nasal cavity and paranasal sinuses, and formaldehyde exposure. *International Journal of Cancer*, **37**, 487–92.

Kromhout, H., Oostendorp, Y., Heederik, D. and Boleij, J.S.M. (1987). Agreement between qualitative exposure estimates and quantitative exposure measurements. *American Journal of Industrial Medicine*, **12**, 551–62.

Rappaport, S.M., Kromhout, H. and Symanski, E.N. (1993). Variation exposure between workers in homogeneous groups. *American Industrial Hygiene Association Journal*, **54**, 654–62.

Schneider, T., Olsen, I., Jorgensen, O. and Lauersen, B. (1991). Evaluation of exposure information. *Applied Occupational and Environmental Hygiene*, **6**, 475–81.

Smith, T.J., Hammond, S.K. and Wong, O. (1993). Health effects of gasoline exposure: I. Exposure assessment for U.S. distribution workers. *Environmental Health Perspectives*, **101**, (Suppl. 6), 13–21.

Stewart, P.A. and Herrick, R.F. (1991). Issues in performing retrospective exposure assessment. *Applied Occu-pational and Environmental Hygiene*, **6**, 421–7.

Stewart, P.A., Lemanski, D., White, D., Zey, J., Herrick, R.F., Masters, M., Rayner, J., Dosemeci, M., Gomez, M. and Pottern, L. (1992). Exposure assessment for a study of workers exposed to acrylonitrile. I. Job exposure profiles: a computerized data management system. *Applied Occupational and Environmental Hygiene*, **7**, 820–5.

CHAPTER 19
Statistics

D. Oakes

SOURCES OF VARIATION

Occupational hygienists spend much of their working lives taking measurements. Unfortunately these can rarely be taken at face value. Consider, for example, a single determination of the concentration of carbon monoxide in a welding plant, made at 3.00 p.m. on a Tuesday in October. Before it can be asserted that this figure represents in any sense the true level of carbon monoxide exposure in that plant, many possible sources of error and variation in that measurement must be considered. Among these are instrument error, calibration error and observer error.

Instrument error. No instrument has been, or can ever be, devised to be perfectly accurate. Technology will always place some limitations on our ability to measure.

Calibration error. An incorrectly calibrated instrument will give measurements that are systematically above or below the true value.

Observer error. The hygienist may make mistakes in reading the instrument. Although with well-designed instruments these will usually be small mistakes, occasionally fatigue or carelessness may cause gross errors.

These are all errors made in the actual measuring process. The hygienist may feel fairly comfortable with these sources of error, since their likely magnitude can be assessed under controlled conditions in a laboratory. But of far greater importance and much less easy to assess are factors relating to the inherent variability of what is being measured. The following factors are among these.

Temporal variation. The determination was made at a specific time on a specific date. The carbon monoxide concentration at other times of day, on other days of the week or in a different month or year will possibly be very different.

Spatial variation. The concentration will vary over the plant according to proximity to sources of exposure and to ventilation systems.

Little ingenuity is needed to think of other possible sources of error or variability. With measurements made on humans, allowance must be made for biological variation and working habits.

Biological variation. People often do not react in the same way to the same external environment. The characteristics and efficiency of the human body viewed as a biological system vary considerably from person to person.

Working habits, too, differ substantially between individuals. Personal sampling of workers side by side on a production line and apparently doing the same job yield very different results.

It is important to distinguish between *random error* (or random variation) and *systematic error* or *bias.* Random variation is a fluctuation of a quantity around its long-term average value. If an instrument sometimes reads too high, sometimes too low, but on the average gives the correct reading then it is exhibiting random error. The effect of random error can be reduced by averaging a series of values. On the other hand, if the instrument is incorrectly calibrated, so that its readings are consistently too high (or consistently too low), then it is exhibiting systematic error. Systematic error is impervious to averaging. The only way to deal with it effectively is to avoid it in the first place, by correct statistical sampling procedures, calibration of instruments and training of observers (see Chapter 17).

Consideration of error and variability is an important part of the planning and execution of any hygiene survey. This chapter shows how appropriate statistical sampling techniques and methods of data analysis can help the hygienist assess the likely magnitude of uncertainty and reduce its effect on the conclusions from a study. Subjects covered in this chapter are: (1) the presentation of series of measurements or counts by histograms and boxplots and various summary measures for describing these distributions; (2) the so-called normal and log-normal distributions and the Poisson distribution; (3) statistical sampling; (4) assessing variability, including an introduction to the term 'standard error'; (5) hypothesis testing, including the much used and abused concept of statistical significance; (5) relations between two variables, concentrating on the technique of linear regression; (7) the analysis of categorized data (contingency tables); (8) some points in the design of experiments, including the technique of randomization; and finally (9) some more advanced statistical techniques and the implications of the increasing use of computers in data processing and analysis.

It is customary to classify statistical methods as either 'descriptive' or 'inferential'. Descriptive statistical methods, as the name implies, concern the concise description and summarization of the data to hand. Inferential methods assess the possible affect of chance variation on the observed results, and thus the extent to which they can be generalized to other similar situations. Boxplots and scatterplots are examples of descriptive techniques; hypothesis tests and confidence intervals are inferential methods.

DISTRIBUTIONS

The first step towards the understanding of a series of measurements is to form a frequency distribution. Consider the list of the forced expiratory volumes (FEV$_1$) measured on 24 fire officers as shown in Table 19.1. (See Chapter 1 for a discussion of the meaning of, and techniques for the measurement of, FEV$_1$.)

It is hard to get any picture of the variability or

average value of these measurements from reading the list in Table 19.1. However, if the data are grouped in 0.5 l class intervals as shown in Table 19.2, a picture does emerge.

Table 19.2 is called a frequency distribution, because it reports the frequency or number of values falling within each class interval. It can be depicted graphically by a histogram as shown in Fig. 19.1. When, as here, the class intervals are of equal width, the frequency for each interval is represented by the height of the corresponding

Table 19.1 Forced expiratory volumes (1.0 s), in litres, of 24 fire officers

4.935	4.383	4.660	3.256	3.329	4.552
4.030	4.372	3.174	3.884	4.017	3.274
4.025	5.176	4.284	3.600	3.226	5.062
2.678	4.201	4.037	4.097	4.410	3.783

Table 19.2 Frequency distribution of forced expiratory volumes (FEV$_1$) given in Table 19.1

Class interval	Frequency
2.500−2.999	1
3.000−3.499	5
3.500−3.999	3
4.000−4.499	10
4.500−4.999	3
5.000−5.499	2
Total	24

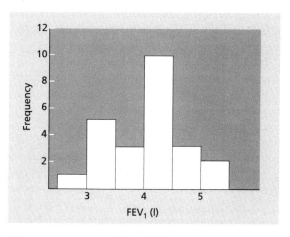

Fig. 19.1 Histogram of the frequency distribution in Table 19.2.

rectangle. The essential features of the distribution of FEV_1 can be seen at a glance from the histogram — the values range from about 2.5 l to about 5.5 l with an average a little over 4.0 l, and with some apparent bunching in the 3.0–3.5 l and 4.0–4.5 l intervals. A full interpretation of these data would require consideration of other variables, for example age, height and smoking habits, which are known to influence FEV_1.

The general picture of a distribution given by a histogram needs to be supplemented by numerical summaries of the major features of the distribution. The most common such measure is the (*arithmetic*) *mean*, obtained by summing all the values and dividing by their total number. From Table 19.1, the mean FEV_1 is:

$$\frac{4.935 + 4.383 + \ldots + 3.783}{24}$$

$$= \frac{96.445}{24}$$

$$= 4.019 \qquad (19.1)$$

where we have used the three dots to avoid writing out all 24 terms in the numerator. If the data values are taken to represent the co-ordinates of unit masses placed along an axis, the centre of gravity of these masses will be at the point represented by the arithmetic mean of the distribution.

An approximate arithmetic mean can be calculated from the grouped data of Table 19.2 by supposing that each value occurs at the midpoint of its class interval. The contribution of each class interval to the total is the product of this midpoint and the corresponding frequency.

The arithmetic mean is a measure of the location (average value, central tendency) of the distribution. Another useful summary of location is the *median* or 'middle value'. To find this, the values must be arranged in order from the lowest to the highest, an operation which although quite straightforward is surprisingly time-consuming for lists of even moderate size. We illustrate this with two simple examples: the median of the five numbers $-1, 0, 4, 3, 1$ is 1 (the ordered list would be $-1, 0, 1, 3, 4$); the median of the four numbers $-1, 0, 4, 3$ is $\frac{1}{2}(0 + 3) = 1.5$. In the latter example, which has an even number of values, as there is no single middle value we take the average of the middle two values.

The enthusiastic reader may check that the median of the values in Table 19.1 is $\frac{1}{2}(4.030 + 4.037) = 4.0335$. The *upper* and *lower quartiles* of a distribution are defined in a similar way. Together with the median they split the data into four equal parts. For the data of Fig. 19.1, the upper quartile is 4.403 and the lower quartile is 3.397.

The distribution shown in Fig. 19.1 happens to be fairly symmetric, and has no wild values (outliers). For such distributions the mean and median will be fairly close together. However, many of the distributions encountered by a hygienist are *skewed*, such as that shown in Fig. 19.2. Distributions of particle sizes and of the levels of a contaminant in an occupational environment typically have this general shape: with a long tail stretching to the right representing the occasional occurrence of values much larger (perhaps by several orders of magnitude) than the typical values near the peak or mode of the distribution. We refer to this shape as 'positive skewness'. 'Negative skewness', which is less common, occurs when the distribution has a long tail stretching to the left. (It is better to avoid the terms 'left-skewed' and 'right-skewed' as they are often confused.) As the median is less influenced than the mean by occasional very high (or very low) values, it is generally preferable to the mean as a measure of location for skewed distributions. However, it may happen that the mean of the distribution is of more intrinsic interest than the median, because the mean exposure level deter-

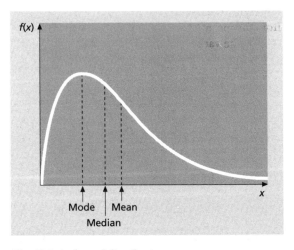

Fig. 19.2 A skewed distribution.

mines the total body burden experienced by a worker or group of workers, and this may be the determining factor as far as implications for the health of the workforce are concerned.

A useful mnemonic holds that for most unimodal (i.e. single peaked) distributions, the mean, median and mode occur in either alphabetical or inverse alphabetical order: the median lying between the mean and mode (see Fig. 19.2).

The second most important feature of a distribution is its spread, scatter or dispersion. Several measures of spread have been proposed. The simplest is the *range*, defined as the largest value minus the smallest value. For the data of Table 19.1 the range is $5.176 - 2.678 = 2.4981$. Although simple to calculate and interpret, the range has serious disadvantages as a measure of spread. Because it is calculated from the two values (largest and smallest) which are, by definition, the least typical, it gives little information about the distribution as a whole. For example, deleting the lowest value of 2.678 from Table 19.1 would change the appearance of Fig. 19.1 only slightly, yet would reduce the range quite noticeably to $5.176 - 3.174 = 2.002$.

A better approach to measuring spread is to ask how far, on average, a typical value is from the mean value. At its simplest, this approach leads to the mean deviation. This is calculated as the arithmetic mean of the differences (without regard to sign) of each value from the mean of the distribution. More convenient technically are the *variance* and the *standard deviation*. The variance represents the mean squared deviation of the values from the mean. The standard deviation is the square root of the variance.

It is convenient to use some algebraic notation. The letter x will denote a value from a distribution. We use a capital Greek sigma Σ to denote the operation of summing (addition) over all values in a distribution, and n to denote the total number of values. The arithmetic mean is denoted by $\bar{x}$ and the formula for its calculation from ungrouped data (as in Table 19.1) is:

$$\bar{x} = \frac{\Sigma x}{n} \tag{19.2}$$

The sample variance, denoted by s^2, is defined by the formula:

$$s^2 = \frac{\Sigma(x - \bar{x})^2}{n - 1} \tag{19.3}$$

In words: subtract from each value the overall mean, square and add. Finally, divide the result by the *degrees of freedom* — calculated as the number of values minus one. The reason for dividing by the degrees of freedom $n - 1$ rather than the sample size n is related to the fact that if the original deviations are summed without first squaring, the result is zero, the positive deviations exactly cancelling the negative deviations:

$$\Sigma(x - \bar{x}) = 0 \tag{19.4}$$

The squaring makes all the deviations non-negative and therefore variances are always positive.

Some calculators have separate keys for calculating a sample variance (with denominator $n - 1$ as above) and the so-called *population variance*, which is calculated with denominator n. The sample variance is usually what is required.

A slightly different, although algebraically equivalent, formula is sometimes used to calculate the variance. This computational formula for s^2 is:

$$s^2 = \frac{\Sigma x^2 - (\Sigma x)^2/n}{n - 1} \tag{19.5}$$

For the data of Table 19.1:

$$\begin{aligned}
\Sigma x^2 &= 4.935^2 + 4.383^2 + \ldots + 3.783^2 \\
&= 24.354 + 19.211 + \ldots + 14.311 \\
&= 397.053 \tag{19.6}
\end{aligned}$$

and

$$\begin{aligned}
s^2 &= \frac{397.053 - (96.445)^2/24}{23} \\
&= \frac{397.053 - 387.568}{23} = \frac{9.485}{23} = 0.412 \tag{19.7}
\end{aligned}$$

If the calculation is done this way, care is needed to keep sufficient decimals to avoid rounding error, since the numerator is found as the difference between two large but similar quantities.

The sample standard deviation is calculated as the square root of the variance. Here $s = \sqrt{0.412} = 0.642$. As for the mean, approximate values of s^2 and s can be calculated from grouped data.

When, as here, all the data are positive (a negative FEV_1 would be somewhat pathological!) it can be

useful to express the standard deviation as a proportion, or percentage, of the mean. The result is
called the *coefficient of variation* (CV). The CV
does not depend on the units in which the data are
measured. Here CV = 0.642/4.019 = 0.160 (16%),
and would be the same if the FEV were expressed
in millilitres instead of litres, for example. The
coefficient of variation is often used to express the
relative precision of different laboratory procedures
for determining concentrations of environmental
contaminants, since the error in such determinations is often approximately proportional to the
magnitude being determined.

A different measure of spread that is less influenced than the standard deviation by the tails of
the distribution is the *inter-quartile range* (IQR).
This is defined as the difference between the upper
and lower quartiles. For example, for the data of
Table 19.1, the IQR is 4.403 − 3.397 = 1.006.

The normal distribution

The *normal* or Gaussian distribution occupies pride
of place in statistical theory and practice. Continuous variables such as height and blood pressure,
and many types of measurement error, are often
found to follow normal distributions. One reason
for this is the central limit theorem (see below).
The characteristic shape of the normal distribution
is the symmetric bell-shaped curve shown in Fig.
19.3. The distribution is fully determined by its
mean (usually denoted by the Greek letter μ) and
its standard deviation denoted by σ. We commonly
use Greek letters such as μ and σ to denote theoretical or population values of quantities or parameters of interest, to distinguish these from values
such as $\bar{x}$ or s that may be calculated from data. For
the distribution shown (of heights in centimetres,
for example) $\mu = 170$ and $\sigma = 5$. The equation of the
curve is:

$$f(x) = \frac{1}{\sqrt{(2\pi)}\sigma} \exp\left[-\frac{1}{2}\left(\frac{x - \mu}{\sigma}\right)^2\right] \quad (19.8)$$

This function, $f(x)$, is called the density of the
distribution. It represents the limiting shape of the
histogram of a large number of values taken from
the distribution when the class intervals are made
arbitrarily small.

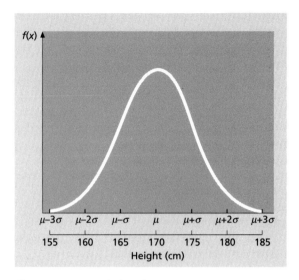

Fig. 19.3 A 'normal' distribution.

The total area under the curve is unity, i.e.:

$$\int_{-\infty}^{\infty} f(x)dx = 1 \quad (19.9)$$

(The proof of this statement is a far from trivial
exercise in calculus.) It can also be shown mathematically that μ and σ represent the mean and
standard deviation of the distribution in the senses
described earlier. The proportion of values falling
between two limits is given by the corresponding
area under the curve. For example, about 68% of
any normal distribution lies within one standard
deviation of the mean (here this would be 165–
175 cm), about 95% within two standard deviations
of the mean (here 160–180 cm) and almost 99.8%
within three standard deviations of the mean (here
155–185 cm). The tails of the distribution decrease
rapidly as $x - \mu$ or its negative becomes large.

The *standard normal distribution* has mean zero
($\mu = 0$) and unit standard deviation ($\sigma = 1$). Tables of
the area under any portion of the standard normal
curve appear in most statistical texts. To use these
tables to calculate areas under other normal curves
we must first standardize the limits. For example,
to find the area under the normal curve of Fig. 19.3
and between limits 160 cm and 175 cm, we convert
each limit to a standard variable z by subtracting the
mean 170 and dividing by the standard deviation 5,
giving:

$$\frac{160 - 170}{5} = -2$$

and

$$\frac{175 - 170}{5} = 1 \qquad (19.10)$$

These standardized limits, sometimes called z-scores, measure the distance of the two values 160 cm and 175 cm, from the mean, in units of the standard deviation. The final step is to read off the area between the limits −2 and +1 from a table of the standard normal distribution. The required area is 0.8185, indicating that 81.85% of the distribution lies between the limits 160 cm and 175 cm.

Boxplots

The *boxplot* is a simple display of the salient features of a distribution. It is particularly useful for visual comparison of several sets of data. It is more immediately informative than numerical summary values such as the mean and median and yet takes up less space than a series of histograms. As an illustration, Fig. 19.4 shows boxplots of repeat samples of dust concentrations from eight locations in a Quebec asbestos mine. The upper and lower sides of the rectangular 'box' for each location give the upper and lower quartiles of the corresponding distribution of values and the middle line corresponds to the median. The 'whiskers' extend from the quartiles to the most extreme observation not further than $1.5 \times \text{IQR}$ from the quartiles. Observations outside this range are marked separately. Figure 19.4 shows the wide variation in both the median levels and the IQR for different locations. It also shows the positive skewness of each distribution – the upper tails are typically longer than the lower tails – and that the variability at each location is greater when the average level is greater.

Figure 19.5 shows the same plots after the data have been transformed by taking natural logarithms. This transformation reduces both the skewness of the distributions and the tendency for the variability to increase with the average level.

The log-normal distribution

Not all distributions are normal. For example, the distribution of the level of contaminant in an occupational environment may well be skewed as illustrated in Fig. 19.2. As illustrated in Figs 19.4 and 19.5, distributions of the logarithms of the concentrations are often much closer to normality. Taking logarithms, or equivalently plotting the level of

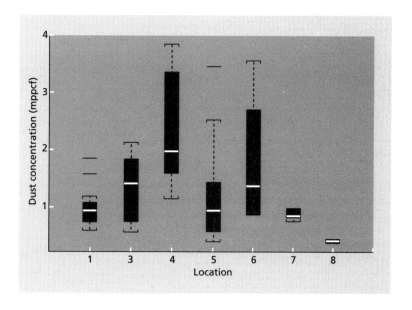

Fig. 19.4 Boxplots of dust concentrations in repeat samples from eight locations in a Quebec asbestos mine. mppcf, millions of particles per cubic foot.

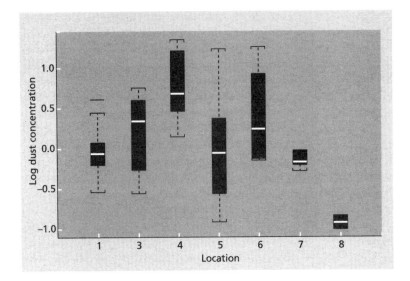

Fig. 19.5 Boxplots of natural logarithms of dust concentrations.

contaminant on log-paper, has the effect of compressing the long right tail of the distribution and expanding the short left tail so that the entire distribution becomes more symmetric, as illustrated in Fig. 19.5. If the transformed data follow a normal distribution, then the original, i.e. untransformed, data are said to follow a *log-normal* distribution, sometimes denoted by $LN(\mu, \sigma^2)$. Here the parameters μ and σ^2 denote the mean and variance of the transformed data. Note that the mean of the original data is not $\exp(\mu)$ as one might expect (the exponential being the inverse transformation to the natural logarithm) but $\exp(\mu + \frac{1}{2}\sigma^2)$. Actually $\exp(\mu)$ corresponds to the *geometric mean* of the original data values. The corresponding quantity calculated from n data values would be the nth root of the product of these values, i.e. of all the values multiplied together. The geometric mean is always less than the arithmetic mean. By analogy, $\exp(\sigma)$ is sometimes called the *geometric standard deviation* (GSD), although this usage has the strange consequence that the geometric standard deviation of a distribution with zero scatter is unity (since $\exp(0) = 1$). It may be shown that, for the log-normal distribution, $GSD \approx 1 + CV$, provided σ is small.

The Poisson distribution

If particles are distributed purely randomly over a microscope slide which is divided into a large number, N, of fields of equal area, then chance will ensure that some fields contain more particles than others. In fact if λ denotes the average (mean) number of particles per field it can be shown that the frequency of fields containing exactly $x = 0, 1, 2, \ldots$ particles will be approximately:

$$f(x) = N \exp(-\lambda) \frac{\lambda^x}{x!} \qquad (19.11)$$

where $x!$ denotes the product of all numbers less than or equal to x, $x! = x \times (x - 1) \times (x - 2) \times \ldots \times 1$. This is the *Poisson distribution*. Figure 19.6 illustrates a hypothetical distribution of particles over a section of slide with 25 fields. The frequencies of fields with 0, 1, 2 and 3 particles are compared in Fig. 19.7 with the frequencies predicted by the Poisson distribution. Here $\lambda = 1$, so there is an average of one particle per field. For example, the predicted number of fields with exactly two particles is:

$$f(2) = \frac{25 \times e^{-1} \times 1^2}{2 \times 1} = 4.60 \qquad (19.12)$$

A surprising property of the Poisson distribution is that its variance is numerically the same as its mean, λ. Its standard deviation is, therefore, $\sqrt{\lambda}$. When λ is large, the shape of the Poisson distribution is similar to that of a normal distribution with mean λ and variance λ.

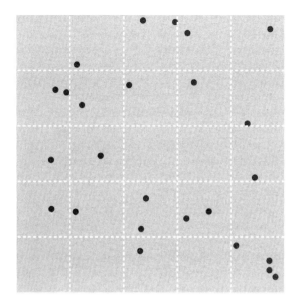

Fig. 19.6 A random distribution of particles on a section of a slide.

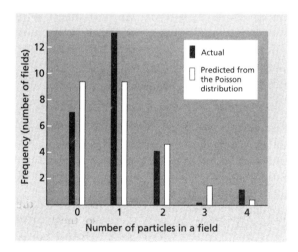

Fig. 19.7 Actual and predicted frequency distribution from Fig. 19.6.

The Poisson distribution has other applications, including describing the occurrence of accidents. If (a big if) each accident which occurs in a plant is equally likely to occur to any worker in the plant, irrespective of how many previous accidents that worker may have had, then the distribution of the number of workers having exactly $x = 0, 1, 2 \ldots$

accidents in a given period will be Poisson. The assumption of *homogeneity* — that all fields have an equal chance of containing a particle, or that all workers are equally likely to have accidents — is crucial to the derivation of the Poisson distribution. If it is not satisfied, other distributions with greater variability must be used, for example the negative binomial.

The Poisson distribution is also used in the analysis of standardized mortality ratios (SMRs) arising from epidemiological studies.

STATISTICAL SAMPLING

Often the hygienist will want to determine the distribution of some characteristic in a population of items, individuals or measurements, but will have the resources to examine only a small fraction of that population.

Example 19.1: the blood lead levels of all 1000 workers in a can-making factory may be of interest, but resources may permit the examination of only 50 workers. How should these 50 be selected?

Example 19.2: as stated above, the level of contaminant in an industrial environment is likely to show considerable temporal fluctuation from day to day, hour to hour or even minute to minute. If continuous monitoring of the environment is not feasible, how should the hygienist select the times to take 20 15 min grab samples so that the distribution of levels of contaminant found from these samples reflects the distribution of levels of contaminant in the environment over a specified week?

Example 19.3: if it is desired to estimate the proportion of firms in the silk-screen printing industry with inadequate ventilation systems, but only a small number of firms can be inspected, how should these firms be chosen?

In Example 19.1 the *target population* (the population of interest) consists of all workers in the factory, in Example 19.2 it consists of all $40 \times 4 = 160$ quarter hour periods in the working week (assuming no overtime or shift work and a 40 h working week) and in Example 19.3 it consists of all establishments engaged in silk-screen printing. We assume that in each case the hygienist wants to choose a representative group or *sample* from the population. One approach, or rather lack of approach, is *haphazard sampling*. We might measure blood lead levels of the first 50 workers who appear, or sample the levels of contaminant at times when it is most convenient to do so. Haphazard sampling gives rise to unknown and possibly substantial biases, since there can be no guarantee that the sample chosen is representative. Indeed it will almost certainly not be.

An alternative approach, which seems attractive, is to sample members of the population who appear to be typical. Unfortunately people are not good judges of who or what is typical and this method of *subjective sampling* is rarely satisfactory.

A further difficulty with both haphazard sampling and subjective sampling is that there is no way of knowing how representative the sample selected is of the population. We would like to place a tolerance, for example, on the difference between the blood lead level of the 50 workers in the sample and of the 1000 workers in the population.

Simple random sampling enables this to be done, as we shall see later. The idea behind simple random sampling is that all the possible samples that might be chosen must have the same probability of selection. This ensures that all members of the population have the same chance of being selected, and that the selection of one member does not influence the chance of selection of any other member. Bias in the selection of the sample is avoided and is seen to be avoided. Simple random sampling is carried out using tables of random numbers. These are specifically devised so that all ten digits 0, 1, ..., 9 appear with equal frequency, all 100 pairs 00, 01, ..., 99 appear with equal frequency and so on. Table 19.3 exhibits a short sequence of random numbers.

To select a simple random sample from a population we first need a list of all members of the population numbered in order. This list is essential; without it no representative sampling strategy is possible. Obtaining such a list can be surprisingly difficult, as the three examples illustrate. In Example 19.1, an up to date and accurate payroll would suffice. In Example 19.2 the actual hours to be worked in the week in question would need to be known. In Example 19.3, itemizing establishments engaged in silk-screen printing would be a major part of the project. Possible sources of information include business directories, trade associations and suppliers of ink and other materials.

Once the list has been obtained, we simply read through the table of random numbers from a predetermined starting point and choose for our sample the corresponding members of the population. The following example illustrates the method. Suppose we want to draw a sample of five from a population of 43 items, and our starting point was determined as row 2, column 9. We require digit pairs, and obtain them, reading from left to right, as follows: 20; 30; 77; 84; 57; 03; 29; 10; 45; etc. To select the sample we choose the first five digit pairs that do not exceed 43. The sample then consists of items numbered: 20; 30; 3; 29; 10. Any number which duplicates one already selected is ignored.

An alternative procedure to simple random sampling is *systematic sampling*. To draw a systematic sample of 50 workers from a population of 5000 we would pick a single random number between 1 and 100 (inclusive), say 73, and select for our sample workers numbered 73, 173, etc., to 4973. Although systematic sampling is usually essentially equivalent to simple random sampling, there is the potential drawback that if some relevant characteristic of the population is periodic, the systematic sampling could hit on that periodicity and give a seriously biased sample.

Stratified random sampling is a variant of simple random sampling in which the population is first divided into sub-populations or strata. The members of each stratum should be as alike as possible. For example, as different tasks lead to different levels of exposure, it might be sensible to group the 1000 workers in the can-making factory of Example 19.1 by the task they perform. A separate random sample is then selected from each stratum. This facilitates comparison between different strata by ensuring that they are each adequately represented in the sample and can also lead to closer tolerances between overall sample and population values.

Table 19.3 Extract from a table of random numbers

27	42	37	86	53	48	55	90	65	72
00	39	29	68	61	66	37	32	20	30
77	84	57	03	29	10	45	65	04	36
29	98	94	07	60	62	93	55	59	33

A stratified random sample may not be representative of the sampled populations, since we may deliberately decide to use a higher sampling fraction (i.e. select a higher proportion of) in one stratum than another. However, the appropriate statistical adjustments to the sample mean to make it a valid estimate of the population mean are quite straightforward, provided we can identify the stratum of each member of the sample.

SAMPLING DISTRIBUTIONS AND STANDARD ERRORS

An important advantage of random sampling as opposed to haphazard or subjective sampling is that the mathematical theory of probability can assess how representative of the population the sample is likely to be. Consider, for example, the 1000 workers of Example 19.1. We want to estimate the mean blood level (μ) in this population. To do this we take a random sample of 50 workers and determine the blood lead level (x) of each worker in this sample. The sample mean $(\bar{x})$ of these 50 values of x estimates the unknown mean μ of the 1000 values in the population. The difference $\bar{x} - \mu$, between the sample mean and the population mean, is called the *sampling error*. The actual amount of this error cannot be determined (unless the population mean (μ) is known, when the entire sampling exercise would be pointless), but we can assess its likely magnitude by appealing to the notion of a *sampling distribution*.

Suppose that we selected not just one but many different random samples of size 50 from the same population of workers and calculated the mean blood level $(\bar{x})$ for each sample. We would then obtain a series of values of $\bar{x}$. The distribution of this series of values is called the sampling distribution of $\bar{x}$. It has three very useful and quite surprising properties.

1 The mean of the sampling distribution of $\bar{x}$ is the same as the mean of the distribution of x in the population.

2 The variance of the sampling distribution of $\bar{x}$ is σ^2/n, where σ^2 denotes the variance of the population distribution of x, and n is the sample size $(n = 50$ in the example). Increasing the sample size decreases the variance of $\bar{x}$. (Notice that, at the risk of some confusion, we telescope the phrase 'variance of the sampling distribution of $\bar{x}$' into the shorter 'variance of $\bar{x}$'.)

3 The sampling distribution of $\bar{x}$ often agrees closely with the normal distribution (see p. 328) even when the distribution of x is markedly non-normal. The larger the sample size, the better the agreement. This fact is a consequence of the famous *central limit theorem* which asserts (roughly) that the sum or average (arithmetic mean) of a large number of quantities, randomly and independently selected from any distribution with finite variance itself, has a distribution whose shape is close to normal.

These three properties are illustrated by Fig. 19.8, showing a hypothetical population distribution which is quite highly skewed and the distribution of means of samples of size $n = 4$ from that population. Even though n is here quite small, the distribution of $\bar{x}$ is much less variable and much less skewed than that of x.

The standard deviation of the sampling distribution of $\bar{x}$ is called the *standard error* of $\bar{x}$. It is usually written as $\text{SE}(\bar{x})$ and from above it can be expressed as:

$$\text{SE}(\bar{x}) = \frac{\sigma}{\sqrt{n}} \qquad (19.13)$$

Provided the sample size n is reasonably large, the approximate normality of the sampling distribution of $\bar{x}$ (property (3) above) leads to quite precise probability statements concerning the sampling error $\bar{x} - \mu$. For example, in only about one in 20 random samples will the sample mean depart from the population mean by more than 1.96 standard errors. Thus for any single random sample, there is a probability close to 0.95 that the sampling error $\bar{x} - \mu$ will be numerically less than $1.96\sigma/\sqrt{n}$. The multiplier 1.96 comes from a table of the standard normal distribution (see above).

Confidence intervals

Strictly, the probability statement applies only before the sample is selected. When the sample has been chosen and $\bar{x}$ determined we refer instead to *confidence levels* or *confidence statements*. For example:

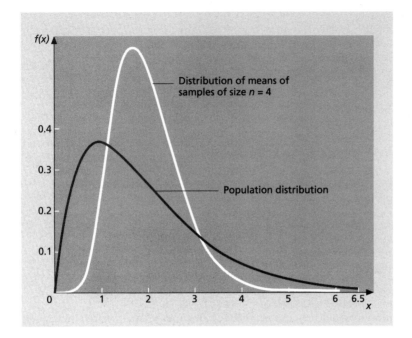

Fig. 19.8 Sampling distribution of means.

$$\left(\bar{x} - 1.96 \frac{\sigma}{\sqrt{n}}, \bar{x} + 1.96 \frac{\sigma}{\sqrt{n}}\right) \quad (19.14)$$

is called a 95% *confidence interval* for the population mean μ. Since 19 out of 20 random samples would lead to confidence intervals which include μ, the confidence interval calculated from any particular random sample is likely to include the population mean μ. Other confidence levels (e.g. 90% or 99%) lead to different multiples of the standard error (1.64 and 2.58, respectively, instead of 1.96), giving narrower or wider intervals compensated by a lesser or greater certainty of including the population value. A practical difficulty in calculating a confidence interval is that the population standard deviation (σ) may also be unknown. Fortunately σ can be estimated from the sample standard deviation (s) as discussed above, but the sampling error between σ and s introduces extra uncertainty. The sample variance (s^2) itself has a distribution with mean equal to the population variance (σ^2). This is why the denominator of s^2 is the degrees of freedom $n-1$ rather than n. With denominator n, s^2 would on average underestimate σ^2. For large n, the sampling distribution of s^2 is approximately normal and is tightly concentrated around σ^2. For samples of small or moderate size

(say, $n < 120$), the distribution of s^2 is appreciably dispersed and for small n it is quite highly skewed.

To allow for the extra uncertainty caused by replacing σ by its sample estimate s, larger multiples must be used to achieve any given level of confidence. These multipliers, which we shall call t^*, are obtained from 'Student's t distribution'. They depend on the degrees of freedom as well as the confidence level. For 9 degrees of freedom (i.e. sample size $n = 10$), the multiplier for a 95% confidence interval is 2.26. When $n = 30$ (29 degrees of freedom) the multiplier is 2.04.

Difference between two means

In comparative work, the hygienist may want to estimate the difference $\mu_1 - \mu_2$ between two population means. A distinction must be made between paired and independent samples. Paired samples arise when two measurements are made on a single individual. In Example 19.1 it might be of interest to see by how much average blood lead levels had changed after the introduction of new methods of work. The blood lead levels of each of the 50 workers would be measured before and after the change. The correct analysis of such data is to calculate the differences, $d = $ 'after' − 'before' for each worker, keeping careful track of signs. The 50 differences (d) would be analysed as a single statistical sample, by computing the mean change $(\bar{d})$ and its standard error as above. A confidence interval for the mean change (Δ) among all 1000 workers could be obtained in the same way. Paired samples arise in epidemiological work when individuals are selected from two different populations (perhaps of 'cases' and 'controls') but the members of one sample are individually selected to have the same sex and age as members of the other sample. This procedure is an example of *matching*. By contrast, we may have two separate samples selected independently from two distinct populations. For example, we might want to compare the blood levels of the 1000 workers in the canning industry with those of another group of workers in a different industry. If random samples, now possibly of different sizes, are selected independently from the two populations, the difference $\bar{x}_1 - \bar{x}_2$ between the two sample means estimates the difference $\mu_1 - \mu_2$ between the population means. (Note that the subscripts 1 and 2 distinguish the two populations.)

Three cases arise in the calculation of the standard error of $\bar{x}_1 - \bar{x}_2$ and of the confidence intervals for the population mean difference $\mu_1 - \mu_2$.

Case a Population variances σ_1^2 and σ_2^2 are both known. The standard error of $\bar{x}_1 - \bar{x}_2$ is:

$$\text{SE}(\bar{x}_1 - \bar{x}_2) = \sqrt{\left(\frac{\sigma_1^2}{n_1} + \frac{\sigma_2^2}{n_2}\right)} \quad (19.15)$$

and multipliers for the confidence intervals are obtained from tables of the standard normal distribution.

Case b Population variances σ_1^2 and σ_2^2 are unknown, but are assumed to be approximately equal. The standard error of $\bar{x}_1 - \bar{x}_2$ is:

$$\text{SE}(\bar{x}_1 - \bar{x}_2) = \sqrt{s^2\left(\frac{1}{n_1} + \frac{1}{n_2}\right)} \quad (19.16)$$

where s^2, the so-called 'pooled estimate of variance', is the weighted average of the two sample variances $(s_1^2$ and $s_2^2)$ with weights proportional to the corresponding degrees of freedom:

$$s^2 = \frac{(n_1 - 1)s_1^2 + (n_2 - 1)s_2^2}{n_1 + n_2 - 2} \quad (19.17)$$

The multiplier for the confidence interval is obtained from tables of Student's t distribution with $n_1 + n_2 - 2$ degrees of freedom.

Case c Population variances are unknown and unequal. Here the standard error is estimated as:

$$\text{SE}(\bar{x}_1 - \bar{x}_2) = \sqrt{\left(\frac{s_1^2}{n_1} + \frac{s_2^2}{n_2}\right)} \quad (19.18)$$

but an exact multiplier for the confidence interval is hard to determine. A simple approximation is to use Student's t distribution with the smaller of $n_1 - 1$ and $n_2 - 1$ as the degrees of freedom. Some computer programs have more sophisticated rules for assigning degrees of freedom.

Assumption of normality

The use of Student's t distribution is strictly valid only when the distributions of x in the parent populations are normal. However, with moderately large sample sizes, slight departures from normality are allowable. If the sample distributions of x are highly skewed, a transformation (e.g. $\log(x)$ or $\sqrt{x}$) may help. For data with outliers (wild values), alternative statistical techniques (known as nonparametric methods) are available.

Sampling distribution of a proportion

Interest may focus on the population possessing some attribute, for example cigarette smoking. Call the proportion of cigarette smokers in the population π and define a new variable x which takes the value 1 for a smoker and 0 for a non-smoker. If the size of the population is N, it will include $N\pi$ individuals having $x = 1$ and $N - N\pi$ individuals having the value 0. The population mean value of x is:

$$\mu = \frac{\Sigma x}{N} = \frac{(1 \times N\pi) + [0 \times (N - N\pi)]}{N} = \pi \quad (19.19)$$

Therefore, the proportion π can be interpreted as the population mean of the new variable x. The population variance of x can also be expressed in terms of π. Since $1^2 = 1$ and $0^2 = 0$, the sum of x^2 is the same as the sum of x, namely $N\pi$. The computational formula for the variance gives:

$$\sigma^2 = \frac{N\pi - (N\pi)^2/N}{N} = \pi(1 - \pi) \quad (19.20)$$

Notice that we have used the divisor N rather than $N - 1$ and called the variance σ^2 rather than s^2 because the calculation is for a population, not a sample. To estimate the proportion (π) of cigarette smokers in the population we select a random sample of size n and determine the proportion (p) of cigarette smokers in the sample. By similar reasoning to that above, the proportion p is the same as the sample mean $\bar{x}$ of the variable x. It follows that the three important properties listed for the sampling distribution of a mean apply also to the sampling distribution of p. This distribution therefore has mean π and variance $\pi(1 - \pi)/n$, whence the standard error of p is:

$$\text{SE}(p) = \sqrt{\frac{\pi(1 - \pi)}{n}} \quad (19.21)$$

Since the population proportion (π) is unknown, we replace it in the formula by the known sample proportion (p). The formula for the estimated standard error of p is then:

$$\text{SE}(p) = \sqrt{\frac{p(1 - p)}{n}} \quad (19.22)$$

If also, n is sufficiently large, the sampling distribution of $p = \bar{x}$ will be approximately normal in shape, even though x is certainly highly non-normal, taking only the two values 0 and 1. This allows a 95% confidence interval for the population proportion π to be derived as:

$$\left(p - 1.96\sqrt{\frac{p(1 - p)}{n}}, \, p + 1.96\sqrt{\frac{p(1 - p)}{n}} \right) \quad (19.23)$$

The multiplier 1.96 is obtained from the normal distribution — Student's t distribution is not used with proportions. For a confidence interval for the difference between two proportions based on estimates from two independent samples the appropriate standard error is the square root of the sum of squares of the standard errors of each proportion:

$$\sqrt{\frac{p_1(1 - p_1)}{n_1} + \frac{p_2(1 - p_2)}{n_2}} \quad (19.24)$$

In comparing proportions from paired samples a slightly different approach is necessary. Consider,

for example, the estimation of the change in proportion of smokers among the same population between 31 January 1992 and 31 January 1993. One approach would be to interview the same people about their smoking habits on the two dates. Therefore, we would choose a single random sample and interview each member on the two dates. Those who were non-smokers on both dates or who were smokers on both dates would not affect the change in the proportion of smokers. If r denotes the number of non-smokers who switched to smoking and s the number of smokers who gave up, the change in the proportion of smokers is:

$$p_1 - p_2 = \frac{(r - s)}{n} \quad (19.25)$$

and can be shown to have approximate standard error:

$$\frac{\surd(r + s)}{n} \quad (19.26)$$

In this formula we do not take the square root of the n in the denominator.

Notes

1 The population size N does not appear in these formulae. (We introduced N in discussing proportions but it was cancelled from expressions.) In fact, the results given are strictly valid only for $N = \infty$. For finite N the standard error formulae should be multiplied by $1 - f$, where f is the sampling fraction and equals n/N. If the whole population is sampled, $n = N$, $1 - f = 0$ and the standard error is 0, as would be expected. But generally the value of N scarcely affects the standard error. With a sample of size $n = 100$ it hardly matters whether the population size is $N = 10\,000$ or $N = 10\,000\,000$; in the first case $1 - f = 0.99$ and in the second $1 - f = 0.99999$. The size of the sample is crucial; the size of the population is almost irrelevant.

2 The notions of a sampling distribution, standard errors and confidence intervals have a much wider application than has been indicated here. For example, measurement errors made in repeat determinations of the same physical quantity are not actually selected from a population, but they can often be regarded as forming a sample from a hypothetical distribution, nature itself, as it were, doing the sampling. To say that the errors form a sample from a population distribution with zero mean is essentially to say that the errors are random and not systematic. If so, standard errors and confidence intervals are useful indicators of the possible effect of chance variation on the estimate obtained. They can be calculated using the techniques of this section, and should be reported.

HYPOTHESIS TESTING: STATISTICAL SIGNIFICANCE

A test of statistical significance is a procedure for testing whether a specific statement about a population is consistent with data observed on a sample from that population.

Example 19.4: to see if the change in working techniques has influenced the mean blood lead levels of the 1000 workers of Example 19.1 we test the *null hypothesis* that the mean population difference between the blood lead levels before and after the change is zero.

Example 19.5: to assert that the time-weighted average concentration of a contaminant in an industrial environment is below the threshold limit value (TLV), the hygienist needs strong evidence against the null hypothesis that the average level is above the TLV.

We use Example 19.4 to illustrate the procedure and language of significance testing.

a State the null hypothesis: $\mu_1 - \mu_2 = 0$.

b Decide on a *test statistic* for rejecting or not rejecting the null hypothesis. The test statistic derives from the sampling distribution of the sample estimate $\bar{x}_1 - \bar{x}_2$ of $\mu_1 - \mu_2$. Here we use the sample estimate divided by its standard error, as estimated above.

c Specify the size, significance level or probability of type 1 error. These three terms all mean the probability that if the null hypothesis were true, it would be rejected. The aim is to keep this probability small, and 0.05 is a conventional choice.

d Use the sampling distribution of the test statistic (the estimate divided by its standard error) to set a criterion for rejecting the null hypothesis. The criterion is the same as the multiplier derived from statistical tables that was used in the calculation of

a confidence interval. For a significance level of 0.05 we use the same value as for a 95% confidence interval. For the paired t test using the sample variance in the formula for the standard error, the criterion value would be $t^* = 2.01$.

Strictly, these calculations should be performed before the sample is chosen and the data collected. After data collection it only remains to:

e Calculate the observed value of the test statistic, compare it with the criterion and accordingly reject the null hypothesis. Supposing that $\bar{x}_1 - \bar{x}_2 = 9 \, \text{mg} \, \text{l}^{-1}$ and $\text{SE}(\bar{x}_1 - \bar{x}_2) = 6 \, \text{mg} \, \text{l}^{-1}$, the test statistic is:

$$\frac{\bar{x}_1 - \bar{x}_2}{\text{SE}(\bar{x}_1 - \bar{x}_2)} = \frac{9}{6} = 1.5 \qquad (19.27)$$

which is numerically less than the criterion value $t^* = 2.01$, so the null hypothesis would not be rejected. If instead $\bar{x}_1 - \bar{x}_2 = 15 \, \text{mg} \, \text{l}^{-1}$ and $\text{SE}(\bar{x}_1 - \bar{x}_2) = 6 \, \text{mg} \, \text{l}^{-1}$ then the ratio:

$$\frac{\bar{x}_1 - \bar{x}_2}{\text{SE}(\bar{x}_1 - \bar{x}_2)} = \frac{15}{6} = 2.5 \qquad (19.28)$$

being numerically greater than the criterion value $t^* = 2.01$ would lead to the rejection of the null hypothesis. Notice that the 95% confidence intervals for $\mu_1 - \mu_2$ in the two cases would be calculated as:

$$9 \pm (2.01 \times 6) \text{ i.e. } (-3.06, 21.06) \quad (19.29)$$

and

$$15 \pm (2.01 \times 6) \text{ i.e. } (2.94, 27.06) \quad (19.30)$$

The first interval includes the value $\mu_1 - \mu_2 = 0$, the second does not. This illustrates a general though not universal relation between significance testing and estimation. The hypothesis of no difference is rejected at the 5% significance level if, and only if, the 95% confidence interval does not include zero. Each of the estimation procedures described in the previous section has its analogue in hypothesis testing. There is a slight modification in the standard error calculation for the difference between two independent sample proportions. To calculate $\text{SE}(p_1 - p_2)$ for the significance test, first determine the pooled proportion:

$$\bar{p} = \frac{n_1 p_1 + n_2 p_2}{n_1 + n_2} \qquad (19.31)$$

and calculate:

$$\text{SE}(p_1 - p_2) = \sqrt{\bar{p}(1 - \bar{p})\left(\frac{1}{n_1} + \frac{1}{n_2}\right)} \qquad (19.32)$$

This formula gives a more accurate estimate of the standard error when the null hypothesis is true, i.e. when the population proportions are equal. An example of the use of this formula is given later.

Notes

1 The null hypothesis is rejected only when the data provide strong evidence against it. Failure to reject the null hypothesis should not be construed as proof that it is true. Indeed in Example 19.4, exact equality of the two population means would be quite implausible.

2 In Example 19.4, a *two-sided test* was used, as the null hypothesis would be rejected if $\bar{x}_1 - \bar{x}_2$ is numerically large, regardless of sign. In Example 19.5, a *one-sided test* should be used since the null hypothesis can only be rejected when the average level of contaminant is below the TLV. This has the effect of reducing the criterion chosen in step (d). For example, a two-sided test concerning a population mean when the population variance is known, would reject the null hypothesis at the 0.05 level of significance if the test statistic were less than -1.96 or greater than 1.96. A corresponding one-sided test would reject at the same level if the test statistic were less than -1.64.

3 Example 19.5 illustrates another point. It may seem perverse to take as the null hypothesis that the average concentration is above the TLV, when we want to demonstrate that it is below the TLV. However, this is the correct formulation, as it places the burden of proof in the right place. If the sample average concentration is slightly higher than the TLV, we certainly do not exonerate the industry. To do this we need a sample average not only lower than the TLV, but low enough to ensure that the difference is not due to sampling variation.

4 After the data have been obtained it is customary to calculate a '*P-value*' or descriptive level of significance. This is the significance level corresponding to exact equality of the criterion and the test statistic. It measures how often, if the null hypothesis were true, a discrepancy as large or larger between the null hypothesis and the sample data would occur purely by chance. The smaller the P-value, the stronger is the evidence against the null hypothesis provided by the data.

5 The P-value is not the probability that the null hypothesis is true. It is unnecessary to quote P-values greater than 0.10, as they simply that the data provide no evidence against the null hypothesis. A simple NS (not significant) will suffice.

Occasionally very low values of the test statistic may occur, leading to P-values close to 1.00. Far from being strong evidence of the truth of the null hypothesis, they are more likely to indicate a mistake in calculation, incorrect choice of test procedure or that the investigator has tidied up (i.e. fudged) or selected data to ensure good agreement with the null hypothesis.

6 Statistical significance is not necessarily the same as practical significance. If sample sizes are large, a small observed difference may be statistically significant because of an even smaller standard error, but a difference of this magnitude may be of no practical use or interest. With small sample sizes, even fairly large observed differences may not lead to rejection of the null hypothesis. The magnitude of a sample estimate, together with its standard error, should be reported, as well as its P-value.

7 In planning a survey, the hygienist must consider the power of the statistical test as well as its level of significance. The power is defined as the probability that when the null hypothesis is false, the test will reject it. Each degree of falsity has its own power. If the null hypothesis is false, but only just false (in Example 19.4, suppose $\mu_1 - \mu_2 = \Delta$ is close to, but not equal to, zero) the test will have very low probability of detecting the difference. But if Δ is large, the probability of rejecting the null hypothesis will be close to unity. The power of a test is like the resolving power of a microscope: it specifies limits on the magnitude of the discrepancy between the null hypothesis and the actual population values that can be reliably discerned. By reducing or increasing the criterion chosen in step (d), we can trade an increased power (good) against an increased significance level (bad) but we cannot simultaneously increase the power and decrease the significance level. This can be achieved only by increasing the sample size or by redesigning the investigation to reduce inherent variability.

8 In view of (7), the choice of sample size becomes vitally important. Statisticians have devised the appropriate formulae, which require specification of:

(a) some estimate of population variability;

(b) the smallest discrepancy from the null hypothesis that the hygienist wishes to detect;

(c) the significance level and power of the statistical test for detecting this discrepancy (0.05 and 0.90 respectively are conventional choices.) One must also specify whether the test is to be one-sided or two-sided.

Often the sample size required will be unrealistically large. The hygienist must then lower his or her expectation or cancel the proposed investigation.

9 A common error, especially when analysing complex sets of data involving many variables, is to choose the hypothesis to be tested in the light of observed data.

Example 19.6: blood lead levels of workers in 10 different firms are compared and any differences noted. With 10 sample means, 45 different comparisons can be made. It would be incorrect to select the largest observed difference and test this for statistical significance, as, even if the 10 population means are identical, we would expect about 5% of the 45 comparisons (say two or three comparisons) to be 'statistically significant' at level 0.05. Clearly, the largest observed sample difference is likely to be among these 'statistically significant' comparisons.

The correct procedure for handling these multiple comparisons is known as 'analysis of variance'. See Armitage and Berry (1987).

10 The earlier comments concerning the assumption of normal distribution in the population from which the samples are drawn applies here also.

RELATIONS BETWEEN TWO VARIABLES: REGRESSION

Often the hygienist is concerned with relations between different variables. Two simple textbook examples of such relations are shown below:

1 Conversion of degree Celsius to degree Fahren-

heit. Multiply the Celsius temperature by 1.8 and add 32. If x denotes the Celsius temperature and y the Fahrenheit temperature, this becomes:

$$y = 32 + 1.8x \qquad (19.33)$$

2 Boyle's law states that for a given mass of gas at constant temperature, pressure × volume = constant. Writing x for the pressure and y for the volume, this can be written:

$$y = \frac{c}{x} \qquad (19.34)$$

where c is the volume of the gas at unit pressure. These equations can be displayed graphically. For a given value of x, the corresponding value of y can be read off the graph. The temperature conversion equation is represented by a straight line and Boyle's law by a curve (in fact a hyperbola). The multiplier or coefficient 1.8 of x in the equation $y = 32 + 1.8x$ is called the slope, as it represents the change in y corresponding to a unit change in x. The constant term or intercept 32 represents the value of y when $x = 0$. Any straight line, except one parallel to the y-axis, can be represented by an equation of the same form but with different numerical values of the slope and intercept.

Although Boyle's law is not linear as it stands, it can be made so by taking logarithms. Supposing that $c = 100$, taking logarithms (to base 10) yields $\log y = 2 - \log x$. This equation represents a linear relation between the new variables $Y = \log y$ and $X = \log x$:

$$Y = 2 - X \qquad (19.35)$$

Taking logarithms is a convenient way of 'straightening' some types of non-linear relations.

Theory may suggest a linear relation between two variables, but practice may indicate that it holds only approximately, if at all. Consider for example the data given in Table 19.4, which were collected on a group of 12 workers exposed to airborne fluoride. The actual fluoride exposure of each worker was measured by personal sampling, as was the difference between the pre-shift and the post-shift urinary fluoride. The first step in the analysis of such data is to form a *scatter plot* as shown in Fig. 19.9. Each point (x, y) on this scatter plot represents the data for a single worker, the x-value being the exposure and the y-value being

Table 19.4 Airborne fluoride exposure and post-shift minus pre-shift urinary fluoride for 12 workers

Airborne fluoride exposure $(\mathrm{mg\,m^{-3}})$	Change in concentration of urinary fluoride (ppm)
0.61	4.8
0.41	2.6
0.84	5.8
0.69	3.7
0.57	2.7
0.87	5.4
0.60	4.3
0.41	2.3
0.90	5.6
0.67	4.1
0.36	2.3
0.93	5.7

the post-shift minus the pre-shift urinary fluoride. Figure 19.9 shows a clear relationship between the exposure x and the response y. Here x is the *independent*, or *stimulus* variable, and y is the *dependent*, or *response* variable.

Suppose we try to fit a linear relation of the form $y = a + bx$, how should the values of the slope (b) and intercept (a) be chosen? One way is by eye, using a transparent ruler or black thread, but different investigators would fit different straight lines to the same data. Linear regression is an objective procedure and yields simple formulae for the values of a and b in terms of the values of x and y

observed. The idea of linear regression can be explained by reference to Fig. 19.10. Here the dashed line represents one possible choice of a regression line (a poor choice as is obvious by eye) and the measured vertical deviations of each value of y from the predicted values from the straight line for the corresponding value of x.

The actual regression line is chosen to make these deviations small. More precisely, since all the deviations cannot be made small simultaneously — there is some element of trade-off of one deviation against another — the sum of squared deviations is made as small as possible. Algebraically, the criterion is to choose a and b to minimize:

$$\Sigma(y - \hat{y})^2 \qquad (19.36)$$

where $\hat{y} = a + bx$ is the value of y predicted by the regression line from the corresponding value of x. It can be shown that this criterion leads to the explicit formula:

$$b = \Sigma\frac{(x - \bar{x})(y - \bar{y})}{\Sigma(x - \bar{x})^2}, \; a = \bar{y} - b\bar{x} \quad (19.37)$$

For example, the data of Table 19.4 give:

$$\bar{x} = 0.655, \qquad \bar{y} = 4.108,$$
$$\Sigma(x - \bar{x})^2 = 0.4369, \qquad \Sigma(x - \bar{x})(y - \bar{y}) = 2.804,$$
$$b = \frac{2.804}{0.4369} = 6.417, \qquad (19.38)$$
$$a = 4.108 - (6.417 \times 0.655) = -0.095$$

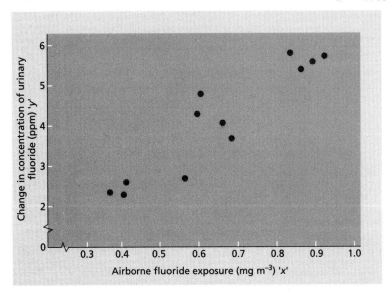

Fig. 19.9 Scatter plot of fluoride data of Table 19.4.

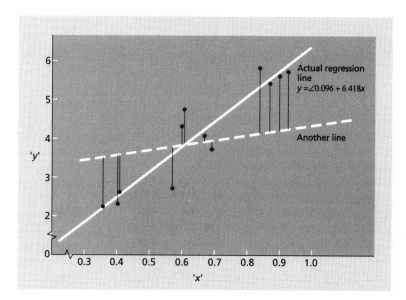

Fig. 19.10 The principle of linear regression.

It can be shown that no matter what the configuration of data points (x, y) (so long as not all the x values are the same), the regression line has the following properties:

1 the sum of the deviations (residuals), taking account of their signs, is zero, i.e.:

$$\Sigma(y - \hat{y}) = 0 \qquad (19.39)$$

2 the regression line goes through the centre of gravity $(\bar{x}, \bar{y})$;

3 points which are far from the centre of gravity, in the sense that $x - \bar{x}$ is large in magnitude, exercise a disproportionate influence on the position of the regression line;

4 paradoxically, points for which the deviation $y - \hat{y}$ is large also exercise a disproportionate influence on the position of the regression line.

Properties (3) and especially (4) can be undesirable and suggest that regression lines should not be indiscriminately calculated without examination of the data to see whether they follow a straight line relationship. After calculation of the regression line, discrepant data points can be identified by inspection of the residuals.

The discussion so far has emphasized the asymmetry of our view of the relationship between the two variables. We seek to explain the response in terms of the exposure, not vice versa. This asymmetry is apparent in the criterion (Equation

19.36) — the residual deviations are to be measured parallel to the response axis, not to the exposure axis. A measure of the strength of the linear relationship between two variables which does not single out either variable in this way is the *correlation coefficient (r)*. This is defined as:

$$r = \frac{\Sigma(x - \bar{x})(y - \bar{y})}{\sqrt{\Sigma(x - \bar{x})^2 \, \Sigma(y - \bar{y})^2}} \qquad (19.40)$$

If the data points happen to be exactly on a straight line, then $r = +1$ or $r = -1$ according to whether the line has positive or negative slope. These are the extreme possibilities: for points which do not exactly lie on a straight line $-1 < r < 1$. For the data of Table 19.4:

$$\Sigma(y - \bar{y})^2 = 20.77,$$

$$r = \frac{2.804}{\sqrt{0.4369 \times 20.77}} = 0.931 \qquad (19.41)$$

indicating a strong linear relation between x and y. A correlation coefficient of $r = 0$ indicates that there is no linear relation between x and y, but does not exclude the possibility of a non-linear (curved) relation between them.

The square of the correlation coefficient has a useful interpretation. It can be shown that the ratio of the variance of the residuals $y - \hat{y}$ to the variance of the original values of y is $1 - r^2$. For this reason

r^2 is often called the coefficient of determination, or (suggestively, if sometimes misleadingly) the proportion of the variance of y 'explained' by x.

Interpretations of the regression equation

A regression analysis can be performed on any collection of values of x and y to calculate the quantities, a, b, r and their statistical significance. Whether the result has any meaning of importance is another issue. It is helpful to distinguish three situations, though the distinctions are not hard and fast.

1 *The control knob model.* The researcher has physical control over x (e.g. angular displacement of the volume knob on a TV set). Changes in x result in changes in y (e.g. decibel level produced by the set) possibly with some random error or distortion.

2 *Spurious or nonsense correlation.* Two variables which really have little to do with each other may still be highly correlated, e.g. salaries of Methodist ministers and rum consumption. Spurious correlations will arise if both variables are increasing over time, or perhaps if they are each related to a third variable.

3 *Indirect relations.* These may be the hardest to interpret. Example: a (fictitious) regression analysis was performed of the heights of married women (y) on that of their husbands (x). The resulting equation was:

$$\hat{y} = 164 + 0.9(x - 174) \qquad (19.42)$$

This equation reflects the biological and sociological facts that men tend to be taller than women and that taller men (women) tend to choose taller women (men) as spouses. It would be an oversimplification to dismiss this relation as 'spurious' — that is, of no real significance. But it clearly does not have a direct causal interpretation: we cannot produce changes in y by changing x. A divorced woman who remarries a man 15 cm taller than her former husband does not thereby increase her own height by $0.9 \times 15 = 13.5$ cm, as would be predicted by the equation, not even 'on average'. Of course this example is extreme — but the same fallacy in other situations can be much harder to recognize.

Several different applications can be made of a regression calculation including prediction, screening, causal inference and multiple regression.

Prediction

The value $\hat{y} = a + bx$ can be used to predict an unknown value of y corresponding to a specified value of x. For example, we could use the value:

$$\hat{y} = -0.095 + (6.417 \times 0.80) = 5.04 \text{ ppm} \qquad (19.43)$$

to predict the change in urinary fluoride for a worker exposed to 0.80 mg m^{-3} of airborne fluoride. The likely error in such a prediction can be gauged from the magnitude of the residuals $y - \hat{y}$ of the observed data points from the regression line.

Depending on whether the specified value of x is within or outside the range of values of x in the data, we speak of interpolation or extrapolation respectively. Extrapolation can be dangerous as there is no guarantee that the linear relation established for the given values of x and y holds also for values of x and y outside the given range.

Screening

Here the interest centres on individuals where their actual response y is very different from their predicted response $\hat{y} = a + bx$ as derived from the regression equation. For example, we may have a regression equation of lung function against age and wish to identify those subjects with especially low lung functions for their age. Both prediction and screening may be carried out whether the relation between the two variables is direct or indirect.

Causal inference

The previous two applications must be distinguished from this, which involves estimating the effect on y of a specified change in x. Strictly, this can only be done when the regression equation represents a direct causal relation between x and y — the control knob model. Our hypothetical example of heights of spouses shows why. The only way to see what happens when you make a change is to actually make the change. To be confident of a direct causal relation we need to do a planned experiment, setting the x-values ourselves and observing the corresponding values of y. We cannot be satisfied with an allocation of (x, y) values that may itself have resulted from a complex amalgam of many other factors.

Multiple regression

Sometimes it is necessary to consider several different explanatory variables simultaneously. For example, lung function is related to height as well as to age. Multiple regression seeks to predict a single y-variable by a linear function of several x-variables. The principles are the same as in linear regression but the algebra is much more complicated and the interpretations can be even more difficult.

Statistical inference for linear regression

Under certain assumptions about the mechanism that generates the data, it is possible to calculate a standard error of the slope b and the intercept a (each regarded as a sample estimate of a population value β or α). For example, in the fluoride example, $\text{SE}(b) = 0.798$ and $\text{SE}(a) = 0.544$. Confidence intervals for β and α may be calculated as:

$$(b - t^*\text{SE}(b), b + t^*\text{SE}(b)), (a - t^*\text{SE}(a), a + t^*\text{SE}(a))$$
$$(19.44)$$

where the multiplier t^* is found from Student's t distribution with $n - 2$ degrees of freedom. In the example $n - 2 = 12 - 2 = 10$, so that for 95% confidence intervals $t^* = 2.228$, giving 95% confidence intervals for the slope of $(6.417 - (2.228 \times 0.798), 6.417 + (2.228 \times 0.798))$, i.e. $(4.64, 8.20)$, and for the intercept of $(-0.095 - (2.228 \times 0.544), -0.095 + (2.228 \times 0.544))$, i.e. $(-1.31, 1.117)$. The confidence interval for the slope does not include zero — these data provide strong evidence that there is a relationship between airborne fluoride exposure and urinary fluoride. The confidence interval for the intercept does include zero, showing that there is no evidence against the hypothesis that the true intercept is zero.

Effect of errors in the explanatory variables

Random errors in the dependent variable y of a linear regression decrease the precision with which slope of the regression line can be estimated, but do not bias the estimate. However random errors in the independent variable do tend to reduce or attenuate the estimate. This is one reason for the importance of accurate determination of exposure levels in epidemiological studies and risk assessment. Although 'corrections for attenuation' are sometimes made to compensate for this tendency, such corrections are not always appropriate.

This issue is related to the fact that the regression line $\hat{y} = a + bx$ of y on x typically differs from the regression line $\hat{x} = a' + b'y$ of x on y, i.e. with the roles of independent and dependent variables exchanged. The interested reader may check from the formulae, or by an example, that the two lines give different predictions for the 'x' corresponding to a specified 'y', i.e.:

$$\frac{y - a}{b} \neq a' + b'y \qquad (19.45)$$

Usually it is the second value $(a' + b'y)$ that is needed.

ANALYSIS OF CLASSIFICATIONS

A common objective of occupational health and hygiene surveys is to relate the exposure to some known or suspected hazard to the presence or absence of a specific disease or medical condition. A survey can ascertain whether each worker is or is not exposed to the hazard, and also whether or not he or she is suffering from the disease. The total population can be cross-classified by exposure category and disease category. Examples of the kind of table that might result are shown in Tables 19.5 to 19.10.

The first step in analysing these tables is to understand the structure of the classification. Except for the last column, all the tables are actual numbers, not proportions or percentages. The next to last column gives the total for that row, and the last column reports the proportion of this total who were 'sick'. In any cross-classification each

Table 19.5 Two exposure categories : two disease categories

	Sick	Well	Total	Proportion
Exposed	15	45	60	0.250
Not exposed	10	80	90	0.111
Total	25	125	150	

Table 19.6 Three unordered exposure categories : two disease categories

	Sick	Well	Total	Proportion
Shop A	20	80	100	0.200
Shop B	10	140	150	0.067
Shop C	30	70	100	0.300
Total	60	290	350	

Table 19.7 Three ordered exposure categories : two disease categories

	Sick	Well	Total	Proportion
Low exposure	5	95	100	0.050
Medium exposure	15	105	120	0.125
High exposure	20	60	80	0.250
Total	40	260	300	

Table 19.8 A three-way classification by gender exposure and disease

	Sick	Well	Total	Proportion
Men				
Exposed	4	36	40	0.10
Not exposed	2	18	20	0.10
Total	6	54	60	
Women				
Exposed	6	4	10	0.60
Not exposed	18	12	30	0.60
Total	24	16	40	

Table 19.9 Data of Table 19.8, aggregated for gender

	Sick	Well	Total	Proportion
Exposed	10	40	50	0.20
Not exposed	20	30	50	0.40
Total	30	70	100	

Table 19.10 Calculation of 'expected' numbers from Table 19.5

	Sick	Well	Total
Exposed	$\dfrac{60 \times 25}{150} = 10.0$	$\dfrac{60 \times 125}{150} = 50.0$	60
Not exposed	$\dfrac{90 \times 25}{150} = 15.0$	$\dfrac{90 \times 125}{150} = 75.0$	90
Total	25	125	150

individual is counted once and once only in the body of the table. For example, in Table 19.5 there were 15 members of the population under study who were both 'exposed' and 'sick'. In Tables 19.5, 19.6 and 19.7, the marginal (that is the row and column) totals and the grand total are also shown. Thus Table 19.5 is the simplest cross-classification, a 2×2 table. By comparing the proportions of sick workers in the exposed and not exposed groups we can detect association between exposure and disease. Here the proportions are $15/60 = 0.25$ in the exposed group and $10/90 = 0.111$ in the not exposed group so there is prima facie evidence that exposure and disease are related.

The classification in Table 19.6 would be appropriate when 'hard' exposure data are unavailable, but when it is suspected that workers in different shops may have different levels of exposure, we might then compare the proportions of sick workers in the three shops. From Table 19.6, these proportions are $20/100 = 0.200$, $10/150 = 0.067$ and $30/100 = 0.300$. The interpretation of these results may be difficult.

Table 19.7, although superficially similar to Table 19.6 is actually quite different. Here each worker has been classified as subject to low, medium or high exposure. If exposure is related to disease, we would expect the proportion sick to increase with the amount of exposure. For the data given, the proportions are $5/100 = 0.050$, $15/120 = 0.125$ and $20/80 = 0.250$, bearing out our expectation. Had the same proportions appeared in a different order (for example 0.050 in the low-exposure group, 0.250 in the medium-exposure group and 0.125 in the high-exposure group), the evidence of relation between exposure and disease would be much less convincing. With data such as that in Table 19.6 it is desirable to rank the 'shop' categories in terms of exposure even if this can be done only informally. To avoid circular reasoning, the ranking must be done using hygiene information, not the medical classification.

Table 19.8 illustrates another issue, that of confounding. In the previous section we commented that association between variables does not necessarily imply the existence of a direct causal relation between them. The association could result from a third variable. If in Table 19.8 we calculate the proportion sick among the exposed and not exposed groups, separately for men and for women, we obtain the values $4/40 = 0.1$, $2/20 = 0.1$, $6/10 = 0.6$ and $18/30 = 0.6$ respectively. Although there is substantial difference between the proportions for men and women, for each gender the rates among the exposed and not exposed groups are the same. These data suggest that exposure does not influence disease.

Ignoring gender leads to the two-way classification shown in Table 19.9. There is a clear difference between the proportion sick in each of the two groups, indicating an association between exposure and disease — in fact suggesting that exposure is beneficial! However, the data of Table 19.8 indicate that this is due to gender differences, and it would be very unwise to draw any conclusion from Table 19.9. In this instance gender would be a confounding factor, as it is related both to disease (women suffering more than men) and to the exposure (fewer women than men being exposed). Confounding factors that are not allowed for in the design or analysis of a study can distort its conclusions.

The appropriate technique for assessing the statistical significance of an observed association between exposure and disease in each of the examples given can be found in textbooks. We shall consider only Table 19.5. The null hypothesis is that the difference between the two proportions ($p_1 = 15/60 = 0.25$, and $p_2 = 10/90 = 0.11$) is due to chance only: the underlying probabilities π_1 and π_2 of becoming sick are the same in the exposed and not exposed groups. Two apparently different, but actually equivalent, tests of this null hypothesis are available.

The first test, based on the difference $p_1 - p_2$ between two sample proportions, was discussed above. The value $p_1 - p_2$ is divided by its standard error, calculated from Equation 19.32, and the result compared with a criterion obtained from a normal approximation to the sampling distribution of $p_1 - p_2$. Here the pooled proportion is:

$$\bar{p} = \frac{15 + 10}{60 + 90} = \frac{25}{150} \qquad (19.46)$$

and calculation with Equation 19.33 gives:

$$\begin{aligned} \text{SE}(p_1 - p_2) &= \sqrt{\frac{25}{150} \times \frac{125}{150} \times \left(\frac{1}{60} + \frac{1}{90}\right)} \\ &= \sqrt{0.003858} \qquad (19.47) \\ &= 0.0621 \end{aligned}$$

The value of the test statistic is:

$$\frac{p_1 - p_2}{\text{SE}(p_1 - p_2)} = \frac{0.25 - 0.11}{0.0621} = 2.24 \quad (19.48)$$

This exceeds the value 1.96 for a two-sided test with significance level 0.05. From a table of the normal distribution, the descriptive level of significance is $P = 0.025$.

The chi-square test has a quite different rationale. It compares the 'observed' numbers of deaths in each cell of the table with the 'expected' numbers calculated as if the null hypothesis were true. These are calculated from the row and column totals as shown in Table 19.10. For example, the top left entry is the total number sick (25) multiplied by the total number exposed (60) divided by the grand total (150). Here the 'expected numbers' are all integers (whole numbers) but generally they will not be and must not be 'rounded off'.

As a check, the totals formed from this table should be the same as those of the original table. More importantly the arithmetic ensures that for the expected numbers, the proportion sick in the exposed group is the same as the proportion sick in the not exposed group.

Observed numbers which differ strongly from the corresponding expected numbers tend to contradict the null hypothesis. The differences among them are summarized by the *chi-square statistic*:

$$\chi^2 = \sum \frac{(O - E)^2}{E} \qquad (19.49)$$

where O stands for the observed or actual number in a cell of the table, E for the corresponding expected number and Σ for summation over all cells in the body of the table (i.e. not the margins). For the data of Tables 19.5 and 19.10:

$$\chi^2 = \frac{(15 - 10)^2}{10} + \frac{(45 - 50)^2}{50} + \frac{(10 - 15)^2}{15}$$

$$+ \frac{(80 - 75)^2}{75} \qquad (19.50)$$

$$= 2.5 + 0.5 + 1.67 + 0.33 = 5.0$$

The approximate sampling distribution of χ^2 when the null hypothesis is true has been tabulated — it is known as the *chi-square distribution* with one degree of freedom. The 5% and 1% points are 3.84 and 6.63, giving statistical significance here at 5% but not at 1%.

Although the chi-square test and the test based on the differences in proportions are quite dissimilar in appearance they are mathematically equivalent in that, within the accuracy of the calculation, they always yield the same descriptive level of significance. The numerical value of the chi-square statistic is the same as the square of the critical ratio calculated from the $p_1 - p_2$ test (thus $5.0 = 2.242^2$). The same is true for the tabulated chi-square and standard normal values for the same level of significance (thus $3.84 = 1.96^2$).

Chi-square does not measure the strength of the association. For example, multiplying all entries in Table 19.5 by 10 leaves the strength of the association (as measured, say by the relative risk — see Chapter 20) between exposure and disease unchanged, but multiplies the value of χ^2 by 10. This increased χ^2 reflects the fact that, if the null hypothesis is true, a large discrepancy between the two sample proportions is much less likely to occur with the larger sample sizes.

Methods for estimation and testing appropriate to Tables 19.6, 19.7 and 19.8 can be found in statistical texts such as Armitage and Berry (1987). In Table 19.6, the chi-square test for heterogeneity is appropriate: Table 19.7 requires a test for trend. Methods for combining information from several contingency tables, as in Table 19.8, have been given by Cochran (1954) and Mantel and Haenszel (1959) — for details see Armitage and Berry (1987).

Statistical analysis of case–control studies

In the previous discussion we have implicitly assumed that the data give a cross-classification of the complete population of interest, or alternatively that independent random samples of workers are available from the different exposure groups. Some epidemiological investigations, for example those of a rare disease or where there is a long latent period between the exposure and disease, compare instead the exposure histories of a sample of subjects who are known to have developed the disease ('cases') with those of a sample of 'controls' who have not developed the disease. Such case–control studies are discussed in Chapter 20. Care needs to be given to the appropriate selection of the two series of subjects and to unbiased ascertainment of exposure histories.

Table 19.11 presents simplified data from one such study, of bladder cancer among smelter workers (Theriault *et al.*, 1984); 85 new cases of bladder cancer were identified over a 10 year period, among current and past workers of a large aluminium smelter. Three controls were selected for each case, by random sampling from a register of other current and past workers, after matching for year of birth, year of starting work in the smelter and length of service at the smelter. Since work in the potroom was known to involve high levels of exposure to aromatic hydrocarbons, the agent of primary research interest, cases and controls were classified by whether they had worked for a year or more in the potroom.

Although Table 19.11 is similar in form to Table 19.5, its interpretation is very different. Since the overall disease rate of $85/(85 + 255) = 0.25$ was fixed by the design of the study, the disease rates among the two exposure groups convey no information in

Table 19.11 Case–control study of smelter workers

	Bladder cancer cases	Controls
Potroom	49	86
Others	36	169
Total	85	255

themselves. It would be more informative to compare the proportions $49/85 = 0.576$ and $86/255 = 0.337$ of potroom workers among the two series of subjects. However a better approach is to calculate the *odds ratio* (OR) or cross-product ratio:

$$\text{OR} = \frac{ad}{bc} = \frac{49 \times 169}{36 \times 86} = 2.67 \quad (19.51)$$

Here $a = 49$, $b = 36$, $c = 86$ and $d = 169$ are just the four entries in Table 19.11. Under certain conditions it may be shown that the odds ratio provides a valid estimate of the relative risk of bladder cancer that would have been obtained in a long-term cohort study of the same population. Thus, these data would suggest that the lifetime risk of developing bladder cancer for a potroom worker would be almost triple that for other smelter workers.

Confidence intervals for the true odds ratio based on these observed data can be obtained from the following formula for the standard error of the log odds ratio:

$$\begin{aligned} \text{SE}\,[\log(\text{OR})] &= \sqrt{\left(\frac{1}{a} + \frac{1}{b} + \frac{1}{c} + \frac{1}{d}\right)} \\ &= \sqrt{\left(\frac{1}{49} + \frac{1}{86} + \frac{1}{36} + \frac{1}{169}\right)} \quad (19.52) \\ &= 0.256 \end{aligned}$$

A 95% confidence interval for the log odds ratio is:

$$(\log(2.67) - (1.96 \times 0.256), \log(2.67) + (1.96 \times 0.256))$$

that is

$$(0.982 - 0.502, 0.982 + 0.502)$$

or

$$(0.480, 1.484) \quad (19.53)$$

This is a confidence interval for the natural logarithm of the odds ratio, and we must exponentiate each value to obtain a confidence interval for the odds ratio itself, i.e.:

$$(\exp(0.480) = 1.62, \exp(1.484) = 4.41) \quad (19.54)$$

Therefore, the data are consistent at a 95% level of confidence with a true odds ratio in the range 1.6 to 4.4. They are not consistent at this level of confidence with an odds ratio of unity, which would imply no influence of potroom work on the risk of bladder cancer. This is another way of saying that the null hypothesis of no association between potroom work and bladder cancer risk would be rejected at the 5% level of significance.

More sophisticated methods of analysis, for example logistic regression, which take account of the individual matching between cases and controls, and which also allow for the influence of other variables, such as smoking, are outside the scope of this chapter. See for example Breslow and Day (1980).

DESIGNED EXPERIMENTS: RANDOMIZATION

Since it is usually desirable to assess the likely consequences of innovations before introducing them on a large scale, the hygienist may need to plan a comparative study of the effects of several different courses of action. For example, the choice may be between two forms of protective gloves, the question being which gloves are more likely to be worn when they should be. The only effective way of answering this question is to give some workers one form of glove, other workers the other form and see which gloves are worn most. Unfortunately, if the participants in this study choose the type of glove themselves they will naturally choose those they prefer and the resulting assessments could well be biased. If hygienists try to overcome this problem by deciding themselves who should get which glove, they still need a procedure for making the allocation, otherwise they may, consciously or subconsciously, give the gloves they prefer to the workers they think need them most or are more likely to wear them. Or they may do the opposite. Either way, comparisons between the two forms of gloves will be biased.

To avoid such selection biases, statisticians devised the procedure known as randomization. The allocation is made to depend on a chance mechanism. A simple form of randomization would be to toss a coin for each worker to decide the type of glove he or she is given — if heads, type A; if tails, type B. Randomized allocation ensures that the two groups of workers are roughly comparable, and that large differences in the performance of the two gloves, should they occur, will not be due to differences between the two groups of workers — in skill, compliancy, seniority or any other factor — but will be due to the gloves themselves.

Randomization, like random sampling, is, in practice, usually carried out with tables of random numbers generated by a computer. Despite the similarity in terminology and execution, the two techniques have different purposes. Random sampling is a procedure for selecting a representative statistical sample from a population. Randomization is a technique for assigning subjects into two (or more) comparable groups.

Randomization is much used in clinical trials of medical innovations. Patients are allocated by randomization into a 'treatment' group and a 'control' (comparison) group. The treatment group receive the new form of treatment; the control group receive the present, standard treatment. Differences between the subsequent performance of the two groups measure the effectiveness of the new treatment as against the standard treatment.

When carried out on human subjects, randomization can raise serious ethical issues. Whichever treatment is actually superior, some subjects will receive the other, inferior treatment. A randomized trial would be unethical if it was known which treatment was better, but where there is genuine uncertainty and the choice of preferred treatment would otherwise depend on fad or fashion rather than knowledge, it may be unethical not to carry out a randomized clinical trial.

An essential prerequisite for randomization is that the investigator can ensure that subjects allocated to a particular group stay in that group. The hygienist, having decided by randomization that Smith should receive type B gloves, must have enough control to ensure that Smith does not subsequently swap with Jones who was given type A gloves. Such swaps would reintroduce the selective biases that randomization is intended to avoid.

Randomization can be used in laboratory investigations involving, for example, the responses of animals to various environmental insults. In fact, it should be used whenever the investigator is ethically and practically able to assign the composition of the experimental and control groups. The units to be assigned by randomization may be entire workplaces, as in a proposed study of the effectiveness of occupational health services staffed by nurses. The factories participating in the study were to be divided into pairs, the members of each pair being selected to be as alike each other as possible. For each pair, a coin toss would determine which factory in the pair should be provided with the new occupational health service.

This example also illustrates the principle of blocking—dividing the experimental units into groups with similar characteristics and then randomizing separately within each group. (Here the groups are the pairs of factories.) The field of experimental design concerns such blocking techniques, which can be mathematically rather sophisticated when several different sources of variation are present.

COMPUTERS

Electronic computers have revolutionized the analysis of survey data. Mathematical calculations which would previously have taken a lifetime to perform can now be completed by a suitably programmed computer in a fraction of a second. This has encouraged the development of sophisticated statistical techniques and has also made possible the analysis of large sets of data involving perhaps thousands of measurements on hundreds of variables. Most of the numerical calculations shown in this chapter would usually be performed by computer.

The evolution of high-level computer languages and packaged programs ('software') is almost as important as that of the computing machines ('hardware') themselves, for it is of little use to be able to carry out a calculation in a fraction of a second if it first takes a statistician or programmer a lifetime to instruct ('program') the machine to do it.

Many packaged programs have been developed to process, edit and analyse statistical data. Commonly available are SAS (Statistical Analysis System), SPSS (Statistical Package for the Social Sciences), BMDP (Biomedical Computer Programs), 'GLIM' and 'SPlus'. 'EGRET' is useful for epidemiological applications. Although little programming skill is needed to master the use of these packages, understanding of statistical principles is essential. The computer does not know what analyses are appropriate to a given set of data. It will faithfully perform any operations it is instructed to do, whether these are relevant or irrelevant, valid or invalid. Responsibility for the validity and relevance of an analysis rests with the investigator, not the computer. Nor can computers magically purify bad data. Although editing programs can aid the investigator to locate missing values, inconsistencies and absurdities in the data, what to do about these is still the investigator's responsibility. As they say: garbage in, garbage out.

An especially useful feature of computers is their ability to link information from several sources. For example, sickness records for an individual can be compared with measurements of exposure to suspected hazards.

These analyses can now be performed on personal computers, even laptops. The wide availability of such machines has led to a booming market in statistical packages, many with facilities for attractive graphical output. Unfortunately not all such packages have been tested properly, and even if they have been they cannot guarantee that statistical techniques appropriate to a given data set have been chosen. However they can take away the drudgery of hand tabulation and calculation.

ACKNOWLEDGEMENT

Preparation of this chapter was facilitated in part by grant R01-CA 61087 from the National Cancer Institute (US).

REFERENCES

Armitage, P. and Berry, G. (1987). *Statistical Methods in Medical Research*, (2nd edn). Blackwell Scientific Publications, Oxford.

Breslow, N.E. and Day, N.E. (1980). *Statistical Methods in Cancer Research*, Vol. 1. *The Analysis of Case–Control Studies*. IARC, Lyon.

Cochran, W.G. (1954). Some methods for strengthening the common χ^2 tests. *Biometrics*, **10**, 417–51.

Mantel, N. and Haenszel, W. (1959). Statistical aspects of the analysis of data from retrospective studies of disease. *Journal of the National Cancer Institute*, **22**, 719–48.

Theriault, G., Tremblay, C., Cordier, S. and Gingras, S. (1984). Bladder cancer in the aluminium industry. *Lancet*, (**i**), 947–50.

FURTHER READING

Clayton, D. and Hills, M. (1993). *Statistical Models in Epidemiology*. Oxford.

Leidel, N.A., Busch, K.A. and Lynch, J.R. (1977). *Occupational Exposure Sampling Strategy Manual*. NIOSH, Cincinnati.

CHAPTER 20
Epidemiology

J.M. Harrington

INTRODUCTION

Definitions

Occupational hygiene is a discipline primarily concerned with the work environment rather than the health of the worker. Nevertheless, as this book has demonstrated, the health of the workforce is heavily dependent upon the control of the environment. Hygienists are thus part of the ill-health prevention process.

Epidemiology may be defined as the study of the distribution and determinants of health-related states or events in specified populations, and the application of this study to the control of health problems. Whenever consideration is given to the health of groups of people — and this is invariably so in occupational health — the principles of epidemiology must be understood. The hygienist, therefore, needs not only to be conversant with the methods of epidemiological investigation, but also to be able to incorporate some of these concepts into his, or her, work. Even if hygienists never wish to undertake an epidemiological study, they must, at the very least, be able to evaluate such studies. This chapter aims to cover these areas.

Consideration of the definition given above implies that epidemiology concerns a study of the distribution of the disease and a search for the determinants of the observed distribution. Hygienists will be concerned mainly with the latter. Once again, the team approach to occupational health studies is vital. If the physician suspects a health risk related to the workplace, further study of the workers may reveal the distribution of this risk — real or apparent — in the health status of the employees. Many variables including age, sex, occupation and race will need to be considered. Collaboration with the hygienist will be necessary to determine the occupational factors that may be involved in the observed ill health, for example, dust concentrations, work cycles, geographical distribution of the disease in the factory, timing of the onset of disease in relation to new or altered processes. All these factors could be important and the hygienist's expertise will greatly enhance the physician's ability to tease out those that are most relevant to the pathological processes underlying the ill health discovered.

The process of elucidating disease causation using epidemiology involves three types of investigation: (1) a description of the current status of health of the 'at risk' group (descriptive epidemiology); (2) *ad hoc* studies to test aetiological hypotheses in order to get closer to the likely cause (analytical epidemiology); and (3) the design and execution of a study that aims to alter exposure to the putative risk factor in order to assess whether this leads to an altered disease rate (experimental epidemiology). The latter type of study is frequently difficult to design and execute for ethical reasons but, in the final analysis, epidemiology is concerned with preventing ill health by establishing the causes of disease and removing them.

Historical development of epidemiology

Like many sciences, epidemiology has developed from a study of the unusual or exotic and then practitioners have sought to establish general principles. It is not nowadays, therefore, a science restricted to the study of epidemics any more than chemistry is confined to searching for the philosopher's stone.

Nor is it just a 'number crunching' exercise. Throughout its history, however, good statistics concerned with population health have been important precursors of epidemiological study. These so-called 'vital statistics' began to be collected in medieval times with the advent in Britain of the Bills of Mortality in 1532. Regular reporting did not commence until 1563, though the accuracy of these weekly records was frequently dubious as their collection was often the prerogative of some venal old widow in the parish! Nevertheless the following extract from the London Bills of 1665 demonstrates that major disease patterns could be discerned.

Executed	21
Flox and smallpox	655
French pox	86
Frightened	23
Overlaid and starved	45
Plague	68 596
Rising of the lights	397
Scurvy	105

Nevertheless, such data are of limited value without information on the population at risk. Formal gathering of such data began in Britain with the establishment of the decennial consensus in 1801 and limited information was collected. Although age was added in 1821, many people could not answer that question accurately until much later, as the registration of births, marriages and deaths did not start until 1836. Occupation was first requested in the sixth decennial census in 1851 and in 1921 Occupational Mortality supplements were started. William Farr, a physician appointed to be responsible for medical statistics in the Office of the Registrar General for England and Wales in 1839, was, perhaps, the founder of modern epidemiology.

These nationally acquired data have proved a fruitful source of research for epidemiologists for many years, but specific epidemiological studies

relating to localized illnesses were being successfully executed by the mid 19th century. John Snow, anaesthetist to Queen Victoria and a pioneer epidemiologist, established that water was the vehicle of transmission for the cholera outbreak of 1854 in Soho, London, long before the micro-organism responsible for the disease had been discovered. (Students of epidemiological history can view some of the memorabilia associated with Snow's classic study by visiting a public house named after him in Broadwick Street, Soho, close to the site of the water pump that caused the disease.)

Early epidemiologists were opportunists: either they described disease patterns in relation to the environment or they gleaned information from natural experiments that occurred around them. For example, the suspected role of air pollution in the causation of respiratory disease received major research impetus when the infamous London 'smog' of 1951, which lasted for 5 days, contributed to the death of over 3000 people.

The collection of accurate mortality data is an essential prerequisite of many epidemiological studies and, although morbidity records are frequently less accurate, these data too are now becoming important sources of information in the continuing quest for causative factors in human disease.

Today, the epidemiologist's desire to record total health surveillance of communities is running into conflict with the individual's desire for privacy. Much of the controversy is politically motivated. In the author's experience, few people refuse to provide health information to a bona fide researcher if they are convinced of the value of the research. Professor MacMahon, late of Harvard University, succinctly summarized the current conflict regarding the divulgence of personal health data: 'maximum confidentiality means minimum epidemiologic information and minimal effectiveness in identifying new cancer hazards .... Most people ... will supply even sensitive information if they believe the cause is reasonable ... the issue of confidentiality becomes more difficult when it is institutionalised or politicised'. This conflict of privacy with epidemiological need continues in the European Union. An unqualified success for the advocates of privacy of personal health data would effectively end many types of epidemiological studies which are already difficult to undertake in many member states.

In occupational health, epidemiology has five main uses.

1 The study of disease causation.

2 The study of the natural history of a disease.

3 The description of the health status of a specified population.

4 The evaluation of intervention in health-related issues.

5 The development of hygiene standards from epidemiological studies of exposure and health outcome.

SOURCES OF DATA

Population census and death registrations were first introduced for political and legal reasons. They have, nevertheless, been a never-ending source of data for the investigation of occupational causes of disease. Pension records, sick benefit schemes and treatment records have likewise been used. In fact, epidemiologists will use almost any source of personal health record to further their researches though few have been collected initially with such researches in mind!

National records (vital statistics)

During an individual's lifetime, major milestones are recorded for various purposes. Birth, marriage, divorce, death are all recorded nationally in developed countries. The registrations are undertaken locally and stored centrally.

Death certificates

Death marks the final event in an individual's health record. It is readily verified and in countries where registration is complete, it provides a reasonably accurate and quantifiable measure of serious illness in the community. Inaccuracies in such countries apply only to the cause of death, not to the fact of death.

In many instances, the cause of death can be incontrovertibly established, but this is not always the case. Every physician has, at one time or another, pondered over what to put on a death certificate. This may be due to the certifying physician's confusion over which of several factors ultimately caused the patient's demise, or ignorance of the preceding illness, or paucity of diagnostic testing pre-mortem. The certifying physician may not have been the patient's attending physician and even if an autopsy is granted to clarify the cause of death, the certificate of death is rarely amended in the light of such post-mortem investigations.

To add to the confusion, the physician has to decide not only what was the final event that killed the patient but also the underlying causes leading to that event. the accuracy of these diagnoses varies with the age and sex of the deceased, the body systems involved, the place and circumstances of death and even the physician's wording of the cause of death.

International agreement now dictates that the underlying cause of death must be given precedence over the immediate cause of death in subsequent classifications; though more recently researchers have been designing methods of allowing for multiple cause coding to be incorporated into analyses of mortality. Every 10 years or so, an international conference is held to establish a numerical code for all the major diseases so that epidemiological studies of mortality can be internationally comparable. This works quite well but cannot easily overcome national (or even regional) differences in disease nomenclature. For years, North American physicians diagnosed emphysema where British physicians presented with the same case would have diagnosed chronic bronchitis. The clinical features were not in dispute, only the name attached to those symptoms and signs.

Having said all that, it has been established with reasonable certainty that if the subsequent epidemiological analysis of mortality data is grouped into broad diagnostic categories, the 'true' cause of death is correctly coded in over 80% of cases. This accuracy varies with the disease — cardiovascular and respiratory disease being notoriously difficult to define, whereas a disease like leukaemia is much more accurately defined, requiring as it does a precise pathological diagnosis prior to the institution of treatment.

Occupation is recorded on the death certificate as the 'last known' occupation. Although uniformly applicable, it leads to a statistic of limited value when studying retired decedents or persons whose death was actually caused by a previous occupation. For example, 'retired', 'housewife' and 'civil servant' are epidemiologically useless occupational categories. Similar inaccuracies are noted when pneumoconiosis is seen to be the cause of death in a car park attendant. This is not due to the dust generated as cars drive in and out of the parking area past the attendant's booth, but due to the fact that the attendant is probably a pensioned-off coal-miner. Such inaccuracies can sometimes be circumvented by using factory pension scheme records (q.v.).

Birth certificates

In the past, these records were primarily used for the establishment of denominators for the calculation of infant disease rates. The recent advent of recording congenital malformations and pregnancy complications, as well as birth weight and duration of pregnancy, has afforded an opportunity of using these records when studying the effects of the mother's as well as the father's occupation. The strictures regarding diagnostic accuracy, are, however, similar to those for death certificates.

Morbidity

Nationally acquired morbidity records regarding health and safety at work are available in some countries. They are less accurate than mortality records and for epidemiological purposes would require supplementation with *ad hoc* recording in order to make them acceptable. In the UK, industrial accidents and certain diseases are reported to the Health and Safety Executive, whilst industrial injury benefit claims and prescribed diseases are reported to the Department of Social Security. Errors in diagnosis, failure to report accidents, illness and injury and incomplete coverage by law all militate against these sources of data as ideal epidemiological tools. Sickness absence data are particularly deficient regarding female employees and notoriously inaccurate except for the broadest

diagnostic groupings. Nevertheless, such national statistics can indicate gross secular changes and may highlight new hazards. For diseases which are not life-threatening, these are crucial measures of occurrence.

Nationally collected statistics such as the General Household Survey and the Hospital In-Patient Enquiry, although of considerable importance to general epidemiology, have less relevance to occupational health.

Local records

These may be acquired through hospitals, family doctors, factories, schools, pension schemes, insurance policies, professional associations and trade unions. All such records have been used at one time or other by occupational health epidemiologists. They are all, however, collected for purposes unrelated to epidemiological study and their accuracy, completeness, comparability and relevance are always doubtful.

Where the occupational group under study tend to stay in the same type of job for a lifetime, such records may prove a major source of information. The author has used such records as the primary source of population enumeration on several occasions when studying occupational groups as disparate as hospital pathologists and sea pilots.

Ad hoc records

Some large industrial organizations are now seeking to maintain continued surveillance of the 'high-risk' workers, not only as they move from job to job within the company, but also if and when they leave or retire. These exposure registers may be of inestimable benefit later on in assessing the health status of workers exposed to various chemicals many years previously. At present, there are few industries in which retrospective exposure data of any worth are available.

Notification and registration of certain specific diseases have been made from time to time. Early examples include various infectious diseases such as whooping cough or measles. More recently, cancer registries have been established in a number of countries. The more efficient ones now boast a diagnostic accuracy in excess of 98%, with a high level of enumeration. Other examples include registers set up to monitor specific diseases, such as mesothelioma, angiosarcoma of the liver, the pneumoconioses, adverse reactions to certain drugs, specific congenital malformations and certain disabilities, such as blindness.

Despite this welter of health records, the epidemiologist frequently has to search several sets to obtain only a portion of the information required regarding an employee's health. It may still be necessary to contact the employee or their next of kin for further data. Even if a total picture of that employee's health from the cradle to the grave is acquired, it may still be too imprecise about possible occupational hazards and their relationship to the worker's health, due to the paucity of exposure data at the factory or factories at which the person worked.

Epidemiologists are frequently accused of being pedants — one can see why!

MEASURES OF EXPOSURE AND HEALTH OUTCOME

Information relating to hazard exposure and health outcome acquired from the above data sources have to be expressed in terms which permit comparisons between and within populations. This section deals with some of those measures and the concepts underlying their use.

Exposure

For the foreseeable future, this will remain the least accurate measure and therefore the weakest link in the chain between cause and effect. The majority of epidemiological studies investigating occupationally related causes of disease falter when it comes to establishing, with any degree of accuracy, the exposure histories of the populations of workers under study. The whole area of retrospective exposure assessment is now a major research priority in occupational hygiene and is described in Chapter 18. This is an area where hygienists can make a major contribution to future occupational health research.

In the final analysis, the ideal epidemiological study will show a dose—response relationship between a suggested cause and the disease outcome. This adds great strength to the association being causative and also materially assists in establishing safe (or relatively safe) working conditions for future generations of employees.

At present, past exposures are frequently classified as low, medium and high, or merely expressed in years of exposure of whatever degree. This is most unsatisfactory. Ideally, past exposure information should be of high quality and measured with great accuracy, using standard or comparable instrumentation. It should not only provide information on the concentrations of the toxic material potentially (and realistically) absorbable by the workers, but also provide accurate data on variations in that concentration during the work cycle, daily, weekly, monthly and its duration. In addition, data should be available on other relevant exposures. These include changes in the physical and chemical formulation of the toxic substance in the worker's immediate environment as well as an assessment of possible interactions between various noxious elements, whether they be additive, multiplicative, synergistic or even negative.

At present such data are rarely available and if available are virtually never complete. Thus, they furnish epidemiologists with a continuing source of major error in their investigations.

The range of possible exposure groupings is:
1 ever/never employed in the industry;
2 length of service in the industry;
3 job categories by precise division or task duties (qualitative);
4 job categories ranked ordinally by exposure intensity;
5 quantitative exposure intensity categories;
6 quantitative dose categories.

Health outcome

It is important, at the outset, to differentiate between ratios, rates and proportions, concerning measures of health outcome. They are not synonymous. Strictly speaking, a 'ratio' relates to a fraction where the numerator and denominator are two separate and distinct quantities, e.g. sex ratio. A 'proportion' is a type of ratio in which the numerator is included in the denominator, e.g. proportion of males in a community. On the other hand, 'rates' are associated with changes in a phenomenon and may be defined as a measure of the change in one quantity (y) per unit of another quantity (x) on which y depends.

Measures of occurrence

In epidemiology the commonest measures of occurrence are the incidence and the prevalence. These are commonly expressed as rates per 'person-periods' (usually person-years). The 'incidence' of a disease relates to the occurrence of new cases and the 'incidence rate' relates to the number of new cases that occur in a given population over a given period of time. (Strictly speaking, the incidence rate (or incidence density) should be distinguished from the cumulative incidence which relates to the proportion of persons developing the disease. Also, incidence (and prevalence) can be expressed as spells of disease rather than persons.)

The 'prevalence' of a disease concerns the existing number of cases of the disease at one point in time or over a period of time. Prevalence is, therefore, in strict terms, a ratio of the number of existing cases by the population at risk at a given time over a given period.

Prevalence and incidence are related to each other with reference to a given disease through the duration of disease. The relationship can be expressed:

$$\text{Prevalence} \propto \text{Incidence} \times \text{Duration} \quad (20.1)$$

Pictorially this can be conceived as a reservoir (Fig. 20.1) supplied with water from streams above and released through the dam below. The quantity of water in the lake (the prevalence) is dependent upon the amount flowing into it from the streams above (the incidence) and the amount of water leaving the lake below the dam (those people with the disease who cease to have the disease — they recover or die).

In practical terms, incidence is an unsuitable measure of occurrence for chronic diseases with a

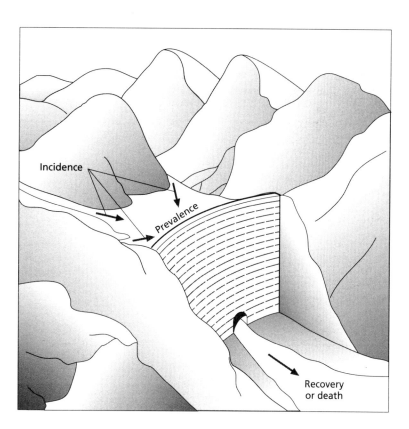

Fig. 20.1 Relationship between incidence and prevalence.

vague or prolonged onset, whereas incidence is a better measure when the disease is acute and has a clearly defined onset.

Measures of frequency

These are rates of one sort or another. Although rates are established to allow comparability between populations, they can be confusing if a clear idea of their limitations is not established. In essence, there are three measures of frequency of a given event (death, disease, accident, etc.) They are:

1 crude;
2 adjusted;
3 standardized.

For illustration purposes, we will concentrate on measuring the frequency of death, but any health-related event can be so measured:

$$\text{Crude death rate} = \frac{\begin{array}{c}\text{Total deaths in the}\\\text{population at risk}\end{array}}{\begin{array}{c}\text{Population at risk}\\\text{in person-years}\end{array}} \quad (20.2)$$

Such a death rate is far from ideal as the deaths relate to both sexes, and, more importantly, all age groups. Comparison of two crude death rates could lead to erroneous conclusions. For example, the crude death rate for town A (an industrial centre) is 12 per 10^6 per year and the crude death rate for town B (a seaside resort) is 15 per 10^6 per year. The implication is that town B is a less healthy place than town A. This is because no account has been taken of the age breakdown of the populations. Town A has a younger population and the age-specific deaths are all higher than town B, but town B has an older population. The way round this dilemma is to compute an adjusted death rate. This removes the latent weighting inherent in the crude rates by another set of weights — in this case, the age-specific rates. If this is done for town A and town B, the comparison now shows town A to have higher age-specific death rates than town B and summary statistics can be calculated to reflect this.

In occupational health, one frequently wishes to compare the mortality experience of an occupational group (the so-called 'index' population) with some other population (the 'standard' population). This procedure produces a summary statistic called the 'standardized mortality ratio' (SMR). Taking the standard population as 1 (or 100%), the mortality experience of the occupational group under study can then be conveniently expressed as a percentage of that standard and appropriate techniques applied to test its statistical significance. An example is given in Table 20.1.

The SMR, though widely used, does have pitfalls in interpretation for the unwary. Firstly, as the

Table 20.1 Calculation of standardized mortality rate (SMR) for agricultural workers (UK) 1949–1953. (Data from Registrar General's Decennial Supplement for England and Wales)

Age	Observed deaths (1949–1953)	Male agricultural population (1951)	National death rate per 1000	Expected deaths*
20–	541	83 400	1.4	116.76
25–	963	133 300	1.6	213.28
35–	1500	131 600	2.9	381.64
45–	3422	117 200	8.2	961.64
55–64	7527	90 600	23.0	2083.52
20–64	13 973	556 100		3756.52

$$\text{SMR} = \frac{13\,973}{5 \times 3756.52} \times 100 = 74$$

* Expected deaths calculated by: $\dfrac{\text{Column 4} \times \text{Column 3}}{1000}$.

technique involves an indirect age adjustment, SMRs calculated for two or more study populations, using the same standard population death rates for calculating expected deaths, cannot themselves be compared with each other. This is because the two index populations may have different age structures.

The second point is that the magnitude of the SMR is dependent upon the choice of the standard population. As the standard population is frequently the national population, it is, by definition, less healthy than a working (occupational) population. This is because the national population contains people who do not work because they are sick, disabled or dying. Therefore, if one assumes that the index population is exposed to no serious occupational hazards, the SMR for that occupational group, calculated using national data as the standard, should be invariably less than 100%. In practice, this 'healthy worker effect' means that an unexposed occupational group, when compared with the national population, should have an SMR of about 80 to 90. In Britain, the Office of Population, Censuses and Surveys is attempting to get round some of this comparison bias by providing national population data for employed persons — the so-called 'Longitudinal Study'.

The third factor is that SMRs gloss over age-specific differences in the working population. Not all workers are exposed equally to the putative hazard — it might be more severe in the youngest group, or more noticeable by its cumulative effect in the older groups. A way round this is to consider age-specific SMRs.

A fourth factor which could be relevant is socio-economic class. There are differences in SMR by socio-economic class and the proportion of each in the two populations compared may not be equal. Allowances can be made for this also. Whilst socio-economic class is a convenient grouping, it is made up of interrelated factors which include income, education, way of life (such as housing and site of house), as well as occupation.

Finally, it is necessary to mention proportionate mortality ratio (PMR). This statistic, though not as robust as the SMR, is useful particularly where populations at risk are not accurately known. The PMR is the proportion of deaths from a given cause in the index population divided by the proportion of deaths from that cause in the standard population.

The relevance of time, place and person

From what has gone before, the reader should, by now, have realized that numbers, the currency in which epidemiologists deal, have to be continually reviewed in the light of factors which could lead to comparison problems. In short, epidemiologists strive to compare apples with apples, not apples with oranges.

Assembling the data for an epidemiological investigation is a bit like piecing together the crucial elements in a criminal investigation. The questions are the same.

1 To whom?
2 Where?
3 When?
4 By what? (Why?)
5 How?

To which can be added the sixth question which is vital to health prevention: so what?

The person, place and time questions were asked by John Snow before discovering that the cholera epidemic of 1854 in Soho affected only people who drank water from the Broad Street pump during a few weeks in August of that year. The great London smog of 1951 (Fig. 20.2) killed the very young and the very old in early December in Central London and most of them died of cardiorespiratory disease or terminal bronchopneumonia upon a serious underlying disease such as cancer. Similarly, a recent study of epidemic adult asthma in Barcelona was linked in time, susceptible person and place to soya bean dust generated in the docks when vessels carrying the beans were unloaded and the wind was blowing in a particular direction.

The main characteristics affecting these three factors are summarized in Table 20.2.

Measures of risk

Risk estimation is primarily a function of data analysis but it can be conveniently considered here. Two measures are commonly used: (1) relative risk; and (2) attributable risk.

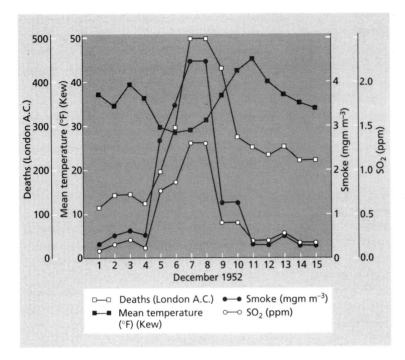

Fig. 20.2 Graph of air pollutants (sulphur dioxide and smoke) and air temperature and their relation to registered deaths for London A.C. for 1–15 December 1952.

Relative risk is the ratio of disease rate in exposed persons divided by the disease rate in non-exposed persons.

Attributable risk is the difference between disease rates in exposed persons and disease in non-exposed persons.

An example of these measures derived from a longitudinal study (q.v.) is given in Table 20.3. Several points regarding these measures should be noted.

1 The magnitude of the relative risk is a measure of the strength of the association between the risk factor and the disease — the magnitude of the statistical significance is not related to this strength.

2 Case–control studies (q.v.) do not usually permit relative and attributable risk values to be obtained as described above, as such studies do not usually permit direct measurement of disease rate, but merely measure the frequency of risk factor exposure. Statistical assessments of such studies are dealt with in Chapter 19.

CAUSATION OR ASSOCIATION

Before considering specific types of epidemiological studies, one further concept needs to be emphasized: the statistical association of a risk factor with a disease does not necessarily prove causation.

Table 20.2 The main characteristics affecting the person, place and time

Person	Place	Time	
Age	Natural boundaries	Day	
Sex	Political boundaries	Month	Secular and
Ethnic group	Urban/rural boundaries	Year	cyclic
Social class	Place of work in factory	Season	
Occupation	Environment		
Marital status	Climate		
Family	Migrant status		
Genes			

Table 20.3 Leukaemia cases diagnosed among Hiroshima residents between October 1950 and September 1966. (Data derived from Atomic Bomb Casualty Commission)

Irradiation dose (Gy)	Exposed population (crude annual incidence per 100 000 persons)	Relative risk	Attributable risk	
			Rate per 100 000	%
Under 0.05	3.0	1.0	0.0	0
0.05−0.19	5.1	1.7	2.1	41
0.2−0.49	20.9	7.0	18.9	90
0.5−0.99	18.3	6.1	15.3	84
1−1.99	41.5	13.8	38.5	93
2−2.99	55.6	18.5	52.6	95
3+	150.5	46.5	137.5	98
Total	7.2	2.4	4.2	58

The association could be spurious or it may be indirect through other known or unknown variables. Epidemiological techniques can never prove A causes B, but they can often provide considerable support (or denial) for a causal hypothesis.

Such support can be conveniently considered under nine headings. (For an elegant exposition of these nine factors, the reader is referred to Bradford Hill (1965).)

1 *Strength of association*: is the disease more common in a particular group of workers? If so, by how much?

2 *Consistency*: has the association been described by more than one researcher and preferably using different methods of enquiry?

3 *Specificity*: is the disease restricted to certain groups of people and to certain sites?

4 *Time*: does the suspect cause always precede the disease and is the time interval reasonable?

5 *Biological gradient*: is there a good dose − response relationship?

6 *Biological plausibility*: does the association seem reasonable or is it absurd?

7 *Coherence*: do all aspects of the causality hang together in a logical and feasible way?

8 *Experimental evidence*: can the causality be tested experimentally or does experimental evidence support causality?

9 *Analogy*: has a similar suspect cause been shown for related causes or effects?

Rarely will all nine points be present in the proof of a hypothesis, nor do they all carry equal weight.

However, the more there are, the stronger the association and the more likely it is that there is a causal relationship. But, as Bradford Hill says in his paper: 'All scientific work is incomplete − whether it is observational or experimental. All scientific work is liable to be upset or modified by advancing knowledge. That does not confer upon us a freedom to ignore the knowledge we already have, or to postpone the action that it appears to demand at a given time'.

Consideration of the design of an epidemiological study requires advance planning. It does not just happen. Having said that, it is usually impossible to stick rigidly to a classic study design as practical considerations will modify such an ideal situation. What is fundamental to all epidemiological studies is the need to have a question which demands an answer.

Study design consideration can be divided into two parts: (1) goals; and (2) options.

Goals

The ultimate aim of an epidemiological study is to obtain accurate information about the object of the study. Practical restrictions present before, during and after the investigation may limit the feasibility of obtaining the most accurate picture. The balance between these two opposing forces can be denoted as the efficiency of the operation as a whole (Fig. 20.3).

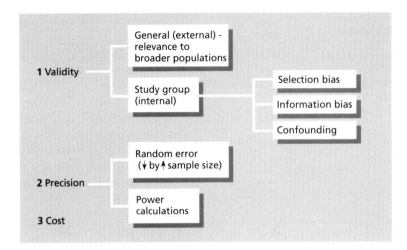

Fig. 20.3 Study design: goals.

Validity

Validity is related to the general (external) and the specific (internal). In the general sense it is concerned with how the study results could be extrapolated in a more general context. For example, if a study showed that farmers in a particular area had a higher prevalence of fractured legs than office workers, can these results be extrapolated to all farmers? Or are there specific circumstances in the study area which show that the farmers, or the landscape, climate, their tractors, whatever, are significantly different from the population of such workers as a whole to militate against such generalizations. (Perhaps the control group is inappropriate and therefore it is the factor that vitiates generalization.)

In a specific sense, the study groups may be biased. Bias can take many forms and some can be controlled at the design stage. Three broad groups can be distinguished.

1 *Selection bias* concerns the way the study populations were assembled and includes the validity of choosing the chosen — for example: were they volunteers?; were they lost to follow up?; were they a survivor population?; did they all come from the same hospital?; district?; and so on.

2 *Information bias* relates to the quality and accuracy of the data gathered. It includes errors by the interviewer or the interviewee, in the diagnosis or the exposure measures and so on.

3 *Confounding* is a factor which independently influences both the exposure and the outcome and thereby suggests a spurious direct relationship between the two. The classic example is age. The older the worker, the more likely he or she is to have been significantly exposed to the occupational hazard and the more likely to have the illness in question — given that most diseases are age dependent.

Precision

Precision is another aspect to be considered. If a study plan, involving a particular size of population (or measurements), were implemented repeatedly and independently an infinite number of times, the results would be grouped about a mean value. Departure from this mean value would give an estimate of random error. A small random error would indicate high precision. Information regarding the precision of the study is augmented by increasing the sample size or by increasing the number of times the measurements are made. Wherever possible, it is valuable to calculate the likelihood of discovering a real effect given the study population size. Formulae are available to undertake these so-called power calculations.

Cost

The cost of the investigation can be measured in terms of time, effort and personnel. The efficiency of the study is a measure of the value of the information gained against the cost of the study.

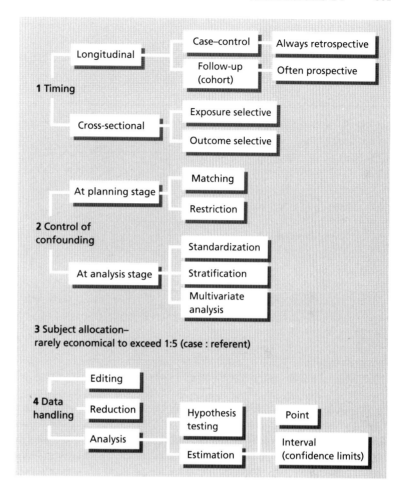

Fig. 20.4 Study design: options.

Options

The goals of rational study design require that certain choices are made in terms of the way the investigation is executed (Fig. 20.4).

Timing

A choice of prime importance is the timing of the investigation. Figure 20.5 depicts the life history of a factory population on a calendar–time/age–time format — and can be used to illustrate these options in timing. Real life events are, of course, more complex than in this example but the principles remain the same. The factory concerned opened in 1945 with a population of workers aged 18–40. The passage of time (horizontal scale) is, of course, accompanied by the ageing of the population (vertical scale). The population is assumed not to alter

and therefore progresses diagonally across the figure. In 1960, a major expansion programme with the advent of new processes necessitates enlarging the workforce with predominantly younger men. This new cohort ages *pari passu* with the extant group. (An alternative model is the introduction and cessation of a particular process in 1945 and 1960 respectively.) If we wish to investigate this process and/or the population, we have several options with regard to timing and the direction of the study. Referring to Fig. 20.5, the study could be cross-sectional (vertically orientated) or longitudinal (horizontally orientated).

Cross-sectional studies

The decision to undertake a cross-sectional study generally means a quick and cheap opportunity to study the problem in hand. These advantages are

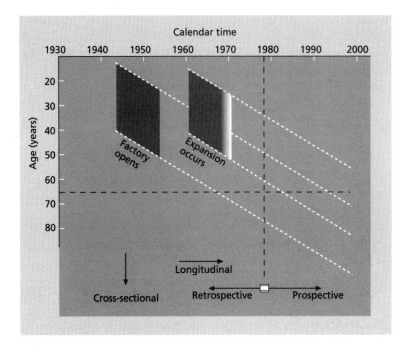

Fig. 20.5 Some age–time factors in study design.

offset by the limitations imposed by having to assess the population at risk in a narrow time frame. The narrowness of the time interval means that the investigators cannot look at exposure and outcome as a time-dependent relationship. The cross-sectional study tends to be outcome- or exposure-selective. All that may be feasible is the estimation of the prevalence of the exposure (or its outcome).

Longitudinal studies

Longitudinal investigations take longer to do and are more expensive but, by virtue of the study being concerned with a period of time rather than an instant, provide an opportunity for looking at an exposure and its outcome as a time-related chain of events. Two types of longitudinal study are commonly employed: (1) the case–control study (or more accurately, case–referent study); and (2) the follow-up study (which includes cohort investigations) (Fig. 20.6).

Case–control studies tend to be retrospective. They begin with a definition of a group of cases and relate these and the non-cases (controls–referents) to the past exposure history. In occupational epi-demiology, the main drawback here is the accurate ascertainment of exposure history going back anything up to 40 years.

Follow-up studies do not necessarily suffer such limitations if the exposure is defined and accurately known, and a group of exposed (and possibly non-exposed) persons are followed up to assess the eventual outcome of such exposure. Such studies are frequently, but not invariably, prospective in directionality. A 'cohort' is a specific type of follow-up study where a population, defined in advance for exposure characteristics, is followed for a period of time and the outcome subsequently measured. Follow-up studies are designed to observe incidence, and, ideally, should span a period of time in excess of the maximum induction period for the exposure factor to produce a putative outcome.

Control of confounding factors

The control of confounding factors can be undertaken at the planning stage or during data analysis. During planning, matching the cases (or exposure group) with persons without the characteristic essential for selection may reduce or eliminate

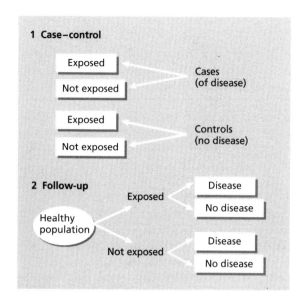

1 Case–control

Exposed

Not exposed

Cases
(of disease)

Exposed

Not exposed

Controls
(no disease)

2 Follow-up

Healthy
population

Exposed

Disease

No disease

Not exposed

Disease

No disease

Fig. 20.6 Longitudinal studies.

such confounders. For example, age matching eliminates the problem of inadvertently comparing old with young. The alternative to matching is the restriction of the cases and their referents to narrow strata, which effectively excludes unwanted confounding. Such stratification without restriction can be done during data analysis, or standardization procedures can be adopted instead. Complex interreactive confounders can be minimized by multivariate analysis.

Subject allocation

Studies are often published in which numbers in the referent (control) group exceed the case by a factor of two or more. This can strengthen the validity of the comparison, and, thereby, the conclusions drawn. The law of diminishing returns, however, begins to operate after the case–referent ratio exceeds 1 to 3, and 1 to 5 is rarely exceeded — largely for reasons of economy.

Data handling

This is dealt with in more detail in Chapter 19. Suffice to say here that three main procedures are employed: (1) the editing of the collected data to a

readily usable form; (2) its reduction to a manageable size; and finally (3) the analysis. Analytical procedures tend to test hypotheses propounded at the outset of the investigation or are employed to estimate various parameters, either to one point or, more commonly, to establish confidence limits for the calculated estimates.

TYPES OF STUDY

In this section the main study types alluded to in the previous section will be described.

Longitudinal studies

For many years, follow-up studies have been considered to be the epidemiological study *par excellence*. Their reputation for accuracy is partly based on their inherently unbiased concept — a group or groups of people are chosen in terms of characteristics manifest before the appearance of the disease in question, and then these individuals are followed over time to observe the frequency of the disease. By definition, however, such studies tend to take a long time to do, and in addition are costly and frequently rather complex. Nevertheless, some epidemiologists nowadays feel that a well-designed and efficiently executed case–control study 'nested' within a cohort carries the advantages of both studies whilst minimizing the disadvantages of each.

The choice between the two is dependent upon the question posed in the exposure/health outcome equation. This can be summarized as follows:

Question	Study type
A causes B?	• Either • Case–control (disease rare) • Follow-up (exposure rare)
A causes B_1, B_2, B_3? A causes?	• Follow-up
B caused by A_1, A_2, A_3? B caused by A?	• Case–control

Follow-up (cohort) studies

Follow-up studies may be undertaken for a variety of reasons. These include not only the desirability of using this method *per se* but also certain attributes in respect of the population. The main selection criteria are listed below.

Special exposure
High levels
Unusual type
Newly suspect agent

Ease of follow-up
Hospital patients
    Obstetric (mothers or babies)
    Specific therapy, e.g. irradiation
Occupational
Insurance policyholders
Pension schemes
Professional societies

Geographical or ethnic groupings
Migrant studies

Examples of such study groups include the investigation of the effects of ionizing radiation. In this example, research has largely centred on groups with specific, high exposures — Japanese atomic bomb survivors, patients receiving radiotherapy and radiation workers. Occasionally, an unusual event occurs which fortuitously — and perhaps tragically — exposes a group of people to an agent: for example, the Seveso disaster in Italy on 10th July 1976. Such an incident needed to be fully investigated as it provided a rare opportunity to follow a group of people heavily exposed to dioxin. Studies were instituted to assess pregnancy outcome, flora and fauna damage, as well as long-term mortality and morbidity investigations of those exposed.

The organochlorine pesticide, chlordane, has been suspected in recent years of causing cancer in experimental animals, though little human research has been undertaken. In March 1976, an unknown quantity of concentrated chlordane entered the public water-supply of part of Chattanooga, Tennessee, resulting in tap water concentrations of up to 0.1%. Acute effects were gauged by surveying the houses linked to that section of water-supply, and long-term studies are feasible of the residents who were identified as having drunk the contaminated water. Environmental hazards are less commonly amenable to such study than occupational exposures because the exposures are usually less marked and are less well characterized. Environmental exposure studies are also often complicated by public opinion — and public perceptions of ill health — particularly as such episodes are usually the result of accidents and there is a concomitant natural desire to blame someone.

It is relatively easy to identify cohorts of exposed workers. Unfortunately, past exposure information is rarely adequate and although current and future exposure data can be collected, the researcher then has to wait for a generation for the final result. Few epidemiologists opt for posthumous publication of their *magnum opus* so case–referent studies are more attractive propositions. These strictures do not apply to studies linking membership of an occupational group with a certain disease if that occupational group can be accurately traced back in time. This is facilitated if the exposed group in question belong to a professional society where membership tends to be lifelong or where pension schemes or insurance policies keep track of the individuals.

For example, the author was once asked by Trinity House sea pilots to investigate the risk of their dying from heart disease as they felt this risk was greater than their non-piloting peers. Pilots join the fraternity at about 35 years of age and rarely leave the occupation before retirement or death. Discussions with Trinity House revealed that not only is there little wastage from the service for reasons other than those stated above, but that the pilots' widow's pension is payable on receipt of a copy of the death certificate. Trinity House, therefore, could provide not only the population at risk but also the 'alive or dead' status of pilots for each year and, if dead, verification of the cause of death. The end result of this study was that the pilots were right!

Tracing a population such as this is the crux of the investigation. The quality and completeness of the follow-up will greatly control the validity of the study results. As follow-up studies require the tracing of a group of people for many years, there is always a serious risk of 'losing' some of the group.

Marriage, moving house, changing job (perhaps for reasons related to workplace exposures) or even frank refusal to collaborate can deplete the study population and put the whole investigation in jeopardy. The reason for this is that the non-responders and the 'drop-outs' may be different in some important way from the responders, and their absence from the final analysis may bias the results disproportionately to their numbers. Studies with response rates in excess of 85% are essential unless the investigators can be sure that the non-responders differ in no significant way from the responders. This might be assessed by acquiring relevant information (age, sex, work, residence) on the non-responders from other sources in an effort to establish this similarity (or otherwise) to the responders.

Decisions also have been made regarding the use of incomplete data on 'drop-outs'. For example, in a mortality study, if 10% of the population cannot be traced to the end of the study period what should be done with the information collected to the time they are lost to follow-up? To exclude them, or to include only the data that is available, could falsely overestimate the mortality rate, whereas to assume that they are alive to the end of the study will falsely underestimate it. The last alternative is frequently chosen as the less misleading alternative.

The corollary to this is that volunteer populations are to be eschewed where possible, as known and unknown factors are at work in the differentiation between those who volunteer and those who do not. Indeed, volunteers are rarely representative of any study population.

Follow-up studies where 'exposure' is merely defined as membership of a particular group are easier to undertake retrospectively than those where exposure is concerned with the measurements of noxious materials present (or absent) in the immediate environment of the worker — for example, lead dust. In these circumstances, the occupational hygiene measurements may be deficient in a number of ways. The readings may be:
- incomplete or absent;
- measured with the wrong equipment;
- measured on obsolete or inaccurate equipment;
- inappropriate to the study aims, i.e. general

environmental levels rather than personal samples, and compliance records rather than routine surveillance.

Under these circumstances researchers cannot rely on the memory of persons working in the factory at the time to recall the missing or deficient data. They may, however, be able to establish, from what records are available and from information regarding working practices at the time, an arbitrary grading system of exposure which may suffice. This subject is discussed in greater depth in Chapter 18. Prospective follow-up studies should not suffer from such data deficiencies.

Comparison groups for a follow-up study population can be selected from within the study population or from without. Within-group comparison can be between sub-groups in different exposure categories, after ensuring that they are otherwise comparable. Comparison groups from outside the study group can come from the general population, local populations or other factory populations similar to the study factory except in the exposures experienced at work. Multiple comparison groups can add considerable strength to the results as they offset design deficiencies that may be present if only one such group is chosen and they will, hopefully, provide additional points on the 'dose–response' graph.

For example, in a mortality of hospital pathologists, the author used both the general population in socio-economic class 1 as well as all medical practitioners to strengthen comparisons with the study group.

Case–control studies

These are also known as case–history, case–comparison and case–referent studies. A case–control study is an investigation in which comparison is made between a group of individuals who have the disease in question and another group or groups who do not have the disease. This comparison is made with respect to past characteristics of both groups. Unlike follow-up studies, the outcome is known and, as a result, a specific hypothesis is tested regarding possible past aetiological factors.

The procedure involved is summarized below.
1 Ascertain cases and verify diagnosis.

2 Select controls, e.g.:
  (a) general population;
  (b) local populations;
  (c) hospital patients;
  (d) other factory workers;
  (e) relatives.
3 Assess possible bias and attempt to reduce it:
  (a) observer;
  (b) subject;
  (c) measurement.
4 Data analysis and interpretation.

It is important that the definition of a 'case' is clearly defined at the outset and that the diagnosis is accurately established using predetermined diagnostic criteria. Newly diagnosed cases are preferable to 'old' cases, as the latter tend to be more complex and may have been exposed to a variety of treatments that could modify the disease or alter their exposure category. In occupational epidemiology, the cases are likely to come from a factory, but they could be derived from hospitals, general practitioner lists or even mortality data. Bias is a potentially serious problem as there may be selective factors at work, determining why a case is in a given hospital, on a given doctor's patient list or working at a particular factory.

In many ways, the most difficult feature of case–control studies is the selection of the control or referent group. In order to select the most unbiased group, the epidemiologist should ask a number of questions.

1 Have I collected information on the comparison with the same zeal as on the cases?
2 Are the response rates from both cases and controls similar?
3 How well are these referents matched to the cases?
4 Have I matched all important potential confounders?
5 Have I 'overmatched'?
6 Do the referents come from a population similar to the cases?
7 Could I choose an equally good comparison group more cheaply or more quickly?

As with follow-up studies, there is much to be said for choosing more than one comparison group. If only one process in the factory is under consideration, another group from the factory could be used

as a comparison. In addition, neighbourhood controls would provide a broader general population-based referent group whilst maintaining similar socio-economic matching. The danger of 'over-matching' comes if the researcher has chosen such a similar group that there is, in effect, no difference between the comparative sets of data — thereby leading to a result which, inadvertently, is bound to show no differences!

Information on past exposure remains a major problem — particularly if the exposure data on the cases is sought with greater enthusiasm than with the comparison group. It is essential, if possible, to avoid using the study participants' memories, as the cases may remember (or recall more readily) their exposure. For example, if a study sought to link occupational factors with subsequent birth defects in working women, the women who had given birth to congenitally malformed children are much more likely to recall real or imagined risk factors than women who had produced normal children. Furthermore, the older the study groups are, or the longer the time interval between the study and the exposure, the less likely it is that accurate recall will be established.

Cross-sectional studies (prevalence studies)

In contrast to longitudinal studies, cross-sectional studies depend on a single examination of a cross-section of the population at a particular point in time. Their aim is primarily descriptive, though screening studies (q.v.) are also cross-sectional in type. Unlike case–control studies, cross-sectional studies tend to estimate the prevalence of a disease or exposure status in a sample of the population to be surveyed. Sampling is dealt with in a number of chapters, in particular Chapter 17. But suffice it to say that some random sampling procedure is essential to ensure that the group surveyed is representative of the whole population. It is important for hygienists to distinguish between hygiene sampling (the procedure of collecting a certain number of samples from a factory environment) and the rather precise procedure of sampling in an epidemiological sense.

The major problem with cross-sectional studies is to determine which came first, the event measured or the circumstances postulated as causing that event. For example, in a medical context, a study of schizophrenics in a sample of the population at large may suggest that such persons come from the lower socio-economic groups. Does this imply that a low socio-economic status predisposes an individual to the illness or that the illness, by compromising the individual's ability to compete in the modern world, results in the disadvantaged sufferer sliding down the socio-economic scale?

A further drawback of cross-sectional studies is that they are an uneconomical way of studying rare phenomena. For example, if researchers wish to study the aetiology of relatively rare conditions such as spina bifida or antimony poisoning, they would be more profitably employed in a case–control study than in attempting to discover such diseases in a survey of the general population.

The design of a cross-sectional (prevalence) study involves the following main stages.

1 *The establishment of precise aims*. It is no use vaguely surveying the population. Such methods produce vague results.

2 *The study population must be defined precisely*. Is it a factory population in one town or all factories employing such persons or processes?

3 *Determination of the sample size*. This is important for the validity of subsequent statistical analysis and depends on the prevalence (or incidence) of the condition, the accuracy of the measurement procedures, an estimate of the error involved and a decision on what level of difference in prevalence the researcher wishes to be able to detect in comparing the study population with some reference group.

4 *The recruitment of the sample*. Having established a population, the researcher must make sure that he or she is capable of picking up all the relevant cases in the sample chosen. Never be satisfied with a volunteer population.

5 *Analysis*. Various procedures can be adopted. Estimated prevalence rates can be related to comparison groups or survey population sub-groups.

Screening tests

It is relevant to consider these tests here as they tend to be cross-sectional investigations. Screening for disease is a procedure much in vogue. It commonly involves surveying large populations to detect early disease which would subsequently be more amenable to treatment than if detection was delayed until overt illness occurred. Screening procedures for cervical cancer, heart disease risk factors and certain congenital diseases are standard practice in many developed countries.

It is beyond the brief of this book to discuss the value of such screening procedures but suffice to say that there is considerable heat generated nowadays when the advantages and disadvantages of such procedures are discussed. In occupational medicine, the routine medical examination (formerly the prerequisite of senior executives) is frequently considered to be a screening technique, but it is of doubtful value in detecting the early stages of diseases and thereby improving the employee's life expectancy.

Nevertheless, screening surveys illustrate certain aspects of epidemiological studies which can be of importance in other areas. In particular the detection of an abnormal state of health or an abnormal biochemical parameter is prone to error. This is partially due to laboratory or observer error but also can be associated with the ability of the screening test to reflect the true picture.

For example, let us assume that a study is designed to detect abnormally high levels of the female sex hormones in men employed in a factory manufacturing such hormones. One way of detecting this would be to measure the blood levels of the hormone in the workers. This is expensive, time consuming and of debatable accuracy. Another way is to measure environmental levels of the hormone in dust collected by personal samplers attached to the worker. This, too, is expensive and subject to considerable analytical error. However, excess female sex hormones in men can produce readily diagnosable enlargement of the male breast. However, not all males respond to a given level of female sex hormone to the same degree. A level which might produce large, painful, even lactating breasts in one man may have no observable effect on the breasts of another man.

A study is thus designed to evaluate the usefulness of blood hormone levels in detecting real effect. A comparison is made between the true diagnosis of feminization (assuming that such a diagnostic procedure is possible) and the blood test in question. Two populations are surveyed: the factory group and a 'normal' or occupationally unexposed group. The value of the screening test can be estimated by its ability to detect 'true positives' — the *sensitivity* of the test — and by its ability to detect 'true negatives' — the *specificity* of the test. Figure 20.7 illustrates that these two measures are related — the higher the specificity, the lower the sensitivity and vice versa.

In the final analysis, the investigator must decide which of the two measures is the more important for the purposes of the study — is it essential to detect all the abnormals (high sensitivity) because the condition is life-threatening or is the proposed treatment of the condition so invasive or dangerous that one will settle for screening out all the normals (high specificity)?

Intervention studies

The studies outlined thus far have been primarily concerned with the description of disease processes or attempts to establish causative factors for established diseases. Epidemiology is more than that. It is a science associated with preventing disease and therefore is concerned with evaluating the effect of altering risk factors and measuring the effect of this intervention on disease outcome. Epidemiological studies are an essential prerequisite to instituting changes in the environment which aim at altering some adverse effect on community health. Some large-scale interventions have been undertaken without such preliminary investigations and can prove costly mistakes. The prohibition of alcohol in the USA might have been avoided if an evaluative epidemiological study had been mounted first!

Some major interventions in public health have

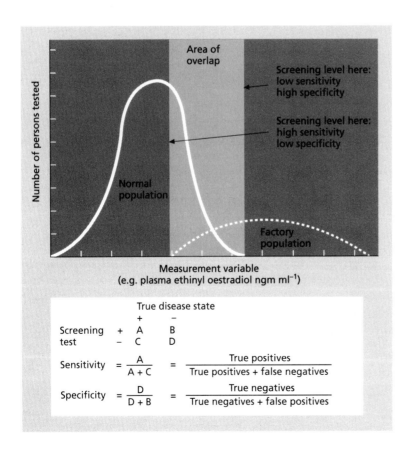

Fig. 20.7 The evaluation of a screening test.

been strenuously resisted despite good epidemio-logical evidence that such intervention would be beneficial. The story of fluoride in drinking water is such a case in point. Having established an aetiological association between dental caries and low fluoride concentrations in drinking water, several large-scale intervention studies were designed to test the effect. In one of these, two carefully matched cities, A and B, were selected, both with low fluoride levels and an estimate was made of dental caries in schoolchildren. Sub-sequently, town A's drinking water had fluoride added to it and the dental health of schoolchildren was followed longitudinally. The rate of caries in the fluoridated town fell dramatically. These researchers, however, were not yet finished. They then removed the fluoride from town A and added it instead to town B. The rate of caries in town A rose again and the rate in town B fell. Few people would dispute the conclusion that the addition of fluoride to drinking water had affected the rate of dental caries.

Similar procedures (admittedly on a smaller scale) are undertaken in drug trials. In such cases, patients are randomly allocated to different treat-ment regimes and the outcome measured by comparing the effect of the new drug with either a placebo or with the best available current treat-ment. Such studies are randomized controlled trials (RCTs). A procedural flow chart of an RCT is illustrated in Fig. 20.8.

Some epidemiologists feel that RCTs are the only way of evaluating anything, but random allo-cation can be difficult to accomplish, either for ethical reasons or for its sheer impracticability in some circumstances. Perhaps because of this, few such studies have been undertaken in the context of occupational medicine or hygiene, though it is not difficult to envisage useful possibilities for this procedure. One occupational example was the large-scale trial of the efficacy of influenza vaccine in a population of British postal workers. The population was selected by area and each area was randomly allocated to receive the vaccine or not. Volunteers were asked for (this was the only ethical way of getting individuals to receive the vaccine) and, after establishing baseline sickness absence data from both treatment and control groups, the

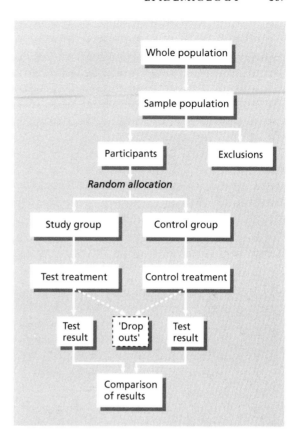

Fig. 20.8 Procedural steps in a randomized control trial.

results of the vaccination were followed during the succeeding winter months. The study was some-what inconclusive and the reasons for this illustrate some of the practical problems of such studies. They include:
1 the use of volunteers;
2 a relatively low response rate from those offered the vaccine;
3 some doubt about the true efficacy of the vaccine;
4 problems relating to the confirmation of true sickness absences;
5 difficulties in establishing precise diagnostic categories for the absence;
6 and last, but not least, the absence, that year, of a major influenza epidemic!

One area where attention has been focusing re-cently is the value, or otherwise, of occupational health services. Despite considerable methodological difficulties, intervention studies could help in establishing whether such services are of use to industry; and if they are, which portions are of greatest benefit and which would be abandoned. To the purist epidemiologist, no opinion, treatment, practice or theory is sacrosanct!

PRACTICAL ASPECTS OF THE FIELD SURVEY

Most hygienists operate in the practical world of the workplace and spend most of their time attempting to measure the environment and controlling the risks they find there. Fieldwork in epidemiology also forms an important part of many of the epidemiological studies discussed above and it might be of value, therefore, to list the steps likely to be required in planning and executing an epidemiological field study.

1 Define study objectives and formulate hypotheses to be tested.

2 Review the literature.

3 Outline the study plan and assess feasibility.

4 Define the study population, preferably with the help of a statistician, especially if the population is large and matching for comparison groups is envisaged.

5 Define study methods: cross-sectional; longitudinal; etc.

6 Decide on timing of the study.

7 Plan data processing and analysis.

8 Assess sample size and costs — including power calculations.

9 Write detailed protocol.

10 Publicize study plan to important, interested parties — especially the workforce — and obtain all necessary agreements (including ethical approval if necessary).

11 Prepare questionnaire, if any.

12 Undertake pilot study to test methods.

13 Recruit and train ancillary staff.

14 Approach study population(s). They should be aware of the aims of the study, the expected benefits, the sponsors and be assured regarding the confidentiality of any personal data they may be asked to provide.

15 Redefine study, if necessary, in the light of previous steps — diagnostic criteria, measurement assessments, questionnaire design, sampling procedures, error assessments, etc.

16 *Main study.*

17 Vigorously minimize 'non-response'.

18 Assess bias and errors.

19 Edit data.

20 Reduce data.

21 Analyse and test hypotheses.

22 Reach conclusions and report results to the participants and in the scientific literature.

23 ?Plan further research in the light of conclusions including any opportunities for preventive action.

Shortcomings in the epidemiological method

By now it will be clear to the reader that the epidemiological method is not without its difficulties! In brief, the main problems can be summarized as follows:

- a healthy worker effect — the comparison group has a different general health status compared with the cases;
- a poor response rate;
- high turnover of study populations — selecting in (or out);
- latency between exposure and effect is longer than the study period;
- insufficient evidence of differing effects by differing exposures;
- poor quality of health effects data;
- poor quality of exposure data;
- multiple exposures;
- no effect of exposure noted — does this imply a true negative result or merely a poor or small study (non-positive result)?

Appraising an epidemiological study

Perhaps the reader has now been finally dissuaded from ever attempting an epidemiological study. That may be so. Indeed it is not an essential part of the hygienist's job description. But it is crucial that hygienists understand what epidemiologists do and equally vital that they can read a report of an epidemiological paper and know whether it is good, bad or indifferent. To help that process, the check-list below summarizes much of what has been described in this chapter:

- question clearly formulated?
- appropriate study design?
- good quality health effects data?
- good quality exposure data?
- valid population choice for cases and control?
- high response rate and good sampling strategy?
- confounders considered and allowed for?
- population large enough to detect an effect if present?
- correct statistical techniques?
- estimates of risk include measures of variability, e.g. confidence intervals?
- cause–association issues addressed?
- non-positive or negative study result reviewed?
- effect of results on current knowledge assessed?

CONCLUSIONS

It is too glib to describe epidemiology as 'common sense made complicated'. It can be (and should be) a science applied to the study of diseases in populations. It is logical but can be complicated. It does not necessarily have to be undertaken by a cast of thousands studying populations of millions for decades. The principles apply equally to smaller-scale, factory-based investigations undertaken by one researcher. Every occupational health specialist should be conversant with the tenets of epidemiology and be capable of executing studies using its methods. It is hoped that a chapter such as this, though seemingly out of place in the eyes of many occupational hygiene specialists, would be viewed by the reader as relevant. Ideally it should stimulate him or her to go back out onto the shop floor and view the workforce anew. The best way of becoming conversant with epidemiological methods is to go out and do it.

REFERENCE

Hill, A.B. (1965). Environment and disease, association or causation? *Proceedings of the Royal Society of Medicine*, **58**, 295–8.

FURTHER READING

Hernberg, S. (1992). *Introduction to Occupational Epidemiology*. Lewis Publishers Inc., Michigan.

CHAPTER 21
Control Philosophy

K. Gardiner

INTRODUCTION

The prevention or reduction of ill health at work relies on the elimination or control of toxic workplace contaminants. Effective measures can range from the simple to the esoteric and this chapter aims to provide a brief review of the hierarchical structure in which these reside and of which ventilation (Chapter 22) and personal protective equipment (Chapter 23) are part. More contaminant-specific means of control are discussed in other chapters (Chapters 9–15).

It is common to split control methods into two groups: (1) software or administrative controls; and (2) hardware or engineering controls. In the main, the hardware or engineering controls are preferable. This is not necessarily due to their effectiveness but more to their longevity. The software and hardware hierarchy are tabulated in Table 21.1.

Table 21.1 Engineering and administrative control techniques

Engineering	Administrative
Appropriate design engineering	Appropriate administrative control by design elimination
Total or partial enclosure	
Local exhaust ventilation	Substitution
Change the process	Isolation or segregation
Shielding	Maintenance and housekeeping
Personal protective equipment	Education and training
	Personal hygiene

CONTROL AT THE DESIGN STAGE

It is much more effective, both in terms of outcome and cost, to instigate control measures when the process or factory is still at the design stage. The following includes a number of the issues that should be considered.

1 Careful a priori selection of the substances for use.

2 Enclosed system from raw material to product.

3 Prevent leakage of raw materials, intermediates, by-products, product and waste from equipment.

4 Vent unwanted contaminants to scrubbers, absorbers or incinerators.

5 Automate the process and control it remotely.

6 Consider the possibility of the amount of work in the workplace increasing over time, such as the installation of additional degreasing tanks, welding bays, sources of noise, etc. This would reduce the possibility of the workplace being radically different from that at the time the controls were designed.

7 'Interactions' between two or more contaminants. For example, chlorinated organic solvents used in degreasing baths may decompose when near to sources of ultraviolet radiation (such as those from welding) and form phosgene (a strong upper respiratory tract irritant).

8 Provide a facility for the removal of residues from the system before opening it.

9 The minimization of maintenance requirements, for example:

(a) continuous leak detection for fugitive emissions;

(b) careful design for infrequent but major tasks,

such as the replacement of filter bags.

10 Chemical specification poses questions related to the following:

(a) is it necessary (are there alternative substances or forms)?

(b) its physical properties (e.g. can it be stored, its temperature and pressure during storage or use, its flammability?);

(c) its chemical properties (e.g. storage, impurities, likely intermediary products, degradation products, etc.?);

(d) its toxicity and occupational exposure limit (OEL);

(e) special handling requirements;

(f) special hazards;

(g) can the plant adequately contain it?;

(h) can the excess or waste material be recovered?;

(i) emergency procedures;

(j) special hygiene or medical requirements.

CONTROL AFTER THE DESIGN STAGE

Generally, however, the occupational hygienist has had little or no influence in the specification of control requirements at the design stage and is therefore left with a number of remedial options. Fortunately, in some forward-thinking companies the occupational hygienist is asked to contribute to the design process and 'sign off' their approval. There are many permutations of control but the majority lie within the broad headings described below.

Elimination

This is the most effective means of control because if the contaminant is no longer present then it can pose no risk. Unfortunately, most contaminants are being used for a specific purpose. However, it is a question one must ask and be sure that a satisfactory answer has been received.

Substitution

Once a contaminant is believed to give rise to an unacceptable level of risk, and it is not possible to eliminate its use, one must look to substitute it for one generating a lower and more acceptable level of risk. If the risk is lower but still unacceptable then other means of control should be used. Care needs to be taken to ensure that a different problem is not created in terms of issues such as flammability or chemical interaction. Figure 21.1 is a flow diagram to assist in the process of substitution. Having identified an unacceptable risk, alternatives should be identified. If none are available then the risks should be managed by other methods. However, if alternatives are available then the consequences of their use, both in terms of the risk to health and their suitability in the process, should be considered. If alternatives appear to be compatible with the process and pose a lower risk to health than the original then they should be compared with each other. The most suitable alternative should be chosen and the change implemented. The effectiveness of this substitution should be evaluated and if found to be acceptable then at regular intervals its used should be reviewed with an aim to substituting again.

Classic examples of substitution include the use of: MDI (methylene bis (4-phenylisocyanate) instead of TDI (toluene-2,4-diisocyanate) (due to its lower volatility); zinc, barium or titanium dioxide instead of white lead in paint (due to their lower toxicity); phosphorus sesquisulphide instead of white phosphorus in matches (due to its lower toxicity); and synthetic mineral fibre instead of asbestos (perceived at the time to be of lower toxicity).

There is also opportunity to substitute the state or form of the same substance for one which gives rise to less exposure. Clearly, a reduction in temperature or increase in pressure will change the physical state of some contaminants with the likelihood that exposure decreases as follows: gas or vapour $\gg$ liquid $>$ solid. In addition, for particulates it is possible to increase their aerodynamic diameter by pelletization or the formation of briquettes, thereby radically reducing the amount of inhalable aerosol.

Changing the process

Significant reductions in exposure can be achieved by quite minor modifications to the process or the

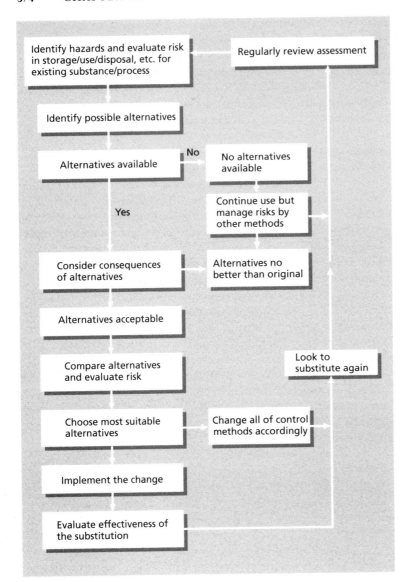

Fig. 21.1 Flow diagram to assist in process of substitution of a contaminant.

conditions under which it operates. The following are a few examples.

• Reduction of the temperature at which a process operates (especially volatile liquids) along with the use of drip trays.

• Reduction of the amount of agitation contaminants receive in a process — such as the liquid surface of a degreasing tank or the movement of bags along a conveyor belt when the rollers are spaced far apart.

• Reduction of the surface area from which liquid evaporation or splashes can occur by covering it with plastic balls or foam which float on the surface.

• Reduction of the pressure at which the process operates. If it is reduced to below that of atmospheric pressure it will ensure that any leaks are inward.

• Increase in the size of the individual solid contaminants from fine particulates to pellets or flakes or if possible to be kept in solution or as a slurry or paste.

• The use of automatic metering systems rather than manual contact with liquids or solids.

- The use of process compatible bags where the bag material itself is either of use or at worst is not detrimental to the process.
- The use of electrostatic spraying or dipping rather than spraying or manual application.
- The order in which work is undertaken.

Ventilation

Ventilation can be used to control a number of different contaminants (gases or vapours, dusts, heat, etc.) and is usually split into three types: (1) general; (2) dilution; and (3) local extract or exhaust ventilation (LEV). Clearly, within the remit of this chapter, LEV is of most importance due to its proximity to the source, however, its complexity in terms of specification and design warrants further explanation (see Chapter 22).

Isolation or segregation

This means of control attempts to remove individuals who are potentially exposed from the proximity of the source. It is simple and can be effective, however, ultimately it does nothing to remove the hazard. There are a number of different means by which the potentially exposed individual can be segregated or isolated from the source of the contaminant and these will be considered in turn.

1 *Total enclosure* of the process (preferably under negative pressure, e.g. shot blasting).
2 *Partial enclosure* of the process with LEV (e.g. fume cupboard).
3 A physical *barrier* can be placed between the source and the receiver, thereby absorbing or reflecting the contaminant, as used for noise (Chapter 9) or ionizing radiation (Chapter 14). This can also be used to reduce the number of workers exposed.
4 The *distance* between the source and the receiver can be maximized (especially where the inverse square ($1/r^2$) law applies for point sources) such as with the thermal environment (Chapter 12), noise (Chapter 9) and ionizing radiation (Chapter 14).
5 The *time* of exposure can be controlled by either minimizing activities in the proximity of the source of exposure or by rotating the workforce, or preferably by ensuring that by examination of the cyclic nature of the process the tasks are carried out when there is no chance of exposure.

6 *Age* may be used as a means of selecting members of the workforce who are capable of carrying out heavy or hot or cold work because of their physical advantage. However, it would be preferable to adapt or control the workplace to such an extent that anyone could work there.

7 *Sex* may be used as a means of selecting members of a workforce who are not, or should not be, allowed to be exposed to certain substances. This is mainly to protect women of child-bearing age and potentially their fetuses. As in the previous example with age, sex may be used as a means of selection for physically demanding jobs — again profound doubts exist about the justification for this, both ethically and morally.

Maintenance and housekeeping

Proactive maintenance schedules minimize the likelihood of breakdown and spills, etc. with the provision of planned shut down periods for major work. As far as possible, residual contaminants should be removed before the system is opened up.

Despite having made every effort to prevent or minimize the release of contaminants into the workplace and the generation of excess and waste material, there will always be the unexpected leak or spill. It is therefore necessary to identify likely sites for fugitive emissions and to instigate well-planned and co-ordinated housekeeping. This relies on: (1) the correct procedure having been identified; (2) the appropriate remedial materials being readily available at the anticipated sites; (3) the personnel being suitably trained; and (4) the waste being correctly removed. However, as with a lot of control techniques it is often the simple technique that is effective, such as: the use of vacuum cleaners rather than brooms or compressed air; the removal of settled particulate from horizontal surfaces before secondary generation; and the immediate disposal of solvent-soaked rags rather than leaving them on bench tops, etc.

In some workplaces, the nature of the contaminants may make it necessary to have facilities to allow the workforce to maintain good personal hygiene. The ability of some contaminants to be rapidly absorbed via the skin, or to interact with it, makes it necessary for the workforce to have access to good washing facilities along with the correct washing media. Care needs to be taken as some surfactants are aggressive to the skin, perhaps exacerbating the defatting action of solvents, etc. (see Chapter 2). It may also be necessary to supply work clothes and ensure that these are changed and washed at whatever frequency is deemed appropriate. The potential for a contaminant to be absorbed by ingestion also necessitates the need for designated areas for eating, drinking and smoking.

Education and training

The provision of information, instruction and training is required to supplement the more permanent means of control. It is necessary for management, supervisors and the individuals undertaking the work to be informed of the relevant information.

Management

Management should be aware of the safety and health hazards in their area (processes, operations and materials) and under what circumstances assistance is required to evaluate and/or control these. Of great importance is that managers and supervisors know everything the workforce have been told and the consequences of non-conformance, both for the individual and the company.

Workforces

In addition to their normal operating instructions, the workforce should be informed about the following:
- the specific means by which they can reduce their own exposure;
- the activities in the workplace where hazardous chemicals are present;
- the means of identifying control defects resulting in the non-routine presence of hazardous chemicals in the workplace;
- potential hazards of non-routine tasks;
- potential health effects;
- how to use the control methods provided and

the consequences of non-use (both the health effects and disciplinary action);
- explanation of the labelling system;
- explanation and location of material safety data sheets (MSDSs);
- reporting defects.

Personal protective equipment

This form of control is often inappropriate and ineffective, and is usually the least desirable for the operative. By the use of this technique, no attempt is made to reduce or eliminate the hazard. It should therefore only be considered or used as a last resort. However, there are four situations in which its use is defensible. Firstly, when it is not technically feasible to control exposure by any other means, for example, for individuals who have to work inside the paint spraying booths at car manufacturers. Secondly, for emergency procedures such as major spillages. Thirdly, for maintenance work where the usual controls have been switched off to facilitate access; and fourthly, where an assessment of the risks to health has shown that there is an immediate risk that needs to be controlled until such time as other means of control can be specified, installed and their effectiveness evaluated.

A great variety of equipment is included under the generic title of personal protective equipment, such as: respiratory protective equipment (RPE); hard hats; safety spectacles; face shields; safety boots; hearing protection (muffs or plugs); overalls (cloth, plastic or chain-mail); gloves; and protective creams and lotions. A comprehensive dissertation is provided in Chapter 23.

Source, transmission and the individual

This philosophy is represented diagramatically in Fig. 21.2. In terms of effectiveness, it is also beneficial to consider the control of an individual's exposure as three distinct components: (1) control at the point of release or source; (2) prevent or control transmission of the contaminant to the individual; and (3) protection of the worker to minimize exposure and absorption. In occupational health terms, control is related to exposure to workplace contaminants, with the magnitude of

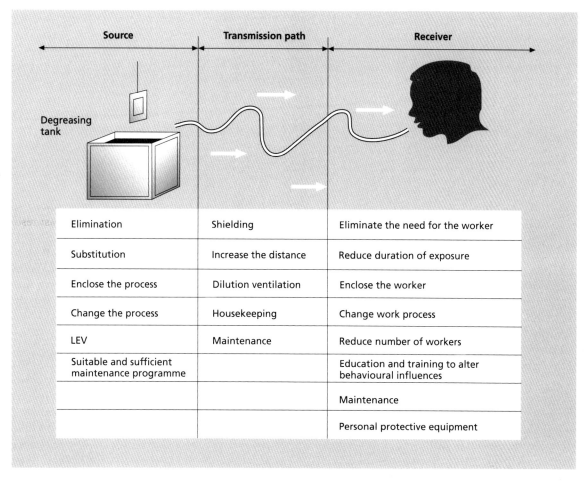

Source	Transmission path	Receiver
Elimination	Shielding	Eliminate the need for the worker
Substitution	Increase the distance	Reduce duration of exposure
Enclose the process	Dilution ventilation	Enclose the worker
Change the process	Housekeeping	Change work process
LEV	Maintenance	Reduce number of workers
Suitable and sufficient maintenance programme		Education and training to alter behavioural influences
		Maintenance
		Personal protective equipment

Fig. 21.2 Movement of a contaminant from source to receiver with control techniques for each component. After Olishitski (1988).

absorption being dictated by the nature of the contaminant, the routes of entry into the body, the concentration and the duration of exposure. Clearly, to reduce this exposure it is necessary to influence one or more of these factors.

SUMMARY

A great many means of controlling exposure exist. It is most convenient to categorize these in terms of engineering and administrative controls, and in terms of the preferred location of control, i.e.

source, transmission path and receiver. Table 21.1 provides a list of engineering and administrative controls and Fig. 21.2 shows the movement of the contaminant from source to receiver with a list of the suitable control techniques for each component.

REFERENCE

Olishitski, J.B. (1988). Methods of control. In *Fundamentals of Industrial Hygiene*, (3rd edn), (ed. B.A. Plog). National Safety Council, Chicago.

CHAPTER 22

Ventilation

F.S. Gill

INTRODUCTION

Ventilation is one of the most powerful tools that the occupational hygienist can employ to control the working environment. It can be used in a variety of ways:

1 to remove toxic or nuisance dusts, or gases or vapours before they reach a level that could constitute a danger to health or a threat to comfort;

2 to dilute to a safe level dusts, gases and vapours that have been allowed to become airborne;

3 to provide sufficient velocity of air over a worker to remove excessive heat from the body surface, thus reducing the risk of heat stress;

4 to become a vehicle for the provision of heating and/or cooling to a workplace;

5 to provide fresh air to the occupants of a workplace that, of necessity, has to be sealed from a surrounding environment for whatever reason;

6 to become a vehicle for the transport of materials from one place to another for production or recovery purposes.

In the applications listed above, energy is required to move the air in quantities and at velocities and temperatures suitable for the task in hand within boundaries set by the constraints of the problem. Furthermore, the cost of installing ventilation and the expense of maintaining its efficiency must be taken into account. This chapter will cover some of the design parameters that are required to make the best use of airflow and will also provide instruction in the measurement of the performance of existing ventilation systems.

Units used

The most common units used in ventilation engineering are given in Table 22.1 in both imperial and Système International (SI) units together with their dimensions and conversions from one system to the other.

Some basic facts on airflow

Whilst the laws governing the flow of fluids are complex, for most ventilation purposes they are simplified by assumptions and approximations, and many of the complex equations used in fluid dynamics can be reduced to charts, nomograms and diagrams. Some precision is lost as a result but this is unimportant when one considers the purposes for which ventilation is provided, that is, to control working environments including criteria and standards which are themselves imprecise and often ill-conceived. Nevertheless, it is necessary to understand some of the basic principles of airflow in order to appreciate the behaviour of currents of air and the capabilities of ventilation systems.

Air density

For most ventilation engineering problems standard air density can be used. The exceptions are if high-temperature air is being dealt with or if the ventilation system is to be used in places where the barometric pressure is substantially different from normal, for example, in deep mines or at high altitudes. Standard air density is taken as $1.2\,\mathrm{kg\,m^{-3}}$ ($0.075\,\mathrm{lb\,ft^{-3}}$) which corresponds to air

Table 22.1 Common units used in ventilation engineering

Unit	Dimension*	Imperial system	SI	Conversion factors
Length	L	foot (ft) or inch (in)	metre (m) or millimetre (mm)	$ft \times 0.305 = m$
Area	L^2	square foot (ft^2)	square metre (m^2)	$ft^2 \times 0.093 = m^2$
Air velocity	$\dfrac{L}{t}$	feet per minute (ft min^{-1}) feet per second (ft s^{-1})	metre per second (m s^{-1})	$ft\,min^{-1} \times 0.0051 = m\,s^{-1}$ or $1\,m\,s^{-1} = 197\,ft\,min^{-1}$ $ft\,s^{-1} \times 0.305 = m\,s^{-1}$
Air volume flow rate	$\dfrac{L^3}{t}$	cubic feet per minute (ft^3 min^{-1}) air changes per hour†	cubic metre per second (m^3 s^{-1}) air changes per hour†	$ft^3\,min^{-1} \times 0.000472 = m^2\,s^{-1}$ or $1\,m^3\,s^{-1} = 2119\,ft^3\,min^{-1}$
Pressure (force per unit area)	$\dfrac{ML}{t^2 L^2}$	pounds force per square foot (lb$_f$ ft^{-2}) inches of water column 1 in H$_2$O $= 5.2\,lb_f\,ft^{-2}$	newton per square metre or pascal (N m^{-2}) (Pa) millibar (mb) $= 100\,Pa$	$lb_f\,ft^{-2} \times 47.9 = N\,m^{-2}$ (Pa) inch water $\times 249 = N\,m^{-2}$ (Pa) NB: newton (N) $= 1\,kg\,m\,s^{-2}$
Power (work done per unit time)	$\dfrac{ML^2}{t^3}$	horsepower $(33\,000\,ft\,lb_f\,min^{-1})$	watt (joule per second) (newton metre per second)	horsepower $\times 746 =$ watt (W)
Air density	$\dfrac{M}{L^3}$	pound per cubic foot (lb ft^{-3})	kilogram per cubic metre (kg m^{-3})	$lb\,ft^{-3} \times 16.02 = kg\,m^{-3}$

* As used in dimensional analysis where: L = length; t = time; and M = mass.
† It is sometimes convenient to express air volume flow rate as air changes per hour: to convert to a usable unit it is necessary to multiply the number of air changes by the volume of the room thus giving the result in cubic feet or cubic metres per hour.

at a barometric pressure of 1013.25 mb (760 mmHg) and at a temperature of 20°C (dry bulb temperature). Any departures from these conditions can be corrected by using the expression:

$$\rho_0 = \rho_s \times \frac{b_0}{b_s} \times \frac{T_s}{T_0} \qquad (22.1)$$

where ρ_0 is air density at the non-standard conditions, ρ_s is standard air density, b_0 is barometric pressure at the conditions, b_s is barometric pressure at standard conditions, T_0 is absolute temperature at the conditions and T_s is absolute temperature at standard conditions.

Reynolds number

In 1883, Osborne Reynolds investigated the loss of energy in a length of pipe through which a fluid is flowing and found it to be dependent upon the type of flow existing in the pipe. At low velocities, a non-turbulent flow exists which is known as 'laminar' flow and in which the energy (E) absorbed is proportional to the velocity (v) of the fluid:

$$E \propto v \qquad (22.2)$$

At higher velocities a turbulent flow exists in which the energy absorbed is proportional to some power of the velocity above unity: $E \propto v^n$, where n is greater than one.

Reynolds showed that the character of the flow is determined by the following variables:

μ = dynamic viscosity of the fluid (dimension M/Lt as defined in Table 22.1);
p = density of the fluid (dimension M/L^3);
v = velocity of the fluid (dimension L/t);
D = diameter of the pipe (dimension L).

These variables were combined together to form a dimensionless number now called Reynolds number (Re) which may be calculated from the equation:

$$Re = \frac{vDp}{\mu} \qquad (22.3)$$

In general, with $Re < 2000$ laminar flow exists and with $Re > 4000$ turbulent flow exists. Between these limits flow conditions are variable (see Chapter 6).

In most engineering applications, $Re > 4000$ and

it is assumed that energy absorbed is proportional to velocity squared, that is: $E \propto v^2$. The main exception to this general statement is in air filtration, where velocities can be very low and Re approaches 2000.

Pressure

Air requires a pressure difference for it to flow and it will always flow from the higher to the lower pressure. The pressure difference can be created by a variety of means, but in ventilation it is normally created naturally, by temperature differences and/or outside wind effects, or artificially, by means of fans or other air movers. Air currents will take the easiest or least resistant route to equalize the pressure difference which is used to overcome the friction of air movement. Thus, pressure is a type of energy which appears in two forms: (1) static pressure (p_s); and (2) velocity pressure (p_v). The sum of these two pressures is known as total pressure (p_t).

Static pressure is the pressure exerted in all directions by a fluid that is stationary, but if it is in motion it is measured at right angles to the direction of flow to eliminate the effects of velocity; it can be positive or negative. On the suction side of a fan the static pressure is negative but on the discharge side it is positive, as shown in Fig. 22.1.

Velocity pressure is the pressure equivalent of the kinetic energy of fluid in motion and is calculated from the following formula:

$$p_v = \rho \frac{v^2}{2} \qquad (22.4)$$

where ρ is the air density and v is the air velocity. Velocity pressure provides the force to move sailing craft and to damage buildings in a high wind. The formula shown above is widely used in the measurement of air velocity and in the calculation of pressure loss in ductwork and fittings. If standard air density of 1.2 kg m^{-3} is used then the expression becomes:

$$p_v = 0.6 \, v^2 \qquad (22.5)$$

and if v is in metres per second, p_v will be in newtons per square metre. Velocity pressure is always positive.

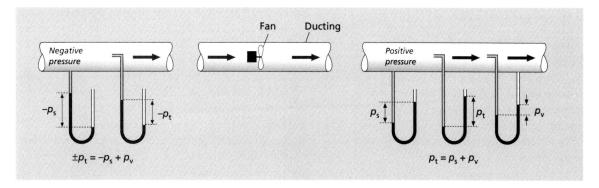

Fig. 22.1 Examples of typical liquid-filled manometer readings on either side of a fan showing the effect of positive and negative pressure.

Volume and mass flow rate

When a quantity of air is moving within a boundary of a duct or a tunnel, the volume flow rate (Q) is calculated from the formula:

$$Q = v A \qquad (22.6)$$

where v in this case is the average air velocity over the cross-section of the duct, and A is the cross-sectional area of the duct at the place where the velocity is taken. If v is in metres per second and A is in square metres, then Q will be cubic metres per second.

The mass flow (M) is related to Q as follows:

$$M = \rho Q \qquad (22.7)$$

where ρ is the density of air. If ρ is in kilograms per cubic metres then M will be in kilograms per second.

The volume flow rate is used when specifying the duties of fans or when calculating the dilution rates of pollutants. Mass flow rates are used to calculate quantities of heat required to temper the air in heating and air-conditioning systems.

Zones of influence at terminals

One important aspect of supply and extract ventilation which has a great influence upon the success or failure of the design, is the behaviour of the airstreams close to the points of entry to and exit from the system (Fig. 22.2). On the supply or discharge side, air leaves the system in a jet which

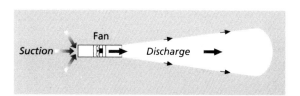

Fig. 22.2 Behaviour of airstreams close to points of entry to and exit from ventilation system.

expands in a narrow conical shape. Thus, if a jet of air is discharged from a parallel-sided duct at a velocity of $20\,\mathrm{m\,s^{-1}}$ the air in the room will be influenced for a considerable distance from the exit. For example, at a distance of 60 diameters from the exit, along the centre line, the air velocity will be $2\,\mathrm{m\,s^{-1}}$. Occupants of the room in direct line of the exit of a ventilation system could feel uncomfortable draughts, and so discharged air should be allowed to mix with room air, either above the heads of the occupants or at a place free of people. On the other hand, the zone of influence on the suction side of the mouth of a system is spherical in shape. As the surface area of a sphere is proportional to the square of the radius the air velocity decays inversely as the square of the distance. Thus within one duct diameter of the mouth the velocity has dropped to approximately one tenth and is virtually non-directional. For this reason extracts points must be placed very close to the source of emission and if possible within one diameter of it.

THE MEASUREMENT OF AIRFLOW

When examining a ventilation system to assess its performance it may be necessary to know:

1 whether it is successfully capturing the pollutants at their point of release;

2 what the velocities of air are at various places in the system;

3 how much pressure or suction the fan is developing; and

4 how much pressure is being absorbed in different parts of the system, in particular, by the filters or dust collectors.

Thus, the technique of measurement involves measuring air velocities, pressure differences and observing the path of the air by means of a tracer such as smoke.

Pressure measurement

The accepted instrument for measuring air pressure is the barometer, but ventilation pressures are low compared with barometric pressure, and often pressure differences are required. Therefore, it is usual to use a gauge and tubing for this purpose.

The simplest of gauges is the U-tube made of glass or transparent plastic half-filled with water. When the limbs of the U-tube are connected to the places where one wishes to discover the pressure difference, the pressure is represented by the difference in levels of the water in the limbs. The pressure measured can be quoted as a column of water, e.g. millimetres of water, or the column can be coverted to an absolute value by means of the simple formula:

$$p = \rho_2 gh \qquad (22.8)$$

where p is the pressure, g is the acceleration due to gravity, h is the height of the liquid column and ρ_2 is the density of the liquid in the column. The units used must be compatible, e.g. if ρ_2 is in kilograms per cubic metre, g is in metres per seconds squared and h is in metres, then p will be in newtons per square metre.

Most pressure gauges of this type are more sophisticated and are called manometers but they are basically U-tubes. Manometers usually have one limb inclined for greater accuracy and often contain a liquid of lower specific gravity than water to allow a longer scale and so give a more precise reading. These instruments can be calibrated in units of length to give the pressure in inches or millimetres of water but scale factors will have to be applied to the result to allow for the angle of inclination and the specific gravity of the liquid. Most of the commercial gauges are calibrated directly in the units of pressure required but some have tubes whose angle of inclination can be varied even to a vertical position. However, care must be taken to ensure that the correct multiplying factor is used to compensate for the different inclinations. Provided these devices are used with the correct fluid and are levelled and zeroed properly, they are accurate within the limits of reading a liquid meniscus along a scale and as such require no further calibration.

The main disadvantages of liquid manometers are the problems of spillage, a presence of bubbles in the liquid often caused by jolting in transit and the application to pressures above their range. They also need to be mounted on a flat surface so that they can be levelled and this may pose problems in some industrial settings. More practical instruments, for convenient use in the field, are available. Mechanical devices using diaphragms linked to an analogue display are suitable for most applications. Electrical instruments using pressure transducers are suitable for non-flammable atmospheres. Their main disadvantage is that they require to be regularly calibrated against a good manometer to be certain of reliable readings.

Smoke tracers

In order to identify airstreams outside the boundaries of ducts, a cloud of smoke is useful. Several methods of smoke generation are in use; commercial smoke tube kits are available which produce a cloud of white smoke. The proprietary ones consist of a glass tube, sealed at either end and filled with a chemical which produces white smoke when the tube ends are broken and air is passed through them. These smoke clouds are at the same temperature as the ambient air and would follow the airflow into which they are introduced, thus the currents can be made visible. It is useful to 'puff' the smoke around the entries to hoods and fume cupboards to identify the flow patterns and the speeds of slow-moving air currents. Leaks in joints and cracks in building work can also be tested using smoke clouds. Cigarette smoke is not suitable for this purpose as it is at a higher temperature than the ambient air and will give a false idea of the flow patterns. In dusty atmospheres the movement of particles can be highlighted using a Tyndall beam apparatus or 'dust lamp'.

Air velocity instruments

Pitot-static tube

This is a device which, in conjunction with a pressure gauge, measures velocity pressure inside a ventilation system irrespective of the static pressure at the point of measurement (Fig. 22.3). The velocity pressure can simply be converted to a velocity using the formula for velocity given above (Equation 22.4). The measuring head consists of two concentric tubes: one facing into the airstream parallel to the flow and the other with peripheral holes which will be at right angles to the airstream when the facing tube is correctly placed. The tubes are connected via flexible tubing to each side of the manometer or pressure gauge so that velocity pressure can be indicated. This device needs no calibration but the airflow measured must be in a

section of duct that is free from obstructions, bends or unnecessary turbulence, i.e. in a straight length of ducting at least 10 duct diameters away from obstructions. As the velocity pressure is proportional to the square of the velocity, the pitot-static tube reading becomes more reliable as the velocity increases. At a speed of $3 \, \text{m s}^{-1}$ the velocity pressure is only $5.4 \, \text{N m}^{-2}$ which is difficult to read on most commercial manometers and therefore readings at this velocity and below are subject to too much error to be reliable.

Rotating vane anemometers

These are like small windmills, usually between 25 and 100 mm in diameter and enclosed in an annular shroud. The rotating vanes are either coupled mechanically or electrically to a meter. Those which are mechanically coupled must be used in conjunction with a stop-watch so that the meter can be read over a known period of time, but they require no power source and are ideal for use in flammable atmospheres. The electrically coupled ones read directly in air velocity units but the meters are battery or mains operated and they may not be used in flammable atmospheres unless intrinsically safe.

The size of most vane anemometers makes them unsuitable for use in narrow ducts or extract slots, although the 25 mm diameter heads can be used

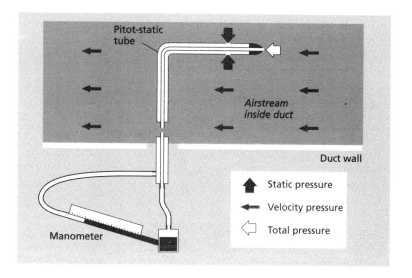

Fig. 22.3 Principle of operation of the pitot-static tube.

in most situations. If the blade settings become altered or the bearings are damaged, due to rough handling or use above the designed velocity, they will give false readings and will require repair and recalibration. They should not be used in very dusty or corrosive atmospheres.

Heated head anemometers

This group of instruments relies on a stream of air to cool a sensitive head consisting of a hot wire, a heated thermocouple or a thermistor. Various electrical means are employed to convert the cooling power, suitably corrected for ambient temperature, to a reading on a meter calibrated in air velocity units. The field version of these instruments consists of a sensing head on the end of a probe with an electrical cable leading to a meter which is usually battery powered. The head is non-directional unless a cowl is fitted, that is, it will sense the airflow in whatever direction it is flowing but the cowl channels it into one direction. The probes and heads are small and can easily be inserted through a small hole in ducting. The air velocities they can measure are in the range $0.1-30\,\mathrm{m\,s^{-1}}$, often in one instrument, but the heads are fragile, susceptible to dust deposits and they require regular calibration. They cannot be used in flammable atmospheres unless they are specifically designed for the purpose.

Calibration

With the exception of the pitot-static tube, all the instruments mentioned above require regular calibration if reliable results are to be obtained. This should be done in a wind tunnel in ideal flow conditions where accurately known air velocities can be produced. Few organizations have such a device, but a small open jet wind tunnel is available which gives sufficiently precise air velocities for calibrating the instruments most often used in the field. An open jet wind tunnel can be purchased at a fraction of the cost of a full one. The calibration can be shown on a chart in the form of a table or graph relating indicated velocity to true velocity or relating a correction value to be added or subtracted from the indicated velocity. This chart should always accompany the instrument.

Techniques for using air velocity instruments

In order to obtain reliable results, not only must the instruments be in good condition and recently calibrated but the reading must be taken in the correct way given the circumstances under which they are used.

The sensing head of the air velocity instrument must be placed in the airstream so that its axis is parallel to the streamlines, as most instruments are sensitive to 'yaw', that is the angle between the axis of the device and the direction of flow at the point of measurement. If the instrument is used at a place where the airstreams are not parallel, it is very difficult to avoid yaw. Some examples of places where it is unlikely that the airstreams will be parallel are given below.

At the discharge point from a ventilation system. Here the airstreams expand in a conical shape, the boundary angle of which is approximately 18°. If the discharge is a grille or diffuser, then the sides may not be axial or parallel and the streamlines will be at an angle greater than 18°.

At the inlet to a ventilation system. Air is being drawn in from all directions from a zone of air movement which is essentially spherical in shape, thus no airstream is parallel to the next.

Inside ductwork. Bends, changes of section, dampers and other obstructions result in the airstreams being distorted for some distance downstream. Nevertheless, airflow in such places has to be measured from time to time to give an indication of satisfactory performance of the system, and so it is important to realize that measurements at such places are inaccurate and should not be used for important design decisions.

In order to obtain reliable readings to establish the volume of air flowing in a system with some confidence, a measuring site must be chosen inside the ductwork where the airstreams are parallel, as far as can be ascertained. Such a site should be in straight, parallel-sided ducting at least 10 duct diameters, downstream of any obstruction or change of direction. Having chosen a suitable site, it will be necessary, in most cases, to drill a hole in the side of the duct of sufficient size to allow the insertion of the air velocity instruments and sensing head, and a plug should be available to block up the hole after taking the readings.

A further complication in the accurate measurement of airflow is the fact that air close to the boundaries of the flow moves at different speeds from that in the centre. In ductwork, the air close to the walls will move more slowly than that in the centre. Therefore, it is necessary to obtain an average velocity from over the whole cross-section of the duct by measuring in more than one place across the duct. In order to ensure that no bias exists in the choice of places, the measuring area must be divided into imaginary sections of equal area and a representative velocity measured in each section. The British Standards Institution in BS 848 Part 1 (British Standards Institution, 1980) suggests ways of dividing the cross-section of a measuring station for both rectangular- and circular-shaped areas (Figs 22.4 and 22.5). Essentially the technique involves dividing the area into equal annuli in circular ducts and according to the log-Tchebycheff rule in rectangular ducts. Velocity measurements are taken at each point and their arithmetic mean calculated. If velocities are measured using the pitot-static tube then it must be remembered that the velocity pressure must be converted to a velocity before taking the arithmetic mean.

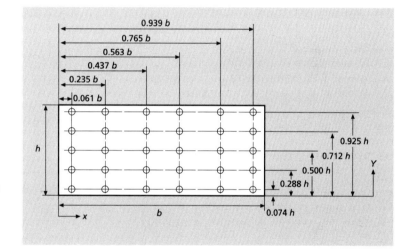

Fig. 22.4 Log-Tchebycheff rule for traverse points in a rectangular duct. To obtain the volume flow rate the true mean air velocity must be multiplied by the area of the measuring cross-section. Based on BS 848 Part I (British Standards Institution, 1980)*.

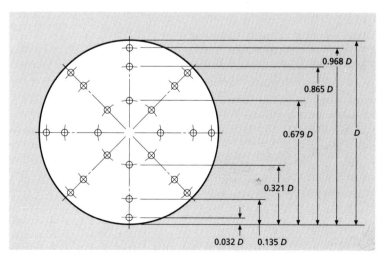

Fig. 22.5 Measuring positions for placing pitot-static tubes in rectangular and circular ducting. Based on BS 848 Part I (British Standards Institution, 1980)*.

* Extracts from BS 848 Part I (1980) are reproduced with the permission of BSI. Complete copies can be obtained by post from BSI Customer Services, 389 Chiswick High Road, London, W4 4AL; tel: 0181 996 7000.

Other volume flow measuring devices and techniques

Orifice plate

This device is installed as part of the ductwork system and is, therefore, not portable. The principle involves measuring a static pressure at points on either side of a disc installed across the duct in the centre of which a circular hole is cut. The size of the hole or orifice depends upon the volume of air likely to be flowing, that is, a larger volume flow rate would require a larger orifice. Details of the dimensions of the orifices and the calculations involved in converting the measured pressure to a volume flow rate is given in the British Standard BS 848 Part 2 (British Standards Institution, 1980). The disadvantage of such a device is that it forms an obstruction to the airflow in the duct by creating an extra resistance to airflow. It also forms a barrier against which airborne dust and particulates could be deposited.

Conical inlet

This device can be fitted to the inlet of a supply ventilation system and, as with the orifice plate, is installed as part of the system and is not portable. It consists of a cone or a bell-mouth shaped inlet to the ductwork with a static pressure tapping upstream of the inlet at a distance of half a duct diameter from the mouth. The theory of this device is that the static pressure measured at the tapping is numerically equal to the velocity pressure at that point (although opposite in sign) multiplied by a factor (C) which is very close to unity (if a good smooth bell-mouth is made then the factor can be assumed to be unity). Thus, to determine air volume flow rate the following formula can be used:

$$Q = AC \left(\frac{2p_s}{\rho}\right)^{\frac{1}{2}} \qquad (22.9)$$

where Q is the volume flow rate, A is the cross-section area of the duct, p_s is the static pressure measured and ρ is the air density. Note that the units must be consistent.

Dilution technique

This method involves the release of a known volume of a tracer gas, such as nitrous oxide or krypton 85, into the airstream over a known period of time and plotting the build-up and decay of the concentration in air against time. The airflow rate can be calculated from the mean dilution of the tracer or from an exponential decay equation. This technique is useful for estimating low flow rates in large spaces and is used for measuring natural ventilation rates in rooms. If krypton 85 is used, a volume of 0.02 ml (74 MBq) of the gas is sufficient for a 100 m³ room. It is a soft beta emitter, but at that concentration is not a health hazard.

EXTRACTION VENTILATION

One of the most useful methods of controlling the airborne concentration of toxic or nuisance pollutants is to extract them at source before they become dispersed into the workroom environment. Extract ventilation can remove gases, vapours, fumes, dust and larger particulates by means of enclosures, hoods or slots (Fig. 22.6) placed as close to the point of release of the pollutant as possible. The volumes of air drawn through these devices can be calculated and depend upon the capture velocity of the substance, the distance of the mouth of the extract from the point of release and the dimensions of the device.

The extract points need to be coupled via ducting, and in many cases the air should be conveyed to an air cleaner connected to a point of discharge which may or may not be outside the building. Fans or air movers are used to provide the motive power unless there is sufficient natural ventilation

Fig. 22.6 (*Facing page*) Extraction ventilation devices: (a) open face hood; (b) slots on tank; (c) booth or enclosure; (d) hood on flexible duct; (e) slot; (f) supplied and extracted enclosure (push–pull); (g) canopy hood; (h) canopy hood on flexible duct; (i) hood with face slots.

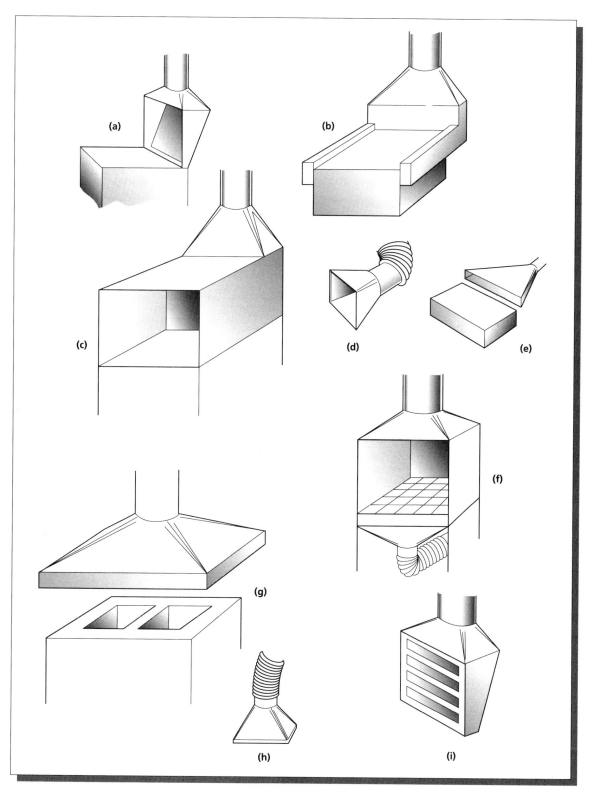

to give an adequate airflow. The design features of these extract devices, together with some simple formulae to calculate the air volume flow rates required to capture the pollutant successfully, are given below. Firstly, however, it is necessary to give some definition of terms used.

Capture velocity   The air velocity required at the source of emission sufficient to cause the pollutant to move towards the mouth of the extract and thus be successfully captured. Table 22.2 gives recommended capture velocities.

Face velocity   The air velocity at the opening of a hood or enclosure.

Slot velocity   The air velocity in slots.

Transport velocity   The minimum air velocity required in all parts of the system, including ductwork and extract devices, to keep collected particles airborne and to prevent them from being deposited on the sides or floor of the system until the collector is reached. Recommended transport velocities are given in Table 22.3.

Plenum   The space behind the face of a hood or slot.

Design features and volume flow rates

Enclosures

The commonest forms of these devices are booths and fume cupboards which contain the process from which the pollutant is released. The mouth of the device provides access for the operator but also provides an escape route for the pollutant. It is necessary, therefore, to maintain an air velocity at the face of the enclosure which is sufficient to prevent the pollutants from escaping. In the case of chemical fume cupboards, the opening area can be varied by raising or lowering a sliding front.

With all these devices it is advisable to enclose as much of the process as possible and to minimize the area of access, compatible with the task being enclosed. In this way the volume of air required can be minimized. If such an enclosure reduces visibility for the operator, then toughened glass or

Table 22.3 Recommended transport velocities

Pollutant	Transport velocity $(\mathrm{m\,s^{-1}})$
Fumes, such as zinc and aluminium	7–10
Fine dust, such as lint, cotton fly, flour, fine powders	10–12.5
Dusts and powders with low moisture contents, such as cotton dust, jute lint, fine wood shavings, fine rubber dust, plastic dust	12.5–17.5
Normal industrial dust, such as sawdust, grinding dust, food powders, rock dusts, asbestos fibres, silica flour, pottery clay dust, brick and cement dust	17.5–20
Heavy and moist dust, such as lead chippings, moist cement, quick-lime dust, paint spray particles	over 22.5

Table 22.2 Recommended capture velocities

Source conditions	Typical situations	Capture velocity $(\mathrm{m\,s^{-1}})$
Released into still air with no velocity	Degreasing tanks, paint dipping, still air drying	0.25–0.5
Released at a low velocity or into a slow moving airstream	Container filling, spray booths, screening and sieving, plating, pickling, low-speed conveyor transfer points, debagging	0.5–1.0
Released at a moderate velocity or into turbulent air	Paint spraying, normal conveyor transfer points, crushing, barrel filling	1.0–2.5
Released at a high velocity or into a very turbulent airstream	Grinding, fettling, tumbling, abrasive blasting	2.5–10.0

perspex can be used for those parts interfering with vision. It may be possible to cover the opening with a flexible curtain to further reduce the face area. Such a curtain could be made of plastic or canvas sheeting hung in narrow overlapping strips to allow the passage of tools or materials with the minimum of disturbance. The front of the enclosure could also be 'washed' by a gentle vertical air curtain.

In order to improve pollutant control it may be possible to supply the enclosure with air in addition to extracting from it. If this is done it will be necessary to extract at least 15% more air than is supplied to prevent the excess air from escaping through the access opening.

If the enclosure covers moving machinery which is producing the airborne pollutant, such as a grinding wheel or circular saw blade, then it is important to take into account the trajectory of any particles released so that the enclosure will capture them. With such an extract, the transport velocity must be maintained in all parts of the system up to the dust collector, including the enclosure itself.

The required volume flow rate is calculated by multiplying the area of the opening by the velocity necessary to prevent the pollutant from escaping. This velocity depends upon the toxicity of the substance and the momentum it has as a result of the way it has been released. For example, if the work being enclosed is being sprayed with paint then particles of paint are likely to rebound from the workpiece with considerable velocity, whereas if the workpiece was being dipped in a tank of paint, only the vapours could escape at a low speed. Thus the face air velocity needs to be much higher in the former than in the latter. As a general rule, face velocities should not fall below $0.5 \, \text{m s}^{-1}$ and for the more toxic pollutants or high-momentum particles, face velocities in excess of $1.5 \, \text{m s}^{-1}$ may be required. Thus an opening of $1 \, \text{m}^2$ area with a face velocity of $1 \, \text{m s}^{-1}$ will require a volume flow rate of $1 \, \text{m}^3 \, \text{s}^{-1}$.

In the case of fume cupboards, the older types had a variable face velocity depending upon the position of the sliding front, such that the wider the opening the lower the velocity and vice versa, but the modern ones have a bypass arrangement or a variable performance fan so that the face velocity remains reasonably constant whatever the position of the front.

Hoods

Often it is not possible to enclose work for reasons of access, for example, workpieces may have to be lowered from above or passed sideways from one process to the next. Therefore hood ventilation, whilst less effective than enclosures, may have to be used. Hoods with a width to length ratio (aspect ratio) of less than 0.2 are called slots and are dealt with separately.

Hoods can be placed over the work like a canopy or at the side or rear of the workplace depending upon the accessibility required. It is inadvisable to place canopy hoods over the top of the work if the operators have to lean over into the path of the air as it rises into the hood. In such circumstances a side or rear hood is more likely to keep the pollutants away from the breathing zone of the worker. When deciding upon the position of a hood it is necessary to take advantage of the natural currents of the substance to be captured. Substances that are hotter than the ambient air temperature or gases which are lighter than air will naturally tend to rise. Therefore, as far as possible, the hood should be sited above the point of release to facilitate capture. Similarly, heavier, cooler substances should be captured from the side. If it is necessary to pull against the natural current of air then a much higher capture velocity must be provided. However, it should be remembered that a concentrated stream of pollutants will obey buoyancy or gravity forces, but if well mixed with air, the mixture will have a density so close to that of air that such forces can be ignored. An example of this concerns vapours from certain cellulose paints which in a concentrated state will be heavier than air but, even at saturation conditions, a mixture of the vapour and air will not be sufficiently different in density from air to have any great effect.

With large hoods, the air velocity distribution across the face can be uneven, being higher close to the duct entrance and lower at the extremities. To overcome this, either the face of the hood can be divided up into a series of slots, or the plenum can be divided by guide vanes or air splitters carefully spaced to ensure even distribution.

In order to minimize the air volume flow rate required the hood should be placed as close as possible to the point of release of the pollutant and it is worth noting that the required quantity varies with the square of the distance.

Slots

For reasons of accessibility even hoods may be too bulky to allow work to flow satisfactorily and it may be necessary for operators to lean over the work on two sides whilst the other two sides are required to be free for the movement of materials or to improve visibility. In these circumstances, hoods with aspect ratios of below 0.2, called slots, can be used, the narrow sides being no more than 50 or 75 mm in width.

Slots are commonly used on degreasing tanks, cleaning baths and electroplating tanks to remove the vapours released from their surfaces. If a wide surface is to be ventilated, it is important to have two slots, one on each side, so that the extraction distance is minimized, as experience has shown that it is difficult to pull the air into a slot from a distance of more than 750 mm. Slots are coupled to the extract ductwork via a manifold or a transformation piece whose position in relation to the slot will influence the distribution of air along the slot. If it is placed at one end, should the slot be too long, very little air will be drawn into the opposite end and then air splitters would be required to improve the flow distribution. Slots which are longer than 2 m require to have more than one connection to the ductwork.

Improvement to the capture can be made by boosting the extract by a supply slot on the opposite side. However, care must be taken not to provide too high an air velocity over the surface of a tank in case the liquid in the tank is unnecessarily evaporated.

Prediction of performance

Fletcher method

The required volume flow rate can be calculated from the formula below given by Fletcher (1977)

which can be applied to both hoods and slots. The formula relates centreline air velocity to the distance from the hood and is dependent upon the aspect ratio of the hood. In order to capture the pollutants successfully, the source should be on the centreline.

$$\frac{VA}{Q} = \frac{V}{V_0} = \frac{1}{0.93 + 8.58\alpha^2} \quad (22.10)$$

where

$$\alpha = xA^{-\frac{1}{2}} \left(\frac{W}{L}\right)^{-\beta}$$

and

$$\beta = 0.2(xA^{-\frac{1}{2}})^{-\frac{1}{3}}$$

where Q is the required volume flow rate, x is the distance of the source from the hood along the centreline, A is the area of the hood, L is the length of the hood, W is the width of the hood, V is the centreline velocity at distance x from the hood and would normally be the capture velocity and V_0 is the mean velocity at the face of the hood. To assist in the numerical solution of the formula a nomogram (Fig. 22.7) is provided which relates: V/V_0, x/A and W/L.

Garrison method

For circular hoods the method described by Garrison (1983) can be used which predicts the centreline velocity at two distances from the end of a circular duct of diameter, d. These distances are: $0.5\,d$ and $1.0\,d$, i.e. half a diameter and one diameter from the mouth of the circular duct. Using the same symbols for velocities and distance as above:

$$V = FV_0 \quad (22.11)$$

When $x = 0$, $F = 1$, i.e. $V/V_0 = 1$. Table 22.4 gives values of F for $x = 0.5\,d$ and $x = 1.0\,d$ for various profiles of duct end. Note that x is measured from the end of the duct not the edge of the profile.

Capture and transport velocities

Capture velocities required to move the pollutants vary with the type of substance and the speed at which it is being released, and can range from $0.25\,\mathrm{m\,s^{-1}}$ up to $10\,\mathrm{m\,s^{-1}}$. For example, the emission

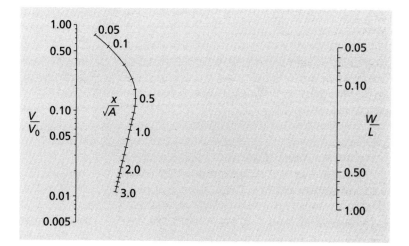

Fig. 22.7 Nomogram to assist in calculation of required volume flow rate. NB: the presence of a flange on the hood can reduce the quantities by 20–25%. Crown copyright is reproduced with the permission of the Controller of HMSO.

Table 22.4 Values of F for various duct ends

Duct end profile (see Fig. 22.8)	F	
	$x = 0.5\,d$	$x = 1.0\,d$
Plain	0.26	0.08
Flanged	0.30	0.10
Flared	0.40	0.18
Rounded	0.69	0.33

of vapour from a degreasing tank is of a low kinetic energy and would be successfully captured by an airspeed of $0.25\,\mathrm{m\,s^{-1}}$, whereas a particle emitted from a grinding wheel or a sand-blasting process would have a high kinetic energy and might require a capture velocity of $10\,\mathrm{m\,s^{-1}}$. Ranges of capture velocities are given in Table 22.2 but it is possible to establish such a velocity for oneself by trial and error with a nozzle of a suction device such as an industrial vacuum cleaner, by bringing the nozzle

closer and closer to the released substance until it becomes captured. The air velocity measured at the point of release is the capture velocity.

The transport velocity is somewhat harder to establish and varies with the size and density of the particle (see Table 22.3). As with capture velocities, several authorities publish values for different substances based on experience. As a general rule, an air velocity in the duct of over $20\,\mathrm{m\,s^{-1}}$ will keep most particles airborne but bends and obstructions inside the duct can cause local changes of velocity which may result in particles being deposited. Care must be exercised in the design of the ductwork system so that local dust deposits are not allowed to build up and accumulate.

DILUTION VENTILATION

This method of ventilation is less positive than extraction and should only be used when extraction ventilation is not practicable, the pollutants have a

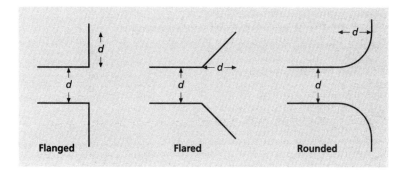

Fig. 22.8 File shapes for ends of round ducts.

low toxicity and the release volume does not fluctuate.

Before calculating the required volume flow rate to dilute the pollutants to an acceptable level it is necessary to establish their rates of release into the space to be ventilated. This may not be easy as the processes involved may be complex. But if the process is in operation it may be possible to sample the concentrations in known flow rates of air, thus establishing the rate of release of the pollutants. It may be necessary to resort to continuously recording instruments and in this way it is possible to establish whether the release of the substances is constant or fluctuating. In some cases, the estimation of the release rate can be related to the consumption of a particular raw material, for example, if a degreasing tank requires to be replenished with a known volume of degreaser in a given time then it is reasonably safe to assume that the amount has evaporated into the air of the workroom and the rate of release can be calculated.

Concentration

Let the rate of emission of the pollutant be r m^{3}s^{-1} and the ventilation airflow rate be Q m^{3}s^{-1}, then the concentration of the substance is given by:

$$\text{Concentration} = \frac{r}{Q} \, \text{m}^3\text{m}^{-3} \qquad (22.12)$$

or

$$= \frac{r}{Q} \times 100\%$$

or

$$= \frac{r}{Q} \times 10^6 \text{ parts per million (ppm)}$$

i.e. all the above are expressed as volume for volume concentrations. If a mass/volume concentration is required then the density of the substance should be used as follows:

$$\text{Mass concentration} = \frac{r}{Q} \times \rho_s \, \text{kg m}^{-3} \qquad (22.13)$$

$$= \frac{r}{Q} \, \rho_s \times 10^6 \, \text{mg m}^{-3}$$

where ρ_s is the density of the substance in kg m^{-3}.

In the case of solvents, it must be remembered that the density of the liquid solvent is not the same as its vapour density. Vapour density can be calculated from the formula:

$$\text{Vapour density at STP} = \frac{M}{24.1} \, \text{kg m}^{-3} \qquad (22.14)$$

where M is the molecular mass of the vapour.

The properties of most liquids and gases can be found in the standard chemistry and physics handbooks.

Required volume flow rates for dilution ventilation

From the above formulae, an expression can be derived from which to calculate the required ventilation airflow rate to dilute the pollutant to a chosen concentration. That concentration could be the occupational exposure limit (OEL) or some other concentration chosen by the designer or his or her advisers. For gaseous emissions the required flow rate (Q) is found by:

$$Q = \frac{r \times 10^6 \times K}{C} \qquad (22.15)$$

where K is a safety factor and C is the chosen concentration in ppm. The units of this expression will be the same as the units of r. That is, if r is in m^{3}s^{-1} then Q will be the same. For vapour emissions, Q is found by:

$$Q = \frac{24.1 \times 10^6 \times K}{M \times C} \, \text{m}^3 \text{ per kg of solvent released} \qquad (22.16)$$

The safety factor (K) depends upon the relationship between the source of pollution and the airflow distribution in the room, the uniformity of the emission and the toxicity of the pollutant. The estimation of K is a matter of judgement and experience and could be as low as one and as high as 10. That is, $K = 1$ would apply to a pollutant of low toxicity emitted at a uniform rate with a ventilation layout that moved the pollutant away from the occupants of the room.

The mode of introducing the diluting air is important. It can be done in one of three ways:

1 allowing the unpolluted diluting air to pass over the worker before reaching the source;

2 ensuring thorough mixing of the diluting air and the pollutant before it reaches the worker;

3 introducing the diluting air at a temperature slightly lower than the rest of the room and at a very low velocity such that the clean air displaces the pollutant and moves it upward towards an extract point.

The choice depends upon circumstances and the layout of the workplace.

DUCTS AND FITTINGS

Fresh air needed to provide satisfactory ventilation, whether it may be for supply or extract, is normally carried in ductwork to and from its source. It is unusual to have a direct route for this purpose, therefore bends and changes of section are required to fit the ventilation system to the needs of the building and the associated plant. The shape and size of the ducts and fittings are determined by the ventilation engineer. Each section of duct or fitting absorbs energy from the air to overcome the friction resulting from the passage of air through it. That energy requires a source of motive power for its generation, either a fan or some other air mover. In order to determine the size and duty of the fan and its associated prime mover, the energy loss for each section of the system is calculated and totalled. The following paragraphs describe these calculations in more detail.

Ducting is usually made of galvanized sheet steel, either in circular or rectangular section, although a variety of other materials, including stainless steel, brick, concrete, PVC, canvas, fibreglass and other plastics, are sometimes used.

Duct sizes

There are several factors which should be considered when deciding upon the cross-sectional area of the duct and usually a compromise is made between them. For a given volume flow rate, the larger the duct the lower the air velocity inside and the less energy absorbed, but the larger the capital cost of the material. A circular cross-section is more economical in material than a rectangular

one, but in some buildings the space available is more suited to the rectangular shape. If a particular transport velocity has to be maintained, once the required volume flow rate is determined the duct cross-section is fixed as the one that provides that velocity.

Pressure losses

The energy losses due to friction are expressed as a pressure loss. These losses can be determined by calculation or by the use of charts and nomograms. As many published texts reproduce these aids there is no need to duplicate them here, but reference should be made to the Chartered Institute of Building Services Engineers (CIBSE) *Guide Book C* (1986), and the British Hydromechanics Association and the British Occupational Hygiene Society (BOHS) publications for further details.

As far as straight lengths of ducting are concerned, pressure losses are quoted per unit length of duct, for example, $N m^{-2}$ per metre run of duct or inches of water per 100 ft of duct. This pressure loss is proportional to the air density and the square of the air velocity and inversely proportional to the fifth power of the duct diameter. As the duct sides are parallel, there is no change in air velocity from one end to the other, therefore the pressure losses calculated are both static and total pressures. The losses in most fittings are calculated by multiplying the velocity pressure (p_v) at a point in the fitting by a factor determined empirically for the geometric shape of that fitting; the resulting pressure loss is in total pressure. It is important to work in total pressures for ventilation calculations as fittings such as expansion pieces have changes in velocity pressure from one end to the other, resulting in gains in static pressure whilst still sustaining a loss in total pressure; working in total pressure throughout avoids any confusion. In the case of expansion pieces, the total pressure loss is calculated by multiplying the difference in velocity pressure between the two ends by a total pressure loss factor. The values of all these factors quoted are given in the texts mentioned previously for a variety of geometric shapes and configurations, but Fig. 22.9 provides some of the more common ones.

Once the pressure loss for each section of the

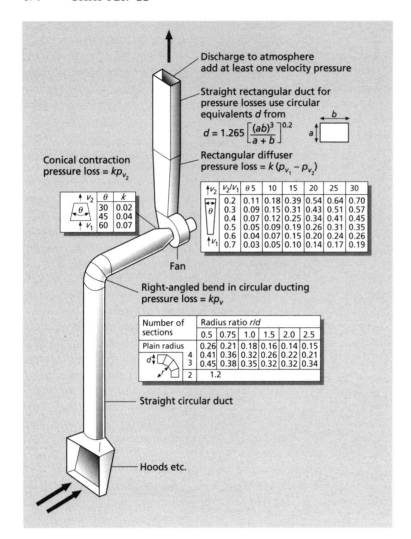

Conical contraction
pressure loss = kp_{v_2}

v_2 θ	θ	k
	30	0.02
	45	0.04
v_1	60	0.07

Discharge to atmosphere
add at least one velocity pressure

Straight rectangular duct for
pressure losses use circular
equivalents d from

$$d = 1.265 \left[\frac{(ab)^3}{a+b} \right]^{0.2}$$

Rectangular diffuser
pressure loss = $k\,(p_{v_1} - p_{v_2})$

v_2	v_2/v_1 θ	5	10	15	20	25	30
	0.2	0.11	0.18	0.39	0.54	0.64	0.70
	0.3	0.09	0.15	0.31	0.43	0.51	0.57
	0.4	0.07	0.12	0.25	0.34	0.41	0.45
	0.5	0.05	0.09	0.19	0.26	0.31	0.35
	0.6	0.04	0.07	0.15	0.20	0.24	0.26
v_1	0.7	0.03	0.05	0.10	0.14	0.17	0.19

Fan

Right-angled bend in circular ducting
pressure loss = kp_v

Number of sections	Radius ratio r/d					
	0.5	0.75	1.0	1.5	2.0	2.5
Plain radius	0.26	0.21	0.18	0.16	0.14	0.15
4	0.41	0.36	0.32	0.26	0.22	0.21
3	0.45	0.38	0.35	0.32	0.32	0.34
2	1.2					

Straight circular duct

Hoods etc.

Fig. 22.9 Pressure loss factors for components of a ventilation system.

ductwork system has been calculated, including any dust collection device, all the total pressures should be added together to determine the overall total pressure loss of the system. Thus the duty of the fan required is computed, i.e. the calculated volume flow rate at the total pressure loss. The velocity pressure of any discharge velocity must be added to the total, as it represents energy that the fan has to provide. If this value is forgotten or ignored it could result in the fan being undersized for the duty it is expected to perform.

A complication arises if more than one offtake is connected to the system, as, for example, when several extract or supply fittings are connected to

one duct leaving the fan. In such cases the fan total pressure required is only that required to move the air between the two extremities of the system, for example, between the fan discharge point and the extract hood furthest from the fan, known as the 'index branch'. Normally there will be sufficient pressure to cater for intermediate branches.

Suggested method of duct sizing and loss calculation

It is first necessary to draw a sketch of the layout of the system (the one shown in Fig. 22.10 is given as an example) in which the volume flow rates for

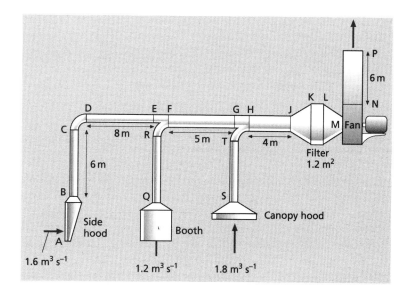

Fig. 22.10 The extract ventilation system used in the text example. The volume flow rates shown here have been arbitrarily chosen but are not untypical. For the purposes of this example, ducting of circular galvanized sheet steel has been taken, carrying air at a velocity of $15\,\mathrm{m\,s^{-1}}$ and at standard density.

each terminal should be marked. In order to identify each section of the system, a symbol should be assigned either to every section or to every junction where the air changes speed or direction. Labelling the junctions rather than the sections facilitates network analysis particularly if analogue or digital computers are used for calculations. Programs are available for this work. In the example given, each junction has been assigned a letter of the alphabet. In order to simplify the calculations, they should be tackled in a tabular form by drawing up a table with the headings as shown in Table 22.5. For each section the appropriate column only need be filled in and the pressure losses calculated. The cumu-

lative pressure loss column enables a running total pressure loss to be maintained from the furthest outlet to the fan so that at any point in the system it is possible to see what the pressure difference is between that point and atmospheric pressure.

With the solution of this example it is necessary to make three decisions which will influence the design.

1 *What velocity should be chosen for the air in the duct?* If there are particles to be carried, the velocity chosen should be the transport velocity for those particles (see Table 22.3), but as transport velocities are high, noise levels from the passage of air in the duct will also be high. If a quiet area is

Table 22.5 Headings for table to be used in designing an extract system

Section	Length (m)	Volume flow rate $(m^3\,s^{-1})$	Duct dimension (mm)	Duct area (m^2)	Air velocity $(m\,s^{-1})$	Velocity pressure (Pa)	Pressure loss factor, k	Pressure loss per metre $(Pa\,m^{-1})$	Section pressure loss (Pa)	Cumulative pressure loss (Pa)
....	....	....	....	....	....	....	....	....	....	....
....	....	....	....	....	....	....	....	....	....	....
....	....	....	....	....	....	....	....	....	....	....
....	....	....	....	....	....	....	....	....	....	....
....	....	....	....	....	....	....	....	....	....	....
....	....	....	....	....	....	....	....	....	....	....
....	....	....	....	....	....	....	....	....	....	....
....	....	....	....	....	....	....	....	....	....	....
....	....	....	....	....	....	....	....	....	....	....
....	....	....	....	....	....	....	....	....	....	....

to be ventilated, the airspeeds should be below $5 \, \mathrm{m \, s^{-1}}$, but in many industrial settings other noises will prevail and higher velocities can be used.

2 *Should the ducting be circular or rectangular in cross-section?* If space is limited then a rectangular section may make better use of what space there is, but if high air velocities are to be carried then circular ducting is better for rigidity and has a lower pressure loss for a given cross-sectional area.

3 *Of what materials should the ducting be made?* Unless corrosive gases or vapours are to be carried, galvanized sheet steel is the normal material for reasons of strength and ease of manufacture of the fittings. Nevertheless, whatever materials are chosen the calculations are carried out as though it was steel and a correction factor is applied depending upon the surface roughness of any other material.

Having worked through the table, section by section, from one extreme end to the other, it is necessary to examine the intermediate branches. It can be seen from Table 22.6 that the cumulative pressure at point F is $236 \, \mathrm{N \, m^{-2}}$, therefore the pressure loss through branch AQRF must be the same, and yet the distance is shorter and the branch happens to be carrying less air than ABCDEF. Likewise, the cumulative pressure at point H is $313 \, \mathrm{N \, m^{-2}}$, therefore branch ASTH must have that pressure loss. If no steps are taken to allow for this, and similar duct sizes are chosen as in the index branch, then, when the system is installed and the fan turned on, the bulk of the airflow will pass through the branch nearest the fan and very little through the one furthest away, thus the system is out of balance. To allow for this, either of the intermediate branches are fitted with controlling dampers, but these can lead to problems of dust accumulation and they are open to interference from uninformed personnel who may tamper with the settings and unbalance the whole system.

In order to size the intermediate branches to balance the pressure losses correctly, equations can be derived which will produce a mathematical solution but it is probably as quick to solve the problem by an iterative 'trial and error' method, i.e. choose a duct slightly smaller than in the index branch and work through the pressure loss calculations. If the pressure loss is too small, choose yet a smaller duct; if too large, choose a larger duct and repeat until the correct duct is arrived at.

In the example, fan manufacturers' catalogues should be consulted to find a suitable fan to provide the duty of $4.6 \, \mathrm{m^3 \, s^{-1}}$ at a total pressure of $1015 \, \mathrm{N \, m^{-2}}$.

Balancing of multibranched systems

If a system has been designed with damper control of intermediate branches, then an initial balance will have to be established and if an existing system is thrown out of balance by injudicious alteration of dampers, rebalancing is required. This task must be undertaken systematically because it should be remembered that the movement of any one damper will alter the airflow rate in every other branch. Thus, a damper set to give the correct airflow rate in one branch will be wrongly set by the time the other branches are adjusted. The correct procedure to follow is laid down in the *CIBSE Commissioning Code: Series A, Air Distribution*. Essentially, the technique involves the adjustment of dampers so that adjacent branches pass the same proportion of the design volume flow rate rather than the correct flow rate. If adjacent branches are balanced together, starting from the index branch and working towards the fan and any one branch only adjusted once, when the branch closest to the fan is reached all branches will be passing the same proportion of their design flows. If this proportion is not close to 100% of design then adjustment is required at the fan.

FANS

There is an infinite variety of shapes and sizes of fans capable of duties ranging from the ventilation of a microcircuit to cooling air for a deep mine, that is from 10 mm up to 10 m in diameter. Each geometric shape of fan has its own characteristics and a family of fans of the same geometric configuration will vary in performance according to diameter and speed of rotation. Each fan consists of a rotating impeller on a shaft to which the power source is connected and a casing which guides the air to and from the impeller. A pressure difference is created between the inlet and outlet

Table 22.6 Duct sizing and fan duty calculation for the example in Fig. 22.10

Section	Length (m)	Volume flow rate (m³ s⁻¹)	Duct dimension (mm)	Duct area (m²)	Air velocity (m s⁻¹)	Velocity pressure (N m⁻² (Pa))	Pressure loss factor, k	Pressure loss per unit length (N m⁻² per m)	Section pressure loss (N m⁻² (Pa))	Cumulative pressure loss (N m⁻² (Pa))	Remarks
A–B		1.6	diam. 370	0.107	15	135	0.25		34	34	Hood
B–C	6	1.6	diam. 370	0.107	15	135		6.5	39	73	
C–D		1.6	diam. 370	0.107	15	135	0.42		57	130	Bend
D–E	8	1.6	diam. 370	0.107	15	135		6.5	52	182	
E–F		1.6	diam. 370	0.107	15	135	0.40		54	236	Junction (through)
F–G	5	2.8	diam. 490	0.187	15	135		4.6	23	259	
G–H		2.8	diam. 490	0.187	15	135	0.4		54	313	Junction (through)
H–J	4	4.6	diam. 625	0.310	15	135		3.3	13	326	
J–K		4.6	angle 60°		ratio 0.21	diff. 129	0.67		87	413	Transformation enlargement round to square
K–L		4.6	1.2 m sq.	1.44	face 3.2	6			420	833	Filter (manufacturer's data)
L–M		4.6	angle 60°		3.2–20	240	0.07		17	850	Transformation contraction square to round
M–N	Fan		inlet diam. 540	0.23	20	240			Fan total pressure		
N–P	6	4.6	600 × 500	0.30	15.3	141		4.0	24	24	Rectangular fan discharge stack
P–A		4.6				141			141	165	Discharge velocity

Total pressure required on suction side of fan = 850 N m⁻² and on discharge side = 165 N m⁻², therefore fan total pressure required = 850 + 165 = 1015 N m⁻². Note that point A represents atmospheric pressure, i.e. anywhere in the room or outside. Note also that it will be necessary to size the straight lengths of duct first before details of the fittings can be designed, thus sections of the system have to be passed over and returned to later.

by the rotation of the impeller. The Fan Manufacturers Association have agreed on the following definitions for fan pressure.

Fan total pressure   The rise in total pressure across the fan equal to the total pressure at the fan outlet minus the total pressure at the fan inlet.

Fan velocity pressure   The velocity pressure based upon the mean air velocity at the fan outlet.

Fan static pressure   The fan total pressure minus the fan velocity pressure.

It is necessary to define two other parameters which occur with regard to the performance of fans: fan power and fan efficiency.

Fan power and efficiency

In engineering terminology, 'power' is work done per unit time and as far as fans are concerned that means the work done on the air to move it against a particular pressure. In dealing with fans there are two components of power: the theoretical power required to move the air; and the actual power required to be provided at the shaft of the fan to achieve the air power. The reason for these two is that fans are not 100% efficient and some power is lost in the turbulence between the blades, the friction of the air as it passes through the casing and the losses in the bearings which support the rotating parts. Air power (P_a) can be calculated from the expression:

$$P_a = Q \times p \qquad (22.17)$$

where Q is the volume flow rate and p is either the fan's static or total pressure. If Q is in cubic metres per second and p is in newtons per square metre then the power is in newton metres per second, which is watts. If imperial units are used, care must be taken to convert inches of water to pounds force per square foot (see Table 22.1); the pressure in pounds force per square foot multiplied by the volume flow rate in feet per minute gives the unit of ft lb$_f$ min^{-1} of which there are 33 000 in 1 horsepower. The resulting units are known as 'air power (static)' if static pressure is used and 'air power (total)' if total pressure is used.

Fan efficiency is obtained from the measurement of the input power to the shaft of the fan using the expression:

$$\text{Fan efficiency} = \frac{\text{Air power}}{\text{Input power at shaft}} \times 100\% \qquad (22.18)$$

As above, if air power (static) is used then the efficiency is known as 'fan static efficiency' and if air power (total) is used then the efficiency is known as 'fan total efficiency'. The efficiency of a fan varies with its duty and is given by the fan manufacturer, if requested, for a particular performance.

Fan characteristic curves

If a fan is run at a constant speed and its volume flow rate is altered by varying the resistance against which it has to operate, curves showing the variation of pressure, power and efficiency can be plotted against a base of volume flow. These curves, known as 'fan characteristic curves', give the performance of the fan over the whole range of resistances for which it is designed. Manufacturers' catalogues quote these curves either as graphs or tables.

Typical characteristic curves are shown in Figs 22.11–22.13 below. Their shape depends upon the geometric design of the fan.

Fan types

Some of the more common types of fan are described below.

Propeller fan

This type of fan (Fig. 22.11) is useful for general ventilation work where there is little resistance to airflow as it is not suitable for use in ductwork or air filtration. It is most commonly used for unit heaters, air cooling on such places as motor-car radiators and refrigeration evaporators and is often seen mounted on an aperture in an outside wall to provide general supply and extract ventilation for rooms, workshops and warehouses. Propeller fans are generally low in efficiency, but as most are low in power this is no great problem. Aerofoil blades fitted to some of the larger ones improve their efficiency from 55% for the sheet steel blades up to 70% for the aerofoil.

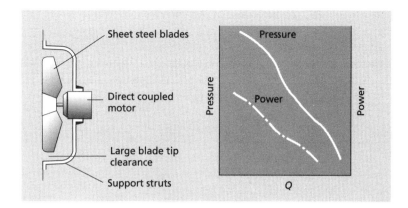

Fig. 22.11 Propeller fan and graph showing its characteristic curves.

Axial flow fan

This type of fan (Fig. 22.12) has a casing which is cylindrical, the shaft of the impeller being at the centre of the casing and running parallel to the sides. The blades of the impeller are usually of aerofoil section and rotate with their tips close to the casing. Whilst similar in principle to the propeller fan, the axial fan produces much higher pressures, up to $1100 \, \text{N} \, \text{m}^{-2}$ (Pa) per stage, although some single-stage fans will produce even higher pressures. Normally, if a higher pressure is required, a second stage is fitted or a centrifugal fan is used.

The performance of the fan can be changed by altering the angle of the blades, as shown in Fig. 22.12. With some axials it is possible to unclamp the blades to reset them at another angle, with others they can be altered whilst in motion.

The rotation of the impeller imparts a swirl to the air which is undesirable from a performance point of view, therefore some form of flow straightener is required to help recover some of the energy due to the rotation. If the fan is to be used close to a finned heat exchanger this is not a problem as the fins act as a flow straightener, but if the fan is to be used on ducting it is advisable to use one fitted with guide vanes. These guide vanes take the form of static blades attached to the casing at an angle sufficient to give a counter-swirl to the air, thus it leaves the fan moving parallel to the casing. If a two-stage fan is necessary, the second stage can be arranged to rotate in the opposite direction to the first to counteract the swirl, thus avoiding the need for static guide vanes. Some axial flow fans available have this facility.

The efficiency of axial flow fans can be as high as 78%. Also in their favour is the fact that they are compact and can fit neatly into a ductwork system, often at the same diameter as the ducting, and if the drive motor is directly coupled to the impeller

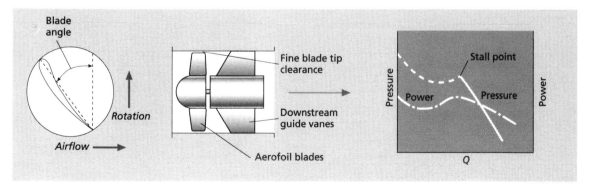

Fig. 22.12 Axial flow fan and graph showing its characteristic curves.

in the airstream, the fan takes up no more space than a short length of ducting.

An axial flow fan has several disadvantages, however, one of which is the high noise levels that are associated with the higher speed, higher pressure fans. Silencers are often necessary to keep noise to an acceptable standard. Another disadvantage is the problem of 'stall' which occurs if the fan is expected to work against a system which has a higher resistance than one for which the fan was designed. Stall condition in a fan is similar to that on an aircraft which is flying at too low a speed to provide the necessary lift to keep it airborne. The symptoms of stall in a fan are: fluctuating fan pressure and power; change in note; and variable flow rate. It is unwise to run a fan in stall condition as the bearings can become damaged. Reducing the blade angle of the fan can move it out of stall condition but the overall performance will be reduced as a result.

It is also unwise to use an axial flow fan with the motor in an airstream where the air is at a high temperature or containing dust or corrosive chemicals. Fans with alternative layouts which put the motor out of the airstream are available and should be used in these situations.

Centrifugal fans

With this type of fan (Fig. 22.13), the air enters the eye of an impeller via a suction sleeve. The rotating impeller, which is not unlike a paddle-wheel, throws the air to its periphery where it is collected by a casing in the shape of a volute. The blades of the impeller can be either forward- or backward-inclined in relation to the direction of rotation, or radial. Each configuration results in a fan with its own idiosyncrasies. All centrifugals can produce high pressures.

The forward-bladed fan (Fig. 22.14(a)) has an impeller with many closely spaced but narrow blades which produces a pressure characteristic which is distinctive in the fact that at a certain pressure three different flow rates are possible, dependent upon the resistance of the system against which it is working. The power characteristic is known as 'overloading' at high flow rates because the curve continues to rise as the volume flow is increased. This type of fan is the most compact of the centrifugals for a given volume flow rate, and is used where space is limited. Because of the shapes of its pressure and power characteristics, the forward-bladed fan should never be run without being coupled to a ventilation system nor should two be coupled together in parallel unless under the guidance of the manufacturer or an experienced fan engineer. Forward-bladed fans are less efficient than the backward-bladed models.

The backward-bladed fans (Fig. 22.14(b)) have fewer, deeper blades than the forward-bladed but are less compact for a given duty. The power characteristic is 'non-overloading' and this family of fans is the most efficient. If aerofoil section blades are used, efficiencies up to 85% have been

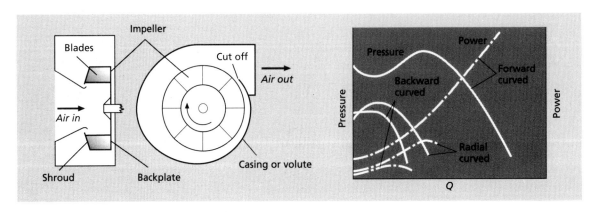

Fig. 22.13 Centrifugal fan and graph showing its characteristic curves.

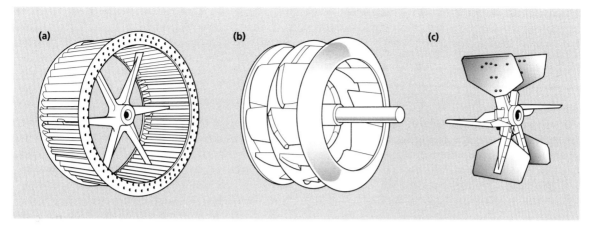

Fig. 22.14 Centrifugal fan impellers: (a) forward-bladed; (b) backward-bladed; (c) radial-bladed.

experienced, particularly on the larger fans. This makes them popular for the high-powered, continuously running operations such as those used on power-stations and deep mines.

Radial-bladed fans (Fig. 22.14(c)) have similar characteristics to the backward-bladed ones but are less efficient. The commonest of this type of fan is the paddle-bladed model where the impeller is made of a number of crude, flat plates riveted or bolted to a central hub. It is used for applications where highly corrosive or abrasive air is handled such that the blades quickly wear or rot away. Replacement blades can be easily fitted to such an impeller which is inherently self-cleaning.

Matching of fan and system

The most efficient part of the pressure characteristic of a fan is just to the right of the peak pressure on the top of the final downward slope (Fig. 22.15). A fan should be chosen so that the duty required lies on that part of the curve. Having calculated the pressure loss of a ventilation system for a given volume flow rate, a point can be plotted and a curve drawn on linear graph paper which represents the system. The curve will be of the form:

$$p \propto Q^2 \qquad (22.19)$$

that is, a parabola and will pass through the origin. If the fan total pressure characteristic is plotted on

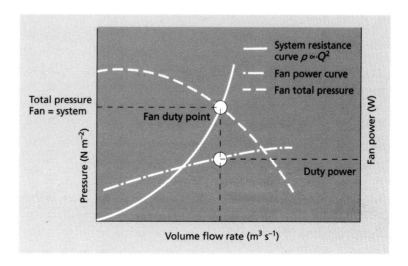

Fig. 22.15 Matching of fan and system.

the same scale, the point of intersection of the two curves will give the duty point that would occur if that fan was installed on that system.

AIR CLEANING AND DISCHARGE TO ATMOSPHERE

It is an infringement of several Acts of Parliament to discharge air into the atmosphere without first rendering it free from pollutants as far as is reasonably practicable. Much of the air that is extracted from workplaces requires some form of cleaning before it is discharged. There are many excellent texts on the engineering control of atmospheric pollution which include the techniques available for removing substances from ventilation air. Therefore, no details will be given here.

If particulates are to be removed from the air, both of which are dry, then dry dust collectors of various types are available. The larger particles can be removed by dry centrifugal methods such as cyclones, whilst bag filters will remove the smaller dusts. Particles that can be easily electrically charged can be collected by electrostatic collectors provided that there is no fire or explosion hazard in the air or the collected material. Dust extracted in humid air or wet or sticky particles must be collected by some wet method such as venturi scrubbers, wet centrifugals or wet orifice collectors. Unfortunately, these devices leave the dust in a sludge which also could become a pollution problem.

Air containing chemicals should be cleaned by absorption or by chemical scrubbing according to the nature of the substance. Whether the air is cleaned or not, it must be discharged into the atmosphere in such a way that it does not re-enter the building or any other building in the vicinity before it has been diluted to negligible concentrations. The best techniques involve discharging the air as high into the atmosphere as possible and at a high velocity. Devices such as cowls and weather caps hinder the upward throw of discharged air and are not recommended. Care should be taken to allow for local wind effects including the turbulence caused by adjacent buildings and any risk of 'blow back' through the ductwork should be prevented.

MAKE UP AIR

Extract ventilation systems can remove very large quantities of air from buildings. This air has to be replaced by outside air which, if not specifically supplied, will find its way in through openings in doors and windows, cracks in the walls and roof and anywhere else that is open to the atmosphere. At certain times of the year, particularly in winter in extreme northern and southern lattitudes, this will result in cold draughts and unsatisfactory working conditions with regard to temperature. Ventilation systems become unpopular as a result and people are tempted to turn them off to minimize cold draughts. Whenever an extract ventilation system is used, a make up system is required where the volume flow of air supplied is equal to that extracted. The supply should be tempered to the correct conditions to suit the comfort of the building occupants.

The provision of adequate heating or cooling is expensive in both capital and fuel costs. The following simple formula will enable a power calculation to be made to estimate the costs of heating or cooling:

$$\text{Heat required} = mc_p\,(t_i - t_o) \qquad (22.20)$$

where m is the mass flow rate of the air, c_p is the specific heat of air $(1.02\,\text{kJ}\,\text{kg}^{-1})$ and t_i and t_o are the temperatures inside and outside the building. From this formula it can be seen that to heat $1\,\text{m}^3\,\text{s}^{-1}$ of air from $0°C$ to $21°C$ requires $25.7\,\text{kW}$ of energy:

$$\text{Heat required} = 1 \times 1.2 \times 1.02 \times 21 = 25.7\,\text{kW}$$
$$(22.21)$$

REFERENCES

British Standards Institution. (1980). *Fans for General Purposes. Part 1: Methods of Testing Performance.* British Standards Institution BS 848 Part 1.

Chartered Institute of Building Services Engineers (1971). *CIBSE Commissioning Code: Series A, Air Distribution.* CIBSE, London.

Fletcher, B. (1977). Centreline velocity characteristics of rectangular unflanged hoods and slots under suction. *Annals of Occupational Hygiene*, **20**, 141–6.

Garrison, R.P. (1983). Velocity calculation for local exhaust inlets — empirical design equations. *American Industrial Hygiene Association Journal*, **44**, 937–40.

FURTHER READING

American Conference of Governmental Industrial Hygienists (1995). *Industrial Ventilation. A Manual of Recommended Practice*, (22nd edn). ACGI, Cincinnati.

Ashton, I. and Gill, F.S. (1992). *Monitoring for Health Hazards at Work*. Blackwell Scientific Publications, Oxford.

British Occupational Hygiene Society (1987). *Controlling Airborne Contaminants in the Workplace*. BOHS Technical Guide No. 7. Science Reviews Ltd, Leeds.

Burgess, W.A., Ellenbecker, M.J. and Treitman, R.D. (1989). *Ventilation for the Control of the Work Environment*. John Wiley, Chichester.

Chartered Institute of Building Services Engineers (1986). *Guide Book C*. CIBSE, London.

Fletcher, B. (1978) Effect of flanges on the velocity in front of exhaust ventilation hoods. *Annals of Occupational Hygiene*, **21**, 265–9.

Fletcher, B. and Johnson, A.E. (1982). Velocity profiles around hoods and slots and the effects of an adjacent plane. *Annals of Occupational Hygiene*, **25**, 365–72.

Harrington, J.M. and Gill, F.S. (1992). *Occupational Health, Pocket Consultant*, (3rd edn). Blackwell Scientific Publications, Oxford.

Miller, D.S. (1978). *Internal Flow Systems*. British Hydromechanics Research Association, Cranfield.

Woods of Colchester Limited (1978). *Woods Practical Guide to Fan Engineering*.

CHAPTER 23

Personal Protective Equipment

R.M. Howie

INTRODUCTION

The objectives of this chapter are to indicate the role of personal protective equipment (PPE) in an overall control programme and to provide advice on setting up and implementing a PPE programme which should enable wearers of PPE to be afforded the required levels of protection without being exposed to either unacceptable stress or discomfort.

PPE such as protective clothing, respiratory protective equipment (RPE) or personal hearing defenders (PHD) is very widely used. This is primarily because PPE is perceived to provide effective and relatively inexpensive protection whereas alternative techniques, such as substitution, segregation or other means of control (see Chapter 21), either cannot be applied or are perceived to be unacceptably expensive.

It is a tenet of good occupational hygiene practice that all possible action should be taken to prevent or reduce risks at source rather than relying on PPE to provide the only protection for the wearer. This is because PPE reduces exposure only for the individual wearer and because competent hygienists have recognized for many years that PPE performance in the workplace is difficult to guarantee and is probably lower than indicated by standard tests. This tenet is enshrined in Article 6 of the European 'Framework' Directive which requires that the employer gives 'collective protective measures priority over individual protective measures' (Commission of the European Communities, 1989a), and is reiterated in Article 3 of the PPE 'Use' Directive (Commission of the European Communities, 1989b). These duties specified in the Commission of the European Communities (CEC) Directives have been incorporated into the national legislation of all member states of the European Community and will similarly be adopted into the national legislation of the member states of the European Free Trade Association.

Notwithstanding the above basic principle, there will be work situations where alternative means of controlling risks are not technically possible and the use of PPE is unavoidable, e.g. during incidents such as chemical spillages, during the period between recognizing a risk situation and implementing prevention or control, during routine maintenance operations and to supplement inadequate controls.

When PPE has to be used it must provide adequate protection without itself leading to any risk or increased risk. To meet these requirements PPE must be selected taking into account the nature and extent of the risk, the wearers' individual characteristics, their jobs and working environments and any other items of PPE which may have to be worn simultaneously.

To ensure that PPE provides effective ongoing protection, it is not sufficient to simply provide nominally adequate equipment. It is necessary to set up a comprehensive programme to ensure that the PPE continues to be correctly used and, if reusable, is maintained in efficient and hygienic condition.

SETTING UP AN EFFECTIVE PPE PROGRAMME

The steps required to establish and run an effective

programme covering PPE such as RPE, PHD, protective clothing, safety helmets, protective foot-wear, gloves or fall arrest harnesses are summarized below.

- Assess risks and identify where control is required.
- Implement all reasonably practicable controls.
- Identify who needs residual protection.
- Inform wearers of consequences of exposure.
- Select adequate PPE to control residual exposure.
- Match PPE to the wearer.
- Ensure that the PPE does not create risk or risks.
- Ensure PPE are mutually compatible.
- Involve wearers in the PPE selection process.
- Provide PPE free of charge.
- Train wearers in the correct use of their PPE.
- Minimize wear periods.
- Supervise wearers to ensure the correct use of PPE.
- Maintain the PPE in efficient and hygienic condition.
- Inspect PPE to ensure it is correctly maintained.
- Provide suitable storage facilities for the PPE.
- Record usage, maintenance and inspection data.
- Monitor programme to ensure continuing effectiveness.

The above subheadings are described in greater detail below.

Assess risks and identify where control is required. The essential first step to achieve effective management of safety and health in any workplace is an assessment to identify any likely occupational hazards and to quantify any risks (see Chapters 7–16). The assessment should identify all unacceptable risks and the individuals at risk and provide the information needed for designing collective and administrative means of prevention or control and for selecting adequate and suitable PPE (see Chapter 21).

Implement all reasonably practicable controls. All reasonably practicable means of prevention or reduction of risk at source must be considered before adopting PPE. Assess whether it is practicable to use less hazardous substances, to adopt less hazardous processes, to enclose any process involving hazardous substances (see Chapter 21)

or to apply local exhaust ventilation to such processes, etc. (see Chapter 22).

Identify who needs residual protection. From the assessment of likely risks and of the effectiveness of any collective or administrative procedures applied to reduce these risks, all persons still potentially at risk should be identified and the level of residual protection still required should be quantified.

Inform wearers of consequences of exposure. To ensure that all workers fully utilize all control measures, they should be made fully aware of the risks to their health and safety in the workplace and the potential consequences if these risks are not adequately controlled. If the correct use of control measures involves inconvenience or reduction in productivity, particularly for those on piece-work, it is possible that the control measures will not be correctly used unless those at risk perceive some benefit to themselves. Similarly, since many types of PPE are inherently uncomfortable, some wearers may refuse to wear such equipment unless convinced that the imposed discomfort can be justified in terms of reduced risk to themselves. To ensure that wearers are aware of the benefit of wearing the PPE provided it is important to ensure that all persons exposed to risk in the workplace have a perception of the risk or risks to which they are exposed.

Select PPE adequate to control residual exposure. The objective should be to select PPE which reduces any risks to the wearer to acceptable levels, e.g. in the case of aerosols of hazardous substances, exposure levels should be reduced to at least below the relevant occupational exposure level (OEL). In the past it was considered that PPE could be selected on the basis of the assumption that the level of protective performance achieved by PPE in the workplace could be adequately predicted from the performance achieved during standard laboratory tests. That is, standards had a central role in the selection procedure for PPE. However, there is now considerable debate about the relevance of laboratory test data to workplace performance for devices such as RPE, PHD or protective clothing.

As a result of this debate, the more responsible PPE manufacturers have carried out studies of their equipments' actual performance in representative workplaces.

In selecting PPE, therefore, potential users should request workplace performance data from a range of relevant manufacturers and only purchase equipment for which suitable workplace data are available.

The role of standards and the specific problems encountered with the use of RPE, PHD or protective clothing are discussed below in the sections on standards and on the reality of PPE performance.

Match PPE to the wearer. When selecting PPE it must be recognized that even in a small workforce there may be large differences in the physical characteristics of PPE wearers and that consequently an item of PPE which fits one person may not fit another. For example, a respirator which correctly fits a large male might not correctly fit a petite female. Although no one would consider that buying safety shoes in only one size would be sensible for a large workforce, many users appear to consider that one size of respirator or earmuff can correctly fit all wearers.

Given the range of differences in body sizes in a typical workforce, the employer should ensure that the equipments provided adequately fit all those required to wear them. It might thus be necessary to provide a range of equipments of different shapes and sizes to ensure that all potential wearers can be adequately protected. Where the potential wearers include persons with non-European characteristics, the supplier should be requested to provide test data demonstrating that the PPE provides such wearers with adequate protection.

For PPE which imposes significant stress on the wearer, e.g. heavy chemical protective suits which can cause heat stress, or breathing apparatus (BA) which may weigh up to 18 kg or which requires the wearer to breathe pure oxygen, it may be necessary to apply tests to ensure that only medically fit and suitable persons will be required to wear the equipment.

Ensure that the PPE does not create risk or risks. Unless selected with care, some types of PPE can create additional hazards for the wearer. For example, eye protectors or full-facepiece respirators can affect the wearer's field of vision, PHD can reduce the ability to hear communication or warning signals or the approach of vehicles, chemical protective clothing can reduce the body's ability to lose metabolic heat, etc. If the required PPE encloses a significant proportion of the area of the body, the possibility of the wearer being at risk due to thermal stress should be addressed and action taken if harmful levels of thermal strain are likely (see Chapter 12).

If the wearers perceive that the consequences of such potential risks are more severe than the risks against which the PPE is provided to protect, they may refuse to wear the PPE. For example, coal-miners traditionally refused to wear PHD because they needed to hear the 'strata creak'. The danger from roof falls was thus perceived to be much more serious than the danger from noise.

Care, therefore, should be taken to ensure that any risks likely to be created by the equipment are fully investigated and reduced to acceptable levels. Where some residual risk remains, action should be taken to minimize the risk created by the PPE at source. For example, if PHD are used where moving vehicles may be present, the vehicles should be fitted with flashing warning lights so that realization of the approach of the vehicles does not rely on aural warning.

For PPE intended to prevent ocular or percutaneous contact, Section 3.10 of Annex 11 of the 'Product' Directive requires the manufacturer to be able to provide guidance on maximum wear periods for forseeable conditions of use (Commission of the European Communities, 1989c). The user should therefore require the potential supplier of such PPE to provide the relevant information. Equipment should only be purchased from manufacturers able to supply the requisite information. If the supplier cannot provide this information, the supplier should be reported to the local trading standards officer who has the duty to enforce the requirements of the 'Product' Directive.

Ensure PPE are mutually compatible. In many work situations where more than one type of PPE has to be worn simultaneously, the different types of PPE can interact to reduce the protection provided by one or both items. For example, if safety helmets are worn with full-facepiece respirators, the facepiece can force the safety helmet to tip backwards, and the front head-harness buckle of some facepieces can reduce the space between the forehead and the helmet, so that an impact on the front of the helmet can force the buckle into the forehead. Other examples of potentially adverse interactions are respirators worn together with eye protectors where the respirator can prevent the correct fitting of the eye protectors, or eye protectors worn with earmuffs where the legs of the eye protectors can prevent a good seal between the head and the muff. In such situations it is essential that each item of PPE provides the required level of protection without affecting the effectiveness of any other item of PPE. It is therefore important that when selecting PPE for such situations, care is taken to ensure that all items of PPE which may have to be worn together are mutually compatible.

While it is important to select items of PPE which do not individually cause unacceptable discomfort, it should be appreciated that wearing two or more items of PPE together can result in previously 'comfortable' equipment being considered 'uncomfortable'. It is therefore essential that where two or more types of PPE have to be worn together, great care is taken to ensure that the overall ensemble is acceptable to the wearers.

The user should therefore seek guidance from the supplier, e.g. ask what type of safety helmet can be worn together with this respirator. While it may be difficult for individual users to ensure mutual compatibility where the various items of PPE are manufactured by different companies, it may be simpler to buy equipments made by the same manufacturer since a manufacturer who produces several types of PPE is required by Annex 11 of the PPE 'Product' Directive to be able to supply information regarding their mutual compatibility (Commission of the European Communities, 1989c).

If suppliers are unable to provide the required information, they should be reported to the relevant enforcing authority, i.e. in the UK, the local trading standards office.

Involve wearers in the PPE selection process. In selecting PPE it must be appreciated that the physical characteristics of wearers can differ and thus an item of equipment which fits one individual may not fit another. In addition, since many types of PPE impose some level of discomfort on the wearer and since the level of discomfort may reflect the degree to which the PPE and the wearer's body have to mutually deform to achieve adequate fit, wearers should be fully involved in the PPE selection process to ensure that the equipment selected does not impose unacceptable discomfort. On a simple psychological basis, involving wearers in the selection procedure and in all aspects of the PPE programme gives them a stake in ensuring the programme's overall effectiveness. The importance of such involvement is recognized in Article 8 of the 'Use' Directive (Commission of the European Communities, 1989b) which requires the 'consultation and participation of workers and/or their representatives'.

Provide PPE free of charge. If the PPE is intended to be used solely for protection against occupational risks, the equipment must be provided and maintained free of any charge to the wearer. Reusable equipment should be provided as a personal issue item unless very thorough cleaning and decontamination procedures will be reliably followed before use by any other wearer.

Where PPE may be used for non-occupational purposes, e.g. for crash-helmets supplied to motorcycle couriers, if agreed between the employer and the user that the PPE may be used for travel to and from the place of work, the employer may levy a charge proportional to the occupational versus non-occupational usage.

Train wearers in the correct use of their PPE. Wearers and their supervisors should be thoroughly trained in how to fit the PPE correctly, how to assess whether the equipment is correctly fitted, how to inspect the PPE to ensure that it has been correctly manufactured and, for reusable equipment, whether it has been adequately cleaned and maintained.

The potential consequences of PPE failure should

be reflected in the thoroughness of the training, i.e. the greater the risk, the more thorough the training. Training should aim to convince wearers that the equipment provided will protect; few people are likely to wear uncomfortable PPE unless they are satisfied that it will protect. Generating such conviction is generally most easily achieved by practical training sessions which allow the wearer to assess how well the PPE can perform when fitted and worn correctly. Where possible the training should involve practical sessions using suitable training tools, e.g. for RPE, using saccharin aerosols to train wearers how to fit and assess the correctness of fit or, for PHD, using noise sources to demonstrate how to fit earmuffs or plugs correctly.

Training should cover the correct use of PPE ensembles, e.g. for RPE and protective clothing ensembles, to fit the RPE first, not to wear the RPE facepiece or headharness over the hood of protective clothing and to remove RPE last after completing all required decontamination procedures. Wearers of RPE should be aware that correct fit may depend on there being no facial hair which can lie between the facepiece and their face and that stubble can be even more damaging than a beard. They should therefore be aware that being 'clean-shaven' means having shaved immediately before the start of each shift during which RPE might have to be worn.

Supervisors should be trained in how to ensure that wearers are likely to be able to fit their PPE correctly, e.g. to ensure that RPE wearers are clean-shaven or that wearers of PHD do not have hairstyles which might prevent earmuffs sealing adequately to the sides of the head. Maintenance and inspection staff should be trained in the relevant procedures with particular emphasis being given to ensuring that they are able to carry out such tasks without placing themselves at risk due to contamination on the PPE, e.g. when cleaning PPE which may be contaminated with asbestos or isocyanates. For highly complex PPE which may be used in situations of acute risk, e.g. breathing apparatus, manufacturers often offer training courses for wearers and for maintenance and inspection staff.

Minimize wear periods. Many types of PPE are inherently uncomfortable. Since the acceptability of a given level of discomfort can decrease with increasing wear time, it can be important to reduce wear times as far as possible. If it is possible to identify those processes which generate most of the risk it could be possible to achieve adequate reduction of exposure by wearing the PPE only during such processes. That is, the imposed discomfort could be reduced, and the likelihood of the equipment being correctly worn increased, if wearers were able to remove their PPE when these processes are not being carried out. Care would have to be taken to ensure that contamination of the wearer or PPE in such circumstances does not itself constitute a risk. The assessment noted above should therefore include identifying whether it is possible to reduce wear durations by identifying periods when the PPE can be safely removed.

Supervise wearers to ensure the correct use of PPE. Supervisors should ensure that PPE is correctly worn at all times when wearers may potentially be at risk, that wearers are correctly prepared for wearing their PPE and that the correct personal decontamination procedures are followed where necessary. The overall effectiveness of any PPE programme can be critically dependent on the actions of shop-floor supervisors who are close enough to the wearers to actively enforce correct usage of PPE and any other control methods adopted. The responsibilities and authority of supervisors in the PPE programme should be specified in the supervisors' job descriptions so that they are fully aware of their role.

Maintain the PPE in efficient and hygienic condition. Reusable PPE will need to be cleaned, serviced and maintained, both to ensure the ongoing efficiency of the equipment and to ensure that the wearer is not exposed to contamination caused by poorly cleaned equipment. It should be appreciated that many wearers will be unwilling to fit obviously dirty or faulty equipment. In setting up a PPE programme, the persons responsible should ask themselves 'would I be prepared to wear the equipment provided?'

The legal duty to maintain equipment is placed squarely on the employer. The employer cannot legally delegate such a responsibility unless the person to whom the responsibility is delegated is 'competent'. Even where competent persons are available, the employer still has the responsibility to ensure that the competent persons carry out their duties in a competent manner.

Inspect PPE to ensure it is correctly maintained. Given that the duty is placed on the employers to ensure that PPE is correctly serviced and maintained, regular inspections and testing of serviced PPE enable them to ensure that the equipment is complete and in good condition.

Provide suitable storage facilities for the PPE. Where reusable PPE has been selected, suitable storage facilities should be provided for the clean PPE since it is clearly inefficient to service and maintain the equipment if it is then going to be left lying around in the wearers' lockers or in dirty locations where it may be stolen, become contaminated or damaged or may be used by unauthorized or untrained persons. Such provision of suitable storage facilities is recommended in some UK guidance, e.g. guidance on the Noise at Work regulations (Health and Safety Commission, 1989a).

Record usage, maintenance and inspection data. Although there is no legal duty to record usage and maintenance data, there is a legal duty to record inspection data, e.g. see Regulation 9 (4) of the COSHH Regulations (Health and Safety Commission, 1989b). Usage records provide the employer with a means of checking if all those who should wear PPE actually do so and to ensure that those who should wear PPE actually do so and to ensure that those who do not are identified so that corrective action can be taken. The maintenance and inspection records provide employers with 'proof' that their legal duties to maintain and inspect relevant items of PPE have been met.

Monitor programme to ensure continuing effectiveness. As with any programme, it is generally inadequate to put a programme into operation and assume that it will continue to function adequately without any further action. It is therefore prudent to routinely check the operation of the programme,

to retrain and 'reindoctrinate' all personnel involved at suitable intervals and to take any remedial action that may be required.

PPE STANDARDS

Almost all PPE, other than that intended to provide only minimal protection, is now designed to meet internationally agreed standards and is manufactured using internationally agreed quality control procedures. Standards thus have a significant effect on the type and nominal performance of the PPE available on the market-place.

Over a period of years, many industrialized countries have developed their own standards for PPE or have adopted the standards of a larger neighbour or of a previous colonial partner. In the European Community it was recognized that the multiplicity of standards among the member states constituted a potential barrier to trade and it was agreed that the individual national standards organizations would develop harmonized standards which would apply in all member states of the Community. Over the past 20 years about 160 European Standards (CEN) for PPE have been developed covering PPE ranging from safety helmets to safety footwear and fall arrest harnesses.

The PPE 'Product' Directive (Commission of the European Communities, 1989c) requires that all PPE crossing internal borders or imported into the European Community after July 1995 must carry the 'CE' mark, demonstrating compliance with the relevant European or national standard. Where no relevant PPE standards are available, the manufacturer or importer must prepare a technical file defining the performance of the PPE before a CE mark can be issued. CE marked equipment must either undergo annual retesting or manufacture must be conducted in accordance with agreed quality systems to ensure that equipment continues to meet the relevant performance criteria.

The adoption of CEN standards has generated a major problem for some users of RPE in that for half and full-facepiece unpowered dust and gas respirators there are no standards for complete devices, there being separate standards for facepieces and for filters. It is assumed that any CE marked filter should be able to be fitted to any relevant CE marked facepiece to yield a correctly functioning respirator. However, some filter and facepiece combinations may never have been tested to demonstrate the correctness of the above assumption. Users should therefore only use filter and facepiece combinations for which the supplier can supply written evidence that the different components do combine to give a correctly functioning respirator.

Although the CEN standards specify minimum performance criteria, the standard tests are intended only to provide manufacturers with a means of assessing the initial and ongoing performance of their products *vis-à-vis* the requirements of a standard. Since the standard tests might either be a poor simulation of actual usage in the workplace (e.g. leakage tests for RPE or attenuation tests for PHD last only about 30 min although equipment in the workplace may have to be worn for many hours) or might not test a critical parameter of performance (e.g. protective clothing is not currently tested for inward leakage at body–garment openings or to assess the potential for generating thermal stress), the results of such standard tests may thus not be a suitable basis on which to select PPE for use in the workplace.

To ensure that the PPE selected is likely to perform adequately in the workplace, only equipment for which relevant workplace data are available should be purchased. As noted above for the provision of information, any supplier unable to provide the required information should be reported to the relevant enforcing authority. In the UK, the relevant authority is the Health and Safety Executive (HSE) since such data should have been generated by the manufacturer or importer to ensure compliance with the requirements of Section 6 of the Health and Safety at Work Act (Health and Safety Commission, 1974).

THE REALITY OF PPE PERFORMANCE IN THE WORKPLACE

For RPE, PHD and protective clothing there is extensive evidence of problems regarding the levels of protection which can realistically be achieved in the workplace. In addition, for these types of PPE there are further concerns regarding how the equip-

ment can be safely used. These problems are addressed below.

Respiratory protective equipment

The performance of RPE is generally expressed in terms of the 'protection factor' (PF) which is the factor by which the in-facepiece contaminant concentration is lower than that in the environment.

In selecting RPE, the required PF is calculated as:

$$\text{Required PF} = \frac{\text{Contaminant concentration}}{\text{OEL}} \quad (23.1)$$

For example, when selecting a respirator for use in a workplace in which the airborne concentration of contaminant is 8 mg m^{-3} and the OEL for the contaminant is 0.5 mg m^{-3}:

$$\text{Required PF} = 8/0.5 = 16$$

For such a workplace, an item of RPE providing a PF of at least 16 could provide adequate protection if the device is matched to the wearers, their jobs and their workplace. Information on the nominal performance which should be achieved by the different types of RPE are obtainable from the standards and from national guidance, i.e. in the UK guidance published by the Health and Safety Executive, from manufacturers' literature and from relevant papers in the literature.

In the past it was generally assumed that the major difficulty with RPE was getting the wearer to wear the equipment. In his 1908 report, the Chief Inspector of Factories reported that his inspectors had instanced 'the old difficulty of getting workers to wear the respirators provided' (His Majesty's Stationery Office, 1908). Many users of today still encounter the 'old' problem of 1908. It was generally assumed that if the RPE would only be worn, the anticipated protection would be obtained.

It was assumed that the 'nominal protection factor' (NPF), the minimum PF which the device was required to achieve during standard laboratory tests to comply with the relevant standard, would be achievable in the workplace if correctly selected equipment was correctly worn by properly trained and supervised wearers. This assumption is enshrined in current UK guidance such as HS(G) 53 (Health and Safety Executive, 1990a) and in CR 529, the CEN report on the selection and use of RPE (Comité Européen de Normalisation, 1993).

However, numerous publications over the past 30 years have demonstrated that the PF achieved by RPE in the workplace, even when correctly worn, is generally markedly lower than the NPF (see review by Sherwood (1991)). For example, Shackleton, Gray and Cottrell (1985) reported PF for full-facepiece dust respirators worn to protect against airborne lead dust of < 3 for these devices which were then approved for use in asbestos concentrations up to 900 times the OEL. Tannahill (1991) demonstrated that for protection against asbestos, similar devices gave PF ranging between 10 and 90. These latter data corroborated similar PF reported by Colton *et al.* (1989).

That is, if these devices had been worn in ambient contamination concentrations towards the upper limits of their approval, the wearers could have been exposed to concentrations substantially above the OEL. In selecting RPE it is therefore essential that only PF which have been shown to be realistically achievable in the workplace are used.

Since few manufacturers are currently able to supply such information no item of RPE should be assumed to be able to provide a PF higher than those shown in EH 53 (Health and Safety Executive, 1990b), the UK guidance note for RPE for use against airborne radioactive substances. The PF cited in this document are summarized in Appendix 23.1. These PF are very similar to those cited in the American Standard 288.2 (American National Standards Institute, 1992), which were derived from a very careful analysis of the publications on the performance of RPE observed in actual workplaces rather than in the laboratory.

For reusable RPE, it will be necessary to change dust and gas filters on a regular basis. Dust filters require to be changed because dust collection can increase airflow resistance, thus increasing breathing resistance in unpowered devices or reducing airflow rates in powered devices. For filters which rely on electrostatic properties of the media, the collection of dusts, oils or some organic solvents can cause filter efficiency to fall substantially. Clear guidance should therefore be sought from the supplier to ensure that the contaminants for which the filter will be used are unlikely to affect filter performance or to find out when filters should be changed.

Gas filters require to be changed regularly because the capacity of such filters is finite and exposure to moisture or other contaminants which are more strongly retained by the filter medium can cause previously retained contaminants to be released.

Gas and combined gas and particulate filters are covered by EN 141 and some special filters are covered by EN 371 and EN 372 (Comité Européen de Normalisation, 1990, 1992a and 1992b). EN 141 has adopted a nomenclature such as 'A2' where the first letter indicates the substances against which the filter should be used and the number indicates the capacity, 1 being the lowest capacity and 3 the highest. Thus an A2 filter is a medium capacity filter for use against organic contaminants with boiling points > 65°C as specified by the manufacturer. The breathing resistance imposed by a gas filter tends to increase with capacity, as does cost. If the filter also provides protection against particulates, the filter nomenclature becomes, for example, 'A2P3', where the 'P3' indicates a high-efficiency particulate filter.

It is not possible to reliably calculate the likely breakthrough time for gas filters in the workplace, even if contaminant concentrations are known, given the complexity of filter chemistry and the possible effects of moisture and other contaminants. Some users who have access to suitable analytical facilities consider it worthwhile to test used filters to determine their residual capacity. This ensures that filter usage is optimized as regards both protective performance and cost.

In all situations where gas filters are to be used, guidance should be sought from the supplier who should be provided with as much information as possible as regards likely contaminant concentrations, any other contaminants likely to be encountered and information on any unusual factors such as unusually high work rates or high ambient temperatures or humidities.

Filters which have previously been exposed to very high contaminant concentrations without breakthrough can release the contaminant on subsequent use. Filters should be changed immediately any odour or other subjective effect is detected by the wearer. Such warning effects should be used to supplement a planned filter replacement regimen and should not be relied upon as the indicator of when to change filters since exposure to some materials can cause olfactory fatigue thereby reducing the sensitivity of subjective detection.

As for users of dust filters, users of gas filters should seek clear, written guidance from the supplier to ensure both that the correct gas filters are selected and that the filters are changed when necessary.

Personal hearing defenders

The current UK guidance for selecting PHD (Health and Safety Commission, 1989c) suggests that the level of attenuation which should be assumed to be achieved in the workplace should be based on subtracting one standard deviation from the mean attenuation at each frequency. However, even if the laboratory attenuations were achievable in the workplace, the 'assumed attenuation' as given above would result in one wearer in six getting less attenuation than the assumed attenuation (if the test data are normally distributed, 16% of results would be less than the mean minus one standard deviation.) If two standard deviations were subtracted, only 2.5% of wearers would obtain less attenuation.

Just as for RPE, many studies have shown that PHD attenuations in the workplace are lower than the laboratory attenuations (see review by Howie (1989)). For example, Hempstock and Hill (1990) reported that by comparison with equivalent laboratory type data, the field attenuations for earmuffs could be 2.5–7.5 dB lower and for ear inserts could be up to 18 dB lower. In addition, they reported that the mean attenuations were lower than in the laboratory and the field standard deviations were larger than in the laboratory. Therefore, had attenuations been based on the mean minus two rather than minus one standard deviation, the relative reduction in the field would have been even larger. Laboratory test data, particularly if based on the mean minus one standard deviation, simply do not provide a secure basis from which to derive likely workplace performance.

Since workplace data are lacking for most items of PHD, it would be prudent to:
1 base the assumed attenuations on subtracting at least two standard deviations from the mean attenuations and;
2 assume that the attenuation thus derived should be halved.
It is of interest that a major ear insert manufacturer who supplies to both the US and European markets recommends the above procedure for devices sold in the US but only the procedure recommended by the HSE for the same devices when sold in the UK market.

A further difficulty with ear inserts is that such devices should be removed and completely refitted at least every 60–90 min because the insert is ejected from the ear canal by jaw movement due to talking, chewing or yawning as highlighted by Abel and Rokas (1986) and by Cluff (1989). Although auto-ejection of ear inserts has been known about for many years, no UK supplier of inserts currently specifies that they should be regularly refitted. The need to regularly refit ear inserts may preclude their use in some workplaces unless good hand washing facilities are available along with supervision to ensure that both the correct refitting and hand washing procedures are followed. For example, in the food industry it might not be acceptable for wearers to remove and refit their inserts given the potential for contaminating food, and where toxic or abrasive substances are involved, it would be unacceptable to risk contamination from the wearers' fingers being transferred into the ear canal.

The available information indicates that the performance of earmuffs can fall rapidly over the first 4 or 6 weeks of usage as discussed by Rawlinson and Wheeler (1987). If the attenuations provided by the earmuffs only marginally achieve the required in-ear noise exposure levels, the muffs should be replaced at least every 4 weeks unless the supplier can provide information demonstrating that a longer replacement frequency is adequate for the given environment.

To ensure that PHD in the workplace do provide adequate protection, routine audiometric testing should be carried out as the 'ultimate' test of their ongoing effectiveness since the legal duty is to protect hearing, not to reduce personal noise exposures.

As for all types of PPE, the supplier should be required to supply sufficient information to enable the user to ensure that the equipment selected will provide effective protection.

Protective clothing

The two major factors which should be addressed when selecting protective clothing are:
1 the overall level of protection afforded;
2 the likelihood of the clothing generating or exacerbating heat stress which could restrict safe periods of wear or preclude the clothing being worn with some types of PPE.
The overall performance of protective clothing is highly dependent on the nature of the challenge against which protection is required. If the challenge is simple physical contact or splash, simple laboratory tests might provide adequate information regarding the likely levels of protection which could be achieved in the workplace. However, if the clothing is required to protect against airborne contaminants, such as aerosols or gases, it is necessary to take account of all routes by which contaminants could breach the protective layer.

For gases or aerosols, the protective layer could be breached by penetration or permeation through the fabrics, seams or fasteners or could leak past seals at body openings such as at the neck, wrists, waist or ankles. The mechanism by which contaminated air can be drawn into protective garments is that movement of the wearer's body creates and destroys voids between the body and the garment; air is drawn inward as the voids are created and expelled outward as the voids are destroyed. A pre-war Home Office document indicated that such 'suction effect produced by movement' could cause the inward leakage of mustard gas to contaminate the inside of protective clothing (His Majesty's Stationery Office, 1938). When selecting protective clothing for use against gases or vapours, the suppliers should be required to supply information regarding the overall protection afforded by their products and not simply information regarding fabric penetration or permeation tests.

Some types of protective clothing may reduce or prevent the body losing heat generated by metabolic processes. For a person working moderately hard, e.g. producing about 100 W of useful work, the body has to lose about 400 W of heat if a body efficiency of about 20% is assumed. If clothing prevents the loss of this heat, heat will be stored in the body leading to an increase in core temperature. For small increases the effect is only discomfort. However, if the storage rate is excessive, the effects can range from heat cramps to death. To limit permissible heat storage to an increase in deep body temperature of 1°C, the USA has produced a threshold limit value (TLV) for heat stress and a correction factor to take account of any heat storage caused by protective clothing. For a highly enclosing chemical protective garment worn during moderate work, the permissible wet bulb globe temperature (WBGT) is reduced by 6°C (American Conference of Governmental Industrial Hygienists, 1995) (see Chapter 12). Until relevant European guidance on controlling heat stress has been produced, it would be prudent to adopt the American Conference of Governmental Industrial Hygienists (ACGIH) TLV and related correction factors to take account of the effects of protective clothing on heat stress.

The effect of protective garments on heat stress was recognized in the 1938 Home Office document referred to above, which indicated that air raid wardens who had to wear heavy anti-gas suits with a full-facepiece respirator and hood might be restricted to three periods of from 30 to 60 min hard work per 24 hours. Since the situation to which the above document refers was that the wearers could be involved in saving life and that lives could be lost if the protected wearers were not available, the limitation was clear recognition of a serious health threat caused by the PPE itself.

Safe wear durations for PPE ensembles to limit the increase in core temperature to 1°C can be determined from the heat storage rate:

$$\frac{\text{Safe wear}}{\text{duration}} = \frac{\text{Body weight (kg)} \times 4200}{\text{Storage rate (W)}} \text{(s)} \quad (23.2)$$

For the purposes of the above equation it is assumed that the specific heat of the body is equal to that of water. The factor of 4200 in the equation is thus the specific heat of water which is approximately $4200\ J\ kg^{-1}\ K^{-1}$.

The storage rate can be calculated by determining how much heat the body must lose *vis-à-vis* how much heat can be lost through the clothing and other PPE and by respiration, i.e. the heat storage rate is a product of two functions:

1 how much heat must be lost;
2 how much heat can be lost.

The approximate heat generation rate can be calculated from information given in the ACGIH TLV booklet (American Conference of Governmental Industrial Hygienists, 1995) or ISO 7243 (International Organization for Standardization, 1982) for given activities if it is assumed that the body is typically about 20% efficient in converting the energy derived from food into external work. (Although the ISO document is easier to use as work rates are given in SI units as against the imperial units used in the ACGIH booklet, more hygienists are likely to have an ACGIH booklet available.) For example, for a person carrying out heavy work with the body, the ACGIH booklet indicates that the total metabolic load would be about $7\ kcal\ min^{-1}$. $7\ kcal\ min^{-1}$ is equal to a total work rate of $7 \times (kcal\ min^{-1} \times 4200/60) = 490\ W$. Assuming 20% efficiency, the external work would be about 100 W and about 390 W would have to be lost as heat.

The insulative value of clothing for dry heat is often expressed in 'clo' units where a value of 1 clo implies a heat conductivity of $6.5\ W\ m^{-2}\ °C^{-1}$. The clo values for typical clothing can be obtained from ISO 9920 (International Organization for Standardization, 1995). If the stagnant air layer on the outside of a garment is assumed to increase its clo value by about 0.5 clo units, the possible heat loss through a coverall type garment for a given ambient temperature can be calculated:

$$\text{Dry heat transfer (W)} = \frac{12 \times (t_{sk} - t_{amb})}{\text{clo value} + 0.5} \quad (23.3)$$

where the constant 12 takes account of the heat transfer coefficient and the effective area of the garment, t_{amb} is the ambient temperature in degrees Celsius and t_{sk} is the skin temperature $= 35°C$. It must be stressed that the above calculation ignores the affects of thermal radiation and heat lost or gained to the air drawn into the body–garment volume by the 'suction effect'. It also incorporates a number of simplifying assumptions and although is thus not a rigorous determination of possible heat loss, provides an indication of realistic garment heat transfer characteristics. For example, the heat loss possible through a 1 clo garment worn in an ambient temperature of 25°C would be:

$$\frac{12 \times (35 - 25)}{1 + 0.5} = 80\ W$$

In practice, some heat could be lost by respiration since the inhaled air is heated and humidified before reaching the deep lung. If it is assumed that heat loss by respiration is typically about 50 W, the total heat loss in the above example would be 80 W through the clothing plus 50 W by respiration which equals 130 W total.

In the above example where the total required heat loss was 390 W, the heat storage rate would be the difference between how much heat had to be lost and the amount of heat which could be lost, i.e. $390 - 130 = 260\ W$.

From Equation 23.2 the wear duration to limit the increase in core temperature for a 65 kg person would be:

$$\frac{65 \times 4200}{260}$$

$$= 1050\ s$$

$$= 17.5\ min$$

The above figure clearly illustrates the potential of protetive clothing for generating heat stress where such stress would not normally be anticipated.

Protective garments often have to be fitted well before potential exposure to contaminants and may require to be worn after exposure while carrying out any decontamination procedures. Since activity levels may differ over the pre-exposure, during and post-exposure periods, the total heat storage rate over the full duration of wear should be calculated.

It is therefore essential that full consideration be given to the possible thermal consequences of the work environment, the wearer's energy expenditure and the PPE ensemble worn.

GENERAL CONCLUSIONS AND RECOMMENDATIONS

In any workplace, the major effort should go into reducing risks as far as possible by means other than by the use of PPE (see Chapter 21). Unless the risks against which PPE is being used are minimal, PPE should only be used as one component of a comprehensive programme to prevent and reduce risks to safety and health.

Where PPE has to be used, the levels of protection assumed should be based on information derived from tests in representative workplaces or from information provided by the supplier. Only if the above information is not available, should equipment be selected on the basis of standard laboratory test data.

Unambiguous written guidance should be sought from the suppliers of any PPE regarding: (1) the protective performance of their product in real workplaces over likely wear durations; (2) any potential problems due to incompatibility with other types of PPE; (3) any risks which may be generated by their product; and (4) relevant servicing and maintenance information. If any suppliers are unable or unwilling to supply the required information, their products should not be bought and their inability to supply such information should be reported to the relevant enforcing authority.

PPE should be selected in conjunction with the wearers to ensure that any equipment selected provides adequate protection without generating either unacceptable risks or discomfort for the wearer. The overall performance of PPE is best summed up by a quotation from the 1988 draft *Approved Code of Practice for Carcinogenic Substances* (Health and Safety Commission, 1988): 'but PPE, particularly RPE, depends for its effectiveness on the wearers willingness to wear it'.

PHD should be selected on the basis of assumed attenuations calculated by subtracting at least two standard deviations from the mean attenuation for each frequency. Until the introduction of European guidance on heat stress, the American heat stress TLV and related correction factors for the effects of protective clothing should be followed when selecting or using protective clothing.

Appendix 23.1 Summary of nominal protection factors (NPF) recommended in EH 53. From Health and Safety Executive (1990b). Crown copyright is reproduced with the permission of the Controller of HMSO

Device and Class	NPF	Wear duration	
		Long	Short
Filtering facepiece			
FFP1	5	—*	—
FFP2	12	3	6
FFP3	50	5	25
Half-facepiece			
P1 dust	5	—	—
P2 dust	12	3	6
P3 dust	50	5	25
Full-facepiece			
P1 dust	5	—	—
P2 dust	17	5	9
P3 dust	1000	100	500
Powered facepiece			
TM1	20	—	—
TM2	100	10	50
TM3	2000	200	1000
Powered hoods			
TH1	10	3	5
TH2	20	5	10
TH3	500	50	250
Fresh air hose			
Half-facepiece	—	5	25
Full-facepiece	—	100	500
Powered fresh air hose			
Half-facepiece	—	10	50
Hood or visor	—	50	250
Full-facepiece or blouse	—	200	1000
Compressed air line			
Not blouse	—	to 500	to 1000
Blouse	—	1000	2000
Self-contained breathing apparatus	2000	1000	2000

* Dashes indicate no standard or not recommended.
NB: short wear periods of 'minutes rather than hours' but only when there are no adverse environmental conditions such as temperatures or humidities or where wearer has a high workload.

REFERENCES

Abel, S.H. and Rokas, D. (1986). The effect of wearing time on hearing protector attenuation. *Journal of Otolaryngology*, **15**, (5), 293–7.

American Conference of Governmental Industrial Hygienists (1995). *Threshold Limit Values for Chemical Substances and Physical Agents and Biological Exposure Indices.* ACGIH, Cincinnati.

American National Standards Institute (1992). *American National Standard for Respiratory Protection.* ANSI Z88.2-1992. ANSI, New York.

Cluff, G.L. (1989). Insert-type hearing protector stability as a function of controlled jaw movement. *American Industrial Hygiene Association Journal*, **50**, (2), 147–51.

Colton, C.E., Johnston, A.R., Mullins, H.E. and Rhoe, C.R. (1989). Workplace Protection Factor Study on a Full-facepiece Respirator. Paper presented at AIHA Conference, St. Louis.

Comité Européen de Normalisation (1990). *Respiratory Protective Devices — Gas Filters and Combined Filters — Requirements, Testing, Marking.* EN 141:1990. CEN, Brussels.

Comité Européen de Normalisation (1992a). *Respiratory Protective Devices — AX Gas Filters and Combined Filters Against Low Boiling Organic Compounds — Requirements, Testing, Marking.* EN 371:1992. CEN, Brussels.

Comité Européen de Normalisation (1992b). *Respiratory Protective Devices — SX Gas Filters and Combined Filters Against Specific Named Compounds — Requirements, Testing, Marking.* EN 372:1992. CEN, Brussels.

Comité Européen de Normalisation (1993). *Guidelines for Selection and use of Respiratory Protective Devices.* CR 529. CEC, Brussels.

Commission of the European Communities (1989a). *Council Directive of 21 June, 1989 on the Introduction of Measures to Encourage Improvements in the Safety and Health of Workers at Work.* 89/391/EEC. CEC, Brussels.

Commission of the European Communities (1989b). *Council Directive of 30 November, 1989 on the Minimum Health and Safety Requirements for the Use by Workers of Personal Protective Equipment at the Workplace* (third individual directive within the meaning of Article 16(1) of Directive 89/393/EEC). CEC, Brussels.

Commission of the European Communities (1989c). *Council Directive of 21 December 1989, on the Approximation of the Laws of the Member States Relating to Personal Protective Equipment.* 89/686/EEC. CEC, Brussels.

Health and Safety Commission (1974). *Health and Safety at Work etc Act, 1974.* HMSO, London.

Health and Safety Commission (1988). *Draft Approved Code of Practice for the Control of Carcinogenic Substances.* HMSO, London.

Health and Safety Commission (1989a). *Legal Duties of Employers to Prevent Damage to Hearing.* Noise at Work Guide No. 1. HMSO, London.

Health and Safety Commission (1989b). *Control of Substances Hazardous to Health Regulations.* HMSO, London.

Health and Safety Commission (1989c). Types and selection of personal ear protectors. Noise Guide No. 5. In *Noise at Work: Noise Assessment, Information and Control.* Noise Guides 3 to 8. HMSO, London.

Health and Safety Executive (1990a). *Respiratory Protective Equipment, a Practical Guide for Users.* Health and Safety Series Booklet HS(G) 53. HMSO, London.

Health and Safety Executive (1990b). *Respiratory Protective Equipment for use against Airborne Radioactivity.* Guidance Note EH 53. HMSO, London.

Hempstock, T.I. and Hill, E. (1990). The attenuation of some hearing protectors as used in the workplace. *Annals of Occupational Hygiene*, **34**, (5), 453–70.

His Majesty's Stationery Office (1908). *HM Chief Inspector of Factories Annual Report.* HMSO, London.

His Majesty's Stationery Office (1938). *Personal Protection Against Gas.* HMSO, London.

Howie, R.M. (1989). Hearing protectors — do they work? In *Proceedings of the Institute of Acoustics Autumn Conference on Industrial Noise.* Vol 11, Part 9, pp. 191–6. Institute of Acoustics, St Albans.

International Organization for Standardization (1989). *Hot Environments — Estimation of the Heat Stress on Working Man, based on the WBGT-index.* International Standard ISO 7243. ISO, Geneva.

International Organization for Standardization (1995). *Ergonomics of the Working Environment — Estimation of the Thermal Insulation and Evaporative Resistance of a Clothing Ensemble.* International Standard ISO 9920. ISO, Geneva.

Rawlinson, R.D. and Wheeler, P.D. (1987). The effects of industrial use on the acoustical performance of some ear muffs. *Annals of Occupational Hygiene*, **31**, (3), 291–8.

Shackleton, S., Gray, C.N. and Cottrell, S. (1985). Field testing of respirator performance during exposure to lead fume in demolition work. In *Abstract of Papers, BOHS Annual Conference.* BOHS, Derby.

Sherwood, R.J. (1991). *Recommendations Concerning the role of Workplace Testing of Respirators as a Condition of Certification.* Report on pre-rulemaking conference on NIOSH assessment of performance levels for industrial respirators and recommendations based thereon. School of Public Health, Harvard University, Cambridge.

Tannahill, S.N. (1991). *Examination of Inter- and Intra-Subject Variability of Workplace Protection Factors Afforded by Negative Pressure Full-facepiece Dust Respirators Against Asbestos Exposure.* Unpublished PhD thesis. University of Strathclyde, Glasgow.

CHAPTER 24

Audit in Occupational Hygiene

S.C. Whitaker and K. Gardiner

BACKGROUND

The purpose of the preceding chapters is to provide information by which to recognize, evaluate and control the working environment; and by so doing, reduce ill health at work. However, this chapter on audit outlines the philosophy and techniques by which the occupational hygienist may seek to determine whether these tenets of occupational hygiene and its ultimate aims are being met.

The term 'audit' unfortunately holds many negative connotations and implies checking up or seeking evidence of fraud or failure. The process is accepted in many commercial ventures as a necessary evil, and, judging by the number of cases of fraud detected each year, perhaps a very necessary one. Nevertheless, it is one which is rarely greeted with enthusiasm. In the context of occupational hygiene, however, we are concerned with the development of an approach to audit which allows professionals to measure and critically to evaluate their own practice, for the specific purpose of improving what it is they do and how they do it. This differs from the more common approach to audit in occupational hygiene (which some have advocated in the past) in so far as it moves beyond quality control or compliance testing (which is largely a reactive process responding to, or searching for, failures), into the realm of continuous quality improvement. Continuous quality improvement seeks to improve the quality of what is done on a continuous basis. This is a proactive process which engages professionals in the systematic critical analysis of their practice as a positive step towards introducing improvements.

Where the concept of punitive investigation through audit exists, we believe that neither the auditors themselves, nor those who are being audited, will be able to function in the manner which is essential to the development of a successful process of audit-led improvement. Therefore, a clear and explicit statement on the underlying philosophy of the type of audit activity which we are describing is made early on in the chapter. In practice, such a clear agreement on this fundamental principle can do much to reassure those who are to be involved in audit and may also help to overcome resistance to change brought about by the process.

Where the ultimate aim of occupational hygiene is accepted to be the reduction of ill health caused by work, the ultimate validator of these efforts is an actual reduction in ill health which can be attributed to the work of the occupational hygienist. However, long-term health outcomes may be difficult to measure, difficult to relate directly to the efforts of any one professional group and may be difficult to attribute solely to the working environment. This chapter explores some of these difficulties in relation to the techniques of audit and offers some suggestions on how occupational hygienists, in everyday practice, might start to evaluate their own work, with the ultimate aim of introducing a system of continuous quality improvement into their practice.

'Quality' has been defined as 'fitness for its purpose' and we believe that it is the professional obligation of all practising occupational hygienists systematically and critically to evaluate their own practice in order to ensure that the highest standards of quality are attained and maintained within their own field.

INTRODUCTION

As has been described in the preceding chapters, occupational hygiene is primarily concerned with the working environment itself, rather than its effect on the health of the workforce. However, because the health of the workforce is so closely related to the degree of control achieved within the workplace, the occupational hygienist may be in the best position, within the occupational health care team, to effect change in order to protect the health of workers. Therefore, occupational hygienists, through their efforts to recognize, evaluate and control hazardous exposures in the workplace, are key participants in the systems designed to protect the health of employees. The contribution which occupational hygiene makes to the overall success of health protection programmes should be evaluated, along with the work of other professional groups, through the process of systematic critical analysis, for the specific purpose of improving practice.

Health programme evaluation has been defined by the World Health Organization as: 'the systematic and scientific process of determining the extent to which an action or set of actions was successful in the achievement of predetermined objectives' (Shaw, 1992). This refers to the end result or outcome of a particular health programme. Some writers in the field of occupational hygiene have drawn a distinction between continuing efforts to 'audit' a programme in operation from that of health programme evaluation. This is on the basis that health programme evaluation is a more complex process and is beset by difficulties encountered in identifying appropriate outcome measures. By contrast, audit is seen as a discrete event within the life of a programme which is used to check compliance with the programme standards. It has been suggested that the results of an audit can be fed back into a programme evaluation, but that the audit is a specific testing action, which can be defined as: 'a methodical examination, involving analyses, tests and confirmations of local procedures and practices leading to a verification of compliance with legal requirements, internal policies and practices' (Corn and Lees, 1983). It would seem that this type of audit would be well suited to verifying that calibration of equipment took place prior to sampling, that only laboratories which were approved for particular types of analysis were used or that company reporting procedures were followed. This approach places 'audit' firmly in the context of quality control and compliance testing, both of which are important functions, but ones which often fail to challenge the professional to think deeper and question why this information is of value.

The process of audit which we are describing goes beyond the concept of quality control or compliance testing and towards a more dynamic process aimed at critical evaluation of what is done, why it is done and what is achieved, with the specific aim of introducing improvements into the practice of occupational hygiene. This may involve working with other specialists, such as occupational health nurses, doctors, safety engineers, etc., in order to maximize the benefit from the audit process. Broadly, it can be defined as an iterative process, where performance is measured and compared to standards, where variations from established standards are identified, the causes of these variations are explored and where necessary changes are introduced to maintain or improve performance. This process will not only assist compliance with existing standards such as the occupational exposure standards (OELs) or company policies to be assessed, but would also require the occupational hygienist critically to evaluate the degree of protection afforded by simple legislative compliance and to consider where improvements in control could be expected to reduce the risk of ill health occurring amongst the workforce still further. This may include seeking ways to change behaviour by education on potential routes of exposure other than by the inhalation of airborne contaminants, by proactively challenging the management systems designed to deal with loss control situations or by closely examining the methods used for sampling complex mixtures or single substances at various temperatures in order to recognize the total exposure to a hazardous substance. This approach places audit firmly in the context of continuous quality improvement as existing professional practice is developed under the influence of critical evaluation.

As professionals, it is necessary not only to repeat what is done with precision (this is the role of a competent technician), but also to consider the accuracy and effectiveness of what is being done, to think beyond the immediate, to conceptualize practice in abstract terms and to bring to bear the knowledge gained through professional experience in other situations to the area of immediate concern.

Clearly, this type of investigation may raise significant questions which are difficult to answer based upon the information which is currently available. For example, where exposure to a respiratory sensitizer is shown to be maintained below the OEL within a particular work site, what is the significance of small decremental changes in lung function observed in groups of exposed workers? Is this a reversible health effect or will it be of clinical significance in later life? Is there a difference between the exposure profiles of those with and without detectable changes? These are questions which are only likely to be answered by epidemiological research, but the initial question on the significance of exposure is often raised by those closest to the sites of exposure. Epidemiologists are thus charged with the task of collecting data, analysing the results and recommending further studies, but their findings within this process often provide significant insight into the relationship between exposure and health effects.

There is a mutually beneficial relationship between audit and research. The audit process can raise questions which will require research projects to answer. The findings of research can be used to set standards for audit. Research into the process of audit can be used to demonstrate in which circumstances the process is most effective. Importantly, the well documented audit programme will provide essential information on the circumstances of work which can then be used in the process of research. All of these activities are designed to improve our knowledge and practice, but the audit process is judged by its ability to improve practice.

In the past, information on actual conditions of work and attempts to improve them have not been recorded in great detail. Therefore, experts in the estimation of retrospective exposure have had the difficult task of trying to categorize exposure groups based upon what many would see as inadequate information. Where the audit records now show the results of compliance testing, this is of some value, but where the audit records show information on compliance testing as well as other routes of exposure, multiple exposures, significant changes in working practices, changes in the workforce, etc., this information will offer a much more valuable insight into the type of occupational exposures which actually occur over a given period of time. This information would support epidemiological investigation by providing the desired degree of detail on actual exposure which is required for accurate assessment (see Chapter 18).

AUDIT PHILOSOPHY

The philosophy of audit is based upon the concept that it is better to know what is actually happening, so far as is possible, than to assume that this is evident. This concept is very much akin to the practice of occupational hygiene in an industrial setting. Audit assumes that accurate information can only be gathered through a process of systematic enquiry and that the information obtained will be utilized in a process of critical evaluation. Without the process of critical evaluation occurring, an audit programme is likely to generate much 'orphan data' which simply accumulates without significant value. Underpinning this approach is the requirement that those who are involved in designing an audit programme and in interpreting the results have some expertise in the field. It is essential that an audit programme is designed to measure what is relevant in the most appropriate way and that the auditors will know not only what to look for, but also the meaning of what they have found.

The philosophical questions on audit arise when one starts to consider why should audit be undertaken. There are several branches of audit which are of relevance to the work of an occupational hygienist, these include health and safety management audit, professional audit by peer review for educational or accreditation purposes, control and compliance audit, etc. Each of these activities may be undertaken for different purposes, but the overall aim of each is to eliminate failures and to achieve acceptable standards. The approach of 'quality control' (detection of errors), 'quality assessment' (designing-out of errors before they occur) and the concept which we are promoting, 'continuous quality improvement', requires that even standards of practice which are currently accepted are subject to critical evaluation in the light of new knowledge on workplace control, research findings and standards of best practice from other industries, in order to recognize the limitations of current standards and to identify areas where improvements can be introduced.

How standards are maintained and improved upon is reliant upon the actions taken as a result of the audit process. Where punitive actions are taken, such as the withdrawal of accreditation or management action taken against individuals, the response to further audit projects can be one of resistance, by limiting the flow of information or producing a deluge of misinformation for the audit team. Both of these make the task of conducting audit much more complex and likely to be subject to error. Where audit results are produced under these circumstances it is almost inevitable that attempts to discredit the process, results or even the audit team will occur. This response can be a manifestation of resistance to change, sometimes brought about by the implied or perceived criticism contained within audit results and the subsequent threat of management action directed towards individuals.

The legitimate use of audit results and the use of the process itself are worthy of consideration before embarking upon data gathering. Where the introduction of a process of audit is intended to involve professionals in critically evaluating their own practice, we believe that an atmosphere of trust is essential. Where improved 'performance' is the aim of audit, many difficulties can be overcome by making an explicit statement on the philosophical basis for conducting audit, such as: 'audit is being undertaken in order to improve professional performance because as professionals it is incumbent upon us to evaluate our own work'. The focus of audit is upon performance, not individuals. The audit process is expected to identify areas where

improvements can be made and this is the purpose of the exercise. Each problem which is identified will be treated as an opportunity for professionals to work together to improve the standards of their professional practice.

This is a fundamental shift in thinking towards a positive approach to the audit process and an effective method of introducing change. Where prior agreement on the value and benefit of this approach can be gained amongst a group of professionals, it is more likely that individuals within the group will be open and honest about current methods of working, and more willing to evaluate their own work critically without feeling that there is any implied criticism or threat involved in the process.

When considering the philosophy of this approach to audit in occupational hygiene — a non-punitive critical examination of practice — it is necessary to be clear about the purpose of conducting this type of audit. This can be broadly divided into two related concepts: (1) of improving efficiency within current practice — can things be done better, communicated more clearly, undertaken more accurately?; and (2) improving effectiveness — are the right things being done, should some other aspect of practice be given a greater priority or should new practices be introduced? The choice of priority between these two aspects of audit is dependent upon the stated aim of the occupational hygiene function. Where this is clear, accurately directed and functioning, the priority will be in terms of the efficiency of the programme to meet the stated aims. Where the aims of the service are vague and/or no longer thought to be appropriate to existing circumstances, the focus of audit activities should be on the effectiveness of the service.

Clearly defining the aims of the service and identifying the standards which will ensure that these aims are met is essential. It is only when clear aims have been identified that progress can be measured. The specific aims of an occupational hygiene programme need to be tailored to the particular industry and conditions of work. The aims need to be agreed and recognized to be of value within the organization if they are to gain support. Company culture, philosophy and commitment to health and safety will influence the choice of aims or degree of excellence with which it is to be pursued. It is the role of the occupational hygienist, along with colleagues in the occupational health and safety teams, to seek to guide and influence company culture and philosophy. The process of audit and the use of results presents an opportunity to exert this influence.

THE AUDIT APPROACH

Choosing an audit topic

In an ideal world, all aspects of occupational hygiene practice would be subject to some form of audit. However, it is not an ideal world and practical considerations will encourage pragmatic choices to be made when first introducing the process of audit. Unless the occupational hygienist and the other professional colleagues who are to be involved have some prior experience of audit it is often wise to select a topic which is small, manageable and of immediate benefit. The choice of audit topic in this instance is driven by the need to gain familiarity with the process, rather than a pressing need to respond to a difficult situation. Early success is a great encouragement, whereas early failure can lead to confusion, future resistance and be wasteful of resources.

When experience has been gained, the choice of utilizing the audit approach in difficult situations will be based upon what is considered to be the most effective strategy within those circumstances. Where the audit process can be introduced as a part of routine practice one of the benefits which could be reasonably expected would be a reduction in the number of hygiene interventions which are driven by difficult circumstances, as the audit process would seek out these potential situations and address them in a proactive manner.

For the audit process to be applied successfully it is necessary to direct its use towards situations where the process could be reasonably assured of achieving the anticipated aim: identification; maintenance; and improvement of standards of practice. In circumstances where the audit approach is favoured, it should be chosen because of its useful application over other approaches, and not simply because it is possible to conduct an audit.

Similarly, the design of an audit should be driven by the answers required, rather than by the possibility of conducting audit in any one particular manner.

Audit is principally concerned with identifying, maintaining and improving standards of practice through a process of systematic, critical analysis based upon information gathered for this purpose. In a narrow sense, audit could be seen as a process of measurement and comparison of findings against standards. However, it would be better to consider audit as a proactive process aimed at introducing improvements to practice on a continuous basis, rather than as a reactive process, identifying failures to meet standards.

The process offers an exciting opportunity for professionals from several disciplines to work together in order to address and improve standards of protection at work. Achieving improved standards of protection based upon advice from an occupational hygienist often requires the efforts of more than one professional group to implement them within the workplace, and we include management professionals in this context. Therefore close collaboration in the process of audit can be used as a catalyst for change and by drawing together all of the relevant professionals it is possible to focus attention on the significance of each of the standards of protection currently being achieved. This is true of each discipline, but particularly relevant to occupational hygiene, as the efforts of the occupational hygienist to recognize, evaluate and control workplace exposures are often particularly dependent upon the actions taken by others. This includes areas of practice such as: (1) operational managers responding to recommendations made by the occupational hygienist on control measures or in establishing management systems which allow early identification of new substances being used within a workplace; (2) health care professionals recognizing the significance of hygiene results and relating these to early signs of health effects; and (3) safety engineers understanding the limitations of sampling techniques and the effective use of hygiene advice rather than reliance upon sampling.

The choice of an audit topic (or use of the audit approach) will be influenced by the membership of this group and careful planning with clear agreement on the aim and purpose of conducting audit of occupational hygiene practice within a mixed group is necessary. This may present a challenge for those concerned, but the process can present a powerful opportunity for change within an organization.

However, audit is not a quick fix and is not an appropriate tool for dealing with all situations. Where evidence exists that there has been a failure adequately to recognize, evaluate or control a workplace hazard, action should not be delayed whilst an audit process is introduced. Immediate action should be taken to establish control and at the same time an audit process can be introduced in order to measure the effectiveness of changes. Some of the considerations which will influence the selection of an area of occupational hygiene practice for audit are given below. This list is intended to be used as a guide and does not include all of the factors which may influence the choice of audit topic within any one site, as corporate culture and the internal demands placed upon the occupational hygienist in a particular industry will influence the decision as to when an aspect of practice should become a priority for audit.

- A high index of suspicion that a problem exists.
- Where the consequences of failure to meet a particular standard of practice may be significant.
- Where the area of practice is frequent.
- Where the area of practice is of high cost.
- Where the area of practice has been recently introduced.
- Where accurate data on exposure, conditions of work or degree of control being achieved are not available.
- Where the findings of current research reveal potential health effects under similar conditions of work.

Audit design

Having selected a topic to audit, one of the primary considerations at this stage must be whether the audit design should be directed towards evaluating the effectiveness or the efficiency of this aspect of practice. Where the effectiveness of a particular aspect of occupational hygiene practice is being considered, it is necessary to be sure that the function is being judged against a stated aim and that the aim remains a valid, desirable and achievable goal. There is little to be gained in ensuring that obsolete standards of practice are maintained or in making the process of achieving those standards more efficient. Where the stated aim of a particular aspect of practice is accepted to be valid, the measurement of progress towards, or achievement of, the aim will be fundamental in evaluating the effectiveness of the function. Where that particular function can be undertaken by improved means, an audit of efficiency can be used to demonstrate this achievement. In both circumstances, opportunities to improve should be sought as an integral part of the audit process.

A process which simply demonstrates achievement of a standard does not go far enough to be considered as a process of continuous quality improvement. Improvement does not only mean expanding areas of practice by choosing ever more complex methods of sampling, training, evaluating or controlling, but also seeking the optimum method of achieving the stated aim. This includes making the most efficient use of hygiene resources. Sometimes the simple approach achieves the same end, and providing that the end-point is accepted to be the most effective in reducing or eliminating ill health effects associated with work, this is acceptable.

It can be useful when considering occupational hygiene practice to utilize the structure, process and outcome model devised by Donabedian (1980). This conceptual framework is not intended to be used for creating artificial rigid boundaries between different aspects of care or practice, but as an operational framework which allows broad areas to be identified and considered separately. This model allows occupational hygiene practice to be conceptualized as discrete components and although few would argue with the logic that in order to practice occupational hygiene it is necessary to have some equipment and facilities (structure), an agreed role in which to undertake a series of functions (process) and that this activity would be directed towards some goal (outcome), what type of facilities are required to produce the desired outcome or to what extent a range of functions contribute towards a desired outcome is often debatable. The role of audit is to try to evaluate these links through a systematic, critical analysis. This is undertaken by identifying standards, measuring practice and seeking ways to improve upon the achievement of desired outcomes. The framework can be applied to the audit of other aspects of occupational health practice (Whitaker, 1993).

Structure

This covers areas such as buildings, facilities, equipment, personnel, training, operational policies, management systems, legal frameworks and recognized sampling strategies. Areas of occupational hygiene which are designed to facilitate accurate recognition, evaluation and control of workplace hazards can be considered under this heading. What is to be done, with what and how? One of the principle uses of audit with regard to structure is in comparing the facilities and organizational arrangements for practising occupational hygiene between various sites or plants with the same degree of risk. Audit could also be used in considering the variations in arrangements between companies or countries. In trying to identify optimum standards for what may be varying circumstances, clearly defined aims for the service will be necessary.

Process

This considers what is actually done in practice, which may include: walk-through surveys; design of sampling strategies; calibration of equipment; sampling; analysis; report writing; management presentations; education and training; and communication with other professionals. It is anticipated in many fields that a good process will automatically lead to the desired outcome, but audit seeks to demonstrate this link and seek evidence of the efficiency of the process itself.

Outcome

This refers to what is achieved, and it is recognized to be the ultimate validator of all efforts. Where the aim is to reduce the actual incidence of work-related illness amongst a workforce, the validator of these efforts would be the actual reduction in ill health which can be attributed to these efforts.

'Outcomes' may be short-term achievements, such as the completion of reports on schedule, achieving control of hazardous exposure, convincing management to invest in intrinsically safe equipment. However, short-term outcome measures are closely related to process measures and are often limited in their usefulness in measuring true outcomes – reduction in total exposure (body dose), reduction in actual health effects, etc.

TECHNIQUES OF AUDIT

There are a variety of audit techniques which can be adopted for use by the occupational hygienist. These include audit as a part of quality control, quality assessment, compliance testing, programme management, programme evaluation and research, all of which may provide valuable information which can be utilized in the audit approach which is referred to here.

Figure 24.1 illustrates the process of audit which we have described: one which aims to promote the use of audit (the systematic, critical analysis of practice) as a part of continuous quality improvement. This is termed the 'audit spiral' in order to convey the impression of a cyclic process where established standards are continually being re-evaluated and improved upon, based upon what has been demonstrated previously. It is a process which occurs over varying time periods depending upon the nature of the audit topic and is strongly influenced by current research, audit results and operational circumstances.

It is not necessary to start with an observation of current practice in all circumstances and the spiral can be entered at any stage. Where good evidence of failure to comply already exists, the audit group may decide to implement changes and then go on

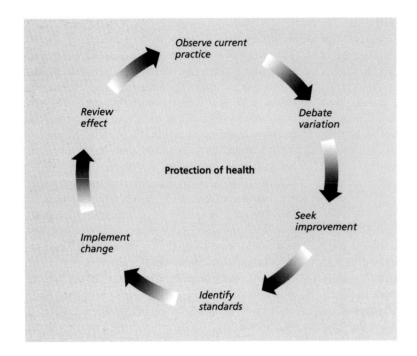

Fig. 24.1 The audit spiral.

to review the effects of these changes, followed by a systematic observation of practice over a specific time period. Similarly, even where no apparent problem exists, a routine audit of that function may provide sufficient information on which to base improvements. The individual steps included in the audit spiral are discussed below in order to inform and guide those who wish to pursue this approach within their own work environment.

Observe current practice

Having chosen the aspect of practice you wish to audit and identified the reasons why the audit is to be performed, it is necessary to focus upon those components of practice which are critical to success and which are of immediate concern to the audit group. It is often impractical and undesirable to try to collect detailed information on each aspect of the practice or particular process being undertaken. By focusing attention on aspects of the activity which are critical to its success and of direct relevance to the audit, it is possible to ensure that efforts are not expended collecting unnecessary information and that the information gathered will

be in sufficient detail to determine the degree to which the critical success factors are being met. It is useful to agree, where this is possible, what degree of achievement is considered to be satisfactory prior to collecting the information on performance (see 'Identify Standards' below).

The information collected should be in sufficient detail and of sufficient degree of accuracy to enable decisions to be based upon it. Clearly there is a relationship between the degree of accuracy required and the level of decision-making which is anticipated. Where significant problems are suspected and the solutions are likely to be expensive, a great deal of attention should be paid to the validity of the results. When dealing with less urgent topics, the resources (time, effort and cost) committed to the process should be balanced against the anticipated benefits.

It is at this stage that the audit design (see above) should be considered. The following factors will influence the choice of approach.

1 Why has this particular topic been chosen as the subject for audit and who should be involved?

2 Have the aims of the audit been made explicit and are these clear to all?

3 Who is likely to be influenced by the results and can they be included in the audit process at the design stage?

4 Do standards exist, or can prior agreement be reached on acceptable standards by the group?

5 What is the sample size required which is likely to yield sufficient information on which to base decisions?

6 Over what period of time is it necessary to collect data in order to reflect practice? This may include the need to consider infrequent events where these are of relevance.

7 Who should be included in the sample, is it important to separate out some of these groups for individual analysis?

8 Are there external events which are likely to influence the results over this time period and can these be controlled for in the analysis?

9 Do the anticipated benefits of conducting the audit in a particular way justify the use of resources?

10 Has any potential link between anticipated improvements to the hygiene function and the protection of health been identified?

Debate variation

When data have been gathered, analysed and the results produced, it is necessary for those with some expertise in occupational hygiene to review these results and to determine the means for their interpretation. Where the views of several professional groups are to be included in the process, clear focus upon the original aims of the audit is essential and a good deal of explanation, education and communication is often necessary at this stage. The process of critical examination needs to be challenging by its nature, but care should be taken by all to ensure that this is directed towards a positive contribution to the audit process. It is performance which is being audited, not individuals, and throughout the process of debate, problems which are identified should be viewed as opportunities for groups of professionals to work together. The limitations of the audit methodology should be made explicit, both for the purposes of current discussions and for future reference when

the information which had been gathered may be used to support research, for further evaluation or in the process of further improvement. Clearly, for this to be of use, the work of an audit group needs to be consistently recorded in a systematic manner. Where recommendations are made, action must be taken to ensure that these recommendations are translated into practice.

The following considerations should be included at this stage.

1 Who can usefully be included in the discussions on these results?

2 Should the interpretation of results involve an external opinion of the relevance of these findings?

3 What is the current state of knowledge in this subject area?

4 Can the audit results be related to other measures of company performance, production rates, sickness absence, morbidity, results from health surveillance or measures of management performance?

5 Where variation from standards exists (occupational exposure standards, company policies or standards of common practice, etc.), what does this variation represent? Are the effects on health (acute and chronic) known?

Seek improvement

A prerequisite to successful audit is the requirement that those who are to be closely involved in the audit process agree that there is a need for it and are willing to consider where improvements can be introduced. Where the need to improve is not recognized or where resistance to change is strong, these factors should be carefully considered before starting to audit. The reason for introducing this type of audit activity is to promote improved practice. Where there are specific concerns about the use of audit in this way, these need to be addressed before significant resources in terms of time, effort and money are committed to the process. Limiting the audit participation to those who are willing, careful choice of a non-threatening topic to audit and the early production of interesting, useful data can prove to be a catalyst for arousing interest.

Identify standards

Standards may be set by an external body, such as a maximum exposure limit (MEL) or the occupational exposure standard (OES). Measurement of performance, in terms of the degree of control which is being achieved, may be compared against these external standards in order to demonstrate compliance or to assess the efficacy of control measures. These limits are designed to be used as a standard throughout a wide variety of workplaces, under different conditions of work, and take account of both technical feasibility and economic factors.

Where no such standard exists, industries or companies may set their own standards. These may be closely related to what can be reasonably achieved, taking into consideration current operating procedures, working practices and economic factors. These standards may not be readily applicable elsewhere, or may in fact represent a lowering of the degree of protection being achieved by a different process or industry. Clearly the practitioner involved in measuring performance against these standards needs to remain aware of the reasoning behind the standard.

Where professional performance is being audited, agreeing what constitutes the 'gold standard' or an 'optimal standard' — which may be achievable under a given set of circumstances only — may be an issue of some debate. However, unless performance is to be evaluated only against the minimum standard which can be agreed, the use of published research, peer reviewed articles and standards agreed by examining bodies should be taken into account. Where broad agreement is arrived at, all concerned may make an a priori agreement to develop standards of practice based upon the findings of the first round of audit results.

The adoption of rigid standards in an audit document is to be viewed with some caution, particularly when considering potential effects on health. One particular standard may not represent the best possible degree of protection for some individuals and careful interpretation of any variation is required. Variations from the norm may in fact represent improvements in practice for some individuals. For instance, where a standard of eye protection is set in relation to the risk of a task, e.g. that eye protection will be worn whilst grinding, this standard may be wholly appropriate for the majority of the workforce. However, an individual with monocular vision could expect a greater degree of protection to be set as a minimum standard, perhaps that eye protection will be worn at all times in the vicinity of grinding operations, because of the increased severity of disability if he or she were to suffer permanent injury to the remaining functional eye. Where the audit process discovered this variation, e.g. that a different standard was being implemented by some worker, it should be recognized that variation in itself does not automatically represent a failure in performance and a critical evaluation of the results would recognize this. Therefore, care should be taken when using simplified scores based upon rigid standards in the audit process in order to take account of the significance of real life variations.

The following considerations should be included at this stage.

1 If a standard exists, how was this arrived at?

2 What degree of protection does compliance with this standard achieve?

3 Have new factors which will affect the validity of this standard been identified from published research, previous audit results, changes in working practices?

4 Is the standard achievable, optimal under certain circumstances or a minimum standard which all should be able to achieve?

5 What other standards are available, either from other companies, industries or countries which may be of relevance to this aspect of practice?

6 What contribution does this standard make to the protection of workers' health in practice?

Implement change

It is important to recognize that all change is not improvement and that some planned interventions do not work in practice. Therefore care should be taken to ensure that where changes are to be introduced these are likely to result in actual improvements in practice which can be related to improved means of recognizing, evaluating and controlling hazardous exposures. It is then necessary to demonstrate, through the process of continued audit, that the changes have been introduced and have resulted in the desired outcome. Where the changes may take some time to implement or the effects may decay rapidly if not supported, these factors should be taken into account in the design of future audit.

Where there has been prior agreement on the purpose of participating in audit this will have included the recognition that change and development are integral to the process; that critical analysis of performance is not the same as criticism of individuals; and that there is a group commitment to introducing improvements wherever possible. These factors will help to overcome the natural resistance to change. Where the management of change needs to be supported by further action (training, communication, improved integration of functions), the audit group should decide upon a strategy which ensures that this support is given and monitored. Target dates may need to be set, action points agreed and further co-ordination of efforts may be necessary.

The following considerations should be included at this stage.

1 It is likely that suggested changes will improve performance?

2 Are changes anticipated to improve the efficiency or effectiveness of this area of practice?

3 Can the anticipated improvements in practice be related to improvements in workplace control, reduction in health effects or more effective use of information.

Review effect

The whole audit process may take some time to complete and require the collection of a broad range of data. However, recently introduced changes often need a speedy evaluation in order to detect initial problems with their introduction. It is useful to conduct a systematic enquiry specifically aimed at evaluating the introduction of changes so that the impact of these is readily apparent. This information can be acted upon to facilitate successful change and fed back into future audit activities.

The following considerations should be included at this stage.

1 When were the changes introduced?

2 Is there a time delay in the anticipated benefits of these changes appearing?

3 To what extent is the Hawthorn effect likely to affect initial results?

4 Are the improvements in practice likely to decay if not supported?

5 Can the findings of the review be supported by evidence from other sources, e.g. health surveillance, symptom reporting, management performance?

Getting started

The outline of the audit process given here may seem much more complicated that it actually is in practice. For those who wish to start conducting audit within their own areas, we would suggest: (1) that some aspect of practice which is relatively uncomplicated and has a clear purpose be chosen; and (2) that a small number of professionals are invited to discuss how this process contributes towards the protection of workers' health and to consider ways in which it may be improved. From these discussions it should be possible to identify the key components of this aspect of practice which are of immediate interest and decide upon a method of measuring how well they are currently being achieved. When this information has been gathered a second meeting can be arranged to discuss the audit results in the light of published research and standards of best practice from other industries. Ways of introducing improvements can be explored and the group will no doubt wish to see if their intervention works in practice. From here it is a short step to a process of continuous improvement.

SUMMARY

It is clear that it is incumbent upon us all critically to evaluate why, what and how we undertake our professional work, and ultimately to assess its impact on the reduction of ill health at work. The process of audit, described here, can assist in the process of answering these fundamental questions as well as providing direction in terms of the continuous improvement of quality. Hygienists are in the ideal position to reduce ill health at work (by prevention rather than cure), as they often have the best understanding of the working environment and the means for effecting changes which are necessary to achieve this aim.

REFERENCES

Corn, M. and Lees, P.S.J. (1983). The industrial hygiene audit: purposes and implementation. *American Industrial Hygiene Association Journal*, **44**, (2), 135–41.

Donabedian, A. (1980). The definition of quality and approaches to its assessment. In *Explorations in Quality Assessment and Monitoring*, Vol. 1. Health Administration Press, Ann Arbor.

Shaw, C. (1992). The background. In *Audit in Action*, (ed. R. Smith), pp. 3–9. BMJ, London.

Whitaker, S. (1993). National audit of pre employment assessment in the NHS. *Occupational Health*, **May 1993**, 173–5.

FURTHER READING

Gifford, P. (1993). Exposure limits and the facts about ACTS. *Occupational Health Review*, **Sept/Oct. 1993**, 34–6.

Moser, R. (1993). Quality management in occupational and environmental health programs. *Journal of Occupational Medicine*, **35**, (11), 1103–5.

Perez, C. and Soderholm, S.C. (1991). Some chemicals requiring special consideration when deciding whether to sample the particle, vapour, or both phases of an atmosphere. *Applied Occupational and Environmental Hygiene*, **6**, (10), 859–64.

Whitaker, S. (1993). PEA: Working towards standards of good practice in the NHS. *Occupational Health*, **Dec. 1993**, 412–3.

Index

Page numbers in *italics* indicate figures or tables.